Clinical Pharmacokinetics

FIFTH EDITION

John E. Murphy, Pharm.D., FASHP, FCCP
Professor of Pharmacy Practice and Science and Associate Dean
College of Pharmacy
Professor of Clinical, Family and Community Medicine
College of Medicine, The University of Arizona, Tucson, Arizona
Honorary Professor, The University of Otago School of Pharmacy
Dunedin, New Zealand

American Society of Health-System Pharmacists®
Bethesda, Maryland

Any correspondence regarding this publication should be sent to the publisher, American Society of Health-System Pharmacists, 7272 Wisconsin Avenue, Bethesda, MD 20814, attention: Special Publishing.

Director, Special Publishing: Jack Bruggeman

Senior Editorial Project Manager: Dana Battaglia

Editorial Resources Manager: Bill Fogle

Cover Design: DeVall Advertising

Page Design: David Wade and Carol Barrer

ISBN: 978-1-58528-254-8

DEDICATION

This fifth edition is dedicated to my students and residents, past and present who continue to inspire me; to our patients for whom we dedicate our professional lives; to my mother and father for their nurturing; to my family for making life interesting and fun; to Mercer University and the University of Arizona for providing me the best jobs I could have ever hoped for; and to the pharmacy profession for giving me opportunities that I never dreamed existed for a guy like me way back when it all started.

PREFACE TO THE FIFTH EDITION

Many studies have been published since the first edition of the *Clinical Pharmacokinetics*. The second, third, fourth, and now the fifth edition authors have taken advantage of advances in understanding to update the chapters. In many cases more judicious monitoring of drug concentrations is suggested compared to the early editions. For some drugs the dosing approaches are radically different now. For others, new prediction approaches are available that have been tested in larger numbers of patients. The impact of drug interactions and the determination of the appropriate dosing weight on pharmacokinetics and pharmacodynamics when patients are overweight can be of great importance to dosing decisions, so the authors have included this information when available. Pharmacogenomic issues are increasingly coming to the forefront in decisions about drug dosing or who should even receive certain drugs, and many chapters have updates regarding what is known about the impact of pharmacogenetic studies on dosing. All of these updates should be helpful to users of the techniques.

This book is largely designed to help predict drug doses to achieve target drug concentrations from doses administered to patients. However, important chapters on rational use of drug concentration measurements, dosing in overweight and obese patients, dosing considerations for a wider variety of drugs used in neonatal, pediatric and geriatric patients, drug dosing in renal disease, and creatinine clearance estimation (the precursor to dose and concentration estimates for a number of drugs), round out the fifth edition. Tables on international and traditional units for drugs and laboratory tests are included as well as specific content on the use of both types of units should allow easier use of the textbook around the world.

I gratefully acknowledge the chapter authors who volunteered a portion of their lives to each of the editions of this book, and to the authors' support staff for their assistance. Finally, without a doubt many thanks are due to the best collaborators in the world—the ASHP staff. I would particularly like to thank the staff editors—Michael Soares (1st edition), Con Ann Ling (2nd edition), and Dana Battaglia (3rd to 5th editions) for their outstanding dedication to making each edition happen. They all did much work and receive little of the credit. But, I know their value and it is tremendous. Thanks.

John E. Murphy
2011

CONTRIBUTORS

Douglas M. Anderson, Pharm.D., BCPS
Senior Director, Medical Affairs
Regeneron Pharmaceuticals, Inc.
Tarrytown, New York

Jacquelyn L. Bainbridge, Pharm.D., FCCP
Professor
Department of Clinical Pharmacy and Department of Neurology
University of Colorado
Anschutz Medical Campus
Aurora, Colorado

Stanley W. Carson, Pharm.D., FCCP
Director Clinical Pharmacology
GlaxoSmithKline Research & Development
Research Triangle Park, North Carolina

William E. Dager, Pharm.D., BCPS (AQ Cardiology), FCSHP, FCCP, FCCM, FASHP
Pharmacist Specialist, U.C. Davis Medical Center
Clinical Professor of Medicine, U.C. Davis School of Medicine
Sacramento, California
Clinical Professor of Pharmacy, U.C. San Francisco School of Pharmacy
San Francisco, California
Clinical Professor of Pharmacy, Touro School of Pharmacy
Vallejo, California

Thomas C. Dowling, Pharm.D., Ph.D., FCCP
Associate Professor and Vice Chair
University of Maryland School of Pharmacy
Baltimore, Maryland

Jeremiah J. Duby, Pharm.D., BCPS
Critical Care Pharmacist
University of California Davis Medical Center
Assistant Professor of Clinical Pharmacy
University of California San Francisco College of Pharmacy
Assistant Professor, Pharmacy Practice
Touro University School of Pharmacy
Sacramento, California

Michael D. Egeberg, Pharm.D.
Clinical Research Fellow, Neurology
University of Colorado School of Pharmacy
Aurora, Colorado

Brian L. Erstad, Pharm.D., FASHP
Professor, Department of Pharmacy Practice and Science
University of Arizona College of Pharmacy
Tucson, Arizona

Patrick R. Finley, Pharm.D., BCPP
Professor of Clinical Pharmacy
University of California at San Francisco School of Pharmacy
San Francisco, California

Christine M. Formea, B.S. Pharm., Pharm.D.
Manager of Pharmacy Research Services
Assistant Professor of Pharmacy, College of Medicine
Mayo Clinic
Rochester, Minnesota

William R. Garnett, Pharm.D., FCCP, FAPHA
Professor of Pharmacy and Neurology
School of Pharmacy
Medical College of Virginia
Virginia Commonwealth University
Richmond, Virginia

Giulia Ghibellini, Ph.D.
Clinical Pharmacology and Pharmacometrics
Alleantis
Research Triangle Park, North Carolina

Barry E. Gidal, Pharm.D.
Professor
School of Pharmacy & Department of Neurology
University of Wisconsin-Madison
Madison, Wisconsin

Sarah L. Johnson, Pharm.D.
Investigator, Initiated Clinical Trials Manager
Rocky Mountain Multiple Sclerosis Center at the Anschutz Medical Campus
University of Colorado Denver, Department of Neurology
Aurora, Colorado

Janet L. Karlix
Medical Director
Autoimmune Division
Elan Pharmaceuticals
San Francisco, California

Kathryn R. Matthias, Pharm.D., BCPS
Clinical Assistant Professor
Department of Pharmacy Practice & Science
University of Arizona
Tucson, Arizona

Gary R. Matzke, Pharm.D., FCP, FCCP, FASN, FNAP
Professor of Pharmacotherapy, Pharmaceutics, and Medicine
Associate Dean for Clinical Research and Public Policy
Director ACCP/ASHP/VCU Congressional Health Care Policy Fellow Program
Schools of Pharmacy and Medicine, Virginia Commonwealth University
Richmond, Virginia

James P. McCormack, B.Sc. Pharm., Pharm.D.
Professor
Faculty of Pharmaceutical Sciences
University of British Columbia
Vancouver, Canada

Susan W. Miller, B.S. Pharm., Pharm.D.
Professor
Mercer University College of Pharmacy and Health Sciences
Atlanta, Georgia

John E. Murphy, B.S. Pharm., Pharm.D., FASHP, FCCP
Professor of Pharmacy Practice and Science, Associate Dean
College of Pharmacy
Professor of Clinical, Family and Community Medicine
College of Medicine
The University of Arizona
Tucson, Arizona
Honorary Professor
The University of Otago School of Pharmacy
Dunedin, New Zealand

Milap C. Nahata, Pharm.D., M.S., FASHP
Professor and Division Chair
Director, Institute of Therapeutic Innovations and Outcomes
College of Pharmacy
Professor of Pediatrics and Internal Medicine
Ohio State University
Associate Director of Pharmacy
OSU Medical Center
Columbus, Ohio

Paul E. Nolan, Jr., Pharm.D., FCCP, FASHP
Professor
Department of Pharmacy Practice and Science
University of Arizona College of Pharmacy
Senior Clinical Scientist
Sarver Heart Center
Tucson, Arizona

Robert E. Pachorek, Pharm.D.
Safe Medication Practice Pharmacist
Sharp Grossmont Hospital
La Mesa, California
Adjunct Assistant Professor of Pharmacy Practice
University of Southern California
Los Angeles, California
Assistant Clinical Professor of Pharmacy
University of California, San Diego and San Francisco
San Diego, California

Robert L. Page II, Pharm.D., MSPH, FCCP, FAHA, FASHP, FASCP, BCPS, CGP
Associate Professor of Clinical Pharmacy & Physical Medicine
Clinical Specialist, Division of Cardiology
University of Colorado, School of Pharmacy
Aurora, Colorado

Vinita Pai, M.S., Pharm.D.
Assistant Professor of Clinical Pharmacy
College of Pharmacy, The Ohio State University
Clinical Pharmacy Specialist
Pediatric Blood and Marrow Transplantation Program
Nationwide Children's Hospital
Columbus, Ohio

Hanna Phan, Pharm.D., BCPS
Clinical Assistant Professor, Department of Pharmacy Practice and Science
University of Arizona College of Pharmacy
Assistant Professor, Department of Pediatrics
University of Arizona College of Medicine
Tucson, Arizona

A. Joshua Roberts, Pharm.D., BCPS
Senior Clinical Pharmacist
University of California-Davis Medical Center
Sacramento, California

Kimberly B. Tallian, Pharm.D., BCPP, FASHP, FCCP, FCSHP
Clinical Pharmacy Manager, Scripps Memorial Hospital
La Jolla, California
Pediatric Neurology Pharmacy Specialist, Rady Children's Hospital
San Diego, California
Associate Clinical Professor, Pharmacy
University of California San Diego and University of California San Francisco
La Jolla, California

Toby C. Trujillo, Pharm.D., BCPS (AQ Cardiology)
Associate Professor
University of Colorado School of Pharmacy
Clinical Specialist, Anticoagulation/Cardiology
University of Colorado Hospital
Aurora, Colorado

Michael E. Winter, Pharm.D.
Professor Emeritus
Department of Clinical Pharmacy
University of California San Francisco School of Pharmacy
San Francisco, California

Ann K. Wittkowsky, Pharm.D., CACP, FASHP, FCCP
Clinical Professor
University of Washington School of Pharmacy
Director, Anticoagulation Services
Department of Pharmacy
University of Washington Medical Center
Seattle, Washington

Christy M. Yeaman, B.S., Pharm.D.
Program Director, Value Metric
Colorado Permanente Medical Group, P.C.
Denver, Colorado

CONTENTS

Dedication iii

Preface to the Fifth Edition v

Contributors vii

Introduction xxix

by John E. Murphy

Section 1: Basic Concepts and Special Populations

Chapter 1. Estimating Creatinine Clearance

by Robert E. Pachorek

Estimating Creatinine Clearance 1

- Factors affecting estimates of glomerular filtration rate 1
- Creatinine assay standardization 2
- Formulas to estimate creatinine clearance in adults 2
- Body weight 5
- Low serum creatinine/elderly patients 6
- Amputations 7
- Spinal cord injury 7
- Chronic renal insufficiency 7
- Dialysis 7
- Liver disease 7
- Pediatrics 7
- Using IDMS calibrated creatinine—enzymatic assay only 8
- Patients with unstable renal function 8

Estimating Time to Steady State Serum Creatinine Concentration 8

Creatinine Clearance Estimation in Unstable Renal Function 9

Chapter 2. Rational Use of Drug Concentration Measurements

by James P. McCormack

Evaluating the Need for a Drug Concentration Measurement 13

- Drug selection 13
- Efficacy issues 14
- Toxicity issues 15
- Adherence issues 15

Approaches to Dosing with Limited Need for Drug Concentration Measurements 15

- Immediate effect required or expected 15
- Immediate effect not required or expected 16
- Titrating the dose up 16

Titrating the dose down 16
Conclusion 17

Chapter 3. Medication Dosing in Overweight and Obese Patients

by Brian L. Erstad

Introduction....19
Obtaining an Accurate Weight 19
Body Composition Changes Associated with Obesity....19
Size Descriptors 22
Pharmacokinetic Considerations....22
Volume of distribution 22
Renal clearance 23
Non-renal clearance 24
Concept of Dose Proportionality 25
Recommendations for Dosing Medication in Obese Patients 25
Loading doses....26
Maintenance doses....26

Chapter 4. Drug Dosing in Pediatric Patients

by Vinita B. Pai and Milap C. Nahata

General Pharmacokinetic Information....30
Absorption—oral....30
Absorption—intramuscular....30
Absorption—percutaneous 31
Absorption—rectal....31
Distribution 31
Elimination....32
Metabolism....33
Factors Influencing Drug Disposition....36
Asphyxia....36
Exchange transfusion 36
Extracorporeal membrane oxygenation 36
Patent ductus arteriosus 37
Cystic fibrosis....37
Human Immunodeficiency Virus (HIV) Infection and Acquired Immunodeficiency Syndrome (AIDS) 38

Chapter 5. Therapeutic Drug Monitoring in the Geriatric Patient

by Susan W. Miller

Physiologic Changes 46
Absorption, distribution, metabolism, and excretion....46
Binding proteins....48

Increased unbound (free) fraction 48

Lean body weight to fat ratio 49

Drug Elimination 49

Metabolism 49

Renal clearance 51

Age-Related Pharmacodynamic Changes Influencing Drug Response 51

Summary of Changes 52

Chapter 6. Renal Drug Dosing Concepts

by Gary R. Matzke and Thomas C. Dowling

Clinical Assessment of Renal Function 73

Mechanisms of Drug Clearance 74

Renal elimination 74

Role of renal drug transporters 74

Nonrenal Mechanisms 75

Metabolism 75

Gastrointestinal absorption 76

Volume of Distribution 76

Drug Dosing Strategies for CKD Patients 77

Hemodialysis and Continuous Renal Replacement Therapy 78

Principles of hemodialysis 78

Dosage regimen adjustment strategies for patients receiving hemodialysis 81

Dosage individualization strategies for patients receiving continuous renal replacement therapies 82

Conclusion 85

Section 2: Specific Drugs and Drug Classes

Chapter 7. Aminoglycosides

by John E. Murphy and Kathryn R. Matthias

Usual Dosage Range in Absence of Clearance-Altering Factors 91

Loading dose 91

Maintenance dose 92

Dosage Form Availability 92

General Pharmacokinetic Information 93

Absorption 93

Distribution 93

Protein binding 94

Elimination 95

Half-life and time to steady state 95

Dosing Strategies 95

Estimating pharmacokinetic parameters—dosing weight and volume of distribution 96

Estimating pharmacokinetic parameters—clearance, elimination rate constant, and half-life 97
Estimating clearance 97
Estimating the elimination rate constant 97
Estimating half-life 97
Using estimated pharmacokinetic parameters to determine dose and interval 97
Standard approaches, nomograms, and algorithms—SDSI and LDEI 98
Traditional SDSI approaches—doses and dosing intervals 98
LDEI dosing—doses and dosing intervals 98
LDEI dosing in adults 99
LDEI dosing in neonates 100
LDEI dosing in children 101
LDEI dosing summary 101
Therapeutic Ranges 102
Therapeutic Monitoring 103
Suggested sampling times and effect on therapeutic range 103
Concentration measurement frequency 103
Initial concentration measurement 104
Follow-up concentration measurements 104
Other approaches to monitoring 105
Assay issues 105
Summary of aminoglycoside concentration monitoring 106
Pharmacodynamic Monitoring 106
Concentration-related efficacy 106
Concentration- or exposure-related toxicity 106
Drug-Drug Interactions 108
Drug–Disease State or Condition Interactions 108
Summary 110

Chapter 8. Antidepressants

by Patrick R. Finley

Usual Dosage Range in Absence of Clearance-Altering Factors 119
Dosage Form Availability 121
General Pharmacokinetic Information 122
Dosing Strategies 123
Therapeutic Range 125
Tricyclic antidepressants 126
Other antidepressants 126
Therapeutic Monitoring 128
Suggested sampling times 128
Further Considerations for Sampling 128

Pharmacodynamic Monitoring ... 128
Drug-drug interactions ... 128
Drug–Disease State or Condition Interactions ... 129
Adolescence ... 129
Advanced age ... 129
Alcoholism, alcoholic liver disease ... 129
Cardiac disease ... 129
Hepatic insufficiency ... 131
Inflammatory disease states ... 131
Nutritional status ... 131
Renal insufficiency ... 131
Smoking status ... 131
Thyroid disease ... 132

Chapter 9. Newer Antiepileptic Drugs
by William R. Garnett, Jacquelyn L. Bainbridge, Michael D. Egeberg, and Sarah L. Johnson
Felbamate ... 135
Gabapentin ... 137
Lamotrigine ... 138
Tiagabine ... 140
Topiramate ... 141
Levetiracetam ... 142
Oxcarbazepine ... 143
Zonisamide ... 145
Pregabalin ... 146
Lacosamide ... 147
Rufinamide ... 148
Vigabatrin ... 149
Use of the Newer Antiepileptic Drugs ... 150
Generic Substitution of AEDs ... 151

Chapter 10. Antirejection Agents
by Christine M. Formea and Janet L. Karlix
Usual Dosage Range in Absence of Clearance-Altering Factors ... 159
Dosage Form Availability ... 159
General Pharmacokinetic Information ... 161
Absorption ... 161
Distribution ... 161
Protein binding ... 162
Elimination ... 162

Half-life and time to steady state ... 162

Therapeutic Range ... 163

Therapeutic Monitoring ... 164

Suggested sampling times ... 164

Pharmacodynamic Monitoring ... 164

Concentration-related efficacy ... 164

Concentration-related toxicity ... 164

Non-concentration-related toxicity ... 164

Drug-Drug Interactions ... 165

Drug–Disease State or Condition Interactions ... 166

Chapter 11. Carbamazepine

by William R. Garnett, Jacquelyn L. Bainbridge, Michael D. Egeberg, and Sarah L. Johnson

Usual Dosage Range in the Absence of Clearance-Altering Factors ... 169

General Pharmacokinetic Information ... 170

Absorption ... 170

Distribution ... 171

Elimination ... 172

Half-life and time to steady state ... 173

Dosing Strategies ... 174

Therapeutic Range ... 174

Therapeutic Monitoring ... 175

Suggested sampling times and effect on therapeutic range ... 175

Pharmacodynamic Monitoring ... 175

Concentration-related efficacy ... 175

Concentration-related toxicity ... 175

Drug-Drug Interactions ... 176

Drug–Disease State or Condition Interactions ... 177

Summary ... 178

Chapter 12. Digoxin

by Robert L. Page II

Usual Dosage Range in Absence of Clearance-Altering Factors ... 185

General Pharmacokinetic Information ... 186

Dosing Strategies ... 187

Estimating digoxin clearance in adults ... 187

Estimating volume of distribution in patients with reduced renal function ... 189

Therapeutic Monitoring ... 189

Therapeutic range ... 189

Suggested sampling times ... 189

Assay issues....189

Pharmacodynamic Monitoring....190

Concentration-related efficacy....190

Concentration-related toxicity....190

Drug-Drug Interactions....191

Drug-Disease/Condition Interactions....192

Chapter 13. Ethosuximide

by William R. Garnett, Jacquelyn L. Bainbridge, and Sarah L. Johnson

Usual Dosage Range in Absence of Clearance-Altering Factors....197

General Pharmacokinetic Information....197

Absorption....197

Distribution....198

Protein binding....198

Elimination and metabolism....198

Half-life and time to steady state....199

Dosing Strategies....199

Therapeutic Range....199

Therapeutic Monitoring....199

Suggested sampling times and effect on therapeutic range....199

Pharmacodynamic Monitoring....200

Concentration-related efficacy....200

Concentration-related toxicity....200

Drug-Drug Interactions....200

Drug–Disease State or Condition Interactions....200

Chapter 14. Unfractionated Heparin, Low Molecular Weight Heparin, and Fondaparinux

by William E. Dager and A. Josh Roberts

Unfractionated Heparin....203

UFH: Usual Dosage Range in Absence of Clearance-Altering Factors....203

UFH: Dosage Form Availability....204

UFH: General Pharmacokinetic Information....204

Absorption....204

Distribution....204

Protein binding....205

Elimination....205

Dosing Strategies....205

Treating venous thromboembolic disease....205

Suspected VTE....205

Confirmed VTE....206

Pharmacokinetic dosing approaches....207
UFH: Therapeutic Range....210
UFH: Therapeutic Monitoring....211
Monitoring....211
Suggested sampling times....212
Assay issues....212
UFH: Pharmacodynamic Monitoring—Concentration-Related Efficacy....212
UFH: Pharmacodynamic Monitoring—Concentration-Related Toxicity....213
Reversing Heparin's Effect....213
UFH: Drug-Drug Interactions....214
UFH: Drug–Disease State or Condition Interactions....215
Summary of UFH Dosing and Monitoring....215
Low Molecular Weight Heparins (LMWHs)....216
LMWH: Usual Dosage Range in the Absence of Clearance-Altering Factors....217
LMWH: Dosage Form Availability....217
LMWH: General Pharmacokinetic Information....217
LMWH: Dosing Strategies....218
Suspected VTE....218
Confirmed VTE....218
LMWH: Therapeutic Range....218
LMWH: Therapeutic Monitoring....218
LMWH: Assay Issues....218
LMWH: Pharmacodynamic Monitoring—Concentration-Related Efficacy....219
LMWH: Pharmacodynamic Monitoring—Concentration-Related Toxicity....219
LMWH: Reversing the Effect of LMWHs....219
LMWH: Drug-Drug Interactions....220
LMWH: Drug–Disease State or Condition Interaction....220
Summary of LMWH Dosing and Monitoring....221
Fondaparinux....221
Fondaparinux: Dosage Range....221
Fondaparinux: Dosage Form Availability....221
Fondaparinux: General Pharmacokinetic Information....221
Fondaparinux: Therapeutic Monitoring....222
Fondaparinux: Reversing the Effect of Fondaparinux....222
Fondaparinux: Drug-Condition Interactions....222

Chapter 15. Lidocaine

by Paul E. Nolan, Jr., and Toby C. Trujillo

Usual Dosage Range in Absence of Clearance-Altering Factors....229
Dosage Form Availability....229

General Pharmacokinetic Information.....231

Distribution.....231

Volume of Distribution.....231

Elimination.....232

Protein binding.....232

Clearance.....233

Half-Life and Time to Steady State.....233

Dosing Strategies.....233

Therapeutic Range.....235

Suggested sampling times and effect on therapeutic range.....235

Pharmacodynamic Monitoring: Concentration-Related Efficacy and Toxicity.....236

Drug-Drug Interactions.....236

Drug–Disease State or Condition Interactions.....237

Congestive heart failure (CHF).....237

Acute myocardial infarction (AMI).....238

Hepatic disease.....238

Renal disease.....238

Morbid obesity.....238

Advanced age (elderly).....238

Severe trauma.....238

Pregnancy and lactation.....238

Chapter 16. Lithium

by Giulia Ghibellini and Stanley W. Carson

Usual Dosage Range in Absence of Clearance-Altering Factors.....243

Acute therapy.....243

Maintenance therapy.....244

Dosage Form Availability.....244

General Pharmacokinetic Information.....244

Absorption.....244

Bioavailability of dosage forms.....245

Distribution.....245

Elimination.....246

Half-life and time to steady state.....247

Dosing strategies.....247

Dose prediction methods.....247

Dosage prediction using the traditional pharmacokinetic method.....247

Dosage prediction by a priori demographics.....248

Dosage prediction by lithium renal clearance estimation.....248

Dosage prediction by population pharmacokinetics and measured concentration(s).....248

Therapeutic Range 249
Therapeutic Monitoring 249
Suggested sampling times and effect on therapeutic range 249
Concentration measurement frequency 250
Assay issues 252
Pharmacodynamic Monitoring 252
Concentration-related efficacy 252
Concentration-related toxicity 252
Drug-Drug Interactions 252
Drug–Disease State Interactions and Special Populations 253
Dialysis 254
Pregnancy 254
Summary 256

Chapter 17. Phenobarbital

by Kimberly B. Tallian and Douglas M. Anderson

Usual Dosage Range in Absence of Clearance-Altering Factors 263
General Pharmacokinetic Information 264
Absorption 264
Distribution 264
Protein binding 265
Clearance 265
Half-Life and Time to Steady State 265
Therapeutic Range 266
Drug Monitoring Assay Considerations 266
Suggested Sampling Times and Effect on Therapeutic Range 267
Pharmacodynamic Monitoring—Concentration-Related Efficacy 267
Pharmacodynamic Monitoring—Concentration-Related Toxicity 267
Drug-Drug Interactions 268
Drug–Disease State or Condition Interactions 268

Chapter 18. Phenytoin and Fosphenytoin

by Michael E. Winter

Usual Dosage Range in Absence of Clearance-Altering Factors 273
Loading dose 273
Maintenance dose 273
Dosage Form Availability 274
General Pharmacokinetic Information 274
Absorption 274
Distribution 275

Elimination 277
Half-life and time to steady state 278
Therapeutic Range 279
Therapeutic Monitoring 279
Suggested sampling times 279
Pharmacodynamic Monitoring 280
Concentration-related efficacy 280
Concentration-related toxicity 280
Non-concentration-related side effects 281
Drug-Drug Interactions 281
Drug–Disease State or Condition Interactions 282
Hepatic disease—cirrhosis 282
Renal failure 282
Obesity 283
Malabsorption 283
AIDS 283
Pregnancy and lactation 283
Critically ill 283

Chapter 19. Procainamide

by Robert L. Page II and John E. Murphy

Usual Dosage Range in Absence of Clearance-Altering Factors 289
General Pharmacokinetic Information 289
Absorption 289
Distribution 289
Metabolism 290
Half-life and time to steady state 291
N-Acetylprocainamide (NAPA) 292
Elimination 292
Dosing strategies 292
Population-based predictors of procainamide clearance 292
NAPA production (the "dose" of NAPA) 293
NAPA clearance prediction 293
Therapeutic Monitoring 293
Therapeutic range 293
Suggested sampling times 294
Assays 294
Pharmacodynamic Monitoring 294
Concentration-related efficacy 294
Concentration-related toxicity 294

Drug-Drug Interactions ... 296

Drug–Disease State or Condition Interactions ... 297

Chapter 20. Quinidine

by Paul E. Nolan, Jr., Toby C. Trujillo, and Christy M. Yeaman

Usual Dosage Range in the Absence of Clearance-Altering Factors ... 300

General Pharmacokinetic Information ... 301

Absorption ... 301

Bioavailability of Dosage Forms ... 301

Distribution ... 302

Elimination ... 302

Renal excretion ... 302

Metabolism ... 302

Protein binding ... 302

Clearance ... 303

Volume of Distribution ... 303

Half-Life and Time to Steady State ... 303

Therapeutic Range ... 303

Dosing Strategies ... 304

Suggested Sampling Times and Effect on Therapeutic Range ... 304

Pharmacodynamic Monitoring—Concentration-Related Efficacy ... 305

Pharmacodynamic Monitoring—Concentration-Related Toxicity ... 305

Pharmacokinetic Drug-Drug Interactions ... 306

Pharmacodynamic Interactions ... 308

Disease state interactions ... 308

Chapter 21. Theophylline

by John E. Murphy and Hanna Phan

Introduction ... 315

Usual Dosage Range in Absence of Clearance-Altering Factors ... 315

Loading dose ... 315

Maintenance dose ... 316

Dosage Form Availability ... 316

General Pharmacokinetic Information ... 316

Absorption ... 316

Distribution ... 317

Protein binding ... 317

Metabolism and elimination ... 318

Clearance ... 318

Half-life and time to steady state ... 318

Dosing Strategies.....318
Therapeutic Range.....321
Therapeutic Monitoring.....322
Suggested sampling times and effect on therapeutic range.....322
Neonates.....322
Infants, children, adults, and geriatrics.....322
Pharmacodynamic Monitoring.....322
Concentration-related efficacy.....322
Asthma or COPD.....323
Apnea or bradycardia in neonates.....323
Concentration-related toxicity.....323
Drug-Drug Interactions.....323
Drug–Disease State or Condition Interactions.....323

Chapter 22. Valproic Acid

by Barry E. Gidal

Usual Dosage Range in the Absence of Clearance-Altering Factors.....327
General Pharmacokinetic Information.....328
Absorption.....328
Distribution.....328
Estimating volume of distribution.....329
Protein binding.....329
Elimination.....329
Half-life and time to steady state.....330
Dosing Strategies.....331
Initial dosing.....331
Dosage Adjustment.....331
Therapeutic Range.....331
Effect of Age and Pregnancy on Therapeutic Range.....332
Therapeutic Monitoring.....332
Suggested sampling times and effect on therapeutic range.....332
Initial and Follow-up Monitoring.....332
Pharmacodynamic Monitoring—Concentration-Related Efficacy.....333
Drug-Drug Interactions.....333
Drug–Disease State or Condition Interactions.....334

Chapter 23. Vancomycin

by Gary R. Matzke and Jeremiah J. Duby

Usual Dosage Range in Absence of Clearance-Altering Factors.....337
Dosing weight.....337

Loading dose....337
Empiric maintenance doses....337
Alternative method of administration: continuous infusion....337
Dosage Form Availability....338
General Pharmacokinetic Information....338
Absorption....338
Volume of distribution....339
Protein binding....339
Elimination....339
Clearance....339
Half-life and time to steady state....339
Dosing Strategies....340
Population Pharmacokinetic Parameters....340
Therapeutic Range....342
Pharmacodynamic Monitoring....343
Minimum inhibitory concentration and efficacy....343
Concentration-related efficacy....343
Concentration-related toxicity....344
Non-concentration-related toxicities....344
Drug-Drug Interactions....344
Drug–Disease State Interactions....345
Dosing and Concentration Monitoring in Hemodialysis Patients....345
Assay issues....346

Chapter 24. Warfarin

Ann K. Wittkowsky

Usual Dosage Range in Absence of Clearance-Altering Factors....352
Dosage Form Availability....352
General Pharmacokinetic Information....353
Absorption....353
Distribution....353
Volume of distribution....353
Protein binding....353
Elimination....353
Half-life and time to steady state....354
Dosing strategies....354
Initiation dosing....354
Average daily dosing method....354
Initiation nomograms that incorporate genetic information....356
Maintenance dosing....357

Therapeutic Range 358

Therapeutic Monitoring 358

Pharmacodynamic Monitoring 360

INR-related efficacy 360

INR-related toxicity 361

Reversing INR-related toxicity 362

Drug-Drug Interactions 362

Drug–Disease State or Condition Interactions 365

Advanced age 366

Pregnancy and lactation 366

Alcoholism 367

Liver disease 367

Renal disease and hemodialysis 367

Congestive heart failure 367

Cardiac valve replacement 367

Nutritional status 367

Thyroid disease 367

Smoking and tobacco use status 367

Appendix A: Therapeutic Ranges of Drugs in Traditional and SI Units 373

Appendix B: Nondrug Reference Ranges for Common Laboratory Tests in Traditional and SI Units 375

Index 377

INTRODUCTION

John E. Murphy

General Pharmacokinetic Principles

Initiating therapy

When therapy is initiated in a patient, a standard dose and interval may be used, or the dose and interval may be individualized by use of population means of clearance or volume of distribution and half-life. These population pharmacokinetic parameters are useful for estimating drug concentrations based on an administered or planned dose and dosage schedule. To adjust therapy, these values then may be compared to actual drug concentration measurements (DCMs) and integrated with the patient's therapeutic outcome.

Using population mean values

Unfortunately, not all patients fit closely to the population means, and some of these means were developed on small samples that do not represent the general population or the patient being monitored. However, for a number of drugs, population means with standard deviations can provide useful information on reasonable ranges of the values to expect.

In any case, a patient's actual pharmacokinetic values (i.e., clearance, volume of distribution, and half-life) may need to be determined to adjust therapy for a desired outcome.

Considering other factors in pharmacokinetic monitoring[1]

In addition to the problems with population pharmacokinetic means, unexpected drug concentration measurements can occur for various reasons. Some patients may be nonadherent with drug therapy, taking either more or less than was prescribed for them. In the institutional setting administration errors can account for unexpected results; a patient may be given the wrong dose of a drug, may be given the drug at the wrong time, or may not receive the scheduled drug at all.

Errors on medication administration records also can occur. For example, it might be indicated that a drug was given at a time other than the actual time it was received by the patient. Furthermore, incomplete drug delivery due to patient problems (e.g., infiltration of an intravenous fluid or clogging of a nasal cannula) can influence drug concentration measurements.

Problems in sample collection can lead to unexpected drug concentration measurements. A blood sample may be drawn at the wrong time, or the wrong collection time may be reported. Samples can be taken from the wrong patient or obtained incorrectly (e.g., through a drug administration line that was inadequately flushed prior to sample withdrawal). In addition, samples may be improperly stored.

Finally, other things to consider include drug or disease state interactions that may influence the prediction of drug concentration measurements and the use of inaccurate assays.

Some reasons drug concentration measurements may fall outside of the range predicted by population estimates

- Patient truly does not well fit the population average values (i.e., falls outside of one standard deviation of the mean).
- The population values used for the predictions were determined in patients unlike the patient being monitored.
- Patient has been nonadherent with therapy (may have taken either more or less than prescribed).
- Nurse did not give the dose at the time prescribed (whether it has been signed off as given on time or not).
- Dose not given at all (whether it is signed off as given or not). Also doses are occasionally administered but not signed off as being given.

- Wrong dose is given (either once or more often).
- Error made in dosing schedule on medication administration record (e.g., every 18-hr schedule is put on record such that patient is given doses 18 and 30 hr apart).
- The complete dose was not administered prior to sample withdrawal due to patient problems (e.g., infiltration of an intravenous line, clogging of nasal cannula).
- Phlebotomist drew blood at a time other than requested and:

  1) Reported that it was collected on time, or (2) Did not report the time of collection and it is incorrectly assumed to have been drawn at the scheduled time.
- The sample was taken from the wrong patient.
- The sample was obtained incorrectly (e.g., through a drug administration line which has been improperly flushed prior to sample withdrawal).
- The sample was not stored properly, leading to artifactual results.
- Assay or assay instrument quality is not satisfactory or the reported result is not accurate.
- A pharmacokinetic drug interaction has occurred, which was not accounted for correctly in estimation of DCMs.
- An in vitro drug interaction occurred, resulting in artifactual results.
- A disease interaction occurred that was not considered, such as reduced absorption rate due to poor blood flow.
- The patient has reduced plasma binding proteins or a drug-drug interaction has displaced the drug from protein (see protein binding issues below)

Protein binding issues

When patients have reduced plasma proteins or highly bound drugs are displaced from plasma proteins by drug or endogenous compound interactions, there may be increased free fraction (unbound concentration/total concentration) and movement of drug out of the bloodstream into tissue. Movement of drug out of the bloodstream can lead to decreases in total (bound and unbound) plasma or serum drug concentrations even when the unbound concentration remains unchanged. Since total concentration is what is usually reported when drug concentration measurements are ordered, this can lead to incorrect assumptions that a dose may need to be increased. Increased unbound fraction can also lead to increased elimination, which will also decrease total concentration. If there is no increase in elimination, the unbound concentration may remain the same as when plasma proteins are normal or no interaction exists, even though the total concentration is decreased. In some cases of highly bound drugs (e.g., phenytoin), an unbound concentration measurement may be warranted if the total concentration is low, to ensure that adequate unbound concentrations exist.

Verifying drug concentration measurements

If measured values fall outside the range estimated using ± one standard deviation of the predicted clearance, volume of distribution, and/or half-life, concentrations should be re-checked before the initially measured concentration(s) are accepted as valid. This step does not preclude changing the dose or interval if such a change would have been made empirically at the start of therapy. If the measured concentrations are far from those predicted, a determination must be made as to whether the measured drug concentrations are reasonable (i.e., within reasonable expectation based on the range of population values) or whether one or more of the problems noted above occurred.

The occurrence of certain problems can be determined with detective work. For example, a patient can be questioned about compliance, past outpatient pharmacy records can be checked, and the nurse administering the drug or the phlebotomist drawing the blood sample can be interviewed. Unfortunately, the validity of the information gathered after the fact may be questionable.

Because of these potential problems, measured drug concentrations may not be a true reflection of the patient's actual drug distribution and clearance. Therefore, an erroneous decision about the dosing needs of the patient can be made. Accurate information is essential to quality therapeutic drug monitoring.

A well-coordinated system of communication is needed between those administering or taking a medication and those collecting blood (or other body fluid or tissue) for analysis. Such a system can prevent many of the problems associated with assessing the validity of reported drug concentrations and dose/sample collection timing. It also can reduce erroneous decision-making based on faulty data as well as the expense of repeating questionable drug concentration measurements. The lack of such a system should be considered a waste of resources and provides the potential for harming patients secondary to a high incidence of debatable data.

After as many causes of discrepancy as possible are eliminated, a decision must be made as to whether the difference between predicted and actual values is due to patient variability from population averages or to erroneous values. If the values are judged to be erroneous, drug concentrations probably should be re-measured, although the need for further evaluation should be as carefully considered as the original decision to monitor (see Chapter 2, "Rational Use of Drug Concentration Measurements").

Determining need for dosage adjustments

Once the drug concentration measurement and dosing information is determined to be as accurate as possible, dosage adjustments are assessed based on pharmacodynamic response and patient outcome. The need for dosage adjustment or the continuation of therapy should be based on patient response relative to measured drug concentration rather than on drug concentration alone.

This approach may not be proper, however, when the disease or symptoms are not continuous or easy to quantify. For example, keeping an anticonvulsant drug within the therapeutic range can be important when seizure activity is infrequent. Without an adequate seizure history, the maintenance of a dosing schedule that produces drug concentration measurements above or below the normal accepted therapeutic range may not be prudent.

Deciding on monitoring frequency

How frequently a patient should be monitored for efficacy or side effects related to drug therapy vary with the drug, the intensity of the disease, the stability of body functions, and other factors. In general, the more severely compromised the patient, the more frequently the patient should be monitored. This is essentially the same as would be recommended for most laboratory tests and monitoring schemes.

Clinicians should be aware of the many factors that can alter a drug's pharmacokinetic and pharmacodynamic activities. Addition or deletion of other drug therapy (or diet) that may interact with the drug being monitored should signal the need for closer inspection. Changes in the function of the primary organs of drug elimination (e.g., liver and kidneys) or in cardiac function also should signal the need for closer monitoring.

Finally, patient (or caregiver) adherence to the treatment regimen must be assessed whenever a decision is based on a drug concentration measurement. Simply assuming appropriate adherence to the prescribed regimen can lead to grave errors in the worst case and a waste of resources in others.

A Basic Pharmacokinetic Glossary

As the science of pharmacokinetic evaluation of drug therapy has progressed, the terminology used has grown as well. Although terms such as half-life and volume of distribution are standardized in most pharmacokinetic texts, a wide variety of terminology is used to describe other basic concepts.

For this reason, an attempt was made to standardize the terminology used throughout this book. The wide collection of studies used to reference the chapters somewhat hindered this effort.

With that understanding, the following terminology is offered as a guideline to interpreting the values and terms in this book.

Selected pharmacokinetic terminology

Actual body weight (ABW)—Patients measured body weight. Equivalent to total body weight.

Average steady state concentration (Css_{av})—Concentration measured approximately halfway between the peak and trough (except for some sustained-release preparations) for a drug administered long enough to be at steady state. Hence, for an intravenous bolus regimen on an every 6-hr interval, the Css_{av} would be at 3 hr after a dose. For a dose requiring absorption that peaks 2 hr after administration, the average would occur at approximately 4 hr on a 6-hr interval.

Ideal body weight (IBW)—Ideal weight for a patient based on their height according to insurance actuarial tables for longevity.

Lean body weight (LBW)—Patients body weight plus some but not all fat weight. It is often used interchangeably with IBW, but LBW increases as patients increase in weight.

Peak concentration (C_{peak})—The peak concentration is the highest or maximum concentration after any type of dosing method. It is the concentration of drug that occurs immediately after an intravenous bolus dose, at the end of a dose infusion, or at a particular time (t_{peak} or t_{max}) after dose administration for a drug requiring absorption. It may also be called C_{max} or Css_{max}. Occasionally the "peak" is considered the concentration measured within 30–60 min after the true peak time (e.g., 30 min after the end of a dose infusion for aminoglycosides); this peak might be considered a "therapeutic peak" for assessment of patient response rather than the actual peak. This time lag before collection in part acknowledges the reality that doses are not always given precisely on time and that blood samples are not always drawn precisely when scheduled for a true peak.

Steady state—Point in time reached after a drug has been given for approximately five elimination half-lives (97% of steady state has been achieved after five half-lives). At steady state, the rate of drug administration equals the rate of elimination, and drug concentration-time curves found after each dose on an even schedule (e.g., every 8 hr) should be approximately superimposable (i.e., if one graph of a drug concentration–time curve were laid on the next dose graph, they would be the same).

Administration of a loading dose can affect the time to steady state if the loading and maintenance doses are matched correctly. If the loading dose provides exactly the amount needed to achieve the steady state concentration that will be achieved by the maintenance dose, then steady state is achieved immediately. If the loading dose is too small or too large relative to attainment of the concentrations that will occur with maintenance doses, five half-lives will be required to achieve 97% of the *difference* between the loading dose concentrations and the final steady state concentrations.

Therapeutic range—Range of concentrations where optimum outcome is expected, based on results of groups of individuals taking the drug. In reality, each person has his or her own therapeutic range for each drug. As concentrations rise to the upper limit of the therapeutic range and beyond, the probability of drug toxicity increases. As concentrations fall to or below the lower limit of the range, the probability of inadequate response increases. This range should be viewed only as an initial target, because patients may respond when below it and may not be toxic when above it. Furthermore, minor toxicity above a therapeutic range might be acceptable to a patient if efficacy increases. Serious toxicity is a definite upper limit to any individual's therapeutic range.

Trough— The trough is the lowest or minimum concentration after a dose given intermittently (also called C_{min} or Css_{min}). It is the concentration that occurs immediately before the next dose for drugs given intermittently in a multiple-dose fashion. However, quite often the "trough" is the concentration measured within 30–60 min of the next dose. This trough might be considered a "therapeutic trough" related to this time in pharmacokinetic and pharmacodynamic studies of the drug. This time period in advance of the true trough also acknowledges variance in compliance with precise dose administration time and phlebotomist arrival time.

Selected pharmacokinetic symbols used in this text

These symbols generally follow the nomenclature suggested by the Committee for Pharmacokinetic Nomenclature of the American College of Clinical Pharmacology.[2] An exception is volume of distribution (V versus V_z).

C = plasma or serum concentration of drug

C_i = initial plasma or serum concentration, the larger of two plasma or serum concentrations in an elimination portion of a concentration-time curve. For example, in Equation 1 (see "General Pharmacokinetic Equations," below), C_i is the largest of two concentrations, C_i and C. Some authors designate the two concentrations as C_1 and C_2.

C_{max} = maximum drug concentration after a dose

Css = plasma or serum concentration at steady state

Css_{max} = maximum drug concentration after a dose at steady state

Css_{min} = minimum drug concentration after a dose at steady state

Css_{av} = concentration approximately halfway between Css_{max} and Css_{min} at steady state. The average steady state concentration.

CL = apparent total body clearance (either in units of volume per time, such as liters per hour, or in units of volume per time per body weight, such as liters per hour per kilogram). $CL = k \times V$.

$CrCl$ = creatinine clearance; the clearance of creatinine (in units of milliliters per minute or liters per hour)

D = dose (in amount, such as milligrams, or amount per patient body weight, such as milligrams per kilogram)

F = bioavailability fraction of a dose (no units). It is the fraction or percent of an administered dose that reaches the systemic circulation.

k = first-order elimination rate constant (in units of 1/time or $time^{-1}$).

$k = 0.693/t½$.

k_a = first-order absorption rate constant (in units of 1/time or time–1).

$k_a = 0.693/t½_a$.

K_m = Michaelis-Menten constant (in units of concentration such as milligrams per liter). It is the concentration at which the metabolic system is one-half saturated.

R_0 = zero-order infusion rate (in amount per time such as milligrams per hour)

S = fraction of a dose that is parent drug (i.e., the drug that is measured in plasma or serum). For example, phenytoin sodium is 92% phenytoin. Thus, S = 0.92 for phenytoin sodium products. No units.

S_{Cr} = serum creatinine (in mg/dl or µmol/L)

t = elapsed time. For example, it is the time between two concentrations, known or estimated, in the elimination phase of a drug following first-order elimination.

t' = time of an infusion (i.e., duration of infusion, usually in hours)

t_{peak} = time to peak (maximum concentration) of a drug that requires absorption (e.g., oral, intramuscular, inhaled, rectal, or buccal). Also called t_{max}.

$t_{1/2}$ = half-life of a drug (in units of time). It is the time needed to reduce the drug concentration or amount of drug in the body by one-half. $t_{1/2} = 0.693/k$.

$t_{1/2a}$ = absorption half-life of a drug product administered in a dosage form requiring absorption (in units of time). $t_{1/2a} = 0.693/k_a$.

T = time elapsed after the *end* of an infusion

Δt = change in time (usually the time between two measured concentrations)

τ = dosage interval (in units of time, usually hours or days)

V = apparent volume of distribution (either in units of volume, such as liters, or in units of volume per body weight, such as liters per kilogram)

V_{max} = (V_m) maximum velocity of drug elimination for a drug following Michaelis-Menten (enzyme saturable) elimination. It is the amount of drug that can be biotransformed per unit of time (in units of amount per time such as milligrams per day or in mg/kg/day).

General Estimating Equations

Like the above terms and symbols, several equations are frequently used in pharmacokinetic calculations and are considered to be standards. Frequently used equations for calculating ideal or lean body weight and body surface area are as follows. Additional information is provided in Chapter 3, "Medication Dosing in Overweight and Obese Patients." Creatinine clearance estimations are provided in Chapter 1, "Estimating Creatinine Clearance."

Calculating ideal body weight (IBW) in ***adults***[3]

$$\text{males} = 50\text{kg} + [(2.3)(\text{H} - 60)]\ \text{kg}$$
$$\text{females} = 45.5\text{kg} + [(2.3)(\text{H} - 60)]\ \text{kg}$$

where H is a patient's height in inches.

Or,

$$\text{males} = 50\text{kg} + [(0.9)(\text{H} - 152)]\ \text{kg}$$
$$\text{females} = 45.5\text{kg} + [(0.9)(\text{H} - 152)]\ \text{kg}$$

where H is a patient's height in cm.

Note: For patients who are less than 60 inches tall (152 cm), the weight should be decreased more conservatively than 2.3 kg/inch (2.3 kg/2.54 cm).

Calculating ideal body weight in ***children*** *aged 1–18* years[4]

For children **less than 5 feet (152 cm)** tall

$$\text{IBW} = 2.05e^{(0.02)(\text{H})}$$

where H is height in centimeters (2.54 cm/inch) and IBW is ideal weight in kg.

For children **5 feet (152 cm) or taller**

IBW (males) = 39 + [2.27(Ht – 60)]

IBW (females) = 42.2 + [2.27(Ht – 60)]

where Ht is height in inches and IBW is ideal weight in kg.

Or,

IBW (males) = 39 + [0.9(Ht – 152)]

IBW (females) = 42.2 + [0.9(Ht – 152)]

where Ht is height in centimeters and IBW is ideal weight in kg.

Calculating surface area (SA) in meters² (m²)

For adults, children, and infants[5]

$$SA = W^{0.5378} \times Ht^{0.3964} \times 0.024265$$

where W is weight in kg and Ht is height in centimeters.

Another simpler approach to determining BSA uses the following formula[6]:

$$BSA = \sqrt{\frac{\text{height} \times \text{weight}}{3600}}$$

where height is in cm, and weight in kg.

Calculating Body Mass Index (BMI) for men and women[7,a]

Metric

BMI = weight (kg) / [height (m)]^2 or [weight (kg) / height (m) / height (m)]

Pounds and inches

BMI = weight (lb) / [height (in)]^2 x 703 or [weight (lb) / height (in) / height (in)] x 703

[a] *BMI is an indicator of body fat and body fat content is related to the risk of disease and death. People are considered underweight if their BMI is <18.5, normal weight if 18.5 to 24.9, overweight if 25 to 29.9, and obese if ≥ 30. There are limits to the use of BMI including the potential to overestimate body fat in athletes and others who have a muscular build and to underestimate body fat in the elderly and in those who have lost muscle mass.*

General Pharmacokinetic Equations

The following equations are used to determine or estimate concentration and other pharmacokinetic parameters. These equations may be manipulated to determine other parameters in the equation when the remaining parameters are known or can be estimated. For example, a dose may be calculated from known or estimated CL, *V*, or *k* values by manipulating the applicable equations to solve for dose (*D*).

1. Concentration at any time *t* after some initial concentration (*Ci*):

$$C = Ci \times e^{-k \times t}$$

2. k from two known drug concentration-time points in the elimination phase:

$$k = \frac{\ln(C_i / C)}{\Delta t}$$

3. Concentration at any time t after a single intravenous bolus dose:

$$C = \left(\frac{S \times D}{V}\right) e^{-kt}$$

4. Concentration at any time t after an intravenous bolus dose given every τ hr (at steady state):

$$C = \frac{S \times D}{V} \left(\frac{\left(e^{-kt}\right)}{(1 - e^{-k\tau})} \right)$$

5. Concentration at any time t after the start of an intravenous infusion at rate R_0:

$$C = \frac{\left(S \times R_0\right)}{CL} (1 - e^{-kt})$$

6. Concentration at steady state of an intravenous infusion at rate R_0:

$$Css = \left(\frac{S \times R_0}{CL}\right)$$

7. Average steady state concentration of a dose given intermittently (by all dosing methods):

$$Css_{av} = \left(\frac{S \times F \times D}{CL \times \tau}\right)$$

or

$$Css_{av} = \left(\frac{S \times F \times D}{k \times V \times \tau}\right)$$

8. Concentration at any time t after a single dose requiring absorption:

$$C = \left(\frac{S \times F \times D \times k_a}{V \times (k_a - k)}\right) (e^{-kt} - e^{-k_a t})$$

9. Time to peak (maximum concentration) of a dose requiring absorption after a single dose:

$$t_{peak} = \frac{\ln\left(k_a / k\right)}{(k_a - k)}$$

10. Concentration at any time t after a dose requiring absorption during steady state conditions:

$$C = \left(\frac{S \times F \times D \times k_a}{V \times (k_a - k)}\right) \left(\frac{\left(e^{-kt}\right)}{(1 - e^{-k\tau})} - \frac{e^{-k_a t}}{1 - e^{-k_a \tau}} \right)$$

11. Time to peak (maximum concentration) of a dose requiring absorption at steady state:

$$tss_{peak} = \frac{\ln\left(k_a\left(1-e^{-k\tau}\right)/k\left(1-e^{-k_a\tau}\right)\right)}{(k_a - k)}$$

12. Concentration at any time T after the end of a single short infusion lasting t' time:

$$C = \left(\frac{S \times D}{k \times V \times t'}\right)(1 - e^{-kt'})e^{-kT}$$

13. Concentration at any time T after the end of a short infusion lasting t' time given every τ hr:

$$C = \left(\frac{S \times D}{k \times V \times t'}\right)\left(\frac{(1-e^{-kt'})}{(1-e^{-k\tau})}\right)\left(e^{-kT}\right)$$

14. Average steady state concentration of a drug that follows Michaelis-Menten elimination:

$$Css_{av} = \left(\frac{\left(\frac{S \times F \times D}{\tau}\right) \times k_m}{V_m - \left(\frac{S \times F \times D}{\tau}\right)}\right)$$

15. Dose to produce desired steady state concentration for a drug that follows Michaelis-Menten elimination:

$$D = \frac{Css_{av} \times V_m \times \tau}{S \times F \times (Css_{av} + k_m)}$$

References

1. Murphy JE, Job ML, Ward ES. Rectifying incorrect dosage schedules. *Am J Hosp Pharm.* 1990;47:2235-6.
2. Committee for Pharmacokinetic Nomenclature. Manual of symbols, equations, & definitions in pharmacokinetics. *J Clin Pharmacol.* 1982;22:1S-23S.
3. Devine BJ. Gentamicin therapy. *Drug Intell Clin Pharm.* 1974;7:650-5.
4. Traub SL, Johnson CE. Comparison of methods of estimating creatinine clearance in children. *Am J Hosp Pharm.* 1980;37:195-201.
5. Haycock GB, Schwartz GJ, Wisotsky DH. Geometric method for measuring body surface area: a height-weight formula validated in infants, children, and adults. *J Pediatr.* 1978;93:62-6.
6. Mosteller RD. Simplified calculation of body surface area. *N Engl J Med.* 1987;317:1098.
7. Anon. Calculate your body mass index. National Heart Lung and Blood Institute: Obesity Education Initiative. Available at: http://www.nhlbisupport.com/bmi/. Accessed November 24, 2010.

Section 1: Basic Concepts and Special Populations

1 Estimating Creatinine Clearance
Robert E. Pachorek

2 Rational Use of Drug Concentration Measurements
James P. McCormack

3 Medication Dosing in Overweight and Obese Patients
Brian Erstad

4 Drug Dosing in Pediatric Patients
Vinita B. Pai and Milap C. Nahata

5 Therapeutic Drug Monitoring in the Geriatric Patient
Susan W. Miller

6 Renal Drug Dosing Concepts
Gary R. Matzke and Thomas C. Dowling

Chapter 1

Robert E. Pachorek

Estimating Creatinine Clearance

The importance of accurate estimations of glomerular filtration rate (GFR), the principal measure of renal function, cannot be overemphasized. Many drugs or active metabolites are eliminated to some extent by renal excretion, creating the need for dosage adjustments as renal function deteriorates, particularly for drugs with a narrow therapeutic range (see Chapter 6, "Renal Drug Dosing Concepts"). In general, decreases in the rate of elimination of drugs primarily excreted unchanged by the kidneys are proportional to decreases in the GFR.

Though determination of inulin clearance and other elaborate clearance methods are available for such assessment, the renal clearance of the endogenously produced amino acid creatinine is the most commonly used estimate of GFR in hospitalized patients. Creatine, a product of protein metabolism, is primarily produced in the liver, pancreas, and kidneys and is actively transported into muscle tissue where it is stored. Creatinine is produced from creatine in muscle tissue proportionally to muscle mass. It is released at a constant rate (approximately 1.5% of the total pool per day) into the general circulation and is distributed to total body water. Creatinine is passively filtered by the glomerulus proportionately to the GFR, although 10% to 40% of the total creatinine found in urine is a result of active renal tubular secretion.[1–4]

The creatinine clearance (CrCl), in milliliters per minute (ml/min), can be directly measured by collecting urine over a period of time (e.g., 24 hr) using the following relationship:

$$\text{CrCl} = \frac{U_{\text{Cr}} \times V_{\text{Cr}}}{S_{\text{Cr}} \times t}$$

where U_{Cr} is the urine creatinine concentration (mg/dl), V_{Cr} is the urine volume collected (ml), S_{Cr} is serum creatinine (mg/dl) measured at the midpoint of the urine collection, and t is the time interval in minutes of the urine collection (e.g., 1440 min for 24 hr).[1,2]

Factors affecting estimates of glomerular filtration rate

Because some creatinine found in the urine is due to tubular secretion, CrCl overestimates the GFR at all levels of renal function. Drugs such as amiloride, cimetidine, trimethoprim, salicylate, triamterene, and spironolactone, which inhibit this secretory function, may increase S_{Cr} and decrease the CrCl estimate without actually affecting the GFR.[2–5] As GFR declines, there is a progressive relative increase in creatinine tubular secretion compared to filtration and a progressive disparity between actual GFR and CrCl. In one study it was noted that when the true GFR was around 100 ml/min, the CrCl overestimates the GFR by about 20%; for a GFR of 60 ml/min, the CrCl was overestimated by about 60%; and for a GFR of 20 ml/min, the CrCl was overestimated by 100% or more.[2–5] In the past this error was partially offset if the laboratory was using an uncorrected Jaffe-based method assay to determine serum creatinine because endogenous serum substances added approximately 0.2 mg/dL to the creatinine value when measured by this common method.[5] The new assay reference standard negates the increase in S_{Cr} seen with the Jaffe-based method and thus reintroduces the error of GFR estimate caused by tubular secretion of creatinine (see Creatinine Assay Standardization, below).[6]

Disease states and aging effects on muscle mass affect creatinine production and turnover. The measured 24-hr CrCl is less likely to be affected than estimates using patient demographics and S_{Cr} to estimate CrCl. Drugs and exogenous or endogenous compounds that interact with the laboratory assays for creatinine may also affect estimates of CrCl. The compounds in Table 1-1 may positively bias the creatinine concentration by interfering with creatinine assays (dependent on the assay system, methodology, and instrument used).

These compounds all have the potential to interfere with the SCr assays though the extent of interference is dependent on the given instrument used. If a patient has a potential for a creatinine–lab assay interaction,

Table 1-1. Compounds that Interfere with Creatinine Assays

Jaffe-based Assays	Enzymatic Assays
Acetoacetate	Flucytosine
Acetohexamide	Lidocaine
Bilirubin	
Cefoxitin, cephalothin	
Other cephalosporins (supratherapeutic)	
Furosemide (supratherapeutic)	
Lactulose	
Methyldopa infusions	
Endogenous serum substances (+ 0.2 mg/dL creatinine unless assay standardized to IDMS reference method)	

clinicians should check with the laboratory for the specific interference with the instrument used. Judicious timing of the drawing of blood for serum creatinine determination (at minimal interfering drug concentration) or using an alternate assay method may be advisable.[2,3,5]

Exogenous creatine supplementation could be thought to affect the creatinine serum concentration since creatine is converted to creatinine. However, a recent review of studies of acute and chronic creatine ingestion in young healthy populations found minimal impact on serum creatinine concentrations.[7]

Creatinine assay standardization

The National Kidney Disease Education Program (NKDEP) of the U.S. National Institute of Health (NIH) recently launched an international program to standardize the creatinine assay calibration in health care laboratories. This will decrease the former positive bias (up to 20%) of the creatinine assay through laboratory instrument recalibration to agree with an isotope dilution mass spectrometry (IDMS) reference method.[6,8] This calibration will lead most of the CrCl estimating equations for adults and pediatrics to give higher CrCl estimates than in the past.[8-10] These differences may not be as clinically important for dosing of a drug with a wide therapeutic index (e.g., cefazolin); however, for drug dosing using pharmacokinetic population estimates in drugs with a narrow therapeutic index (e.g., aminoglycosides) this change may have important clinical implications. Laboratories using the IDMS reference method can provide specific mathematical conversion factors to adjust creatinine values to results similar to those obtained using their previous method of calibration.[8] These adjusted creatinine values can be used in CrCl estimating equations developed in the past.[8]

Formulas to estimate creatinine clearance in adults

Collecting urine for 24 hr for a creatinine measurement is tedious and must be done accurately with no missed collections and accurate measurement of urine volume to properly measure the CrCl. Because this is difficult and time consuming, formulas have been derived that use the serum creatinine and patient demographics to estimate GFR.

The many equations for rapid estimation of CrCl published over the last 25 years generally produce similar values. Two well-validated and commonly used equations for *adult* patients when S_{Cr} is at steady state are the Cockcroft/Gault equation and the Jelliffe equation.[11-13] Cockcroft/Gault is the equation usually included in drug product labeling (package inserts) for individualizing drug dosages for renally cleared drugs when an equation is mentioned.[14] Another more recently developed equation is being used to estimate GFR in adult patients with chronic kidney disease (MDRD Study equation; discussed later); however, at this time its use for drug dosing purposes has been questioned.[14]

Cockcroft/Gault equation:

$$\text{CrCl (males)(ml/min)} = \frac{(140 - \text{age})(W)}{(72)(S_{\text{Cr}})}$$

$$\text{CrCl (females)} = \text{CrCl (males)} \times 0.85$$

where S_{Cr} is in milligrams per deciliter (mg/dl) and *W* is weight (kg). The International Systems conversion is:

$$\text{CrCr (males)} = \frac{1.23 \times (140 - \text{age}) \times (W)}{S_{\text{Cr}}}$$

$$\text{CrCl (females)} = \text{CrCl (males)} \times 0.85$$

where S_{Cr} is in micromoles per liter (µmol/L) and *W* is weight (kg).

Jelliffe equation:

$$\text{CrCl (males)(m1/min/1.73 m}^2\text{ BSA)} = \frac{98 - [0.8(\text{Age} - 20)]}{S_{\text{Cr}}}$$

where BSA is body surface area and S_{Cr} is in mg/dl.

The International Systems conversion is:

$$\text{CrCl (males)(m1/min/1.73 m}^2\text{ BSA)} = \frac{8863 - [70.7(\text{Age} - 20)]}{S_{\text{Cr}}}$$

where S_{Cr} is in µmol/L.

CrCl (females) = CrCl (males) x 0.9 for both versions.

Because creatinine is produced in muscle tissue, weight in the Cockcroft/Gault equation is preferably ideal body weight (IBW) or actual body weight (ABW) if it is less than IBW. However, there are many important considerations in these generalizations (see section on body weight). The original authors used ABW in developing their equation, but other researchers have examined the impact of obesity on predictability. IBW is estimated by the following[15]:

IBW (males) (kg) = $50 + [2.3(H - 60)]$

IBW (females) (kg) = $45.5 + [2.3(H - 60)]$

where *H* is height in inches, or,

IBW (males) (kg) = $50 + [0.9(H - 152)]$

IBW (females) (kg) = $45.5 + [0.9(H - 152)]$

where H is height in centimeters (cm).

In the Jelliffe equation, the CrCl is normalized to an average adult body surface area (BSA) of 1.73 m^2 and the units are ml/min/1.73 m^2. If the patient does not have a BSA of 1.73 m^2 then the result needs to be converted to their actual CrCl in ml/min. To calculate the CrCl (in ml/min), the result is multiplied by the patient's BSA and then divided by 1.73.[16] BSA may be determined from the following equation.

$$\text{BSA (m}^2\text{)} = W^{0.5378} \times H^{0.3964} \times 0.024265$$

where W is weight (kg) and H is height (cm)

The Cockcroft/Gault and Jelliffe equations work reasonably well for most adults with S_{Cr} at steady state because they allow for declining muscle mass (and creatinine production) often associated with reduced weight and advancing age and are adjusted for the average smaller muscle mass of females. The Cockcroft/Gault equation is the most commonly used and recommended equation for CrCl estimation for drug dosing and is discussed in greater detail in the following sections. The Jelliffe equation is still used by some clinicians and is reasonably accurate for use when height and weight are not available in average size patients.[13] The accuracy of these equations in predicting CrCl is often limited in patients with various disease states or conditions. These include the elderly, the malnourished, the obese, patients with amputations or spinal cord injuries, those with chronic renal insufficiency, acutely changing renal function, those with liver disease, critically ill patients, and pediatric patients.[1–3,17–42] Other, possibly more accurate methods and equations for rapid prediction of renal function will continue to evolve as more patients and larger subgroups are studied.[17,43]

The National Kidney Disease Education Program (NKDEP) has recommended using one of the Modification of Diet in Renal Disease (MDRD) Study equations for estimation of GFR in adults as a screening tool for kidney disease, and is encouraging clinical laboratories to report this estimated GFR (eGFR) along with the patient's serum creatinine. An MDRD Study equation eGFR result may be seen in this situation, as they do not require the patient's weight. The NKDEP has suggested use of the eGFR or the Cockcroft/Gault equation for drug dosing.[9] In the U.S., many of the drugs that have FDA approved product labeling for drug dosing in patients with renal dysfunction, have dosing guidelines specifically indexed to CrCl and some note use of the Cockcroft/Gault equation.[14] For this reason use of the eGFR for drug dosing has been questioned, and it was recently reported in one survey that pharmacy clinicians did not substitute eGFR for CrCl.[14]

Abbreviated MDRD Study equations:

Non-IDMS lab-calibrated creatinine[9]:

$$\text{GFR (ml/min/1.73 m}^2\text{)} = 186 \times (S_{Cr})^{-1.154} \times (\text{age})^{-0.203} \times (0.742 \text{ if female}) \times (1.21 \text{ if African American})$$

IDMS lab-calibrated creatinine[9]:

$$\text{GFR (ml/min/1.73 m}^2\text{)} = 175 \times (S_{Cr})^{-1.154} \times (\text{age})^{-0.203} \times (0.742 \text{ if female}) \times (1.21 \text{ if African American})$$

where S_{Cr} is in milligrams per deciliter (mg/dL). For conversion to International Systems using S_{Cr} in μmol/L, change both of the S_{Cr} equation terms to:

$$(S_{Cr})^{0.1}$$

The rest of the equations remain the same.

Both of these equations provide values that are automatically normalized to ml/min/1.73 m^2. When using these equations in very large or very small patients, the result in ml/min/1.73 m^2 should be converted to ml/min.[9] To calculate the actual eGFR (in ml/min), the result is multiplied by the patient's BSA and then divided by 1.73 m^2.

The MDRD Study equation, though created from a large group of patients, has not been validated in many population groups including: children, the elderly (>70 years), patients with serious comorbid conditions, body size extremes, muscle mass extremes, severe malnutrition, pregnant patients, ill hospitalized patients, amputees, and patients with near normal renal function.[8,44] The equation is not weight based but is affected by obesity and other factors that affect creatinine production.[6,8,44] As noted above, the NKDEP is currently recommending eGFR reporting by laboratories along with serum creatinine to aid in the detection, evaluation, and management of patients with chronic kidney disease. They recommend reporting exact actual values for eGFRs of 60 ml/min/1.73 m^2 and below, but for values above 60 ml/min/1.73 m^2 they recommend reporting it as "> 60 ml/min/1.73 m^2." The rationale for this is: 1) the equation was more extensively studied in patients with chronic kidney disease, 2) the imprecision of creatinine assays have the greatest effect on near normal renal function, and 3) quantification of GFR below 60 mL/min/1.73 m^2 has more clinical implications from a disease progression point of view.[6]

Adjustments in the weight and/or creatinine variables based on a patient's clinical condition are commonly made in the Cockcroft/Gault equation in attempts to improve predictive performance. Clinicians should carefully assess the patient's clinical status and importance of an accurate assessment of renal function and modify these variables or use another more suitable equation or a timed CrCl measurement if necessary. In general, the following subgroup reviews pertain to adult patients (see section on pediatrics for CrCl estimation in children).

Body weight

Creatinine production is dependent on muscle mass, and the use of IBW in the Cockcroft/Gault equation appears to produce reliable results in patients whose ABW is not far from IBW. For patients who are malnourished or cachectic with an ABW less than their IBW, the ABW should be used.[1–3,15,18] For adult patients less than 1.52 m (60 inches) tall, use of the lesser of ABW or IBW (males = 50 kg, females = 45.5 kg) has been proposed.[19] Other methods of predicting IBW are provided in the Introduction and Chapter 3, "Medication Dosing in Overweight and Obese Patients."

Obesity (defined as >20% over IBW or BMI > 30) is another factor that affects the Cockcroft and Gault CrCl estimation. Obese patients appear to have a larger muscle mass than would be predicted when using height in the IBW equation. Using IBW is still preferable to using ABW; however, using an adjusted body weight (BW_{adj}) between IBW and ABW may be more accurate. Use of a factor of 40% or 20% of the difference between ABW and IBW has been proposed.[3,17,19]

$$BW_{adj} = IBW + 0.4(ABW - IBW)$$

$$BW_{adj} = IBW + 0.2(ABW - IBW)$$

The notion of "correct" weight to use in the prediction equations is an interesting one. As mentioned earlier, Cockcroft and Gault used ABW to develop the equation. Many authors have studied and suggested the use of IBW or one of the BW_{adj} for patients who weigh more than their IBW. Intuitively such approaches seem reasonable since creatinine is produced in muscle, not fat tissue. One suggestion that might help in determining a reasonable weight is to avoid use of only standards and to visually examine the patient. For example, a 180 cm (5'11") body builder who weighs 100 kg (220 lb) would clearly be expected to produce more creatinine daily than a sedentary individual of the same height and weight. Both patients would be estimated to have the same IBW and both are considered obese by definition (ABW > 20% above IBW). It would seem reasonable to anticipate that the former patient should have creatinine clearance estimated using ABW, since the additional weight will be creatinine producing, while the latter would be best estimated using BW_{adj} (or even IBW if they were extremely sedentary with little additional muscle mass associated with the adiposity). Finally, it should be expected that the more the patient differs from the patients used in the studies to develop the equations, the greater the potential that predictions might not match actual measured CrCl.

Another method of CrCl estimation may have better predictive ability in the obese patient (see Salazar-Corcoran equation below) but is a bit more complicated to use.[3,17,20] Methods of adjusting body weight in the morbidly obese (BMI > 40) have recently been reviewed.[36]

$$\text{CrCl (males)} = \frac{(137 - \text{age}) \times [(0.285 \times W) + (12.1 \times H^2)]}{(51 \times S_{Cr})}$$

$$\text{CrCl (females)} = \frac{(146 - \text{age}) \times [(0.287 \times W) + (9.74 \times H^2)]}{(60 \times S_{Cr})}$$

where W is weight in kg, H is height in **m**, and S_{Cr} is in mg/dl.

In international units where S_{Cr} is in μmol/L, the equations would be:

$$\text{CrCl}_{\text{(males)}} = \frac{(137 - \text{age}) \times [(0.285 \times W) + (12.1 \times H^2)]}{0.58 \times S_{Cr}}$$

$$\text{CrCl}_{\text{(females)}} = \frac{(146 - \text{age}) \times [(0.287 \times W) + (9.74 \times H^2)]}{0.68 \times S_{Cr}}$$

Low serum creatinine/elderly patients

It is a fairly common practice for clinicians to round measured S_{Cr} concentrations that are less than 0.8 or 0.9 mg/dl to a higher value in elderly or underweight adult patients before using the estimating equations. The S_{Cr} is inversely proportional to CrCl and using an unrealistically low S_{Cr} value in an elderly or other patient with significantly decreased muscle mass or creatinine production may overestimate the CrCl, leading to the use of higher drug doses. The use of a value of 1 mg/dl as the lower limit of S_{Cr} in these equations has been popular with some clinicians; however, underprediction of CrCl may also occur. Using 0.8 or 0.7 (or less) as the lower limit of S_{Cr} may be more appropriate.[21–24] Intuitively, it would seem to make sense that a patient's muscle mass would give some guide to how much "fudging" should be done in setting a lower limit of S_{Cr}. That is, in a patient with obviously limited muscle mass it might be more reasonable to adjust the S_{Cr} upward than in a patient with average muscle mass. Also, it seems reasonable to assume that the larger the degree of "fudging" of the S_{Cr} upward to some minimum value, the greater the likelihood of poor prediction. That is, changing a measured S_{Cr} from 0.3 to 0.7 might result in a poorer prediction of actual CrCl than changing from 0.6 to 0.7. Further, it also seems logical that the same conditions (elderly with decreased muscle mass) present in a patient with an S_{Cr} of 1 or more would lead to a need to increase the S_{Cr} arbitrarily in order to avoid overestimating CrCl. However, this has not generally been recommended and there is little data to support such approaches. The use of a percentage increase in S_{Cr} might be more logical and would be an area for study.

Amputations

Estimation of CrCl in patients with amputated limbs poses a dilemma for IBW calculation. A reasonable approach would be to determine the height-based IBW before the amputation, then subtract the percent of the missing limb based on data from a body segment percentage table.[25] The weight used would be the lesser of this adjusted IBW or the ABW. The average weight of body segments of a 68-kg (150-lb) man are: upper limb, 4.9%; entire lower limb, 15.6%; thigh, 9.7%; leg (below knee), 4.5%; foot, 1.4%. This suggested method for IBW calculation in amputees has not been validated for its utility in predicting CrCl in these patients.

Spinal cord injury

CrCl estimation in patients with spinal cord injury appears to be unpredictable because of the changes in muscle mass that occur over time after the injury. Accuracy has been reported in some patient populations (paraplegics with good renal function); however, the 24-hr CrCl measurement should be used in patients with spinal cord injuries if accuracy is necessary.[26,39]

Chronic renal insufficiency

As already noted, with declining renal function S_{Cr} may become a less accurate indicator of renal function (GFR) due to the increasing percentage of tubular secretion of creatinine in relation to the total urinary excretion. That is, as renal function decreases, tubular secretion becomes a larger part of creatinine elimination. In addition, there appears to be an extrarenal route of creatinine elimination via the GI tract in uremic patients. These patients may have a poor dietary intake and reduced muscle mass as well.[2,17] Use of oral cimetidine (800 mg every 12 hours for three doses) to inhibit tubular secretion of creatinine prior to urine collection or S_{Cr} measurement has been advocated to improve estimation of GFR.[27,38,40] Ranitidine and famotidine have not been shown to inhibit the tubular secretion of creatinine and should not be used for this purpose.[38] Again, if the CrCl is being used to determine doses, it may not be necessary to make such changes for estimating GFR, since drug dosing studies have traditionally used CrCl estimates.

Dialysis

Estimating creatinine clearance in patients receiving dialysis is problematic and not recommended. A patient without functioning kidneys has no glomerular filtration. Thus, the S_{Cr} concentration becomes primarily a function of the dialysis procedure rather than the patient's kidney function. Because no urine output indicates no renal function, monitoring residual urine output gives some idea whether the patient's kidneys have any potential role in drug elimination.

Liver disease

Estimation of renal function in patients with cirrhosis presents certain dilemmas. Estimates of GFR using CrCl estimations (Cockcroft/Gault) and 24-hr CrCl measurements may be unreliable as shown by inulin clearance tests. These patients should have their drug therapy monitored more carefully, particularly for drugs with a narrow therapeutic index, where drug concentration monitoring is recommended whenever possible.[28–31,41,42]

Pediatrics

Creatinine clearance measurements in children have been shown to accurately predict GFR. Because a measured 24-hr CrCl is as difficult and time consuming as in adults, equations have been developed for rapid estimation based on a patient's height and weight. These estimates appear most accurate for patients of average weight for their size. The equations use S_{Cr} and height (body length) to estimate the normalized CrCl (as if BSA was 1.73 m^2). The correlation of a child's muscle mass with his or her height helps factor in the relationship between muscle mass and creatinine production. However, these estimations may be less accurate for children who are significantly under- or overweight for their height and in the first week of life when the serum creatinine of an infant still reflects maternal serum creatinine and renal function is immature.[33]

A commonly used equation (the first equation in Table 1-2) for *children 1–18 years* of age was developed by Traub and Johnson.[32] For *infants, children, and adolescents*, specific equations shown in Table 1-2 have been used.[33] For institutions that have moved to the IDMS creatinine calibration, use of this standard with the Jaffe method introduces a potentially unacceptable amount of error, i.e., the CrCl appears higher than it actually is. The following equation can only be used if the lab is employing the enzymatic assay.[45-47]

Using IDMS calibrated creatinine—enzymatic assay only[45-47]

GFR (ml/min/1.73m^2) = 0.413 (H/S_{cr})

where SCr is in mg/dl and H in cm.

In international units where S_{Cr} is in µmol/L, the equation would be:

GFR (ml/min/1.73m^2) = 36.5 (H/S_{cr})

All of these equations provide values that are automatically normalized to 1.73 m^2. To calculate the actual CrCl (in ml/min), the equation result is multiplied by the patient's BSA and divided by 1.73.[16]

Table 1-2. Creatinine Clearance Estimation in Children (Using Non-IDMS Calibrated Creatinine Assay)

Age Range	Standard Units[a]	International Standardized Units[b]
1 to 18 years[32]	$\text{CrCl (ml/min/1.73 m}^2\text{ BSA)} = \frac{(0.48)(H)}{S_{Cr}}$	$\text{CrCl (ml/min/1.73 m}^2\text{ BSA)} = \frac{(42.4)(H)}{S_{Cr}}$
< 1 year[33]		
Preterm Infant	$\text{GFR (ml/min/1.73m}^2) = \frac{(0.33)(H)}{S_{Cr}}$	$\text{GFR (ml/min/1.73m}^2) = \frac{(29.2)(H)}{S_{Cr}}$
Full Term Infant	$\text{CrCl (ml/min/1.73 m}^2\text{ BSA)} = \frac{(0.45)(H)}{S_{Cr}}$	$\text{CrCl (ml/min/1.73 m}^2\text{ BSA)} = \frac{(39.8)(H)}{S_{Cr}}$
1 to 12 years[33]	$\text{CrCl (ml/min/1.73 m}^2\text{ BSA)} = \frac{(0.55)(H)}{S_{Cr}}$	$\text{CrCl (ml/min/1.73 m}^2\text{ BSA)} = \frac{(48.6)(H)}{S_{Cr}}$
13 to 21 years girls[33]	$\text{GFR (ml/min/1.73m}^2) = \frac{(0.55)(H)}{S_{Cr}}$	$\text{GFR (ml/min/1.73m}^2) = \frac{(48.6)(H)}{S_{Cr}}$
13 to 21 years boys[33]	$\text{GFR (ml/min/1.73m}^2) = \frac{(0.70)(H)}{S_{Cr}}$	$\text{GFR (ml/min/1.73m}^2) = \frac{(61.9)(H)}{S_{Cr}}$

[a]SCr is in mg/dl and H in cm.
[b]SCr is in µmol/L and H in cm.

Patients with unstable renal function

The discussed equations for CrCl estimation are based on patients with stable renal function with S_{Cr} at steady state. In patients with changing renal function, S_{Cr} may not reflect the current function for several days. Using a value of S_{Cr} that is not at steady state to calculate a CrCl may significantly over- or underestimate the patient's renal function and result in inappropriate drug dosing.

Estimating Time to Steady State Serum Creatinine Concentration

The time to a steady state S_{Cr} value increases as the patient's renal function declines. The time to 95% of steady state has been estimated to be 0.92, 1.85, and 4.5 days as a patient's renal function rapidly declines to 50%, 25%, and 10% of normal, respectively. It is estimated that if the S_{Cr} changes by more than 0.2 mg/dl in 12 hr, steady state probably has not been reached.[34]

Determining a rough estimate of the half-life and time to steady state of creatinine in a specific adult patient may be made by assuming that the Cockcroft/Gault equation is accurate in estimating CrCl, that the patient's volume of distribution (*V*) of creatinine is approximately 0.6 L/kg of IBW[34,35] and making the following calculations:

1. Estimate the patient's CrCl (ml/min) based on the Cockcroft/Gault equation.
2. Convert the patient's CrCl in milliliters per minute (ml/min) to liters per hour (L/hr) by multiplying by 0.06 (because of the following conversion):

   $$\frac{60\text{ min}}{1\text{ hr}} \times \frac{1\text{L}}{1000\text{ ml}} = 0.06 \text{ (units will cancel appropriately below)}$$

   Thus, ml/min × 0.06 = L/hr.

3. Use the relationship $K = CL/V$ to calculate K, the elimination rate constant, where CL is the creatinine clearance in liters per hour (L/hr), and V is the volume of distribution of creatinine in liters (0.6 L/kg × IBW).
4. Use $t½ = 0.693/K$ to estimate the half-life.
5. Approximately 4 times the estimated half-life equals time to steady state (94% achieved).

Creatinine Clearance Estimation in Unstable Renal Function

Several equations for use in patients with unstable renal function are available and may be useful for initial drug dosing; however, estimating CrCl in a patient with changing renal function can be problematic and drug concentration monitoring is recommended for drugs with a narrow therapeutic index.[1-3,34,35] For 24-hr CrCl measurements in patients with changing renal function, use the midpoint (12th hr) S_{Cr} or the average of the S_{Cr} at the beginning and the end of the 24-hr urine collection.[35] The following equation has been used to estimate CrCl in patients with unstable renal function[37]:

$$\text{CrCl (males)} = \frac{[[293 - 2.03(age)] \times [1.035 - 0.01685(S_{Cr1} + S_{Cr2})]] + [49(S_{Cr1} - S_{Cr2})/\Delta t]]}{S_{Cr1} + S_{Cr2}}$$

where Δt is the change in time in number of days between measurement of S_{Cr1} and S_{Cr2}.

CrCl (females) = CrCl (males) × 0.86

References

1. Lam YW, Banerji S, Hatfield C, et al. Principles of drug administration in renal insufficiency. *Clin Pharmacokinet.* 1997;32:30-57.
2. Duarte CG, Preuss HG. Assessment of renal function—glomerular and tubular. *Clin Lab Med.* 1993;13(1):33-52.
3. Robert S, Zarowitz BJ. Is there a reliable index of glomerular filtration rate in critically ill patients? *DICP Ann Pharmacother.* 1991;25:169-78.
4. Stevens LA, Levey AS. Measurement of kidney function. *Med Clin N Am.* 2005;89:457-73.
5. Ducharme MP, Smythe M, Strohs G. Drug-induced alterations in serum creatinine concentrations. *Ann Pharmacother.* 1993;27:622-33.
6. Myers GL, Miller WG, Coresh J, et al. Recommendations for improving serum creatinine measurement: a report from the Laboratory Working Group of the National Kidney Disease Education Program. *Clin Chem.* 2006;52:5-18.
7. Pline KA, Smith CL. The effect of creatine intake on renal function. *Ann Pharmacother.* 2005;39:1093-6.
8. National Institute of Health. National Kidney Disease Education Program. Laboratory Professionals. Clinical Laboratories. Creatinine Standardization Recommendations. Available at: http://www.nkdep.nih.gov/labprofessionals/Clinical_Laboratories.htm. Accessed November 14, 2010.
9. National Institute of Health. National Kidney Disease Education Program. Health Professionals. CKD and Drug Dosing: Information for Providers. Available at: http://www.nkdep.nih.gov/professionals/drug-dosing-information.htm. Accessed January 2, 2011.
10. Levey AS, Coresh J, Greene T, et al. Using standardized serum creatinine values in the Modification of Diet in Renal Disease Study equation for estimating glomerular filtration rate. *Ann Intern Med.* 2006;145:247-54.
11. Cockcroft DW, Gault MH. Prediction of creatinine clearance from serum creatinine. *Nephron.* 1976;16:31-41.

12. Lott RS, Hayton WL. Estimation of creatinine clearance from serum creatinine concentration—a review. *Drug Intell Clin Pharm.* 1978;12:140-50.
13. Jelliffe RW. Creatinine clearance: a bedside estimate. *Ann Intern Med.* 1973;79:604-5.
14. Dowling TC, Matzke GR, Murphy JE, et al. Evaluation of renal drug dosing: Prescribing information and clinical pharmacist approaches. *Pharmacother.* 2010;30:776-86.
15. Devine BJ. Gentamicin therapy. *Drug Intell Clin Pharm.* 1974;7:650-5.
16. Haycock GB, Schwartz GJ, Wisotsky DH. Geometric method for measuring body surface area: a height-weight formula validated in infants, children, and adults. *J Pediatr.* 1978;93:62-6.
17. Spinler SA, Nawarskas JJ, Boyce EG, et al. Predictive performance of ten equations for estimating creatinine clearance in cardiac patients. Iohexol Cooperative Study Group. *Ann Pharmacother.* 1998;32:1275-83.
18. Boyce EG, Dickerson RN, Cooney GF, et al. Creatinine clearance estimation in protein-malnourished patients. *Clin Pharm.* 1989;8:721-6.
19. Sawyer WT, Canaday BR, Poe TE, et al. Variables affecting creatinine clearance prediction. *Am J Hosp Pharm.* 1983;40:2175-80.
20. Salazar DE, Corcoran GB. Predicting creatinine clearance and renal drug clearance in obese patients from estimated fat-free body mass. *Am J Med.* 1988;84:1053-60.
21. Reichley RM, Ritchie DJ, Bailey TC. Analysis of various creatinine clearance formulas in predicting gentamicin elimination in patients with low serum creatinine. *Pharmacotherapy.* 1995;15:625-30.
22. Smythe M, Hoffman J, Kizy K, et al. Estimating creatinine clearance in elderly patients with low serum creatinine concentrations. *Am J Hosp Pharm.* 1994;51:198-204.
23. O'Connell MB, Dwinell AM, Bannick-Mohrland SD. Predictive performance of equations to estimate creatinine clearance in hospitalized elderly patients. *Ann Pharmacother.* 1992;26:627-35.
24. Bertino JS Jr. Measured versus estimated creatinine clearance in patients with low serum creatinine values. *Ann Pharmacother.* 1993;27:1439-42.
25. Brunnstrom S. *Clinical Kinesiology.* 4th ed. Philadelphia, PA: F.A. Davis Co.;1983:56.
26. Mohler JL, Ellison MF, Flanigan RC. Creatinine clearance prediction in spinal cord injury patients: comparison of 6 prediction equations. *J Urol.* 1988;139:706-9.
27. Walser M. Assessing renal function from creatinine measurements in adults with chronic renal failure. *Am J Kidney Dis.* 1998;32:23-31.
28. DeSanto NG, Anastasio P, Loguercio C, et al. Creatinine clearance: an inadequate marker of renal filtration in patients with early posthepatitic cirrhosis (Child A) without fluid retention and muscle wasting. *Nephron.* 1995;70:421-4.
29. Papadakis MA, Arieff AI. Unpredictability of clinical evaluation of renal function in cirrhosis. *Am J Med.* 1987;82:945-52.
30. Hull JH, Hak LJ, Koch GG, et al. Influence of range of renal function and liver disease on predictability of creatinine clearance. *Clin Pharmacol Ther.* 1981;29:516-21.
31. Pachorek RE, Wood F. Vancomycin half-life in a patient with hepatic and renal dysfunction. *Clin Pharm.* 1991;10:297-300.
32. Traub SL, Johnson CE. Comparison of methods of estimating creatinine clearance in children. *Am J Hosp Pharm.* 1980;37:195-201.
33. Schwartz GJ, Brion LP, Spitzer A. The use of plasma creatinine concentration for estimating glomerular filtration rate in infants, children, and adolescents. *Pediatr Clin North Am.* 1987;34:571-90.
34. Winter ME. Creatinine clearance. In: Winter ME. *Basic Clinical Pharmacokinetics.* 3rd ed. Vancouver, WA: Applied Therapeutics;1994:93-103.
35. Chow MS, Schweizer R. Estimation of renal creatinine clearance in patients with unstable serum creatinine concentrations: comparison of multiple methods. *Drug Intell Clin Pharm.* 1985;19:385-90.
36. Demirovic JA, Pai AB, Pai MP. Estimation of creatinine clearance in morbidly obese patients. *Am J Health Syst Pharm.* 2009;66:642-8.
37. Brater DC. Drug use in renal disease. Balgowlah, Australia: ADIS Health Science Press;1983:22-56.
38. Kemperman FAW, Krediet RT, Arisz, L. Formula-derived prediction of the glomerular filtration rate from plasma creatinine concentration. *Nephron.* 2002;91:547-58.
39. Thakur V, Reisin E, Solomonow M, et al. Accuracy of formula-derived creatinine clearance in paraplegic subjects. *Clin Nephrol.* 1997;47:237-42.
40. Ixkes MCJ, Koopman MG, van Acker AC, et al. Cimetidine improves GFR-estimation by the Cockcroft and Gault formula. *Clin Nephrol.* 1997;47:229-36.

41. Lam NP, Sperelakis R, Kuk J, et al. Rapid estimation of creatinine clearances in patients with liver dysfunction. *Dig Dis Sci*. 1999;44:1222-7.

42. Orlando R, Floreani M, Padrini R, et al. Evaluation of measured and calculated creatinine clearances as glomerular filtration markers in different stages of liver cirrhosis. *Clin Nephrol*. 1999;51:341-7.

43. Seronie-Vivien S, Delanaye P, Pieroni L, et al. Cystatin C: current position and future prospects. *Clin Chem Lab Med*. 2008;46:1664-86.

44. National Institute of Health. National Kidney Disease Education Program. Laboratory Professionals. When Not To Use the MDRD. Available at: http://www.nkdep.nih.gov/labprofessionals/estimating_gfr.htm. Accessed January 2, 2011.

45. National Institute of Health. National Kidney Disease Education Program. Laboratory Professionals. Guidelines for laboratories: calculating estimated GFR for children. Available at: http://www.nkdep.nih.gov/labprofessionals/labgfr_children.htm. Accessed January 2, 2011.

46. Schwartz GJ, Munoz A, Schneider MF, et al. New equations to estimate GFR in children with CKD. *J Am Soc Nephrol*. 2009;20:629-37.

47. Staples A, LeBlond R, Watkins S, et al. Validation of the revised Schwartz estimating equation in a predominantly non-CKD population. *J Am Soc Nephrol*. 2010;25:2321-6.

Chapter 2

James P. McCormack

Rational Use of Drug Concentration Measurements

For the vast majority of medications, drug concentration monitoring is unnecessary. In contrast a thorough efficacy and monitoring plan should be developed for every drug a patient receives. The value of drug concentration monitoring in achieving desired therapeutic outcomes and patient well being for those drugs where concentration monitoring is generally considered useful is often debated. Some suggest that concentration monitoring is excessive and, when concentrations are measured, they are frequently used inappropriately. Others consider it a routine part of outcome assessment for a number of important drugs with narrow therapeutic ranges.

Clinicians who consider using drug concentration monitoring should always ask themselves the following questions:

- Is the patient already responding appropriately to the drug therapy?
- Is the patient having any toxicity from the drug therapy?
- Is the efficacy and toxicity of this drug better predicted by measuring drug concentrations or evaluating the clinical response?
- Will obtaining a drug concentration change the clinical management of the patient?

Clinicians should also carefully establish goals of therapy and monitor whether or not they are achieved, even when drug concentrations are used as an adjunct to regimen evaluation.

For drugs where concentration monitoring is fairly routinely used but the desired effect of the drug can be easily and quickly measured clinically the value of measuring its concentration is limited or even potentially harmful if one spends time measuring concentrations at the expense of proper clinical assessment. Where the signs and symptoms of benefit and toxicity can be assessed easily and quickly (within hours or in some cases days), appropriate dosage adjustments can usually be based on the clinical response of the patient rather than on drug concentrations. When drug concentration monitoring adds to the predictability of response over monitoring the patient clinically, a number of key issues should be considered before ordering a drug concentration measurement. Figure 2-1 is a graphic representation of the decision-making process involved in considering those issues.

Evaluating the Need for a Drug Concentration Measurement

Drug selection

Before considering the need for drug concentration monitoring, the first consideration for all drug therapy is appropriateness of the selected drug for obtaining the desired outcome in the specific patient. For instance, evidence suggests the addition of aminoglycosides to other safer antibiotics in patients with sepsis or with febrile neutropenia doesn't improve a patient's outcome but does increase the chance of nephrotoxicity.[1,2] Clinicians should ask themselves whether there are potentially equally effective, less toxic, or less expensive alternatives that should be considered (e.g., cephalosporins instead of aminoglycosides for non-life-threatening infections with susceptible organisms; valproic acid instead of phenytoin for certain types of epilepsy, inhaled corticosteroids instead of theophylline for asthma). After it is deemed necessary to use a drug that may require drug concentration monitoring, it is important to determine if efficacy and toxicity are related to drug concentrations in the particular situation. For example, valproic acid in the treatment of infrequent seizures may necessitate the use of concentration measurements, while its use for migraine headache prophylaxis would not.

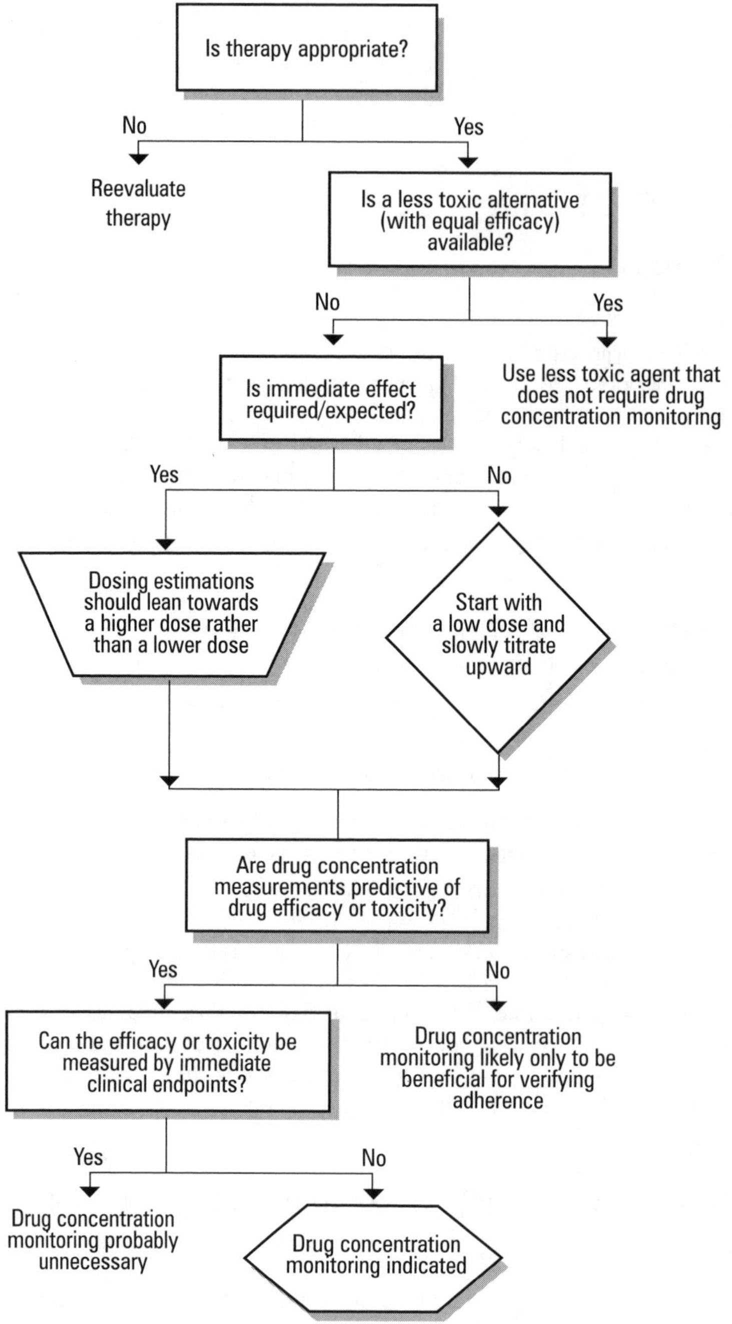

Figure 2-1. Decision-making process for using drug concentration measurements.

Efficacy issues

When therapeutic and toxic end points cannot be readily and quickly determined clinically, drug concentration measurements may be useful if research has shown them to be predictive of therapeutic or toxic effects. For instance, in a patient started on an antiepileptic medication for relatively infrequent (every 2–3 months) seizures, improved seizure control may not become apparent for several months. Ensuring that the patient's concentrations are in the generally accepted population therapeutic range may be the best and likely only approach to determining an appropriate dose and schedule.

Clinicians should always ask themselves whether patient outcomes are better predicted by an established "therapeutic range" or by the individual clinical response. If the clinically important event occurs infrequently (e.g., seizures or arrhythmias), is life threatening, or if the beneficial effect of the drug may be delayed (e.g., resolution of depression), the drug concentration found to be effective in similar patients can be used as an initial goal. However, depending on the drug used and the disease state treated, population-based therapeutic ranges may only be weak predictors of therapeutic success because the concentration-effect relationship is variable between individuals. Dosage adjustments should be made based on the clinical response whenever possible, using drug concentrations as a guide.

For many patients, there likely exist specific threshold concentrations (assuming the drug will be effective or toxic at some point) above which a desired effect will be achieved and another where toxicities will start to be seen. Some clinicians have recommended measuring the drug concentration associated with therapeutic success to serve as a benchmark for subsequent therapy, and that subsequent failure of therapy could be evaluated based on whether concentrations have fallen below this established benchmark. This approach assumes that the threshold for efficacy does not change with time. Because physiologic and pathophysiologic conditions can change with time, this assumption may not be valid in all cases.

Toxicity issues

When patients exhibit signs or symptoms of toxicity, the practitioner should first determine if the dosage could likely be decreased or stopped empirically without loss of benefit. If the patient is at risk for toxicity or develops toxicity that is likely caused by the drug rather than other potentially confounding aspects of the patient's diseases or other drug therapies, the dose should be empirically decreased or the drug stopped. If this cannot be done because of concerns over the loss of therapeutic benefit or inability to differentiate potential causes, a drug concentration measurement may help to determine if the drug is the likely cause. This situation is only appropriate if drug concentrations have been shown to predict toxicity.

Drug concentration measurements may also be useful in patients who develop dysfunction in the primary organ of clearance for the drug (e.g., liver or kidney) or in whom an interacting drug was started or stopped after the patient was stabilized on the initial drug. Measurements are not required if empiric reduction or increase in the drug dosage is possible.

Adherence issues

Lack of adherence by patients to medication regimens is a frequently occurring problem. When a patient is suspected of not adhering to his or her medication regimen, drug concentration monitoring may be a useful tool, along with evaluation of pharmacy records or the medication administration record, to help establish whether or not adherence is an issue.

Approaches to Dosing with Limited Need for Drug Concentration Measurements

Immediate effect required or expected

If a patient requires treatment for an immediate life-threatening illness, the initial dosage should be selected based on avoidance of underdosing, not overdosing. The largest dose usually associated with efficacy and acceptable toxicities should be chosen to ensure the greatest chance of a positive outcome. When concentrations are not measured, concern for toxicity, if it occurs acutely, may be assessed clinically (if possible) and evaluated on the basis of the benefits versus risks of continued therapy at the selected dosage.

For drugs such as the aminoglycosides, vancomycin, and phenytoin that may be used for life-threatening illness, severe toxicity usually does not develop until after at least a few days of therapy (e.g., renal/ototoxicity from aminoglycosides/vancomycin) or the acute toxicities are minor (nystagmus, or ataxia with phenytoin). The acute treatment of life-threatening infections with aminoglycosides or vancomycin should be accomplished with dosages known to produce effective clinical results, while concerns over possible toxicity should be relevant but secondary. The initial dosage selected for the life-threatening infection does not have to be the dosage used for continued therapy. Dosage adjustment can be guided by drug concentration measurements, when appropriate, based on all other considerations. However, before clinicians routinely measure concentrations for a particular drug or class of drugs they should review the available evidence for the therapeutic range. The evidence is often not very persuasive.[34]

Immediate effect not required or expected

For the vast majority of conditions treated with medications, an immediate response is not needed. In these cases the dosing can be approached in one of two ways.

Titrating the dose up

In conditions that do not require an immediate response, it may be possible to gradually titrate the dose up to the usual recommended starting dose with the understanding that the medicines that can extend or improve a patient's quality of life can also produce a number of side effects. A strategy of using ¼ to ½ the usual starting dose could minimize side effects by identifying the lowest effective dose. This may also provide cost-savings to the patient. Such a dose titration approach will likely require more time for the clinician to monitor patient outcomes as well as more time for clinician-patient discussion, as the patient often needs to be made aware of how to monitor for efficacy and toxicity. Patients should be told that the dose titration process takes time and that an immediate effect is not necessarily expected or necessary based on selection of this approach. The patient should be made to understand that the time spent in determining the appropriate dose may prevent unnecessary adverse effects and may reduce drug product expense.

Taking this approach may be justified from the perspective that many clinical trials begin with fairly aggressive doses to establish efficacy. Studies are often not conducted on lower doses until after the product has been on the market for a considerable length of time.[5]

As an example, if one wanted to start theophylline in a patient, given the caveat the evidence that theophylline produces a useful clinical response is limited, start with a 100-mg sustained release product twice daily for 1 week, evaluate for any important clinical changes (less shortness of breath, signs and symptoms of toxicity), and then if there is limited or no response after 1 week the dose should be increased to 200 mg twice daily. Evaluate again in 1 week. If there has been only limited response, increase the dose to 300 mg twice daily. If there is little or no response at this dose it is unlikely that there will be any response from further increases and the drug can just be stopped, assuming that the patient has been adherent to the recommended regimen, there were no identifiable problems with absorption, and the patient was not on a drug that was enhancing the metabolism of the theophylline. If one wished to increase the dose further, measuring concentrations may be useful if for no other reason than to justify doses greater than those typically used. If the concentration comes back and is not consistent with estimates, other reasons for uncharacteristic drug concentrations should be considered (see Introduction). In a similar fashion, low doses of some of the antiepileptic medications could be used initially when these agents are being used for the treatment of chronic neuropathic pain and the dose could be titrated up slowly over a period of a few days to a week. This approach also decreases a clinician's need to worry about potential drug interactions that impact the anticonvulsant's pharmacokinetic parameters as one is starting with a low dose. However, clinicians need to keep in mind that even low dose anticonvulsants may still have a clinically important impact on other drugs the patient is receiving.

Titrating the dose down

A second approach that may be used to determine the lowest effective dose is to begin therapy with the product monograph recommended dose (empirically adjusted on the basis of kidney and/or liver function and drug-disease interactions), assess response, and gradually reduce the dose according to the response of the patient (weighing beneficial and toxic effects). The advantage of this approach is that an effect will likely be seen more quickly than by titrating upward. However, titrating down may not lead to finding the lowest effective dose because clinicians and patients may be unwilling to decrease the dose once benefits are being achieved. It is important to remember that higher than necessary doses increase the chance of adverse effects, may increase the frequency of dosing and thereby compromise adherence, and usually increase the cost of therapy. Even in the face of drug efficacy without signs of toxicity, there may be value in tapering to the lowest effective dose over time to determine if the correct diagnosis was made, if the disease state is fluctuating, or if non-drug factors such as lifestyle changes have made a difference.

The approaches of titrating up or down apply to many medical conditions for which clinical end points are frequent and easily measurable (e.g., asthma and hypertension). However, when the clinical end points are infrequent (e.g., seizures) or life threatening (e.g., arrhythmias), this approach may be of less value.

Conclusion

Drug concentration monitoring should only be considered as a tool to supplement proper clinical assessment of patient response. Appropriate drug selection (based on the best available evidence) and proper initial dosage selection, along with the clinical monitoring of response are the most crucial components of pharmacotherapy.

References

1. Paul M, Benuri-Silbiger I, Soares-Weiser K, Leibovici L. Beta lactam monotherapy versus beta lactam-aminoglycoside combination therapy for sepsis in immunocompetent patients: systematic review and meta-analysis of randomized trials. *Br Med J.* 2004;328:668.
2. Paul M, Soares-Weiser K, Leibovici L. Beta lactam monotherapy versus beta lactam-aminoglycoside combination therapy for fever with neutropenia: systematic review and meta-analysis. *Br Med J.* 2003;326:1111.
3. McCormack JP, Jewesson PJ. A critical re-evaluation of the therapeutic range of aminoglycosides. *Clin Inf Dis.* 1992;14:320-39.
4. McCormack JP. An emotional-based medicine approach to monitoring once-daily aminoglycosides. *Pharmacotherapy.* 2000;20:1524-7.
5. McCormack JP, Allan MG, Virani AS. Is bigger better? An argument for "very" low initial doses. *J Can Med Assoc.* 2010;83:1.

Chapter 3

Brian L. Erstad

Medication Dosing in Overweight and Obese Patients

Introduction

The increasing prevalence of obesity, and particularly extreme obesity, is a major public health issue that presents a number of challenges for health professionals caring for these patients. Among these is the difficulty of designing medication dosing regimens that take into account the body composition alterations and disease states associated with excess weight. If these factors are not considered the patient may incur toxicity when medications are dosed based on mg/kg of actual body weight (ABW) when ABW is not the most appropriate size descriptor to use, or therapeutic failure when some form of adjusted body weight in mg/kg or standard dosing in mg is used. The purpose of this chapter is to describe important considerations for designing dosing regimens for overweight and obese patients. Much of the discussion will pertain to patients with more extreme forms of obesity since they are the most difficult to dose given the paucity of published literature.

The terms *overweight* and *obesity* are most commonly defined by body mass index (BMI) calculations. Adult subjects with a value of 25.0 to 29.9 are considered overweight, while subjects with a value of 30.0 and above are considered obese.[1] For purposes of this paper, unless specified otherwise, adult subjects with BMI values above 40 are termed extremely obese. BMI calculations can also be used for screening children and teens for weight problems, but the values require adjustment based on growth charts. The calculations and references for other size descriptor terms used in this paper are listed in Table 3-1.

Obtaining an Accurate Weight

Research has shown that ABW recordings documented in nursing records in both ICU and non-ICU settings are frequently inaccurate. Therefore, clinicians should try to ensure that ABW is measured using an accurate and reliable device when feasible and that the measurement is appropriately documented in the patient's medical records. This means that weighing devices must be periodically checked and calibrated to ensure appropriate function and accuracy. Measurement of weight may not be possible in some patients due to the type of injury (e.g., head injury), which may preclude an immediate determination. While estimates of patient weight by health care personnel may be used in such situations, they are often inaccurate. Self-reporting of weight by adult subjects has been shown to be reasonably accurate in some investigations but may not be possible depending on the type of injury or disease state. When multiple weights are documented in medical records, the clinician should look for clues to inaccurate estimates or measurements as might be seen when values vary greatly from day to day in the absence of substantial fluid gains or losses. In light of all of these considerations, the process for obtaining measured or estimated ABW and other size descriptor data should be standardized as much as possible.

Body Composition Changes Associated with Obesity

When accurate recordings of height and weight are available, the subject's body composition is another factor that must be considered when dosing medications. The most basic body composition model has two compartments, fat and fat-free mass; but more complex models (atomic, molecular, cellular, functional, and whole body) have been studied.[2] While the simpler models are easier to study and require fewer assumptions, the multi-compartmental model reflects more the complexity of the human body and has the potential to yield a better understanding of compositional changes associated with obesity and medication disposition in obese

Table 3-1. Body Size Descriptor Equations[a]

		Units	Intended Age (Sex)	Ref
General Body Size Descriptors				
Body mass index (BMI) =	(ABW in kg) / (Height in m)^2	kg/m^2	adult	4
	(ABW in kg) / (Height in m)^2 adjust by growth charts for age and sex	percentile	child	5
Body surface area (BSA) =	[(ABW in kg)$^{0.425}$ × (Height in cm)$^{0.725}$] × 0.007184	m^2	adult	6
	SQRT [(Height in cm) × (ABW in kg) / 3600]	m^2	child/adult	7
	[(ABW in kg)$^{0.5378}$ × (Height in cm)$^{0.3964}$] × 0.024265	m^2	infant/child/adult	8
Lean Body Mass Descriptors				
Ideal body weight (IBW)[b] =	50 kg + 2.3 kg [(Height in inches) – 60]	kg	adult (male)	9
	45.5 kg + 2.3 kg [(Height in inches) – 60]	kg	adult (female)	9
	2.05 $e^{0.02\ (\text{Height in cm})}$	kg	child < 5 feet	10
	39 kg + 2.27 kg [(Height in inches) – 60]	kg	child ≥ 5 feet (male)	10
	42.2 kg + 2.27 kg [(Height in inches) – 60]	kg	child ≥ 5 feet (female)	10
Lean body weight (LBW) =	[1.1 × (ABW in kg)] – {120 × [(ABW in kg)/ (Height in cm)]^2}	kg	adult (male)	11
	[1.07 × (ABW in kg)] – {148 × [(ABW in kg)/ (Height in cm)]^2}	kg	adult (female)	11
Fat-free mass (FFM) =	[0.285 × (ABW in kg)] + [12.1 × (Height in m)^2]	kg	adult (male)	12
	[0.287 × (ABW in kg)] + [9.74 × (Height in m)^2]	kg	adult (female)	12
	[9,270 × (ABW in kg)] / [6,680 + (216 × BMI)]	kg	adult (male)	13
	[9,270 × (ABW in kg)] / [8,780 + (244 × BMI)]	kg	adult (female)	13
Adjusted Body Size Descriptors				
Adjusted body weight =	(IBW in kg) + {[(ABW in kg) – (IBW in kg)] × 0.2 to 0.6}[c]	kg	adult	14–16[d]
Predicted normal weight =	[1.57 × (ABW in kg)] – [0.0183 × BMI × (ABW in kg)] – 10.5	kg	adult (male)	17
	[1.75 × (ABW in kg)] – [0.0242 × BMI × (ABW in kg)] – 12.6	kg	adult (female)	17

ABW = actual body weight; SQRT = square root. BMI = body mass index; IBW = ideal body weight.

[a]There are a number of variations of these formulae but only the most commonly cited and recently introduced versions are listed. This table is for illustration purposes only. Some of the equations are inappropriate or have not been validated for use in more extremely obese patients so the references need to be pulled and reviewed prior to use.

[b]Although ideal body weight was originally used as a target weight for life insurance tables, it has since been used as a surrogate for lean body mass, albeit based on tenuous assumptions.

[c]Various adjustments for various medications have been reported where the adjustment adds 20% to 60% of the difference between ABW and IBW to the IBW for medications not as well distributed into adipose tissue.

[d]These are some of the first citations of this formula with a correction factor (i.e., 0.3 to 0.6), but a number of variations of the correction factor were subsequently studied, so a range is listed in the table.

subjects. The importance of body composition is illustrated by a hypothetical example using three patients of the same age, sex, height, and weight. One patient weighing 100 kg has 20 liters of excess body fluid from over-resuscitation. A second patient weighing 100 kg has 20 kg of excess fat weight. The third patient weighing 100 kg is a body builder with a very low percentage of body fat. If dosed simply by body weight, it is easy to see how medications with varying physicochemical characteristics could result in substantial pharmacokinetic and pharmacodynamic differences in these three patients.

The anticoagulant heparin provides a useful example for illustrating how body composition and choice of size descriptor complicates dosing in a patient with excess weight relative to height. Heparin is commonly dosed by weight-based regimens in hospital settings. Typical recommendations for the treatment of venous thromboembolism include a load of 80 units/kg followed by a continuous infusion of 18 units/kg/hr. This raises the question as to which weight should be used in overweight or obese patients. Table 3-2 illustrates the range of size descriptors available for an assumed 70-inch tall male even when factors such as age, sex, race and co-morbidities are presumed to be similar. Using data from this table and the heparin dosing guidelines above, a 70-inch tall male could receive an intravenous loading dose of heparin as low as 4,640 units using a fat-free mass weight of 58 kg for a normal-weight 73 kg patient, to a high of 12,800 units using ABW for an extremely obese 160 kg patient. The continuous infusion dose for these same weights would range from a low value of 1044 units/hour to a high value of 2880 units/hour. When deciding which weight to use the clinician must consider the thromboembolic consequences of under-dosing such as pulmonary embolism, versus the potentially fatal hemorrhage that can occur with over-dosing.

There is no high level evidence to guide decisions on the most appropriate choice of weight for the extremely obese patient. One group has recommended the use of an adjusted body weight that adds 30% to 40% of the excess weight to IBW for heparin dosing, but prospective studies need to be conducted to evaluate this approach.[3] Unfortunately, this example of the difficulty of designing a dosing regimen for heparin is common to other medications. Therefore, approaches used to dosing the more severely obese patient require a careful risk/benefit assessment based on data often extrapolated from studies of more normal-weight subjects.

Table 3-2. Examples of Output from Size Descriptor Equations for Patients of Different Weights but Similar Height, Age, Sex, Race, and Co-Morbidities[a]

Equation	Extremely Obese	Moderately Obese	Mildly Obese	Overweight	Normal	Reference
ABW =	160 kg	120 kg	100 kg	80 kg	73 kg	-
BMI =	50.61 kg/m^2	37.96 kg/m^2	31.63 kg/m^2	25.31 kg/m^2	23.10 kg/m^2	4
BSA =	2.66 m^2	2.35 m^2	2.18 m^2	1.99 m^2	1.90 m^2	6
BSA =	2.81 m^2	2.43 m^2	2.22 m^2	1.99 m^2	1.90 m^2	7
BSA =	2.90 m^2	2.48 m^2	2.25 m^2	2.00 m^2	1.90 m^2	8
IBW =	73.00 kg	73.00 kg	73.00 kg	73.00 kg	73.00 kg	9
LBW =	78.82 kg	77.34 kg	72.04 kg	63.71 kg	60.07 kg	11
FFM =	83.85 kg	72.45 kg	66.75 kg	61.05 kg	59.06 kg	12
FFM =	84.22 kg	74.76 kg	68.61 kg	61.05 kg	57.99 kg	13
Adj (20%) =	90.40 kg	82.40 kg	78.40 kg	74.40 kg	73.00 kg	14–16
Adj (60%) =	125.20 kg	101.20 kg	89.20 kg	77.20 kg	73.00 kg	14–16
PNWT =	92.51 kg	94.54 kg	88.62 kg	78.05 kg	73.25 kg	17

ABW = actual body weight; BMI = body mass index; BSA = body surface area; IBW = ideal body weight; LBW = lean body weight; FFM = fat-free mass; Adj = adjusted body weight; PNWT = predicted normal weight.

[a]Each patient is assumed to be a 70-inch tall male. This table is for illustration purposes only; some of the equations are inappropriate or have not been validated for use in more extremely obese patients, so the references need to be pulled and reviewed prior to use.

Size Descriptors

The limitations of using ABW for dosing medications with different physicochemical characteristics in patients with varying body compositions have fostered research in the area of size descriptors.[4-17] A listing of size descriptors and the equations used to calculate them is contained in Table 3-1. Equations for allometric scaling, which deals with relationships between body function and body size, are not included since the body weight used to develop allometric equations is presumed to be of normal body composition.[18] Note that only a few of the equations in Table 3-1 take into account all the common factors (age, sex, height, and weight) that are likely to be needed in a size descriptor equation used to adjust the dose of a medication for obesity, and none take into account potential factors such as race that might further improve dose individualization.[19] Of importance, the equations for adults should not be used for infants or children who may have substantially different body composition and medication disposition compared to adults.[20]

BMI has primarily been used to define subjects at risk from the complications of excess body weight and has not been found to be useful as a size predictor for adjusting medications in obese patients. Body surface area (BSA) is commonly used to adjust doses in infants and young children, as well as patients receiving chemotherapy, but BSA has not been validated for dosing medications in obese patients. In fact, doses are often capped when used to dose chemotherapeutic agents due to toxicity concerns. Of the equations used to estimate lean body mass, the IBW calculation by Devine (and subsequent minor modifications) has been most frequently used in pharmacokinetic investigations and for adjusting loading doses of medications with small volumes of distribution (e.g., < 15 liters in an adult) or with limited fat distribution (e.g., digoxin) in the clinical setting. But, as previously stated, more recent equations with better approximations of lean body weight have been evaluated in modeling calculations in patients with obesity.[13] These newer equations are intended to account for the portion of lean weight that is associated with increases in adipose tissue weight; these equations also incorporate weight in addition to the sex and height parameters used in more traditional IBW equations. Strictly speaking, fat-free mass and lean body weight are not equivalent since lean body weight takes into account fat in cell membranes, bone marrow and central nervous system, but the difference as a percent of ABW is small (usually less than 3% to 5%).[13] More accurate estimations of fat-free mass are possible with various devices (e.g., bioelectrical impedance, dual energy x-ray absorptiometry), but such devices require the equipment and technical expertise to perform and interpret the measurements, in addition to being costly.

Adjusted body weight equations were originally developed in pharmacokinetic investigations of the aminoglycoside antibiotics in extremely obese patients (i.e., patients whose ABW is at least twice their IBW). The equations were subsequently evaluated in the pharmacokinetic dosing of beta-lactam antimicrobials, where it was found that, similar to aminoglycosides, they have distribution volumes based on weight (L/kg) that is best reflected by using an adjusted body size descriptor somewhere between IBW and ABW. There has been little attempt to prospectively evaluate adjusted weight equations for their predictive dosing potential in patients with varying degrees of obesity.

Pharmacokinetic Considerations

Obesity is now known to be a chronic inflammatory state that has the potential to affect most major organ systems in the body.[21] Therefore, not only the isolated effects of increased body size (along with other traditional covariates such as age and sex) on the body's disposition of medications, but also the effects of any organ dysfunction related to long-term obesity must be considered. With respect to pharmacokinetics, potential alterations in the distribution and clearance of medications administered by the intravenous route have been most studied in patients with obesity. Less information is available on the pharmacokinetics of orally administered medications and those injected by intramuscular or subcutaneous routes although, based on the limited studies available, oral absorption does not appear to be substantially affected by obesity.

Volume of distribution

The primary factors affecting the distribution of a medication into fat and fat-free mass are the relative size of the compartments and binding competition between fat, blood, and lean tissues. The binding competition is a function of the medication's lipophilicity, which determines binding to adipose tissue, and its chemical structure (e.g., polarity and ionization in body fluid pH), which determines binding to lean tissues. Blood flow affects the rate of distribution.[22]

The degree of medication lipophilicity is often expressed by the octanol:water partition coefficient or more commonly the logarithm of the partition coefficient (log P). However, a high log P (e.g., > 2) is not synonymous with extensive adipose tissue disposition as exemplified by a number of basic lipophilic medications such as desipramine (log P of approximately 4) that have extensive lean rather than adipose tissue binding. From a practical standpoint, this means that the loading doses of medications that are highly lipophilic are not necessarily dosed on ABW. Digoxin is a case in point. Digoxin has a log P of approximately 2 and a large volume of distribution (6 to 7 L/kg in patients with normal renal function); however, studies in obese subjects have found that digoxin should be dosed on some form of lean body mass (not ABW) due to minimal distribution into adipose tissue and no change in clearance compared to normal weight subjects.[23] This illustrates the complex nature of the factors affecting distribution.

While information concerning tissue binding of medications usually must be inferred, changes in plasma protein binding can be measured and have been investigated in obese patients. Unfortunately, few generalizations are possible other than the concentrations of albumin and alpha-1-acid glycoprotein do not appear to be substantially altered in obesity. Although not well studied, binding and displacement changes associated with elevations in free fatty acid and lipoprotein concentrations are possible in obese subjects.[24]

Equations have been developed for predicting the volumes of distribution of medications in patients with obesity.[25] These equations take into account the various physicochemical characteristics of both the medication and body tissues. However, the equations are limited by assumptions concerning lean and adipose tissue mass, tissue binding changes, and the inability to find characteristics such as partition coefficients for newer medications. Most importantly, the equations have not been tested prospectively in patients with varying degrees of obesity.

Renal clearance

Since its publication in 1976, the Cockcroft-Gault equation has become the most common method used to predict creatinine clearance for dosage adjustments of renally eliminated medications.[26] The choice of weight for use in this equation was controversial since its inception when the authors suggested the use of an IBW or lean weight in patients with excess adipose tissue (or fluid) even though such patients had not been studied in adequate numbers. Five years after publication of the Cockcroft-Gault equation the first study to investigate creatinine clearance estimations in extremely obese subjects was published.[27] In addition to age, sex, and serum creatinine both IBW and ABW were evaluated. None of the methods of creatinine clearance estimation was found to be an accurate predictor of measured clearance; furthermore, the use of IBW led to under-estimations and ABW to over-estimations of clearance. During the 5 to 10 years following the publication of the Cockcroft-Gault equation, more widespread availability of assays for aminoglycosides and vancomycin led to pharmacokinetic investigations of potential dosing regimens for extremely obese patients. Although the kidneys primarily eliminate aminoglycosides and vancomycin, results of the latter studies suggested a need for a different approach to dosing recommendations. For the aminoglycosides, volume of distribution and clearance appeared to increase proportionately to each other, but not to the increase in weight of the extremely obese patients.[14-16] This led to the recommendation for use of an adjusted body weight for dosing aminoglycosides to avoid the under-dosing that would likely occur with the use of an IBW and the over-dosing that would likely occur with the use of ABW. For vancomycin, clearance, but not volume of distribution, increased proportionately to ABW as evidenced by the shorter terminal half-life in the extremely obese compared to normal-weight patients.[28] The initial volume of distribution (i.e., volume of the central compartment) was similar as expressed in liters in the extremely obese and normal-weight patients, which suggests that loading doses should not be based on ABW. The apparent proportionality between vancomycin clearance and ABW in patients with more severe forms of obesity is an unusual finding, particularly for medications with a high fraction of renal elimination. Pharmacokinetic studies involving most other antimicrobials for example, have had findings similar to those from the aminoglycoside studies (i.e., increased, but non-proportionate changes in volume of distribution or clearance relative to ABW).

The inherent inaccuracies associated with creatinine clearance determinations by the Cockcroft-Gault method in obese patients led to the development of predictive equations for male and female subjects based on estimated fat-free body mass. The so-called Salazar-Corcoran equations were developed to predict creatinine clearance and medication clearance in obese male and female subjects.[29] These equations were based on the same weight-height formula (i.e., Quetelet's index) used to calculate body mass index. Salazar-Corcoran has been used for creatinine clearance estimations in some important pharmacokinetic studies. For example, it was used to estimate creatinine clearance in extremely obese patients who received vancomycin for severe infections.[30] Vancomycin clearance determined by pharmacokinetic parameters derived from measured vancomycin concentrations was found to correlate with ABW (r = 0.948, $p < 0.0001$) and was similar to the creatinine clearance calculated by Salazar-Corcoran (197 mL/min vs. 209 mL/min, respectively). This study is important because it confirmed the results of the earlier vancomycin trial that demonstrated a proportional increase in vancomycin clearance relative to ABW in extremely obese patients. As in the earlier vancomycin study, volume of distribution did not increase proportionately to ABW.

More recent investigations of creatinine clearance by urine collections or glomerular filtration rate measurements using accurate techniques such as inulin clearance or technetium-99m-labelled diethylenetriamine penta-acetic acid (^{99m}Tc DTPA) radionuclide scanning have found that use of lean body weight in Cockcroft-Gault improves predictive accuracy in obese and normal-weight subjects.[17,31,32] The lean body weight used in these studies was determined by accurate methods such as bioelectrical impedance or dual X-ray absorptometry (DXA), rather than older IBW equations of unclear origin and limited validation. A study evaluating different size descriptors for estimating creatinine clearance in extremely obese patients gives further support to the use of a lean weight.[33] In this study, the creatinine clearance estimations from eight equations (six variations of Cockcroft-Gault, Salazar-Corcoran, and MDRD4) were compared to measured creatinine clearance determinations. The Cockcroft-Gault equations using fat-free weight determined by bioelectrical impedance, or lean weight by a more recent equation were the least biased and provided the most accurate estimates of creatinine clearance.

There is no consensus as to which equation should be used for estimating creatinine clearance or which size descriptor should be used in any given equation. Some have argued for more recent versions of the MDRD equation since it is already being used in hospitals to estimate glomerular filtration rate and detect chronic kidney disease. However, the MDRD equations were developed to predict glomerular filtration rate and not creatinine clearance that also takes into account secretion processes in the kidney; furthermore, the MDRD involves standardization based on body surface area, but dosing of medications in pre-approval investigations or in the clinical setting is usually not standardized in this manner. Others have argued for the use of Cockcroft-Gault with a specific type of size descriptor such as lean weight, or a combination of equations depending on the specific patient (e.g., Salazar-Corcoran or Cockcroft-Gault with an adjusted weight for obesity, Cockcroft-Gault with ABW for normal-weight patients). However, there is little prospective evaluation of either of these approaches in obese patients, particularly more severely obese patients. If anything the situation has become even more complicated with reporting of serum creatinine based on an IDMS-traceable standard.

Until consensus develops, important concepts to apply in the clinical setting for creatinine clearance estimations are practicality and consistency. When a high degree of accuracy of renal function is needed such as glomerular filtration rate determination in potential kidney donors, measurements using gold standards such as inulin or DTPA should be performed rather than relying on estimations from equations.[34] Currently, the FDA in its guidance to industry states that Cockcroft-Gault may be used for creatinine clearance estimation in studies although no particular weight is recommended. Therefore, Cockcroft-Gault using ABW is most commonly used for weight-based dosing in pre-approval studies that typically involve more normal-weight patients. Additionally, the Cockcroft-Gault equation is the most common equation used in the clinical setting. Therefore, a strong argument can be made for the continued use of Cockcroft-Gault for estimating creatinine clearance in order to adjust doses of renally eliminated medications. As for a size descriptor, a good argument can be made for the use of ABW for more normal-weight patients (e.g., within 130% of IBW) since the estimation of creatinine clearance by either lean weight or ABW is likely to be fairly similar and differences are likely to be small in comparison to sources of error such as weight estimation. For more obese patients, an adjusted or lean weight is more likely to reflect actual clearance of renally eliminated medications and is a reasonable approach to use in the clinical setting.

Non-renal clearance

Much less information is available regarding non-renal elimination (e.g., liver, lungs, gastrointestinal tract) or mechanisms (e.g., Hofmann degradation, esterase elimination). For many medications the amount eliminated by the kidneys is determined in pharmacokinetic studies and the amount not accounted for by renal elimination is considered "non-renal," occasionally without further investigation, though these pathways might be affected by obesity. Some of the assumptions of non-renal elimination do not always appear to be accurate when more in-depth investigations are performed. For example, vancomycin is often stated to have 15% to 30% non-renal elimination, presumably through the liver, which would suggest dose adjustments might be needed for more severe forms of liver dysfunction. But, when this issue was investigated in patients with cancer, liver failure did not influence vancomycin clearance.[35] As with renal clearance, the overall effect of obesity on hepatic metabolism appears to be an increase or no change in phase I and phase II metabolic processes.[24] The clearance by some hepatic metabolic pathways (e.g., glucuronidation) appears to be more consistently increased than others based on a limited number of medications that have been studied. From a practical standpoint, for the majority of medications that are titrated to clinical effect or that use blood concentration determinations as a surrogate marker, any alterations due to obesity are likely to be mitigated. Perhaps the ability to dose medications cleared by hepatic processes may improve with advancements in pharmacogenomics and body composition assessments.

Concept of Dose Proportionality

The use of ABW for weight-based dosing of a medication in an obese patient presumes that pharmacokinetic parameters such as volume of distribution and clearance increase proportionately with the excess weight. In other words, if ABW increases by a certain percent, volume of distribution and clearance not adjusted for weight will increase by the same percent. However, this is often not the case and should not be assumed, particularly for patients with extreme forms of obesity. Even assuming there is data to suggest dose proportionality with increasing weight for a particular medication, there may be other reasons to avoid the use of ABW for initial dosing. For example, assume that an intravenously administered antihypertensive agent has recently become available that was dosed using ABW in clinical trials involving small numbers of patients with relatively normal body weights. This agent is now being considered for use in a severely obese patient with postoperative hypertension, but no organ dysfunction attributable to the increased pressure. In this example, the risk of hypoperfusion of organs associated with rapid decreases in blood pressure would more than offset the benefit of acute pressure reduction in a patient who does not have a hypertensive emergency. If blood pressure reduction with this new antihypertensive agent was needed more quickly in the case of a hypertensive emergency, other options such as a series of mini-boluses administered over a relatively short period of time may be safer while accomplishing the same purpose as the administration of one large bolus loading dose.

Recommendations for Dosing Medications in Obese Patients

Product information from the pharmaceutical industry typically lacks details regarding dosing in obese patients, which is not surprising since the investigators in pre-approval clinical trials of a medication usually strive to obtain a homogeneous patient population in order to ensure internal validity. Subjects in these trials almost always receive fixed doses or mg/kg doses based on ABW, although this is often not explicitly stated in the published methodology. Furthermore, extremely obese subjects are either limited in numbers or specifically excluded. Many pharmacokinetic studies are single-dose evaluations involving small numbers of patients that are unlikely to be obese; nevertheless, they may provide useful information for initiating therapy. Therefore, the first step in developing a dosing regimen for a medication in an obese patient begins with a search of the literature for applicable studies. In the absence of specific investigations or therapeutic alternatives with more dosing-related information, there is little choice but to dose obese patients using pharmacokinetic and pharmacodynamic data that are available.

Many medications used in adults are not dosed by bodyweight but rather started at a set dose and titrated to clinical effect (see Chapter 2 for additional discussion of this approach). This is a reasonable approach for dosing non-critically ill adult patients with less severe forms of obesity. Designing a weight-based dosing regimen for hospitalized adults and children with more severe forms of obesity is challenging given the lack of information available in common resources such as manufacturers' product information, and the unstable nature of more severely ill patients, no matter what their weight might be. The latter problem is illustrated by a study of the pharmacokinetics and pharmacodynamics of vancomycin in critically ill patients, where the volume of distribution was found to be double the usual 0.6 to 0.7 L/kg often cited in published literature, and standard dosing was found to be inadequate in one third of patients.[36]

Loading doses

Given the difficulties in choosing an appropriate size descriptor for weight-based dosing in obese patients, particularly in patients with more severe forms of obesity, the first question to ask is whether a loading dose is needed. For example, many of the vasoactive medications administered to critically ill patients must be given by continuous intravenous infusion due to their onset and offset of effects that often occurs within a few minutes. For such medications, loading doses may be replaced by rapid titration of the infusion to clinical effect. For other medications that take days or weeks to reach therapeutic or steady state concentrations, loading doses may be needed. In these situations the loading dose is primarily a function of the medication's volume of distribution, so the literature should be evaluated for evidence that the volume of distribution increases proportionally to increased ABW before considering ABW for dosing.

Maintenance doses

Clearance is the more important parameter to assess for dose proportionality in obese patients when starting maintenance regimens of medications given by regularly scheduled intermittent doses or by continuous infusions. With a few notable exceptions (e.g., vancomycin), most hydrophilic medications eliminated by the kidneys do not have clearance increase in proportion to excess bodyweight, so use of ABW for dosing patients with more severe forms of obesity could lead to toxicity. Even when dose proportionality appears to exist, a risk/benefit assessment of using ABW compared to a lean or adjusted weight should be performed.

Figure 3-1 provides a conceptual framework for initiating the dosing of medications in obese patients, particularly patients with more severe forms of obesity. The step-by-step process contains the major scenarios likely to be encountered in clinical practice, but cannot account for every possible scenario and does not replace sound clinical judgment backed by available evidence. Furthermore, pharmacokinetic parameters may change relatively quickly in any patient in settings such as the intensive care unit, which may necessitate dosing adjustments. When feasible, it is preferable to titrate a medication to desired clinical effect, possibly in conjunction with pharmacokinetic monitoring, rather than relying solely on estimated pharmacokinetic parameters derived from previous studies of drug monitoring to predict a dosing regimen.

References

1. Centers for Disease Control and Prevention. About BMI for Adults. Available at http://www.cdc.gov/healthyweight/assessing/bmi/adult_bmi/index.html. Accessed November 24, 2010.
2. Ellis KJ. Human body composition: In vivo methods. *Physiol Rev.* 2000;80:649-80.
3. Myzienski AE, Lutz MF, Smythe MA. Unfractionated heparin dosing for venous thromboembolism in morbidly obese patients: Case report and review of the literature. *Pharmacother.* 2010;30:105e-112e.
4. Keys A, Fidanza F, Karvonen MJ, et al. Indices of relative weight and obesity. *J Chronic Dis.* 1972;25:329-43.
5. Centers for Disease Control and Prevention. About BMI for children and teens. Available at: http://www.cdc.gov/healthyweight/assessing/bmi/childrens_bmi/about_childrens_bmi.html. Accessed November 24, 2010.
6. Du Bois D, Du Bois EF. Clinical calorimetry. Tenth paper. A formula to estimate the approximate surface area if height and weight be known. *Arch Intern Med.* 1916;17:863.
7. Mosteller RD. Simplified calculation of body-surface area. *N Engl J Med.* 1987;317:1098.
8. Haycock GB, Schwartz GJ, Wisotsky DH. Geometric method for measuring body surface area: A height weight formula validated in infants, children and adults. *J Pediatr.* 1978;93:62-66.
9. Devine BJ. Case number 25: Gentamicin therapy. *Drug Intell Clin Pharm.* 1974;8:650-5.
10. Traub SL, Johnson CE. Comparison of methods of estimating creatinine clearance in children. *Am J Hosp Pharm.* 1980;37:195-201.
11. Cheymol G. Effects of obesity on pharmacokinetics: Implications for drug therapy. *Clin Pharmacokinet.* 2000;39:215-31.
12. Garrow JS, Webster J. Quetelet's index (W/H^2) as a measure of fatness. *Int J Obesity.* 1985;9:147-53.
13. Janmahasatian S, Duffull SB, Ash S, et al. Quantification of lean bodyweight. *Clin Pharmacokinet.* 2005;44:1051-1065.
14. Blouin RA, Mann HJ, Griffen WO, et al. Tobramycin pharmacokinetics in morbidly obese patients. *Clin Pharmacol Ther.* 1979;26:508-12.
15. Bauer LA, Blouin RA, Griffen WO, et al. Amikacin pharmacokinetics in morbidly obese patients. *Am J Hosp Pharm.* 1980;37:519-22.

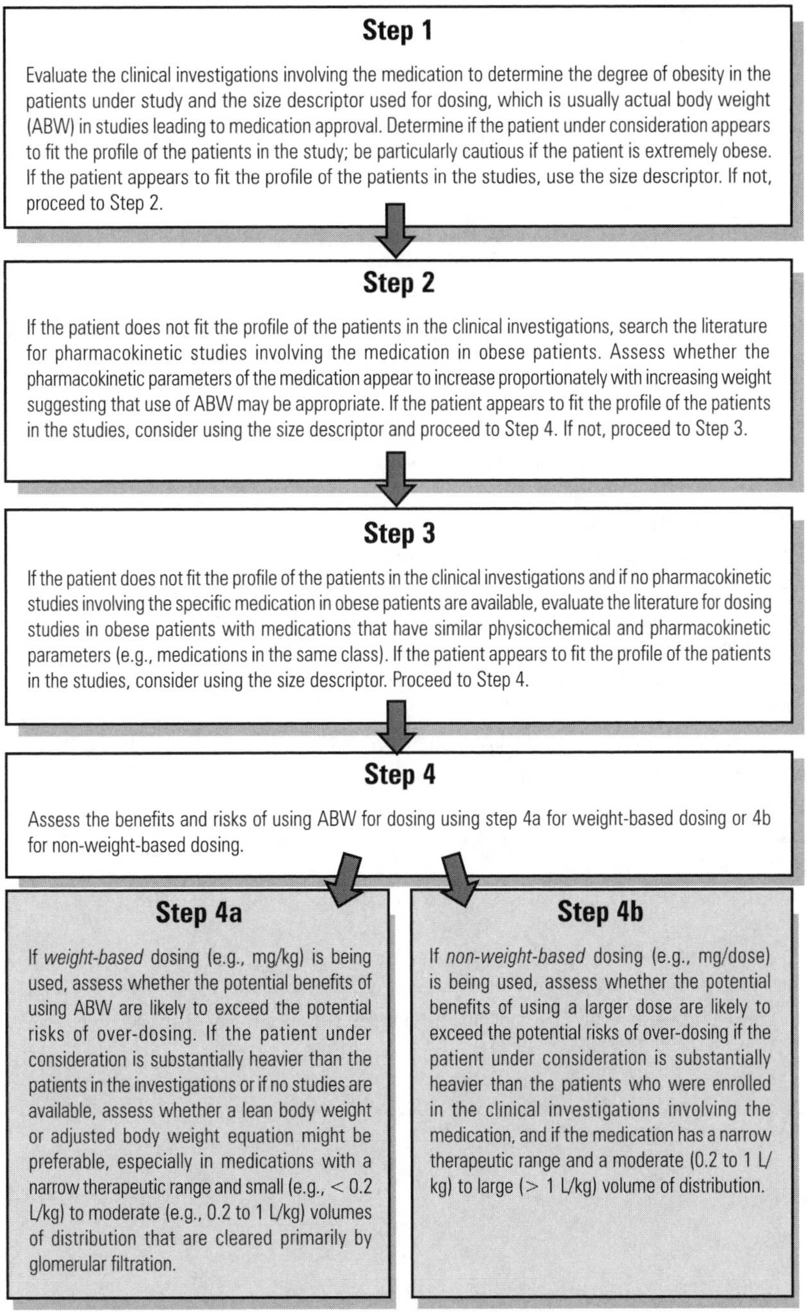

Step 1

Evaluate the clinical investigations involving the medication to determine the degree of obesity in the patients under study and the size descriptor used for dosing, which is usually actual body weight (ABW) in studies leading to medication approval. Determine if the patient under consideration appears to fit the profile of the patients in the study; be particularly cautious if the patient is extremely obese. If the patient appears to fit the profile of the patients in the studies, use the size descriptor. If not, proceed to Step 2.

Step 2

If the patient does not fit the profile of the patients in the clinical investigations, search the literature for pharmacokinetic studies involving the medication in obese patients. Assess whether the pharmacokinetic parameters of the medication appear to increase proportionately with increasing weight suggesting that use of ABW may be appropriate. If the patient appears to fit the profile of the patients in the studies, consider using the size descriptor and proceed to Step 4. If not, proceed to Step 3.

Step 3

If the patient does not fit the profile of the patients in the clinical investigations and if no pharmacokinetic studies involving the specific medication in obese patients are available, evaluate the literature for dosing studies in obese patients with medications that have similar physicochemical and pharmacokinetic parameters (e.g., medications in the same class). If the patient appears to fit the profile of the patients in the studies, consider using the size descriptor. Proceed to Step 4.

Step 4

Assess the benefits and risks of using ABW for dosing using step 4a for weight-based dosing or 4b for non-weight-based dosing.

Step 4a

If *weight-based* dosing (e.g., mg/kg) is being used, assess whether the potential benefits of using ABW are likely to exceed the potential risks of over-dosing. If the patient under consideration is substantially heavier than the patients in the investigations or if no studies are available, assess whether a lean body weight or adjusted body weight equation might be preferable, especially in medications with a narrow therapeutic range and small (e.g., < 0.2 L/kg) to moderate (e.g., 0.2 to 1 L/kg) volumes of distribution that are cleared primarily by glomerular filtration.

Step 4b

If *non-weight-based* dosing (e.g., mg/dose) is being used, assess whether the potential benefits of using a larger dose are likely to exceed the potential risks of over-dosing if the patient under consideration is substantially heavier than the patients who were enrolled in the clinical investigations involving the medication, and if the medication has a narrow therapeutic range and a moderate (0.2 to 1 L/kg) to large (> 1 L/kg) volume of distribution.

[a]Always take into account potential co-morbidity confounders such as renal or liver dysfunction when determining dosing regimens.

Figure 3-1. Conceptual framework for dosing medications in obese patients.[a]

16. Bauer LA, Edwards WA, Dellinger EP, et al. Influence of weight on aminoglycoside pharmacokinetics in normal weight and morbidly obese patients. *Eur J Clin Pharmacol.* 1983;24:643-7.

17. Duffull SB, Dooley MJ, Green B, et al. A standard weight descriptor for dose adjustment in the obese patient. *Clin Pharmacokinet.* 2004;43:1167-78.

18. Holford NH. A size standard for pharmacokinetics. *Clin Pharmacokinet.* 1996;30:329-32.

19. Green B, Duffull SB. What is the best size descriptor to use for pharmacokinetic studies in the obese? *Br J Clin Pharmacol.* 2004;50:119-33.

20. Kearns GL, Abdel-Rahman SM, Alander SW, et al. Developmental pharmacology-drug disposition, action, and therapy in infants and children. *N Engl J Med.* 2003;549:1157-67.

21. Haslam DM, James WP. Obesity. *Lancet.* 2005;366:1197-1209.

22. Bickel MH. Factors affecting the storage of drugs and other xenobiotics in adipose tissue. *Adv Drug Res.* 1994;25:55-86.

23. Abernathy DR, Greenblatt DJ, Smith TW. Digoxin disposition in obesity: Clinical pharmacokinetic investigation. *Am Heart J.* 1982;102:740-4.

24. Blouin RA, Warren GW. Pharmacokinetic considerations in obesity. *J Pharm Sci.* 1999;88:1-7.

25. Ritschel WA, Kaul S. Prediction of apparent volume of distribution in obesity. *Meth Find Exp Clin Pharmacol.* 1986;8:239-47.

26. Cockcroft DW, Gault MH. Prediction of creatinine clearance from serum creatinine. *Nephron.* 1976;16:31-41.

27. Dionne RE, Bauer LA, Gibson GA, et al. Estimating creatinine clearance in morbidity obese patients. *Am J Health-Syst Pharm.* 1981;38:841-4.

28. Blouin RA, Bauer LA, Miller DD, et al. Vancomycin pharmacokinetics in normal and morbidly obese subjects. *Antimicrob Agents Chemother.* 1982;21:575-80.

29. Salazar DE, Corcoran GB. Predicting creatinine clearance and renal drug clearance in obese patients from estimated fat-free body mass. *Am J Med.* 1988;84:1053-60.

30. Bauer LA, Black DJ, Lill JS. Vancomycin dosing in morbidly obese patients. *Eur J Clin Pharmacol.* 1998;54:621-5.

31. Anastasio P, Spitali L, Frangiosa A, et al. Glomerular filtration rate in severely overweight normotensive humans. *Am J Kid Dis.* 2000;35;1144-8.

32. Janmahasatian S, Duffull SB, Chagnac A, et al. Lean body mass normalizes the effect of obesity on renal function. *Br J Clin Pharmacol.* 2008;65:964-5.

33. Demirovic JA, Pai AB, Pai MP. Estimation of creatinine clearance in morbidly obese patients. *Am J Health-Syst Pharm.* 2009;66:642-8.

34. Lim WH, Lim EE, McDonald S. Lean body mass-adjusted Cockcroft and Gault formula improves the estimation of glomerular filtration rate in subjects with normal-range serum creatinine. *Nephrology.* 2006;11:250-6.

35. Aldaz A, Ortega A, Idoate A, et al. Effects of hepatic function on vancomycin pharmacokinetics in patients with cancer. *Ther Drug Monitor.* 2000;22:250-7.

36. del Mar Fernandez de Gatta Garcia M, Revilla N, Calvo MV, et al. Pharmacokinetic/pharmacodynamic analysis of vancomycin in ICU patients. *Intensive Care Med.* 2007;33:279-85.

Chapter 4

*Vinita B. Pai and Milap C. Nahata**

Drug Dosing in Pediatric Patients

Pediatric patients have been labeled "therapeutic orphans" because of the lack of pharmacokinetic, pharmacodynamic, efficacy, and safety data necessary to provide safe and effective drug therapy to this population. Efficacy and safety trials of new drugs are initially conducted in adult patients, most often excluding infants, children, and pregnant women. Many drugs routinely used in pediatric patients do not have pediatric labeling. Rather, safety and efficacy data in the pediatric population may come from trial and error approaches with use of these drugs.

Children should not be considered miniature adults; adult doses scaled down based on body weight may not be as safe or effective in the pediatric population as in adults. As neonates develop into toddlers and young adolescents, physiologic events occur that change the body composition and organ function. Changes in body water, body fat, plasma proteins, hormonal composition, and renal and hepatic function all occur and influence drug disposition.

Table 4-1 shows the classification of the pediatric population into distinct age groups and provides selected birth age terminology.[1] Physiological changes resulting in growth and development of a human body do not strictly remain in these age-related boundaries and are often not linearly related to age. Drug disposition in pediatric patients may change due to certain intrinsic factors such as sex, race, heredity, inherited diseases, and certain extrinsic factors such as acquired diseases, diet, and prior exposure to drug therapy. To provide safe and effective drug therapy to pediatric patients, it is important to gain knowledge of the pharmacokinetic and pharmacodynamic properties of each drug and the effect of development on its disposition. Within the pediatric population, neonates (especially premature neonates) exhibit marked differences in body composition and organ function when compared to each other and to the rest of the pediatric population. This chapter focuses on the influence of growth and maturation on drug disposition and pharmacodynamic response to drugs in the pediatric population, ranging from neonates to adolescents.

Table 4-1. Age Groupings of Children and Birth Age

Terminology	Age Grouping
Neonates	Birth to 4 weeks of age
Premature neonate	Gestational age of 37 weeks or less at birth
Full-term neonate	Gestational age of 38–41 weeks at birth
Post-term neonate	Gestational age of 42 weeks or more at birth
Infant	1 to <12 months of age
Child	1–12 years of age
Adolescent	13–18 years of age
Pediatric	Birth to 18 years of age
Birth Age Terminology	
Gestational age (GA)	Number of weeks from the first day of the last normal menstrual period to birth
Postnatal age (PNA) or chronological age	Age since birth
Postconceptional age (PCA) or postmenstrual age	Gestational age plus postnatal age, in weeks

*The authors acknowledge Ana M. Lopez-Samblas, Kamal Behbahani, Jorge Chivite, and Helena Wang for allowing us the use of information from their chapter, which was included in the third edition of this book.

General Pharmacokinetic Information

Absorption—oral

Most drugs administered by the oral route are absorbed by passive diffusion. Gastric pH, gastric and intestinal motility, pancreatic enzyme activity, bacterial colonization of the intestines, bile salt production, blood flow to the gastrointestinal (GI) tract, and the surface area of absorption affect the rate and extent of GI absorption.[2,3] These factors undergo considerable maturational changes as a neonate grows into an adult. Newborns of <32 weeks GA rarely have any gastric acid production, while the gastric pH in a newborn at term is alkaline (pH 6–8) but becomes acidic over the next 24 hr (pH 1.5–3).[4-6] Over the next few months of life, gastric acid production may remain low. The volume and acid concentration of the gastric fluid are dependent on age and approach the lower limit of normal adult values by 3 months of age; but reach adult values only after 2 years of age.[5,8] The rate and extent of absorption for drugs that are weak acids or bases may depend on their partition coefficients and gastric/intestinal pH. Gastric pH may change with ingestion of certain foods. For example, orange juice, cranberry juice, and carbonated beverages decrease the gastric pH causing acidic drugs such as itraconazole to be absorbed more readily (increased bioavailability) since an acidic gastric pH is necessary for complete absorption. H_2-antagonists such as ranitidine can raise pH and reduce absorption of drugs such as itraconazole. Absorption of acidic drugs may decrease when given with milk or infant formula due to increases in gastric pH.[11]

Gastric emptying rate is considerably delayed in infants, only reaching adult capacity by 6–8 months of age.[12,13] Since most drugs are absorbed in the small intestine, the rate of drug absorption may be decreased due to delayed (lengthened) gastric emptying time, but bioavailability of the drugs may increase due to slower intestinal transit. The rate and extent of drug absorption may be significantly altered in patients with acute changes in the GI tract. Decreased and delayed absorption of ampicillin and nalidixic acid was observed in infants and children treated with these drugs for acute shigellosis. In another study involving use of ampicillin in the treatment of gastroenteritis in children, mean concentrations of ampicillin were lower in the children with gastroenteritis than in children without the malady, possibly due to malabsorption.[14] In infancy and beyond, differences in GI maturation and absorption between the different age groups may not be significant enough to impact oral dosing recommendations for most drugs.

Pancreatic enzymes increase the bioavailability of oral drug dosage forms that require intraluminal (GI) hydrolysis prior to absorption such as oral liquid ester formulations of clindamycin and chloramphenicol palmitate.[8] Pancreatic enzyme activity is low at birth.[15] Amylase activity remains low (approximately 10% of adult values) even after the first month of life.[8] Lipase activity is present by 34 to 36 weeks GA and increases 5-fold during the first 7 days of life to 20-fold during the first 9 months after birth. Trypsin secretion in response to pancreozymin and secretin is decreased at birth but develops during the first year of life.[15-17] Bile salts may influence the absorption of certain fat-soluble drugs and nutrients. Bile salt metabolism matures postnatally within the first few months of life and continues to mature during the first year of life.[18] After infancy, neither pancreatic enzymes nor bile salts activity should be expected to affect dosing recommendations in normal children.

Composition and rate of GI colonization by bacterial flora depend more on diet than on age; however, the effect of bacteria on intestinal motility and drug metabolism is not completely known.[19] For example, the GI bacterial flora approaches adult composition by 4 years of age, and intestinal colonization by oral digoxin-reducing anaerobic bacteria approaches adult values by 2 years of age; however, the reduction of digoxin by these bacteria that is observed in adults may not be achieved until adolescence.[20] Therefore, when compared to adults, higher digoxin bioavailability can be anticipated in infants and children below 2 years of age.

Absorption—intramuscular

The surface area over which the injected drug volume can be distributed, blood flow to the site of injection, ease of penetration through the endothelial capillary walls, and muscle activity may all influence the absorption of drugs after intramuscular administration. Intramuscular absorption is variable in premature newborns as they have a small percentage of body weight that is skeletal muscle and subcutaneous fat compared to older infants, children, and adults. Circulatory insufficiency, hypoxia, and exposure to a cold environment may also decrease the rate or extent of intramuscular (IM) absorption in newborns, particularly those who are premature. For example, the IM administration of *aminoglycosides* in premature neonates is discouraged due to inconsistent serum concentrations, but it may be employed in full-term, otherwise healthy, infants. Drugs administered by this route are generally well absorbed in infants and children. Obviously, IM injections can be a painful route of administration and should be used only when oral administration is not indicated or intravenous access is unavailable. The IM route is more commonly used for administration of vaccines.

Absorption—percutaneous

Greater skin hydration, thinner and/or immature stratum corneum, and greater body surface area to weight ratio increase percutaneous drug absorption in pediatric patients.[21] Percutaneous absorption is pronounced in the premature neonate because the epidermal barrier is thin and often poorly developed.[22,23] Toxic effects have been reported with topical agents such as EMLA (eutectic mixture of lidocaine and prilocaine) and hexachlorophene solution.[24,25] Topical drugs with limited safety experience in neonates should be employed cautiously. Since percutaneous absorption is increased through damaged skin, application of high-potency corticosteroids to diaper rashes with severe perianal inflammation should be avoided.[26]

Absorption—rectal

With proper formulation, the rectal route of administration is a useful alternative when oral, intravenous, or intramuscular administration is not possible (e.g., nausea, vomiting, seizures, preparation for surgery, lack of injectable products). Due to limitations in availability of different doses, suppositories are often impractical for drugs with narrow therapeutic ranges since dosing requirements in neonates are often based on body weight. In addition, cutting suppositories may result in an unpredictable dose because the drug is not always uniformly dispersed throughout the preparation. The rate and extent of absorption of certain drugs such as diazepam may be improved when solutions are used rather than suppositories for rectal administration.[27] For example, diazepam concentrations attained after rectal administration of solution have been comparable to those attained after intravenous administration. However, rectal administration is often erratic or incomplete compared to oral or IV administration. Delay in onset of action and failure to reach minimal effective concentrations for some drugs make the rectal route of administration inferior to the oral and intravenous routes.

Distribution

Factors such as the relative proportion of body water and body fat and differences in protein binding determine the differences in drug distribution between infants and adults. The total body water decreases from approximately 92% of body weight in a premature newborn, to 75% in a full-term newborn to 60% (25% is extracellular water and 35% is intracellular) by one year of age.[8,28] Total body water approaches adult values of 50%–60% (20% extracellular and 40% intracellular) by 12–13 years of age.

Hydrophilic drugs such as the aminoglycoside antibiotics and linezolid largely distribute into the extracellular fluid and thus have larger volumes of distribution in neonates compared to older infants and children.[29-31] Larger volumes of distribution require larger milligram-per-kilogram doses of aminoglycosides to achieve similar peak concentrations. However, caution should be exercised in using actual body weight in calculating aminoglycoside doses in obese children due to the relatively lower percentage of extracellular water in obesity.

On average, total body fat increases from 12%–16% of body weight at full-term to 20%–25% at 1 year of age. It then increases between 5 and 10 years of age, followed by a decrease in boys around age 17. At puberty, there is a rapid increase in percent body fat in females, approaching twice the value compared to males.[28,32] Lipophilic drugs will have a larger volume of distribution relative to body weight in children and adults than neonates and infants due to higher percentage of body fat.[33] Obesity in any age group will generally increase volume of distribution of lipophilic compounds compared to normal weight patients.

The binding of drugs to circulating plasma proteins depends on multiple factors such as total amount of proteins, the number of binding sites, the binding affinity, and the presence of pathophysiologic conditions (e.g., change in blood pH) or endogenous compounds (e.g., bilirubin, free fatty acids) that may alter the drug-protein interaction. Albumin, alpha-1-acid glycoprotein, and lipoproteins are the important drug-binding proteins; albumin comprises an average of 58% of all plasma proteins.[34] The plasma protein binding of various drugs is less in the neonate compared to other patient populations because of lower total plasma protein concentration and lower drug-protein binding capacities.[35] Total protein concentration including serum albumin and alpha-1-acid glycoprotein as well as their function and binding capacity approach adult values by the first year of age and remain consistently stable in healthy children between 2 and 18 years of age.[33,36] Conditions that decrease plasma proteins may increase the free, active fraction of highly protein-bound drugs.

Acidic and neutral drugs such as beta-lactam antibiotics, warfarin, and digoxin exhibit great binding affinity for albumin; basic compounds such as propranolol and alprenolol bind to alpha-1-acid glycoprotein, lipoproteins, and beta-globulins.[37] Several endogenous substances such as bilirubin and free fatty acid compete for the albumin binding sites and influence the drug–protein binding capacity. For example, bilirubin is often increased in neonates secondary to increased red cell destruction and limited liver capacity to conjugate it. The binding capacity of bilirubin to plasma albumin is decreased in newborn infants but approaches adult values by 5 months of age. Drugs highly bound to the plasma proteins, such as the sulfonamides, may displace bilirubin and contribute to kernicterus in neonates.[38] The pharmacological action of a drug moiety is attributed to the free (unbound) form of the drug, so increased free concentrations can lead to enhanced effect or toxicity.

Elimination

Most drugs or their water-soluble metabolites are excreted through the kidneys. Glomerular filtration, tubular secretion, and reabsorption all impact the renal elimination of drugs. The anatomical development of nephrons (nephrogenesis) in a fetus continues until 36 weeks GA with significant glomerular maturation occurring between 34 and 36 weeks GA.[39] After 36 weeks GA, the increase in renal mass is predominantly due to renal tubular growth. The overall functional capacity of the kidney increases with age up to early adulthood.

Glomerular filtration of drugs depends on the functional capacity of the glomerulus, the integrity of renal blood flow, and the extent and strength of drug-protein binding. The glomerular filtration rate (GFR) increases with increases in renal blood flow and decreases with increasing protein binding of a drug. There is a positive correlation between GA and GFR in newborns between 27 and 43 weeks of GA. Renal blood flow approaches adult values by approximately 5–12 months of age.[2,3] The GFR dramatically increases from birth and approaches adult values by approximately 3–5 months of age.[40] The GFR undergoes postnatal increases ranging from 10–15 ml/min/ 1.73 m^2 in a full-term newborn to 20–30 ml/min/ 1.73 m^2 by 1–2 weeks of life and approaches adult values of 73–127 ml/min/1.73 m^2 by 3 months of age.[40-42]

GFR can be assessed by determining or estimating creatinine clearance (CrCl). Determining CrCl requires a 24-hr urine collection that is difficult to obtain in infants and children wearing diapers. Incomplete collections will lead to inaccurate results; complete collection may require catheterization of the patient, making the process more invasive. Creatinine clearance may not be the most accurate estimate of GFR, especially in neonates and infants since creatinine is not only filtered by the glomerulus but also secreted by the renal tubules.[43] In the early postnatal period, the serum creatinine value reflects maternal values. Creatinine clearance can be estimated from single serum creatinine values by using nomograms or mathematical formulas, which are most convenient but potentially less accurate (see Chapter 1).[44] The Schwartz formula is commonly used to determine CrCl in the pediatric population. It uses serum creatinine (Scr) as a surrogate marker of GFR and the concept of body height or length as a measure of body muscle mass. The formula is GFR (ml/min/1.73 m^2) = k x L/ Scr, where L is height or length in centimeters, Scr is in mg/dL, and k is an empirical constant. This constant is determined by comparing L/Scr ratio against measured GFR. The value of k is 0.45 for term infants through first year of life, 0.55 for children and adolescent girls, and 0.7 for adolescent boys.[57] However, this method of CrCl measurement invariably overestimates GFR in children, especially in those with mild to moderate chronic kidney disease. The k values used in this formula are more specific to the colorimetric method used to assay Scr. However, by the end of 2010, all clinical laboratories in the US will use the new standardized Isotope Dilution Mass Spectrometry (IDMS) method to measure serum creatinine.[45] The IDMS method appears to underestimate Scr when compared to older methods and hence increases estimates of CrCl by 20 to 30%. A new equation has been developed taking into account this change in assay methodology. This new equation was developed in children with chronic kidney disease (CKD) with a median GFR of 41.3 ml/min/1.73 m^2 using iohexol plasma disappearance measurements as gold standard.[46] The bedside formula recommended in this group of patients is GFR (ml/min/1.73 m^2) = 0.413 x (L/Scr), where L is height or length in centimeters and Scr is in mg/dl. This formula has not been evaluated in children with normal renal function and additional studies are required. GFR determined by the original and the updated Schwartz formula were compared to GFR measured using the technetium 99 diethylenetriaminepentaacetic acid as gold standard.[47] These measurements were conducted in pediatric patients prior to their hematopoietic stem cell transplantation and had a mean (± standard deviation) GFR of 107 ± 28 ml/min/1.73 m^2. Only 53% of the GFR values estimated using the original Schwartz formula were within 30% of the corresponding DTPA-Tc99m determined GFR, compared to 77% of the GFR values estimated using the updated Schwartz formula. The new formula classified normal GFR as reduced. Hence the updated formula performed marginally better compared to the original formula but may not be accurate enough for routine use. The updated formula was developed for pediatric patients with mild to moderate CKD; however, the patients in this study had near normal GFR. In patients receiving aminoglycosides, renal clearance of the aminoglycoside approximates creatinine clearance, since >90% of the dose is filtered through the glomeruli and minimal excretion occurs in the form of tubular secretion.[48,49] Because of this, aminoglycoside clearance has also been used to estimate GFR.

Significant anatomical and functional immaturity of the renal tubules exists at birth. This affects passive reabsorption, active secretion, and active reabsorption processes. The tubular secretory function does not mature at the same rate as the GFR because the proximal convoluted tubules are small relative to their corresponding glomeruli at birth.[50] Tubular function approaches adult values by 1 year of life, thus affecting drugs eliminated by tubular secretion in addition to glomerular filtration. The renal tubules of a neonate have less surface area and urine concentrating ability and pH is lower compared to infants, children, and adults.[51]

Dosing recommendations for renally excreted drugs, especially those with a narrow therapeutic range, should be based on the patient's renal function to avoid toxicity due to decreased elimination and increased accumulation when renal function decreases. Monitoring parameters such as urine output, creatinine clearance, and serum creatinine can help in the assessment of renal function. However, urine output varies with fluid intake, hydration status, renal solute load, and urine concentrating capabilities and may not accurately reflect renal clearance of drugs primarily excreted through the kidneys, especially drugs eliminated by tubular secretion rather than glomerular filtration.

Table 4-2 lists physiologic changes that occur with aging in children and some examples of the pharmacokinetic consequences that can result from the changes.

Metabolism

Drug metabolism primarily occurs in the liver; however, the kidneys, intestines, lungs, and skin may also be involved.[55] Most drugs that are metabolized are converted to more water-soluble compounds for excretion from the body by the kidneys. Active parent compounds may be transformed into inactive or active metabolites and pharmacologically inactive compounds or prodrugs may be converted to their active moiety.

Hepatic blood flow, extraction efficiency, binding affinity, and enzyme activity can affect hepatic drug metabolism. Of these factors, enzyme activity is greatly dependent on patient age. Two primary enzymatic processes, phase I (nonsynthetic) reactions and phase II (synthetic) reactions, are involved in drug biotransformation. Phase I reactions include oxidation, reduction, hydrolysis, and hydroxylation. These reactions introduce or reveal a functional group within the substrate that will serve as a site for a phase II conjugation reaction.

The activity of the oxidizing enzymes is greatly reduced at birth, resulting in prolonged elimination of drugs such as phenytoin and diazepam.[2,3,56,57] The hepatic mono-oxygenase system approaches and exceeds adult capacities by approximately 6 months of age.[58] Alcohol dehydrogenase activity, detectable at ≤3%–4% of adult activity at 2 months of age, approaches adult capacity after 5 years of age.[59] Demethylation activity may not be seen until 14–15 months of age and may increase thereafter. Hydrolytic activity reaches adult values within the first few months of life. Quantitatively, cytochrome P450 isoforms are the most important phase I enzymes with CYP1, CYP2, and CYP3 genes being important in human drug metabolism (see Table 4-3).[60-68]

In phase II reactions, the substrate may be conjugated with endogenous agents such as sulfate, acetate, glucuronic acid, glutathione, and glycine, resulting in a more polar, water-soluble compound that can be eliminated easily by the renal and/or biliary systems. The phase II enzymes consist of glucuronosyltransferases, sulfotransferases, arylamine *N*-acetyltransferases, glutathione *S*-transferases, and methyltransferases, all of which play an important role in biotransformation of drugs (Table 4-4).[69] Important differences exist between children and adults, and phase II enzymes do not all follow the same developmental patterns.

Table 4-2. Age-Dependent Differences in Physiologic Functions and Drug Disposition

Physiologic Variability	Neonate	Infant	Child	Adolescent	Pharmacokinetic Consequence
ABSORPTION					
Gastric pH	(>5)	(2–4)	(2–3)	↔	Increase in bioavailability of acid-labile drugs, e.g., penicillin G in neonates and infants compared to children and adults; decreased bioavailability of weak organic acids, e.g., phenobarbital.[9,10]
Gastric and intestinal emptying time	↑	↑	↔	↔	Specific examples influencing drug pharmacokinetics not available.
Biliary function	↓	~ ↔	↔	↔	Reduced absorption of fat and fat-soluble vitamins D and E in neonates compared to infants and children.[18]
Pancreatic function	↓	~ ↔	↔	↔	Reduced hydrolysis and bioavailability of oral liquid ester formulations of clindamycin and chloramphenicol in neonates compared to infants and children.[8]
Gut microbial colonization	↓	~ ↔	↔	↔	Increased bioavailability of digoxin in neonates and infants compared to adults due to lack of microbial gut colonization with an oral digoxin-reducing anaerobic bacteria.[20]
Intramuscular absorption (rate and extent)	↓	↑	↑ to ~ ↔	↔	Benzathine penicillin G more rapidly absorbed in children compared to adults since no measurable activity was detected in children 18 days after the injection.[52]
Skin permeability and percutaneous absorption	↑	↑ (extent)	~ ↔	↔	EMLA (eutectic mixture of local anesthetics lidocaine and prilocaine) should be used with caution in patients less than 3 months of age due to risk of methemoglobinemia from increased percutaneous absorption of prilocaine and decreased methemoglobin reductase, especially in combination with other methemoglobinemia-inducing agents.[24]
DISTRIBUTION					
Total body water and extracellular water	↑	↑	↓ ~ ↔	↔	Increase in mean apparent volume of distribution (*V*) for hydrophilic drugs, e.g., gentamicin.[29,30]
Total body fat	↓	↓	Increases by ages 5-10 yr	↔	Mean apparent *V* for lipophilic drugs increases from infants to adults, e.g., diazepam. 1.3–2.6 L/kg in infants vs. 1.6–3.2 L/kg in adults.[33]
Total plasma proteins	↓	↓ or ~ ↔	↔	↔	Increase in *V* and unbound phenytoin fraction in infants and children.[53]
RENAL ELIMINATION					
Glomerular filtration	↓	↔	↔	↔	Famotidine—renal clearance reduced in neonates but equivalent to adults by 1 year of age.[54]
Tubular secretion and tubular reabsorption	↓	~ ↔	↔	↔	Penicillins—increased half-life due to decreased excretion both by glomerular filtration and tubular secretion, therefore, lengthened dosing interval in infants compared to children and adolescents.[8]

↔ = similar to adult capacity, ~↔ = near adult capacity, ↑ = increased compared to adult capacity, ↓ = decreased compared to adult capacity.

Table 4-3. Age-Dependent Differences in Activity of Important Phase I Drug Metabolizing Enzymes and Drug Metabolism

Enzyme	Fetus	Neonate	Infant	Child	Adolescent	Pharmacokinetic Consequences
CYP1A2	No activity	↓	↓; 50% of adult activity by age 1 year	↔ after 1 year of age	↔	Theophylline has a long half-life and low systemic clearance in newborns.[60-62]
CYP2C9	10% of adult activity	30% of adult activity	↔ (reached by age 1–6 months)	↑ (peak activity at age 3–10 years)	↔ (decreases to adult value at puberty)	Vm values for phenytoin decreased from 14 mg/kg/day in infancy to 8 mg/kg/day in adolescence as a function of progressively decreasing CYP2C9 activity.[63]
CYP2C19[55]	10% of adult activity	30% of adult activity	↔ (reached by age 6 months)	↑ (peak activity at age 3–4 years)	↔ (decreases to adult value at puberty)	Diazepam half-life increased in young infants (25–100 hr) compared to children (7–37 hr) and adults (20–50 hr) due to decreased oxidative activity.[57,64]
CYP2D6	Minimal activity	↓ 30% of adult activity[58]	Maturation completed by 1 year of age[55]	↔	↔	O-demethylation of codeine to morphine decreased in infants resulting in lack of efficacy and poor pain control.[65]
CYP2E1	10%–30% of adult activity[79]	No data	30%–40% of adult activity[79]	↔ by 10 years of age[79]	↔	Caffeine, acetaminophen, and certain toxic substances such as cigarette smoke and alcohol metabolized by this pathway.[66]
CYP3A4	10% of adult activity	↓ 30%–40% of adult activity[74]	Adult pattern (by age 1 year)[74]	↑ (between age 1–4 years then progressively decreases)	↔ (at puberty)	Midazolam systemic clearance and metabolism to one of its primary metabolites 1′-hydroxy–midazolam reduced in premature infants but increases 5-fold by 3 months of age.[67,68]

↔ = similar to adult capacity, ~ ↔ = near adult capacity, ↑ = increased compared to adult capacity, ↓ = decreased compared to adult capacity.

Table 4-4. Age-Dependent Differences in Activity of Important Drug-Metabolizing Phase II Enzymes and Drug Metabolism

Enzyme	Fetus	Neonate	Infant	Child	Adolescent	Pharmacokinetic Consequences
Uridine 5′-diphosphate glucronosyl transferase (UGT)	10%–20% of adult activity[69]	↓	25% of adult activity by 3 months of age[70]	↔ present by age 6 months to 3 yr	↔	The ratio of glucuronide conjugate to sulfate conjugate of acetaminophen increases with age as the enzyme system matures; newborn 0.34; child (3–10 yr) 0.8; adolescent 1.61; and adult 1.8–2.3.[71]
N-acetyl-transferase-2	↓	↓	↓	↔ past 1 year of age	↔	Decreased acetylation of sulfapyridine (sulfasalazine metabolite) results in increased side effects of nausea, headache, and abdominal pain.[72]
Methyltransferase		↑	↔	↔	↔	Specific drug example not available.
Sulfotransferase		↓	↑ for specific substrates	↑ for specific substrates	↔	Specific drug example not available.

↔ = similar to adult capacity, ~ ↔ = near adult capacity, ↑ = increased compared to adult capacity, ↓ = decreased compared to adult capacity.

Factors Influencing Drug Disposition

Asphyxia[73-75]

The elimination of aminoglycosides, phenobarbital, and theophylline in neonates asphyxiated at birth is markedly reduced due to decreased renal and liver perfusion during severe hypoxia. The Apgar score, used as a measure of viability in the newborn, is the total score of five objective neonatal assessment signs performed at different time intervals shortly after delivery (maximum score is 10 and scores <3 reflect severe respiratory depression). In neonates with Apgar scores of <3 at 1 or 5 min or with cardiac and respiratory arrest requiring resuscitation, concentrations of drugs with narrow therapeutic windows should be closely monitored. Dosage requirements for some drugs might need to be decreased by up to 50%. Since the duration of this effect is not well established, close follow-up is warranted.

Asphyxiated neonates receiving phenobarbital or theophylline can be initially empirically dosed with half the usual maintenance dose, followed by drug concentration monitoring for dosage adjustment (no adjustment is needed for loading doses). For neonates receiving aminoglycosides or vancomycin, urine output should be evaluated to assess the need for dosing interval adjustments. Urine output can serve as an early indicator of decreased renal clearance due to hypoxia.

Exchange transfusion[76-78]

Information regarding the effect of exchange transfusions on concentrations of drugs commonly administered to neonates is limited and often controversial. Drug loss has varied from 1% to 55%, depending on the medications, study design, and timing and frequency of procedures. The magnitude of the decline in drug concentrations is greatest when the procedure is performed shortly after dose administration (since concentrations are higher) and can be considered clinically inconsequential at the end of the dosing interval. The effect is augmented by the number of blood volumes exchanged (on the same dose) and the rate used.

When exchange transfusions are at the beginning of the dosing interval and a drop in concentration might be clinically consequential, drug concentrations may be obtained to assess drug loss and to calculate a "replacement" dose. Concentrations obtained following exchange transfusions should not be employed for routine pharmacokinetic calculations since they do not reflect steady state conditions.

Extracorporeal membrane oxygenation (ECMO)[79-93]

Extracorporeal membrane oxygenation provides prolonged cardiopulmonary bypass and thus, supports infants with life threatening cardiac and/or respiratory failure. Drug disposition during ECMO is influenced by the following factors: (1) priming volume of the circuit that may exceed the blood volume of the neonates and lead to an increased volume of distribution for water soluble drugs; (2) membrane oxygenator and PVC tubing that provides a large surface area for drug adsorption and subsequent leakage (binding occurs to a greater extent with a new circuit and declines when the circuit has been used over several days); (3) site of administration (administration post-reservoir minimizes the effects of ECMO on drug disposition but bypasses the benefit that occurs with pre-reservoir administration of bolus injections—the trapping of air bubbles that can lead to cerebral emboli); and, (4) flow rate <250 ml/min that can lead to drug pooling at the reservoir for medications administered pre-reservoir. As a result of these physiologic and mechanical variables, determining pharmacokinetic parameters and appropriate dosing regimens during ECMO is difficult.

In neonates on ECMO, the apparent volume of distribution for gentamicin is increased, and the elimination half life is prolonged as compared to values observed off ECMO, as well as when compared to term neonates.[79-82] For an infant on ECMO, a gentamicin dose of 2.5–3 mg/kg administered every 18–24 hr to achieve a peak serum concentration between 5–10 mg/L and trough serum concentrations of 0.5–1 mg/L is empirically recommended.[80] Similar modification in extension of dosing interval can be made for other aminoglycosides such as tobramycin and amikacin. For vancomycin, the data are conflicting.[83,84] Most studies report similar variability in pharmacokinetic parameters among neonates on or off ECMO and thus suggest no need for vancomycin dosing adjustments. Others suggest extending the interval to assure troughs within the therapeutic range. Pharmacokinetic studies of midazolam used for sedation in neonates on ECMO offer conflicting data and interpretation.[86,87] The studies reported a significant increase in volume of distribution and a prolonged half-life from the onset of ECMO. However, one study reported a 3-fold increase in the clearance of midazolam and 1-hydroxymidazolam in the first 5 days after start of ECMO.[87] The clearance of hydroxymidazolam glucuronide, the metabolite, remained constant.

A constant 10% of sedation was provided by 1-hydroxymidazolam, but sedation provided by hydroxymidazolam glucuronide increased from 12% to 34% over the course of 7 days, due to rising concentrations. The authors of this study recommend increasing the infusion rate of midazolam after 5–7 days to compensate for the increased clearance of midazolam and 1-hydroxymidazolam to achieve a target midazolam concentration of 400 mcg/L. The authors of the second study believe that the initial increase in the volume of distribution is due to reversible sequestration of midazolam by the ECMO circuit.[86] Therefore, increased plasma concentrations of midazolam during the later phases of ECMO were observed. Hence, the need for a higher initial dose of midazolam followed by a decrease in dose rate, to prevent high concentrations is recommended. Both studies found large interpatient variability in the volume of distribution and clearance; careful dose titration based on sedation scores and adverse effects is recommended. Dosing during ECMO should take into account site of administration and flow rate and should be individualized based on drug concentrations.[88] An increased volume of distribution and prolonged elimination rate with large interpatient variability was noted when bumetanide was administered to neonates on ECMO.[89] Extensive non-renal elimination of bumetanide was hypothesized to be mainly due to loss of the drug in the ECMO circuit. A pronounced diuresis was observed during the early period after drug administration (6 hr). Due to insufficient data, specific dosing and interval recommendations cannot be made; however, additional doses of the drug may be needed to offset the shorter duration of action. Higher doses of morphine and fentanyl were required in neonates on ECMO to induce prolonged sedation and analgesia.[90-93] The reason for increased dose requirement during ECMO is unclear. Clearance also increases once the infants are taken off ECMO, which may result in opioid withdrawal. Despite a possible higher dose requirement in these infants, both drugs should be initiated at standard doses and titrated as needed to obtain pain control and sedation without toxicity. A slow taper can prevent opioid withdrawal after discontinuation of ECMO.

Patent ductus arteriosus (PDA)[94-96]

In fetal circulation, the ductus arteriosus (DA) connects the pulmonary artery to the descending aorta allowing blood to bypass the lungs. At birth, with clamping of the umbilical cord and aeration and expansion of the lungs, the ductal PaO_2 rises to approximately 100 mmHg. Concurrently, the amount of circulating prostaglandin (PG) and the sensitivity of the ductus to the circulating PG is lowered and the DA constricts and closes. When the DA fails to close, it is called patent ductus arteriosus (PDA).

Significant differences in the volume of distribution (depending on whether the ductus arteriosus is open or closed) have been shown for several drugs including gentamicin, indomethacin, and vancomycin. The calculated volume of distribution decreases after PDA closure, potentially changing dosing requirements that were previously adequate. When using indomethacin for the pharmacological closure of the PDA, its nephrotoxic effects may decrease renal clearance of aminoglycosides, digoxin, and vancomycin.

Cystic fibrosis (CF)

Cystic fibrosis is an autosomal recessive disease, predominantly seen in the Caucasian population, affecting approximately 30,000 children and young adults in the United States and 70,000 worldwide.[97] About 1000 new cases are diagnosed each year in the U.S. with 70% diagnosed by 2 years of age. More than 45% are ≥18 years of age and the predicted median age of survival was almost 37 years in 2005. Mutation of a single gene on chromosome 7 encoding the CF transmembrane conductance regulator leads to abnormalities affecting multiple organs; this mutation impacts all aspects of drug disposition.[98] Factors such as lower rate of absorption, larger apparent volume of distribution, and greater metabolic and renal clearances may alter drug disposition and will result in lower drug concentrations after administration of age-appropriate doses of many drugs in patients with CF when compared to normal patients.

Drug absorption in patients with CF may be decreased due to altered GI physiology such as gastric acid hypersecretion, bile acid malabsorption, and proximal small intestinal mucosal injury.[99,100] However, changes do not always occur.

Alteration in protein binding of drugs due to hypoalbuminemia and hypogammaglobulinemia in patients with CF can alter the distribution volume.[101] The choice of units using body surface area (L/m^2) and body weight (L/kg) may affect the apparent volume of distribution because body weight is affected much earlier than would be expected from linear growth during the course of CF. A higher volume of distribution has been reported for cloxacillin, theophylline, and ceftazidime in patients with CF compared to healthy individuals when expressed by units of body weight.[102-104] For drugs such as methicillin and ticarcillin, the distribution volume was not significantly different when expressed per unit of body surface area (BSA).[104] It has been recommended that volume of distribution should be normalized by lean body mass (LBM) rather than BSA in CF patients.[105,106] However, the appropriateness of one approach over another is still unknown.

Hepatobiliary dysfunction, increases in hepatic enzymes, and reduced synthesis of proteins is reported in approximately 30%–40% of patients with CF.[107,108] Hepatic clearance of drugs is largely influenced by the hepatic blood flow and activity of liver enzymes. Evidence of an increase in portal venous blood flow in CF patients is conflicting. Age, severity of CF disease, and extent of hepatic dysfunction may influence the hepatic blood flow.

Hepatic biotransformation of drugs by phase I and II reactions may either be increased or remain unchanged in patients with CF compared to healthy individuals. Disease-specific alterations in hepatic biotransformation in patients with CF are not limited to the mono-oxygenase system. Ibuprofen is mainly metabolized by glucuronosyltransferase to a glucuronide conjugate for example.[109] A significant increase in the apparent total clearance of ibuprofen was observed after oral administration in children with CF compared with healthy children, suggesting that glucuronidation is enhanced in CF.[110] Both in vitro and in vivo data showed increased metabolic clearance of unbound sulfamethoxazole to *N*4-acetylsulfamethoxazole and thus confirmed that the intrinsic activity of *N*-acetyltransferase (NAT1) was significantly increased in patients with CF.[111,112]

Results from studies measuring renal function, i.e., GFR and tubular clearance, are conflicting with both parameters either increased or unchanged in patients with CF. These conflicting results are possibly attributed to differences in age and severity of the CF disease, e.g., glomerulomegaly and hyperfiltration. The renal clearance of ceftazidime was significantly increased in patients with CF compared to healthy adults due to increased glomerular filtration.[113,114] Aminoglycosides are primarily eliminated by glomerular filtration; however, they are also reabsorbed by the proximal tubule. Studies comparing renal clearance of amikacin to inulin and tobramycin to iothalamate indicated that the glomerular filtration of aminoglycosides is not altered in patients with CF.[115,116] Therefore, a decrease in tubular reabsorption and/or clearance into the respiratory tract was speculated to be the cause of increased plasma clearance of the aminoglycosides. Despite faster clearance in the pediatric CF population, extended-interval once daily dosing (EID) of aminoglycosides is a recommended option for treatment of acute pulmonary exacerbations.[117] In tobramycin naïve patients, a starting dosage of 10 mg/kg/day given once daily may be appropriate.[118] The therapy should be individualized for the patient by drawing two tobramycin concentrations; one drawn at least 2 hours after the dose has been administered followed by the second measurement drawn 8 to 12 hours after the dose. These concentrations can be drawn after the first or second dose. Dose recommendations should be made to achieve extrapolated peak concentrations of 20–30 mg/L, troughs of less than 1 mg/L or area under the concentration-time curve of 100 mg × hr/L. In amikacin naïve patients, therapy can be started at 30–35 mg/kg/day given once daily. Extrapolated peak amikacin concentrations of 73 to 121 mg/L, trough less than 1 mg/L and area under serum concentration-time curve of 235–287 mg × hr/L can be expected with such doses. If the patient has received aminoglycosides dose given every 8 hours in the past with pharmacokinetic dosing adjustments, that total daily dose can be administered as a single daily dose. Tubular secretion of penicillin derivatives such as cloxacillin, methicillin, and ticarcillin that are primarily eliminated renally by tubular secretion was significantly higher in patients with CF compared to healthy individuals.[104,119,120]

Altered drug disposition in patients with CF can impact drugs with a narrow therapeutic index and drugs that demonstrate a large degree of variability in their pharmacokinetic parameters. Therefore, the normal age-appropriate drug doses may need to be altered in CF patients based on the results of measured drug concentrations.

Human Immunodeficiency Virus (HIV) Infection and Acquired Immunodeficiency Syndrome (AIDS)

Children aged 18 months to <13 years are categorized as HIV infected if they have a positive result from a screening test for HIV antibody confirmed by a positive result from a supplemental test for HIV antibody or positive result for or a detectable quantity of HIV nucleic acid, HIV p24 antigen, or HIV isolation.[121] Alternatively they are considered HIV positive if they are diagnosed by a physician or qualified medical-care provider based on the laboratory criteria and documented in a medical record.[121] They are categorized as having AIDS if they meet the criteria for HIV infection and have at least one of the 24 AIDS-defining conditions such as Pneumocystis jiroveci pneumonia. An estimated 9,349 children (<13 years at diagnosis) were living in the US with an AIDS diagnosis in 2008.[122] There were an estimated 41 AIDS diagnoses among children in 2008, compared to 195 in 1999 and 896 in 1992.[122]

Disposition of antiretroviral therapy is affected by differences in developmental changes in HIV infected children. Absorption of oral antiretrovirals can be affected by the presence and type of food in the gastrointestinal tract. This can be a significant problem in infants who have to feed regularly, thus making administration of antiretrovirals on an empty stomach difficult. Infants may not be able to tolerate feeds with high fat content necessary for absorption of certain antiretroviral drugs such as nelfinavir. At recommended doses, children <2 years of age may exhibit lower nelfinavir concentrations when compared to older children due to decreased bioavailability secondary to the inconsistency in the quantity and the type of food with which it is administered.[123] The higher pH in the stomach of the newborns and infants may also decrease the bioavailability of the weakly acidic nelfinavir. Decreased albumin content and reduced drug binding capacity in newborns and neonates may lead to increased unbound drug concentrations of highly protein bound anti-HIV drugs causing increased efficacy and toxicity. Enfuviritide, a fusion inhibitor anti-HIV drug is highly protein bound (92%), primarily to albumin, and to a lesser extent to alpha-1 glycoprotein.[124] Weight-based dosing of enfuvirtide in HIV patients between 5 and 16 years of age yielded similar AUC when compared to adult patients receiving the standard milligram dose. However, no data are available regarding the dosing of enfuvirtide in newborns and neonates given the effect of changes in protein binding in this population.[125] Metabolism of antiretroviral drugs, especially protease inhibitors and non-nucleoside reverse transcriptase inhibitors, shows variability with age among children and also when compared to adults. Due to this variability in metabolism, fixed-dose combinations of antiretrovirals usually recommended for adults cannot be routinely used in children. These combinations may lead to subtherapeutic concentrations of one antiretroviral but overdosing of another. The use of fixed doses containing lamivudine, stavudine, and nevirapine, intended for adults and available outside of the U.S., resulted in low nevirapine trough concentrations and virologic failure due to increased metabolism of nevirapine in the younger children compared to the adults.[126] Nevirapine is primarily metabolized by CYP3A4 and CYP2B6 isoenzymes. Anti-retroviral drugs eliminated primarily by glomerular filtration or tubular secretion are affected by maturation of renal function. For example, lamivudine is 70% excreted unchanged in the urine with a renal clearance exceeding the glomerular filtration rate indicating that lamivudine is also excreted by renal tubular secretion.[127] Since GFR and renal tubular secretion are reduced in neonates and adults compared to older children, the lamivudine dosing recommendation for neonates <28 days of age is 2 mg/kg/dose twice daily compared to 4 mg/kg/dose twice daily for infants 28 days of age and older.[128]

References

1 Committee on Fetus and Newborn. American Academy of Pediatrics Policy Statement: Age terminology during perinatal period. *Pediatrics*. 2004;114:1362-4.

2. Besunder JB, Reed MD, Blumer JL. Principles of drug disposition in the neonate: a critical evaluation of the pharmacokinetic-pharmacodynamic interface. Part I. *Clin Pharmacokinet.* 1988;14(4):261-86.

3. Besunder JB, Reed MD, Blumer JL. Principles of drug disposition in the neonate: a critical evaluation of the pharmacokinetic-pharmacodynamic interface. Part II. *Clin Pharmacokinet.* 1988;14(5):189-216.

4. Keene MFL, Hewer EE. Digestive enzymes of the human fetus. *Lancet*. 1929;1:767-9.

5. Agunod M, Yomaguchi N, Lopez R, et al. Correlative study of hydrochloric acid, pepsin and intrinsic factor secretion in newborns and infants. *Am J Dig Dis.* 1969;14(6):400-14.

6. Euler AR, Byrne WJ, Cousins LM, et al. Increased serum gastrin concentrations and gastric acid hyposecretion in the immediate newborn period. *Gastroenterology*. 1977;72:1271-3.

7. Hess AF. The gastric secretion of infants at birth. *Am J Dis Child.* 1913;6:264-76.

8. Reed MD, Besunder JB. Developmental pharmacology: ontogenic basis of drug disposition. *Pediatr Clin N Am.* 1989;36:1053-74.

9. Huang NN, High RH. Comparison of serum levels following the administration of oral and parenteral preparations of penicillin to infants and children of various age groups. *J Pediatr.* 1953;42:657-68.

10. Wallin A, Jalling B, Boreus LO. Plasma concentrations of phenobarbital in the neonate during prophylaxis for neonatal hyperbilirubinemia. *J Pediatr*. 1974;85(3):392-8.

11. Pinkerton CR, Welshman SG, Glasgow JF, et al. Can food influence the absorption of methotrexate in children with acute lymphoblastic leukaemia? *Lancet*. 1980;2(8201):944-6.

12. Cavell B. Gastric emptying in preterm infants. *Acta Paediatr Scand.* 1979;68(5):725-30.

13. Grand RJ, Watkins JB, Torti FM. Development of human gastrointestinal tract: A review. *Gastroenterology.* 1976;70(5PT1):790-810.

14. Elliot RB, Stokes EJ, Maxwell GM. Ampicillin in paediatrics. *Arch Dis Child.* 1964;39:101-5.

15. Kearns GL, Reed MD. Clinical pharmacokinetics in infants and children: a reappraisal. *Clin Pharmacokinet.* 1989;17(Suppl. 1):29-67.

16. Hadron B, Zoppi G, Shmerling DH, et al. Quantitative assessment of exocrine pancreatic function in infants and children. *J Pediatr.* 1968;73(1):39-50.

17. Zoppi G, Andreotti G, Pajno-Ferrara F, et al. Exocrine pancreatic function in premature and full-term neonates. *Pediatr Res.* 1972;6:880-6.

18. Heubi JE, Balistreri WF, Suchy FJ. Bile salt metabolism in the first year of life. *J Lab Clin Med.* 1982;100(1):127-36.

19. Yoshioka H, Iseki K, Fujita K. Development and differences of intestinal flora in the neonatal period in breast-fed and bottle-fed infants. *Pediatrics.* 1983;72(3):317-21.

20. Linday L, Dobkin JF, Wang TC, et al. Digoxin inactivation by the gut flora in infancy and childhood. *Pediatrics.* 1987;79(4):544-8.

21. Shear NH, Radde IC. Percutaneous drug absorption. In: Radde IC, MacLeod SM, eds. *Pediatric Pharmacology and Therapeutics.* St. Louis, LA: Mosby;1993:377-83.

22. Nachman RL, Esterly NB. Increased skin permeability in preterm infants. *J Pediatr.* 1977;79:628-32.23.

23. Harpin VA, Rutter N. Barrier properties of the newborn infant's skin. *J Pediatr.* 1983;102:419-25.

24. Nilsson A, Engberg G, Henneberg S, et al. Inverse relationship between age-dependent erythrocyte activity of metahemoglobin reductase and prilocaine-induced methemoglobinemia during infancy. *Br J Anaesth.* 1990;64(1):72-6.

25. Powell H, Swarner O, Gluck L, et al. Hexachlorophene myelinopathy in premature infants. *J Pediatr.* 1973;82:976-81.

26. Feinblatt BI, Aceto T Jr, Beckhom G, et al. Percutaneous absorption of hydrocortisone in children. *Am J Dis Child.* 1966;112(3):218-24.

27. Dhillon S, Ngwane E, Richens A. Rectal absorption of diazepam in epileptic children. *Arch Dis Child.* 1982;57(4):264-7.

28. Friis-Hansen B. Body water compartments in children: changes during growth and related changes in body composition. *Pediatrics.* 1961;28:169-81.

29. Semchok WM, Shevchuk YM, Sankaran K, et al. Prospective randomized controlled evaluation of a gentamicin loading dose in neonates. *Biol Neonate.* 1995;67(1):13-20.

30. Shevchuk YM, Taylor DM. Aminoglycoside volume of distribution in pediatric patients. *Drug Intell Clin Pharm.* 1990;24(3):273-6.

31. Kearns GL, Jungbluthy GL, Abdel-Rahman SM, et al. Impact of ontogeny on linezolid disposition in neonates and infants. *Clin Pharmacol Ther.* 2003;74:413-22.

32. Milsap RL, Hill MR, Szefler SJ. Special pharmacokinetic considerations in children. In: Evans WE, Schentag JJ, Jusko WJ, eds. *Applied Pharmacokinetics: Principles of Therapeutic Drug Monitoring.* Vancouver, WA: Applied Therapeutics Inc.;1992:10-1-32.

33. Divoll M, Greenblatt DJ, Ochs HR, et al. Absolute bioavailability of oral and intramuscular diazepam: effects of age and sex. *Anesth Analg.* 1983;62:1-8.

34. Wilkinson GR. Plasma and tissue binding considerations in drug disposition. *Drug Metab Rev.* 1983;14(3):427-65.

35. Strolin Beneditti M, Baltes EL. Drug metabolism and disposition in children. *Fundam Clin Pharmacol.* 2003;17:281-99.

36. Pacifici GM, Viani A, Taddeucci-Brunelli G, et al. Effects of development, aging, and renal and hepatic insufficiency as well as hemodialysis on the plasma concentration of albumin and alpha 1 acid glycoprotein: implications for binding of drugs. *Ther Drug Monit.* 1986;8(3):259-63.

37. Piafsky KM. Disease-induced changes in the plasma binding of basic drugs. *Clin Pharmacokinet.* 1980;5(3):246-62.

38. Walker PC. Neonatal bilirubin toxicity: A review of kernicterus and the implications of drug-induced bilirubin displacement. *Clin Pharmacokinet.* 1987;13(1):26-50.

39. Haycock GB. Development of glomerular filtration and tubular sodium reabsorption in the human fetus and newborn. *Br J Urol.* 1998;81:Suppl. 2:33-8.

40. Leake RD, Trygstad CW. Glomerular filtration rate during the period of adaptation to extrauterine life. *Ped Res.* 1977;11:959-62.

41. Heilbron DC, Holliday MA, al-Dahwi A, et al. Expressing glomerular filtration rate in children. *Pediatr Nephrol.* 1991;5:5-11.

42. Aperia A, Broberger O, Elinder G, et al. Postnatal development of renal function in pre-term and full term infants. *Acta Paediatr Scand.* 1981;70:183-7.

43. Manzke H, Spreter von Kreudenstein P, Dorner K, et al. Quantitative measurements of the urinary excretion of creatinine, uric acid, hypoxanthine and xanthine, uracil, cyclic AMP, and cyclic GMP in healthy newborns. *Eur J Pediatr.* 1980;133:157-61.

44. Schwartz GJ, Brion LP, Apitzer A. The use of plasma creatinine concentration for estimating glomerular filtration rate in infants, children and adolescents. *Pediatr Clin N Am.* 1987;34(3):570-90.

45. Myers GL, Miller WG, Coresh J, et al. Recommendations for improving serum creatinine measurement: a report from the Laboratory Working Group of the National Kidney Disease Education Program. *Clin Chem.* 2006;52:5-18.

46. Schwartz GJ, Muñoz A, Schneider MF, et al. New equations to estimate GFR in children with CKD. *J Am Soc Nephrol.* 2009;20:629-37.

47. Qayed M, Thompson A, Applegate K, et al. Is the updated Schwartz formula appropriate for assessing renal function prior to hematopoietic stem cell transplantation? *Pediatr Blood Cancer.* 2010;55:199-201.

48. Koren G, James A, Perlman M. A simple method of estimation of glomerular filtration rate by gentamicin pharmacokinetics during routine drug monitoring in the newborn. *Clin Pharmacol Ther.* 1985;38:680-5.

49. Zarowitz BJ, Robert S, Peterson EL. Prediction of glomerular filtration rate using aminoglycoside clearance in critically ill medical patients. *Ann Pharmacother.* 1992;26:1205-10.

50. Fitterman GH, Shuplock NA, Phillip FJ. The growth and maturation of human glomeruli and proximal convolutions from term to childhood. *Pediatrics.* 1965;35:601-19.

51. Morselli PL. Clinical Pharmacology of the perinatal period and early infancy. *Clin Pharmacokinet.* 1989;17 Suppl 1:13-28.

52. Ginsburg CM, McCracken GH, Zweighaft TC. Serum penicillin concentrations after intramuscular administration of benzathine penicillin G in children. *Pediatrics.* 1982;69(4):452-4.

53. MacKichan JJ. Influence of protein binding and use of unbound (free) drug concentrations. In: Evans WE, Schentag JJ, Jusko WJ, eds. *Applied Pharmacokinetics: Principles of Therapeutic Drug Monitoring.* Vancouver, WA: Applied Therapeutics Inc.;1992:5-1-5-48.

54. James LP, Marshall JD, Heulitt MJ, et al. Famotidine pharmacokinetics and pharmacodynamics in children. *J Clin Pharmacol.* 1996;36(1):48-54.

55. Litterst CL, Mimnaugh EG, Reagan RL. Comparison of in vitro drug metabolism by lung, liver, and kidney of several common laboratory species. *Drug Metab Dispos.* 1975;3(4):165-259.

56. Nitowsky HM, Matz L, Berzofsky JA. Studies on oxidative drug metabolism in the full term newborn infant. *J Pediatr.* 1966;69(6):1139-49.

57. Morselli PL, Principi N, Tognoni G, et al. Diazepam elimination in premature and full-term infants and children. *J Perinat Med.* 1973;1(2):133-41.

58. Neims AH, Warner M, Loughman PM, et al. Developmental aspects of the hepatic cytochrome P450 mono-oxygenase system. *Ann Rev Pharmacol Toxicol.* 1976;16:427-45.

59. Pikkarainen PH, Raiha NCR. Development of alcohol dehydrogenase activity in the human liver. *Pediatr Res.* 1967;1(3):165-8.

60. Sonnier M, Crestiel T. Delayed ontogenesis of CYP1A2 in the human liver. *Eur J Biochem.* 1998;251:893-8.

61. Tateishi T, Nakura H, Asoh M, et al. A comparison of hepatic cytochrome P450 protein expression between infancy and postinfancy. *Life Sci.* 1997;61:2567-74.

62. Hendeles L, Weinberger M. Theophylline. A state of the art review. *Pharmacotherapy.* 1983;3:2-44.

63. Chiba K, Ishizaki T, Miura H, et al. Michelis-Menten pharmacokinetics of diphenylhydantoin and application in pediatric age patient. *J Pediatr.* 1980;96:479-84.

64. Hines R, Mccarver G. The ontogeny of human drug-metabolizing enzymes: Phase I oxidative enzymes. *J Pharmacol Exp Therap.* 2002;300:355-60.

65. Mortimer O, Persson R, Ladona MG, et al. Polymorphic formation of morphine from codeine in poor and extensive metabolizers of dextromethorphan. Relationship to the presence of immunoidentified cytochrome P 450 IID1. *Clin Pharmacol Ther.* 1990;47(1):27-35.

66. Vieira I, Sonnier M, Cresteil T. Developmental expression of CYP2E1 in the human liver. Hypermethylation control of gene expression during the neonatal period. *Eur J Biochem.* 1996;238:476-83.

67. Burtin P, Jacqz-Aigrain E, Girard P, et al. Population pharmacokinetics of midazolam in neonates. *Clin Pharmacol Ther.* 1994;56:615-25.

68. Payne K, Mattheyse FJ, Liebenberg D, et al. The pharmacokinetics of midazolam in paediatric patients. *Eur J Clin Pharmacol.* 1989;37:267-72.

69. Pacifici GM, Franchi M, Giulani A, Rane A. Development of the glucuronyltransferase and sulphotransferase towards 2-naphthol in humans fetus. *Dev Pharmacol Ther.* 1989;14:108-14.

70. Coughtrie MW, Burchell B, Leakey JE, et al. The inadequacy of perinatal glucuronidation: immunoblot analysis of the developmental expression of individual UDP-glucuronosyltransferase isoenzymes in rat and human liver microsomes. *Mol Pharmacol.* 1988;34:729-35.

71. Miller RP, Roberts RJ, Fischer LJ. Acetaminophen elimination kinetics in neonates, children and adults. *Clin Pharmacol Ther.* 1976;19(3):284-94.

72. Buratti S, Lavine JE. Drugs and the liver: advances in metabolism, toxicity, and therapeutics. *Curr Opin Pediatr.* 2002;14:601-7.

73. Friedman CA, Parks BR, Rawson JE. Gentamicin disposition in asphyxiated newborns: relationship to mean arterial blood pressure and urine output. *Pediatr Pharmacol.* 1982;2:189-97.

74. Gal P, Toback J, Erkan NV, et al. The influence of asphyxia on phenobarbital dosing requirements in neonates. *Dev Pharmacol Ther.* 1984;7:145-52.

75. Gal P, Boer HR, Toback J. Effect of asphyxia on theophylline clearance in newborns. *South Med J.* 1982;75:836-8.

76. Assael BM, Caccamo ML, Gerna M, et al. Effect of exchange transfusion on elimination of theophylline in premature neonates. *J Pediatr.* 1977;91:331-2.

77. Kliegman RM, Bertino JS, Fanaroff AA, et al. Pharmacokinetics of gentamicin during exchange transfusions in neonates. *J Pediatr.* 1980;96:927-30.

78. Roberts RJ. *Drug Therapy in Infants: Pharmacologic Principles and Clinical Experience.* Philadelphia, PA: W.B. Saunders; 1984.

79. Southgate WM, DiPiro JT, Robertson AF. Pharmacokinetics of gentamicin in neonates on extracorporeal membrane oxygenation. *Antimicrob Agents Chemother.* 1989;33:817-9.

80. Bhatt-Mehta V, Johnson CE, Schumacher RE. Gentamicin pharmacokinetics in term neonates receiving extracorporeal membrane oxygenation. *Pharmacotherapy.* 1992;12:28-32.

81. Cohen P, Collart L, Prober CG, et al. Pharmacokinetics of gentamicin in neonatal patients undergoing extracorporeal membrane oxygenation. *Pediatr Infect Dis.* 1990;9(8):562-6.

82. Dodge WF, Jellife RW, Zwischenberger JB, et al. Population pharmacokinetic models: effect of explicit versus assumed constant serum concentration assay error patterns upon parameter values of gentamicin in infants on and off extracorporeal membrane oxygenation. *Ther Drug Monit.* 1994;16:552-9.

83. Hoie EB, Swigart SA, Leushen MP. Vancomycin pharmacokinetics in infants undergoing extracorporeal membrane oxygenation. *Clin Pharm.* 1990;9:711-5.

84. Amaker RD, Dipiro JT, Bhatia J. Pharmacokinetics of vancomycin in critically ill infants undergoing extracorporeal membrane oxygenation. *Antimicrob Agents Chemother.* 1996;40(5):1139-42.

85. Buck ML. Pharmacokinetic changes during extracorporeal membrane oxygenation: Implications for drug therapy of neonates. *Clin Pharmacokinet.* 2003;42:403-17.

86. Mulla H, McCormack P, Lawson G, et al. Pharmacokinetics of midazolam in neonates undergoing extracorporeal membrane oxygenation. *Anesthesiology*. 2003;99:275-82.

87. Ashman MJ, Hanekamp M, Wildschut ED, et al. Population pharmacokinetics of midazolam and its metabolites during venoarterial extracorporeal membrane oxygenation in neonates. *Clin Pharmacokinet.* 2010;49:407-19.

88. Hoie EB, Hall MC, Schaap LJ. Effects of injection site and flow rate on the distribution of injected solutions in an extracorporeal membrane oxygenation circuit. *Am J Hosp Pharm.* 1993;50:1902-6.

89. Wells TJ, Fasules JW, Taylor BJ, et al. Pharmacokinetics and pharmacodynamics of bumetanide in neonates treated with extracorporeal membrane oxygenation. *J Pediatr.* 1992;121:974-80.

90. Caron E, Maguire DP. Current management of pain, sedation, and narcotic physical dependence of the infant on ECMO. *J Perinat Neonatal Nurs.* 1990;4:63-74.

91. Arnold JH, Truog RD, Orav EJ, et al. Tolerance and dependence in neonates sedated with fentanyl during extracorporeal membrane oxygenation. *Anesthesiology.* 1990;73:1136-40.

92. Arnold JH, Truog RD, Scavone JM, et al. Changes in the pharmacodynamic response to fentanyl in neonates during continuous infusion. *J Pediatr.* 1991;119:639-43.

93. Burda G, Trittenwein G. Issues of pharmacology in pediatric cardiac extracorporeal membrane oxygenation with special reference to analgesia and sedation. *Artif Organs.* 1999;23:1015-9.

94. Watterberg KL, Kelly WH, Johnson JD, et al. Effect of patent ductus arteriosus on gentamicin pharmacokinetics on very low birth weight (<1500 g) babies. *Dev Pharmacol Ther.* 1987;10:107-17.

95. Spivey J, Gal P. Vancomycin pharmacokinetics in neonates. *Am J Dis Child.* 1986;140:859.

96. Zarfin Y, Koren G, Maresky D, et al. Possible indomethacin-aminoglycoside interaction in preterm infants. *J Pediatr.* 1985;106:511-3.

97. Cystic Fibrosis Foundation. About cystic fibrosis. Available at: http://www.cff.org/AboutCF/. Accessed February 1, 2011.

98. Collins FS. Cystic fibrosis: molecular biology and therapeutic implications. *Science.* 1992;256(5058):774-9.

99. Cox KL, Isenberg JN, Ament ME. Gastric acid hypersecretion in cystic fibrosis. *J Pediatr Gastroenterol Nutr.* 1982;1(4):559-65.

100. Fondacaro JD, Heubi JE, Kellogg FW. Intestinal bile acid malabsorption in cystic fibrosis: a primary mucosal cell defect. *Pediatr Res.* 1982;16(6):494-8.

101. Strober W, Peter G, Schwartz RH. Albumin metabolism in cystic fibrosis. *Pediatrics.* 1969;43(3):416-26.

102. Spino M, Chai RP, Isles AF, et al. Cloxacillin absorption and disposition in cystic fibrosis. *J Pediatr.* 1984;105(5):829-35.

103. Blumer JL, Stern RC, Yamashita TS, et al. Cephalosporin therapeutics in cystic fibrosis. *J Pediatr.* 1986;108(suppl):854-60.

104. de Groot R, Smith AL. Antibiotic pharmacokinetics in cystic fibrosis: differences and clinical significance. *Clin Pharmacokinet.* 1987;13:228-53.

105. Prandota J. Drug disposition in cystic fibrosis: progress in understanding pathophysiology and pharmacokinetics. *Pediatr Infect Dis J.* 1987;6(12):1111-26.

106. Morgan DJ, Bray KM. Lean body mass as a predictor of drug dosage: implications for drug therapy. *Clin Pharmacokinet.* 1994;26(4):292-307.

107. Kearns GL. Hepatic drug metabolism in cystic fibrosis: recent developments and future directions. *Ann Pharmacother.* 1993;27(1):74-9.

108. Isenberg JN. Cystic fibrosis: its influence on the liver, biliary tree and bile salt metabolism. *Semin Liver Dis.* 1982;2(4):302-13.

109. Albert KS, Gernaat CM. Pharmacokinetics of ibuprofen. *Am J Med.* 1984;77(1A):40-6.

110. Konstan MW, Hoppel CL, Chai BL, et al. Ibuprofen in children with cystic fibrosis: pharmacokinetics and adverse effects. *J Pediatr.* 1991;118(6):956-64.

111. Hutabarat RM, Unadkat JD, Sahajwalla C, et al. Disposition of drugs in cystic fibrosis I: Sulfamethoxazole and trimethoprim. *Clin Pharmacol Ther.* 1991;49(4):402-9.

112. Hutabarat RM, Smith AL, Unadkat JD, et al. Disposition of drugs in cystic fibrosis VII: Acetylation of sulfamethoxazole in blood cells: in vitro-in vivo correlation and characterization of its kinetics of acetylation in lymphocytes. *Clin Pharmacol Ther.* 1994;55(4):427-33.

113. Prandota J. Clinical pharmacology of antibiotics and other drugs in cystic fibrosis *Drugs.* 1988;35(5):542-78.

114. Pechere JC, Dugal R. Clinical pharmacokinetics of aminoglycoside antibiotics. *Clin Pharmacokinet.* 1979;4(3):170-99.

115. Levy J, Smith AL, Koup JR, et al. Disposition of tobramycin in patients with cystic fibrosis: a prospective controlled study. *Pediatrics.* 1984;105(1):117-24.

116. Finkelstein E, Hall K. Aminoglycoside clearance in patients with cystic fibrosis. *J Pediatr.* 1979;94(1):163-4.

117. Flume PA, Mogayzel PJ Jr, Robinson KA, et al. Clinical Practice Guidelines for Pulmonary Therapies Committee. Cystic fibrosis pulmonary guidelines: treatment of pulmonary exacerbations. *Am J Respir Crit Care Med.* 2009;180:802-8.

118. Prescott WA, Jr., Nagel JL. Extended-interval once-daily dosing of aminoglycosides in adult and pediatric patients with cystic fibrosis. *Pharmacotherapy.* 2010;30:95-108.

119. Yaffe SJ, Gerbracht LM, Mosovich LL, et al. Pharmacokinetics of methicillin in patients with cystic fibrosis. *J Infect Dis.* 1977;135(5):828-31.

120. Jusko WJ, Mosovich LL, Gerbracht LM, et al. Enhanced renal excretion of dicloxacillin in patients with cystic fibrosis. *Pediatrics.* 1975;56(6):1038-44.

121. Centers for Disease Control. Revised surveillance case definitions for HIV infection among adults, adolescents and children aged <18 months for HIV infection and AIDS among children age 18 months to <13 years—United States, 2008. *MMWR.* 2008;57(RR10):1-8.

122. Centers for Disease Control and Prevention. Basic Statistics. Available at: http://www.cdc.gov/hiv/topics/surveillance/basic.htm#aidsage Accessed February 1, 2011.

123. Hirt D, Urien S, Jullien V, et al. Age-related effects on nelfinavir and M8 pharmacokinetics: a population study with 182 children. *Antimicrob Agents Chemother.* 2006;50:910-6.

124. Patel IH, Zhang X, Nieforth K, et al. Pharmacokinetics, pharmacodynamics and drug interaction potential of enfuvirtide. *Clin Pharmacokinet.* 2005;44:175-86.

125. Bellibas SE, Siddique Z, Dorr A, et al. Pharmacokinetics of enfuvirtide in pediatric human immunodeficiency virus 1-infected patients receiving combination therapy. *Pediatr Infect Dis J.* 2004;23:1137-41.

126. Ellis JC, L'homme RF, Ewings FM, et al. Nevirapine concentrations in HIV-infected children treated with divided fixed-dose combination antiretroviral tablets in Malawi and Zambia. *Antivir Ther.* 2007;12:253-60.

127. van Leeuwen R, Lange JM, Hussey EK, et al. The safety and pharmacokinetics of a reverse transcriptase inhibitor, 3TC, in patients with HIV infection, a phase I study. *AIDS.* 1992;6:1471-75.

128. Panel on Antiretroviral Therapy and Medical Management of HIV-Infected Children. Guidelines for the Use of

Antiretroviral Agents in Pediatric HIV Infection. August 16, 2010; pp 1-219. Available at: http://aidsinfo.nih.gov/ContentFiles/PediatricGuidelines.pdf. Accessed February 1, 2011.

Chapter 5

Susan W. Miller

Therapeutic Drug Monitoring in the Geriatric Patient

The complex process of aging is characterized by progressive loss in the functional capacities of organs, a reduction in mechanisms of homeostasis, and altered response to receptor stimulation.[1] These changes combine to increase the susceptibility of elderly individuals to environmental and physical stressors as well as the effects of medications. The prevalence of diseases increases with advancing age, and this increase is accompanied by an increase in the use of medications.[2] Medication therapy is among the most widely used and highly valued interventions for acute and chronic diseases of older adults, yet the use of drug therapy in the geriatric patient is one of the most difficult aspects of patient care.[3,4] The unexpected or exaggerated response to drug therapy exhibited by a geriatric patient compared with a younger patient of the same sex and body weight can frequently be explained through pharmacokinetic or pharmacodynamic changes.[5] Older patients take more medications than younger persons, yet major drug studies are performed primarily on individuals younger than 55 years of age.

The effects of aging on drug metabolism are complex and difficult to predict. These effects depend on the pathway of drug metabolism in the liver, on environmental factors, and on cardiac function.[6] Although many irreversible changes occur with aging, it is now well recognized that individuals age at different rates (chronological and biological age are not necessarily synonymous). Frailty, a biological syndrome in the geriatric patient, is recognized as a confounding factor when considering the impact of aging on drug disposition.[2,7] The frailty of a geriatric patient can alter drug metabolism, and this effect appears to vary from drug to drug. The frail elderly (those that are vulnerable and are at the highest risk for adverse health outcomes) have been shown to have reduced drug metabolism.[8] Frail older adults are identifiable as those at high risk for dependency, institutionalization, falls, injuries, acute illness, hospitalizations, slow recovery from illness, and mortality.[9] Markers for inflammation, such as tumor necrosis factor [TNF-α], interleukin-6 [IL_6], and C-reactive protein, may serve as biochemical markers for frailty and may prove to be a method to characterize an individual's biological age.[10] Because of the frailty of elderly patients, it is important that the first medication prescribed be the most effective choice for the best chance at an optimal clinical outcome.[11] To make the most effective choice, clinicians should take into consideration both personalized pharmacokinetic changes in drug metabolism and pharmacodynamic responses of individual patients, when selecting drug therapies for geriatric patients.

Pharmacokinetic studies comparing young and older adults are often difficult to accomplish due to the problems associated with recruiting healthy older individuals to compare with healthy younger individuals, however they are increasing in number.[12-28] Problems have been identified with the selection of patient participants and reporting of the results of clinical trials to assess age-related pharmacokinetic differences in drugs.[29] Often, participants are the healthy (younger) geriatrics and not the very old (over the age of 85 and/or frail) geriatric patients. The extrapolation of dosages and possible side effects in the very old population may or may not be appropriate.[29] Physiological differences, pathophysiological changes, altered protein binding, and/or concomitant use of medications may account for the altered pharmacokinetics displayed by older patients.[30]

The following examples illustrate the variability of changes that occur in the elderly. There is evidence to show that increased age may delay absorption of transdermal *opioids* but not affect the maximum and steady state concentrations. [31] An infusion of morphine into older patients showed a rapid distribution, followed by a slower elimination when compared to younger patients.[32] Recent pharmacokinetic studies have reported no need for dosage changes in the elderly for proton-pump inhibitors, or 3-hydroxy-3-methylglutaryl-coenzyme A (HMG-CoA) reductase inhibitors.[33-35] Data show that the angiotensin converting enzyme inhibitors *trandolapril* and *moexipril* should be initiated at lower doses in geriatric patients, but no overall dosage modifications are necessary.[36] Other data show that, in the presence of renal impairment, plasma concentrations of ACEIs increase and doses should be adjusted based on renal function.[37] The SERMs (selective estrogen receptor modulators) have variable pharmacokinetic changes associated with aging, with *tamoxifen* and *toremifene* exhibiting increased plasma concentrations with increased age; tamoxifen greater than toremifene; however, neither drug has accompanying package insert recommendation for dosage alterations. No age-related differences in *raloxifene* pharmacokinetics have been identified, but cautionary dosing is advised in both moderate-to-severe renal impairment and in hepatic impairment.[38] Nonsteroidal anti-inflammatory drugs (NSAIDs) exhibit reduced renal clearance in the presence of renal impairment.[39]

Decreased clearance and prolonged half-life of *sertraline* suggest that steady state concentrations would be higher and achieved later during long-term administration to geriatric patients.[40] A reduced clearance for *fosphenytoin*, *ticlopidine*, and *ropinirole* has been shown in geriatric patients, with the clinical significance of this reduced clearance unknown.[41-43] The fluoroquinolone antibacterials, including *ciprofloxacin*, and *levofloxacin* require dosage adjustments based on their predominant renal elimination.[44] The antiepileptic drugs, *felbamate*, *gabapentin*, *lamotrigine*, *levetiracetam*, *oxcarbazepine*, *tiagabine*, and *topiramate,* all exhibit a decrease in apparent oral clearance in elderly patients when compared to non-elderly adult controls.[45] Studies measuring the pharmacokinetics of the cholinesterase inhibitors *tacrine, donepezil, rivastigmine*, and *galantamine* in geriatric patients report some changes in pharmacokinetic parameters, but these are not considered clinically significant and no dosage changes are suggested unless patients are in severe renal impairment (*galantamine* and creatinine clearance < 9 ml/min).[46] Due to hepatic toxicity, *tacrine* and *galantamine* are not recommended for use in patients with severe hepatic impairment.[46]

Information regarding dosage alterations based on the pharmacokinetic profiles of drugs in geriatric patients is very important to the clinician as current dosing in geriatric patients is often based on broad generalizations such as "use one third to one half the usual dose," or anecdotal data—not on solid pharmacokinetic or pharmacodynamic studies. Pharmacokinetic and/or pharmacodynamic differences in older patients may account for either the toxic or subtherapeutic response that often occurs.

Adverse drug reactions or events (ADEs) and drug-drug interactions (DDIs) occur more frequently in geriatric patients, in part because this population is most likely to be using complex drug therapies.[47-53] The estimated annual rate of ADEs for individuals aged 65 years or older has been measured at more than twice the rate for those younger than 65 years of age.[54] Additional data have shown that for persons 65 years of age and older, the estimated annual rate of ADEs requiring hospitalization was nearly seven times the rate for persons younger than 65 years. Although considerable evidence suggests that an ADE will not occur simply because a patient is elderly, pharmacokinetic and pharmacodynamic changes in the elderly may significantly alter drug disposition and must be considered as contributing to ADEs.[55-57] Symptoms of ADEs can be extremely subtle in an elderly patient and may be manifested by increased frequency of falls, increased confusion, excessive sedation, constipation, urinary retention, decreased oral intake, or a general failure to thrive.[58]

Significant ADEs are most likely observed with drugs having a narrow therapeutic index or saturable hepatic metabolism (e.g., *phenytoin*, *warfarin*, and *theophylline*) or when elimination is via a single mechanism or pathway. A study of emergency department visits for ADEs showed that drugs that commonly require regular outpatient monitoring to prevent toxicity (*antidiabetic agents, warfarin, several anticonvulsants, digitalis glycosides, theophylline*, and *lithium*) were involved in the most unintentional overdoses.[54] The patients most at risk usually have multiple disease states or compromised organ function, and they receive multiple drug therapy. Complicated drug therapy, poor compliance, and altered pharmacokinetics are among the many possible causes of ADEs and DDIs.[47,48,52,57-59]

Physiologic Changes

Absorption, distribution, metabolism, and excretion

The processes of absorption, distribution, metabolism, and excretion determine the amount of drug present at any given time within the body's various tissue and fluid compartments.

Pharmacokinetic parameters represent a composite of both genetic and environmental effects.[60-63] The physiologic changes produced by aging that may have important implications for altered pharmacokinetics are summarized in Table 5-1.

Age-related physiologic changes in the gastrointestinal (GI) tract include elevated gastric pH, delayed gastric-emptying, and decreases in GI motility, intestinal blood flow, and absorptive surface area. Reduced gastric secretion of acid can reduce tablet dissolution and decrease the solubility of basic drugs.[64]

Table 5-1. Physiologic Changes with Aging that May Affect Pharmacokinetics[6,62]

Process	Physiologic Effect
Absorption	Reduced gastric acid production Reduced gastric-emptying rate Reduced GI motility Reduced GI blood flow Reduced absorptive surface
Distribution	Decreased total body mass Increased percentage of body fat Decreased percentage of body water Decreased plasma albumin Disease-related increase in alpha-1-acid glycoprotein Altered relative tissue perfusion Altered protein binding
Metabolism	Reduced liver mass Reduced liver blood flow Reduced hepatic metabolic capacity Reduced enzyme activity Reduced enzyme induction
Excretion	Reduced renal blood flow Reduced glomerular filtration Reduced renal tubular secretory function
Tissue sensitivity	Alterations in receptor number Alterations in receptor affinity Alterations in second messenger function[a] Alterations in cellular response Alterations in cellular nuclear response

[a]A chemical (e.g., cyclic AMP or Ca^{++}) inside the postsynaptic neuron released by a first messenger (e.g., a neurotransmitter) and responsible for downstream regulation of a pathway or gene expression.

The delay in gastric emptying allows more contact time in the stomach for

- Potentially ulcerogenic drugs such as the NSAIDs and bisphosphonates.
- Antacid drug interactions due to an increased opportunity for binding.
- Increased absorption of poorly soluble drugs.

A higher incidence of diarrhea and a delay in onset action of weakly basic drugs also result from this physiologic effect.

One study reported a three-fold decrease in *levodopa* availability in the elderly because delayed gastric emptying allowed the increased degradation by GI dopa-decarboxylase to dopamine.[65] Differences in gastric emptying might help explain the unpredictable and inconsistent responses to levodopa in individual patients.[66] The increased degradation of *levodopa* by dopa-decarboxylase occurs when *levodopa* is used alone (not in combination with a dopa-decarboxylase inhibitor such as *carbidopa*). *Levodopa* is only used in combination therapy as an anti-Parkinson's agent.

Clorazepate, a benzodiazepine, is converted by acid hydrolysis in the GI tract to an active metabolite, desmethyldiazepam. Desmethyldiazepam concentrations have been reported to be lower in both elderly and gastrectomized patients compared with younger adults. This decrease in active metabolite levels is presumed to be a result of a decreased conversion from the parent drug.[67]

Age influences the active transport mechanisms involved in the absorption of nutrients such as sugars, vitamins (e.g., *thiamine* and *folic acid*), and minerals (e.g., *calcium* and *iron*). In elderly patients, this absorption is often reduced.[68] Age-related physiologic changes alone apparently do not influence the passive transport mechanisms by which most drugs are absorbed.

Some drugs with high intrinsic clearance in the liver are metabolized during their passage from the portal vein through the liver to the systemic circulation, thus reducing their oral bioavailability. Drugs with potentially *increased* bioavailability in the elderly, presumably due to a decrease in first-pass metabolism, are shown in Table 5-2.[69,70]

Drugs that undergo first-pass metabolism and may have *decreased* bioavailability in older patients include *clorazepate,*[22] *digoxin,*[71] and *prazosin.*[72] The decrease in bioavailability may be the result of a combination of reduced blood flow to the hepatic system and slowed GI motility that allows for drug degradation in the GI tract prior to absorption.

Although the total amount of absorbed drug reaching the systemic circulation is affected for only a few drugs, age-related physiologic changes can alter the absorption rate, resulting in an erratic and sometimes inconsistent pharmacologic response. The clinical effect of this is a delay in the time to peak or maximum concentration, which is more problematic with therapies where a high peak or short time to peak is important. Clinical factors such as acute congestive heart failure (CHF), achlorhydria, and unusual dietary patterns may occasionally necessitate the intravenous route of administration because of the incomplete absorption via oral and intramuscular routes. The absorption of intramuscularly administered drugs decreases in bedridden elderly patients, perhaps because of changes in regional blood flow. In geriatric patients, percutaneous absorption of transdermal medications can be affected by reductions in the water and lipid layers of the aged skin. Lipophilic medications such as *testosterone*, *estradiol*, and *fentanyl* have shown reduced absorption in geriatric patients.[73] Considerations involved in using controlled-release dosage formulations include age-related changes in GI transit time, motility, and pH.[74]

Table 5-2. Drugs with Increased Bioavailability in the Elderly

Amitriptyline	Lidocaine
Chlordiazepoxide	Metoprolol
Cimetidine	Metronidazole
Desipramine	Propranolol
Imipramine	Quinidine
Labetalol	Trazodone
Levodopa	Verapamil

Binding proteins

Age can alter the distribution of drugs throughout the body and to target organs. Although total protein generally is unaffected by aging, the plasma albumin portion has been shown to decrease from 4 g/dl in young adults to approximately 3.5 g/dl in patients over 80.[75] The mean serum albumin of nursing facility residents has been found to be 3.0 g/dl or lower.[76] The two major plasma proteins to which medications can bind are albumin and alpha-1-acid glycoprotein (AAG), and concentrations of these proteins may change with concurrent pathologies seen with increasing age. Plasma protein binding is a major determinant of drug action, particularly for drugs that are highly protein bound and changes in protein binding can have clinical implications.[30] If albumin is decreased, a compensatory increase in unbound (active) drug occurs if the percentage of the bound drug is 90% or more; however, this is often compensated by increased distribution or clearance, so little or no clinical effect is experienced. In addition to age, disease states such as cirrhosis, renal failure, and malnutrition can lower albumin concentrations.

AAG, an acute phase reactant, binds mostly to lipophilic basic drugs and tends to increase with age and in response to acute illness. The binding of drugs to AAG increases during acute illness and can return to normal after several weeks or months when the acute stress passes and AAG decreases.[77,78] Medications that bind to AAG and are commonly associated with adverse effects in geriatric patients are *lidocaine, meperidine,* and *propranolol.*[30] Though protein binding may be altered in aging, physiological changes and pathophysiological disorders also occur and these changes usually have greater clinical significance than changes in drug plasma protein binding.[30]

Increased unbound (free) fraction

Increases in the free fraction of *naproxen*, *diflunisal*, and *salicylates* have been found in the elderly, presumably as a result of the decrease in albumin protein binding.[79] Increased concentrations of NSAIDs have been associated with a higher incidence of gastric bleeding from peptic ulcers.[80] Whether the increase in gastric bleeding is due to changes in protein binding or the increased drug concentration is not known.

Decreased protein binding (as well as the resultant increased free fraction) is also seen with *phenytoin*, which is cleared from the plasma more rapidly because of an increase in free phenytoin.[81] Seizure control may be seen at lower measured total (bound plus unbound) phenytoin concentrations in the elderly whose unbound fraction has increased. Although the increase in the free fraction of phenytoin with age is statistically significant, it is unlikely to warrant a compensatory change in dose unless the patient has a total phenytoin concentration that is near the upper limit of the therapeutic range and/or that is sufficient to saturate metabolizing enzymes. With *meperidine*, binding to red blood cells decreases with age, thus increasing the amount of free meperidine available in the elderly patient.[82] Meperidine is considered an inappropriate drug for use in the elderly.[83-85]

Although higher concentrations and the resulting therapeutic effects of some drugs may be beneficial, the accompanying risks of toxicity are problematic in the geriatric patient. Doses of most highly protein-bound drugs (>90% protein bound) should be reduced initially and increased slowly if there is evidence of decreased serum albumin (i.e., <3.5 g/dl). If several highly protein-bound drugs are used together, the chance of a drug interaction increases. Table 5-3 shows the impact of age on the protein binding of select drugs.

Lean body weight to fat ratio

Changes in the ratio of lean body weight to fat also can alter drug distribution leading to changes in pharmacologic response. In the average elderly patient, total body water is decreased and total body fat is increased. These changes influence the onset and duration of action of highly tissue-bound drugs (e.g., *digoxin*) and water-soluble drugs (e.g., *alcohol*, *lithium*, and *morphine*). The dosages of most water-soluble drugs are based on estimates of lean or ideal body weight. If a patient's actual weight is less than the estimated lean body weight, the actual weight should be used in most dosage calculations.

Between ages 18 and 85, total body fat increases on average in both females and males; lean body mass eventually decreases in both groups as well. With increasing age, the volume of distribution of lipophilic drugs may increase as a result of diminished protein binding and an increased fat to lean muscle ratio. Fat-soluble drugs (e.g., most *tricyclic antidepressants*, *barbiturates*, *benzodiazepines*, *calcium channel blockers*, and *phenothiazines*) may have a delayed onset of action and can accumulate in adipose tissue, prolonging their action sometimes to the point of toxicity.[86,87] All of these drugs are considered inappropriate in the elderly due to safer alternatives.[83-85]

Drug Elimination

Drugs are primarily cleared from the body by metabolism in the liver, excretion by the kidneys, or some combination of the two processes. A decrease in total body clearance results in higher drug concentrations and an enhanced pharmacologic response, which can lead to toxicity.[86]

Metabolism

For some drugs, hepatic metabolism is highly dependent on blood flow. Liver blood flow can decrease significantly with increasing age and is further compromised in the presence of congestive heart failure (CHF). With drugs that are highly dependent on hepatic metabolism (e.g., most *beta-blockers*, *lidocaine*, and *narcotic analgesics*), a decrease in hepatic clearance can increase the drug concentration and lead to toxicity.

In addition to altering hepatic blood flow, age influences the rate of hepatic clearance by causing changes in the intrinsic activity of selected liver enzymes. This age-related process has been found in the Phase I enzymatic pathway. Common drugs using this pathway and having the potential for metabolism influenced by age include the longer acting benzodiazepines such as *diazepam*, *chlordiazepoxide*, and *clorazepate*. The enzymatic demethylation of *nortriptyline*,[88] *imipramine*,[89] *thioridazine*,[90] and *theophylline*[91] also decreases in the elderly. All of these drugs are considered inappropriate for use in the elderly except *imipramine*.[83-85]

Drugs that undergo hepatic Phase II enzymatic biotransformation (e.g., *lorazepam*, *oxazepam*, and *temazepam*) do not appear to be adversely affected by age; therefore, they are preferred agents for older patients.

At all ages, drug metabolism can be affected by genetics, smoking, diet, gender, comorbid conditions, and concomitant drugs. The cytochrome P (CYP) 450 enzyme system, primarily a part of the Phase I hepatic metabolism pathway, can be affected by many drugs. Of the more than 30 CYP 450 isoenzymes identified to date, the major ones responsible for drug metabolism include CYP3A4, CYP2D6, CYP1A2, and the CYP2C subfamily. Newer evidence in geriatric patients has shown a reduction in CYP2C19 activity, no reduction in

Table 5-3. Effects of Age on Plasma Protein Binding of Select Drugs in Geriatrics

Drugs with decreased protein binding (increased free fraction)	
Acetazolamide[b]	Lorazepam[a]
Carbenoxolone	Meperidine[a,b]
Ceftriaxone[a]	Naproxen
Clomethiazole	Phenytoin[a]
Desipramine[a]	Salicylate[a]
Desmethyldiazepam	Temazepam
Diazepam[a]	Theophylline
Diflunisal	Tolbutamide
Fluphenazine	Triazolam[a]
Flurazepam	Warfarin[a]
Lidocaine[a]	
Drugs with increased protein binding (decreased free fraction)	
Amitriptyline[a,b]	Flurazepam
Benazeprilat	Haloperidol[a]
Ceftriaxone[a]	Ibuprofen[a]
Chlorpromazine[a]	Lidocaine[a]
Clomethiazole[a]	Naproxen
Disopyramide[a]	Nortriptyline[a]
Enalaprilat	Propranolol[a]
Etomidate	
Select drugs with no change in protein binding	
Alprazolam	Metoprolol
Amitriptyline[a,b]	Midazolam
Atropine	Nadolol
Caffeine	Nitrazepam[a]
Oxazepam	Nortriptyline[a]
Chlordiazepoxide	Penicillin
Chloroquine	Phenobarbital
Desipramine[a]	Phenytoin[a]
Desmethyldiazepam	Piroxicam
Diazepam[a]	Propranolol[a]
Disopyramide[a]	Quinidine
Donepezil	Risperidone
Etodolac	Salicylate[a]
Fentanyl	Sotalol
Furosemide	Sulfadiazine
Haloperidol[a]	Sulfamethoxazole
Ibuprofen[a]	Thioridazine[b]
Imipramine	Triazolam[a]
Lorazepam[a]	Trimethoprim
Maprotiline	Vancomycin
Meperidine[a,b]	Verapamil
Methadone	Warfarin[a]
Methotrexate	

[a]Conflicting data have been reported.
[b]Drugs considered to be inappropriate for use in the elderly.

CYP2D6 activity, and marked variability with little change in the CYP1A2, CYP2C9, CYP2E1, and CYP3A4 isoenzymes.[73,92] CYPs are increasingly being identified in extrahepatic organs such as the intestine, kidney, brain, and skin. The full effect of aging on these enzyme systems is yet to be determined.[93] Unlike renal function, no accurate laboratory tests directly measure liver function for drug dosage adjustment. Nonspecific tests to monitor liver function include ALT, plasma albumin, and prothrombin time.

Renal clearance

Consistent with the behavior of many drugs, pharmacokinetic data from elderly patients are similar to that of patients with mild renal compromise, in that most age-related declines in drug clearance can be explained by reductions in renal function.[94] Age-related physiologic changes in the kidneys influence drug response and elimination more than hepatic changes in the geriatric patient. Between ages 20 and 90, the glomerular filtration rate (GFR) may decrease as much as 50% (average decline of 35%). The average CrCl of elderly nursing facility residents has been found to be about 40 ml/min.[95] Serum creatinine is frequently used to monitor kidney function, but this test alone is of limited utility in estimating the GFR of the geriatric patient. Serum creatinine does not increase significantly unless kidney function deteriorates greatly. The production of creatinine, which is dependent on muscle mass, decreases in the elderly; therefore, an apparently normal serum creatinine in a geriatric patient may not be a valid predictor of renal function and drug elimination. Blood urea nitrogen (BUN) also is not a useful predictor of renal function because it can be affected by hydration status, diet, and blood loss.

The most accurate, readily available estimation of GFR in the elderly is creatinine clearance (CrCl), which correlates well with both GFR and tubular secretion. The CrCl can be estimated using a standard equation that considers age, body weight, and serum creatinine in patients with stable renal function (see Chapter 1). Of course, mathematical equations are simply estimates of an individual's actual renal function. Even the best methods for estimating creatinine clearance may result in suboptimal dosing for many elderly patients. For geriatric patients with low serum creatinine <1.0 mg/dl, (88.4 µM/L SI), the practice of rounding the serum creatinine to 1.0 mg/dl (88.4 µM/L SI) may result in underestimation of creatinine clearance and suboptimal dosing.[96]

Dosages of drugs that are primarily renally excreted should generally be adjusted if the patient has lost more than 50% of kidney function. If creatinine clearance is less than 50 ml/min, major dosage adjustments may be necessary to avoid drug toxicity. Some common drugs with a narrow therapeutic range that are excreted primarily unchanged by the kidneys are shown in Table 5-4.

Age-Related Pharmacodynamic Changes Influencing Drug Response

With increasing age, the tolerance to drugs decreases as a result of altered pharmacodynamic responses at target organs. Pharmacodynamics governs the type, intensity, and duration of drug action. The clinical manifestation of this altered sensitivity may range from an insignificant response, to an adverse drug reaction, or to therapy failure.

Table 5-4. Select Narrow Therapeutic Range Drugs with Primary Renal Excretion

Acetazolamide[a]	H2-antagonists (e.g., cimetidine)
ACE inhibitors	Lithium
Amantadine	Methotrexate
Aminoglycosides	Penicillin
Cephalosporins	Procainamide
Chlorpropamide[a]	Quinidine
Digoxin	Tetracycline
Disopyramide[a]	Vancomycin
Ethambutol	

[a]These drugs are considered inappropriate for use in the elderly.

Qualitative differences in drug response also may occur. Pharmacodynamic alterations are often unpredictable and can lead to toxicity. Altered response may be due to changes in receptor number or affinity, depletion of neurotransmitters, disease, or physiologic changes. With aging, there is evidence of:

- Decreased acetylcholine, dopamine, and serotonin
- Decreased enzymatic degradation of monoamine oxidase
- Impaired baroreceptor response to blood pressure changes
- Decreased responsiveness of beta-adrenergic receptors
- Increased pain tolerance
- Decreased antibody response to vaccination
- Decreased *insulin* sensitivity
- Decreased cortisol suppression
- Enhanced responsiveness to the anticoagulants *warfarin* and *heparin*
- Enhanced responsiveness to thrombolytics

Altered end organ sensitivity may result in exaggerated pharmacologic response, as seen with *barbiturates* and *benzodiazepines*, or diminished pharmacologic response, as seen with *beta-blockers*, *beta-agonists*, and *calcium channel blockers*. Other affected drug classes include the *narcotic analgesics*, *antihypertensive agents*, *antiparkinson drugs*, *phenothiazines*, and *antidepressants*. The incidence and irreversibility of tardive dyskinesia are increased in the elderly and may be due to age-related imbalances in neurotransmitters.[97]

Dosing adjustments are usually necessary since many of these same drugs are also influenced by age-related physiologic changes, especially drug distribution and elimination. The net effect in an individual patient is often difficult to predict. For example, elderly patients have increased bioavailability of *beta-blockers* but decreased responsiveness at the receptor site level (a variable effect is seen with *propranolol*). Another example is that *theophylline's* inotropic effect increases with age but its bronchodilator effect decreases.[98] Drugs that may exhibit an increased pharmacologic response in the geriatric population include *halothane, hydroxyzine*, *metoclopramide, warfarin*, and the *calcium channel blockers*.[98] Age related peripheral and central pharmacokinetic changes may contribute to age-related sensitivity to *antipsychotic agents*, but pharmacodynamic mechanisms may play the most significant role in a geriatric patient's response to any dose of an antipsychotic agent.[99]

More than one in six elderly patients is taking prescription drugs that are not suited for geriatric patients and may lead to physical or mental deterioration and possibly death.[100] Recently strategies have been developed in attempts to foster appropriate prescribing of medications in the geriatric population overall. The explicit criteria for determining potentially inappropriate medication use by elderly patients, labeled the "Beers Criteria," were originally published in 1992, and have since been twice updated.[83-85] These criteria are listed in Table 5-5.

These criteria were developed through a consensus panel of experts in geriatric care, geriatric pharmacology, geriatric psychopharmacology, and nursing home care. These experts reached agreement on criteria defining inappropriate drug use in nursing home residents. The criteria relate to certain drugs that should not be used and doses and durations of therapy of some drugs that should not be exceeded in the older patient who is a resident of a nursing facility.[84] These criteria have since been applied and evaluated in geriatric patients in various levels of care, including assisted living facilities, community dwelling, receiving care from office-based physician practices, and emergency departments.[101-108]

A study of use of these medications in a very large group of hospitalized senior patients showed that about half of geriatric patients received a medication deemed inappropriate according to Beers List criteria.[109] Practitioners may extrapolate these recommendations to the geriatric patient population at large, keeping in mind that they are not meant to regulate practice in a manner to which they supersede the clinical judgment and assessment of the practitioner.[85] Refined Beers Criteria, to include preferred medications for use in geriatric patients or those with the greatest benefit-to-risk ratio for use in geriatric patients, are in development.[110]

Summary of Changes

Table 5-6 is a compilation of the pharmacokinetic and pharmacodynamic literature available on the dosing of drugs in the geriatric population. However, dosing of any drug in a specific patient should be based on that patient's response and ability to clear the drug.[111-112]

Table 5-5. Explicit Criteria for Inappropriate Medication Orders[83-85]

Medications that should (generally) be avoided in geriatric patients

- Sedative or hypnotic agents
  - Long-acting benzodiazepines
    - Chlorazepate
    - Chlordiazepoxide
    - Diazepam
    - Flurazepam
    - Quazepam
    - Meprobamate
  - Short-acting benzodiazepines
    - Alprazolam
    - Lorazepam
    - Oxazepam
    - Temazepam
    - Triazolam
- Antidepressants
  - Amitriptyline
  - Combination antidepressants-antipsychotics
  - Doxepin
  - Fluoxetine (daily)
- Antihypertensive agents
  - Clonidine
  - Doxazosin
  - Ethacrynic acid
  - Guanethidine
  - Hydrochlorothiazide
  - Methyldopa
  - Nifedipine (short-acting)
  - Reserpine
- Nonsteroidal anti-inflammatory drugs
  - Indomethacin
  - Ketorolac
- Oral hypoglycemic agents
  - Chlorpropamide
- Analgesic agents
  - Propoxyphene (single product and combination)[a]
  - Pentazocine
  - Meperidine
- Platelet inhibitors
  - Dipyridamole (short-acting)
  - Ticlopidine
- Muscle relaxants or antispasmodic agents
  - Carisoprodol
  - Chlorzoxazone
  - Cyclobenzaprine
  - Methocarbamol
  - Metaxalone
  - Orphenadrine
  - Oxybutynin

Table 5-5. (Continued)

Gastrointestinal antispasmodic agents
Dicyclomine
Belladonna alkaloids combination
Thioridazine
Digoxin
Cimetidine
Ferrous sulfate (greater than 325 mg/day)
Trimethobenzamide
Antiarrhythmics
Disopyramide
Amiodarone
Anticholinergics and antihistamines
Chlorpheniramine
Cyproheptadine
Dexchlorpheniramine
Diphenhydramine
Hydroxyzine
Promethazine
Tripelennamine
All barbiturates (except phenobarbital)
Amphetamines and anorexic agents
Long-term use of full-dosage, longer half-life non-COX-selective NSAIDs
Naproxen
Oxaprozin
Long-term use of stimulant laxatives
Bisacodyl
Cascara sagrada
Neoloid (except in the presence of opiate analgesic use)
Nitrofurantoin
Methyltestosterone
Mineral oil
Desiccated thyroid
Estrogens (not in combination with progestins)

[a]Withdrawn from the U.S. market in November 2010.

Table 5-6. Pharmacokinetic Parameters and Average Doses of Drugs Commonly Used in Geriatric Patients[a,110,11]

Drug	Volume of Distribution	Clearance	Half-Life	PB (%f)	Time to Peak	Dynamics	Dose (mg/day)	Comment
Acarbose		D					75-300	Use is not recommended in significant renal dysfunction (Scr >2 mg/dl)
Acetaminophen	D	D	I		D		1500–3000	Hepatic metabolism not significantly altered; no dosage adjustment necessary unless patient is taking chronic high doses
Alendronate	D						10	No dosage adjustment necessary in elderly; use not recommended in CrCl < 35 ml/min
Alprazolam	D	D	I	NC	D	**	0.75–2	
Amantadine	D		I				200	Dosage reduction in renal impairment
							CrCl (ml/min/1.73 m^2)	Dose
							≥80	100 mg twice daily
							60–79	200 mg/100 mg on alternate days
							40–59	100 mg once daily
							30–39	200 mg twice weekly
							20–29	100 mg three times weekly
							10–19	200 mg/100 mg alternating every 7 days
Amikacin	I	D	I				***	Dose conservatively based on CrCl of measured concentrations
Aminophylline	I	NC	I	NC			0.4 mg/kg/hr	
Amitriptyline	I	D	I	D*	I		10–150	Prolonged half-life; evaluation of therapeutic effect to be delayed; increased bioavailability
Amlodipine	NC	D	I			**	2.5–10	Elderly may experience greater hypotensive response
Amoxicillin							750–1500	Dosage reduction in moderate to severe renal impairment
Ampicillin	NC	D	I		I		500–2000	Dosage reduction in moderate to severe renal impairment
Aripiprazole							7.5–30	Dosage adjustments not routinely indicated on basis of age, gender, race, or renal or hepatic impairment status
Aspirin	I	D	I	I*	I		1300–4000	
Atenolol	I	D	I				25–150	

Table 5-6. (Continued)

Drug	Volume of Distribution	Clearance	Half-Life	PB (%f)	Time to Peak	Dynamics	Dose (mg/day)	Comment
Azathioprine	No data	D	I	I	No data		1.5–2.5	If CrCl <50ml/min give 75% of dose; if CrCl < 10 ml/min, give 50% of dose
Azithromycin	NC	NC	NC	NC	No data		250-500	If CrCl < 10 ml/min, use with caution
Benazepril	NC	I	NC	NC	Exaggerated		5–40	Preferred class in comorbid CHF, DM, HTN
Bleomycin	NC	*	I	*				If CrCl <50 ml/min give 75% of dose; if CrCl < 10 ml/min, give 50% of dose
Bupropion		D					100–300	SE profile allows use in patients intolerable to TCAs. A single and multiple dose pharmacokinetic study suggested that accumulation of bupropion and its metabolites may occur in the elderly.
Buspirone	NC	D	I	NC	NC	I	10–60	Slow titration to avoid side effects in hepatic failure; reduced sedation advantageous
Busulfan	NC			D				
Candesartan							8–32	Use lower doses in mildly impaired hepatic and renal function; stronger effect on blood pressure at any dose
Captopril		D	I			I	12.5–250	In renal impairment monitor K+; see benazepril
Cefadroxil			I	NC	NC		1–2 g/day	Base dose on renal function and severity of infection
Cefaclor	NC	D	I	NC	NC		750–1500	If CrCl <50 ml/min, use 50% of dose twice daily
Cefamandole	NC	D	I	NC	NC		4–12 g/day	If CrCl <50 ml/min, reduce dose and increase dosage interval
Cefazolin	NC	D	I					Dosage reduction in renal impairment; all adults receive loading dose of 500 mg
							CrCl (ml/min)	Dose
							≥55	Usual adult dose
							35–54	Usual adult dose every 8 hr
							11–34	One-half usual adult dose every 12 hr
							≤10	One-half usual adult dose every 18–24 hr
Cefdinir	NC	NC	NC	NC	NC		300–600	Reduce dose by 50% in renal impairment
Cefepime	NC	D	I	NC	NC		0.5–4 g/day	Base dose on renal function and severity of infection

Cefixime	NC	D	I	NC	NC	400	If CrCl 21–60 ml/min, give 75% of usual dose; < 20 give 50%
Cefoperazone	NC	D	I	NC	NC	2–12 g/day	Reduce dose in hepatic failure; sodium content is 1 g (1.5 mEq)
Cefotaxime	I	D	I	NC	NC	2–12 g/day	If CrCl = 10–50 ml/min, give every 8–12 hr; if < 10 mg/min, give every 24 hr; a significantly greater increase in t ½ and decrease in CL is reported in patients > 80 years of age
Cefotetan	NC	D	I	NC	NC	1–6 g/day	If CrCl <30 ml/min, increase dosing interval
Cefoxitin	I	I	I	D		3–8 g/day	Dosage reduction in severe renal impairment (may need to give every 12–48 hr)
Cefpodoxime	NC	D	I	NC	NC	200–800	If CrCl <30 ml/min, give every 24 hr
Cefprozil	I	D	I	NC	NC	500–1000	Administer for ≥10 days
Ceftazidime	D	D	I	D	NC	*	*Base on renal function; minimum interval is 12 hr
Ceftizoxime	I	D	I	NC	NC	1.5–12 g/day	If CrCl <80, reduce dose
Ceftriaxone	D	D	I	I		500–2000	No dosage reduction with impaired renal or hepatic dysfunction; in severe renal impairment or in both hepatic and substantial renal impairment (maximum dosage of 2 g daily)
Cefuroxime	NC	D	I	NC	NC	0:250 mg–1 g/day P: 3–6 g/day	If CrCl <20 ml/min, reduce dose
Celecoxib						200–400	Use lowest recommended dose in patients weighing <50 kg
Cephalothin	I	D	I		I	3–6 g/day	Dosage reduction with concurrent renal and hepatic dysfunction
						CrCl (ml/min)	Dose
						>50–80	2 g every 6 hr
						>25–50	1.5 g every 6 hr
						>10–25	1 g every 6 hr
						2–10	500 mg every 8 hr
Cephradine							Dose based on degree of renal impairment, severity of infection, and susceptibility of causative organism
						CrCl (ml/min)	Dose
						>20	500 mg every 6 hr

Table 5-6. (Continued)

Drug	Volume of Distribution	Clearance	Half-Life	PB (%f)	Time to Peak	Dynamics	Dose (mg/day)	Comment
							5–20	250 mg every 6 hr
							<5	250 mg every 6 hr
Chlorambucil	NC	*	*	*	*			
Chlordiazepoxide	I	D	I	NC*			10–40	Not a drug of first choice in the elderly
Chlorpromazine	I	D	I	D			10–800	
Chlorpropamide							100–750	Inactive metabolite excreted via urine; avoid in elderly
Cholestyramine	Not absorbed*	*	*	*	*		16–24 g/day	
Cimetidine	D	D	I				300–600	If CrCl <30 ml/min/1.73 m^2, 300 mg every 12 hr (intravenous or oral); further dosage reduction in concomitant hepatic impairment. Half-life dependent on urine pH
Ciprofloxacin		D	I					If CrCl = 30–50 ml/min/1.73 m^2, 250–500 mg every 12 hr (intravenous or oral); if CrCl = 2–25 ml/min/1.73 m^2, 250–500 mg (oral) every 18 hr or 200–400 mg every 24 hr
Cisapride	NC	NC	NC	NC	NC		40–80	Css higher, no clinical effect; use restricted due to QTc/ Torsade de Pointe
Cisplatin	*	*	*	*	*			Hydrate to prevent toxicity. If CrCl <50 ml/min, give 75% of dose; if CrCl < 10 ml/min, give 50% of dose
Citalopram	*	D	I	*	I		20–40	Avoid in CrCl < 20 ml/min
Clarithromycin							500 - 1000	If CrCl < 30 ml/min, give 50% of dose or every 24 hrs
Clonidine		D					0.1–1.2	Potential for adverse CNS effects
Colestipol	Not absorbed*	*	*	*	*		13–30 g/day	
Clorazepate	I	D	I	I	I	**	15–30	
Cyclophosphamide	I	D	I			**		If CrCl < 10 ml/min, give 75% of dose; risk of hemorrhagic cystitis
Daunorubicin	*	*	*	*	*			
Desipramine		I	I*				20–150	Prolonged half-life; evaluation of therapeutic effect to be delayed
Diazepam	I	D	I	I*		**	2–20	

Diclofenac	NC	NC	NC	NC	NC		50–150	High risk for GI bleed or CNS effects; reduce dose in CrCl <50 ml/min
Diflunisal	NC	D	I	NC	NC		500–1500	High risk for GI bleed or CNS effects
Digoxin	D	D	I				0.125–0.25	Conservative dosing based on IBW and CrCl
Diltiazem	NC	D	I			**	120–480	Initiation with low dose because of significantly reduced clearance; see amlodipine
Diphenhydramine	NC	D	I				25–50	Elderly more sensitive to anti-cholinergic and sedative effects
Donepezil	I	NC	I					No dosage adjustments suggested
Doxepin			I				25–150	Prolonged half-life; evaluation of therapeutic effect to be delayed
Doxorubicin	NC	NC	NC	NC	NC			Risk of acute renal failure and nephritic syndrome
Doxycycline	NC	D	I				50–100	Tetracycline drug of choice in severe renal impairment
Enalapril	D	D	I				2.5–40	See benazepril
Erythromycin		D	I				1–4 g/day	
Eplerenone							50–100	
Eprosartan							400–800	Monitor BP and volume status
Escitalopram			I				10	34% increase in maximum concentration; 50% increase in AUC
Esomeprazole	NC	NC	NC		NC		20–40	No dosage adjustment in renal insufficiency or mild to moderate hepatic dysfunction; maximum dose of 20 mg in severe hepatic dysfunction
Ethanol	D							Increased concentrations due to lowered volume of distribution; additive effects with other sedatives
Etodolac	NC	NC	NC	NC	NC		400	High risk for GI bleed or CNS effects
Ezetimibe							10	Plasma concentrations higher in geriatric patients in multiple-dose study. Bioavailability increased in severe renal and hepatic impairment
Famotidine							CrCl (ml/min)	Dose
							>60	Usual adult dose 40 mg
							30–60	20 mg
							<30	10 mg

Table 5-6. (Continued)

Drug	Volume of Distribution	Clearance	Half-Life	PB (%f)	Time to Peak	Dynamics	Dose (mg/day)	Comment
							<10 mg	4 mg
Fentanyl		D	I		?	I		Increased age may delay absorption from transdermal system
Felodipine						**	2.5–10	In hepatic impairment, use initial dose of 2.5 mg/day; avoid doses >10 mg/day; see amlodipine
Fenoprofen	NC	NC	NC	NC	NC		1.2–4 g/day	High risk for GI bleed or CNS effects
Fexofenadine			I				60–180	Peak plasma concentrations 99% higher in elderly; however, no adverse effects observed
Fluorouracil	NC	NC	NC	NC	NC			
Fluoxetine							20–40	SE profile allows use in patients who can't tolerate TCAs
Flurazepam				I		**	15	Dose-related drowsiness from drug accumulation
Flurbiprofen	NC	NC	NC	NC	NC		200–300	High risk for GI bleed or CNS effects
Flutamide	*	*	*	*	*		450	Gynecomastia; antiandrogenic
Fluvastatin	NC	NC	NC	NC	NC		2–10	No dosage reduction in reduced CrCl
Fosphenytoin	NC	D						Lower and less frequent dosing required
Fosinopril							5–40	See benazepril
Furosemide	D	D	I	NC		**	40–2000	
Gabapentin		D						Dosage reduction in renal impairment; base dose on calculated CrCl
							CrCl (ml/min)	Dose
							30–60	200–700 twice daily
							16–29	200–700 daily
							15	100-300 daily
							<15	Dose appropriately
Gatifloxacin		D	I	I	NC	I	200–400	Dose-dependent QT prolongation; assess renal function
Gemfibrozil		NC	NC	NC			1200	
Gentamicin	I	D	I			**		Conservative dosing based on weight and CrCl or measured concentrations; interpatient variation

Glimepiride						**	1–8	Rapid and prolonged hypoglycemia >12 hr reported
Glyburide	I	NC	I				2.5–20	Reduce dose in CrCl <10 ml/min/1.73 m^2
Haloperidol			I	D*			0.25–4.0	Elderly more susceptible to side effects; prolonged half-life
Heparin						**		Increased age may increase risk of major bleeding
Hydralazine						**	20–200	
Hydrochlorothiazide		I					25–50	Not effective in CrCl<30 ml/min
Hydrocodone	I	D	I	NC	NC	I	10–30	Enhanced CNS effects and constipation noted
Hydroxyurea		*	*	*	*			If CrCl <50 ml/min give 50% of dose; if CrCl < 10 mg/min, give 20% of dose
Ibuprofen	NC	NC, D	NC	NC	NC		800–3200	High risk for GI bleed or CNS effects
Imipramine			I	NC			30–150	Prolonged half-life; evaluation of therapeutic effect to be delayed
Indomethacin			I				50–200	Other NSAIDs preferable due to efficacy and lower toxicity
Irbesartan							150–300	See eprosartan
Isoniazid	D	D					200–300	Dosage adjustment in slow acetylator patients
Isradipine						**	5–10	See amlodipine
Ketoprofen	I	D	I				150–300	
Ketorolac	NC	D	I	NC	NC		60–120	High risk for GI bleed or CNS effects; reduce dose because of decreased clearance
Labetalol		D	I				200–2400	Initiation with lower doses because of increased bioavailability with age
Lamotrigine		*					100-500	If CrCl 10–50 ml/min give 75% of dose; if CrCl < 10 ml/min, give 100 mg every other day
Lansoprazole		D	I				15–30	No dosage reduction in reduced CrCl
Levetiracetam							1000–3000	Essential to base dose on calculated CrCl
							O/P	
							CrCl (ml/min) Dose	
							50–80	500–1000 every 12hr
							30–50	250–750 every 12 hr
							<30	250–500 every 12 hr

Table 5-6. (Continued)

Drug	Volume of Distribution	Clearance	Half-Life	PB (%f)	Time to Peak	Dynamics	Dose (mg/day)	Comment
Levodopa	D	D	D		I			Decreased bioavailability possibly due to slowed gastric emptying
Levofloxacin		D	I				250–500	Dosage reduction based on renal impairment. If CrCl = 20–49 ml/min/1.73 m^2, 250 mg every 24 hr (after initial dose of 500 mg). If CrCl 10–19 ml/ min/1.73 m^2, 250 mg every 48 hr (after initial dose of 250 mg for renal infections and 500 mg for others)
Lidocaine	I	D	I	D		**		Decreased clearance in presence of CHF or liver disease
Lisinopril		D	I				2.5–40	See benazepril
Lithium		D	I				150–900	One-half initial dose because of susceptibility to volume depletion; dose based on drug concentrations (0.4–0.7 mEq/L)
Loratadine			*				10	Wide variation in half-life is a consideration in initiating dosing
Lorazepam	D	D	I	I*	**		1–3	
Losartan			I				25–100	See eprosartan
Lovastatin		NC	NC	NC			20–80	
Maprotiline							25–75	
Meclofenamic acid		NC	NC	NC	NC		150–400	High risk for GI bleed or CNS effects
Mefenamic acid		NC	NC	NC			1000	High risk for GI bleed or CNS effects
Melphalan		D	I				6	If CrCl <50 ml/min, give 75% of dose; if CrCl < 10 ml/min, give 50% of dose
Meperidine	I	D	I	I*		**	150–500	Dosage reduction because of increased sensitivity; elderly more susceptible to side effects
Metformin		D	I				850–2500	Lower dosages and frequent monitoring are recommended
Methotrexate	NC	D	I	NC	NC		5–10 mg/week	For rheumatoid arthritis; if CrCl <50 ml/min, give 50% of dose; if CrCl < 10 ml/min, avoid; refer to specific disease protocols for neoplastic disease
Methyldopa		D	I				250–3000	May be inappropriate due to side effect profile
Metoclopramide	NC	D	I	I	NC	I	0:10–20 P:10–20	Geriatrics more likely to develop dyskinesias

Metoprolol		NC, I	NC, I	NC	D		25–300	
Miglitol							75–300	
Mirtazapine		D	I			I	15–45	Dosage reduction in mild to moderate hepatic and renal impairment
Misoprostol			I				0.1–0.4	Routine use as prophylaxis not justified
Moexipril	I				I		3.75–30	Initiate at lower dose; no overall reduction in total daily dose
Morphine	D	D	D				20–100	Dosage reduction because of increased sensitivity; elderly more susceptible to side effects
Moxifloxacin	NC	NC	NC	NC	NC		400	
Nabumetone	NC	NC	NC	NC	NC		1–2 g/day	High risk for GI bleed or CNS effects; reduce dose if CrCl <50 ml/min
Nadolol				NC			40–320	
Naproxen	I	D	I	I	I		500–750	Avoid use in CrCl <30
Nateglinide	No data						60–360	
Nefazodone	NC	D	I	NC	NC	–	100–400	Conflicting pharmacokinetic data reported in single-dose vs. multiple-dose studies
Nicardipine	NC	D	NC				30–60	See amlodipine
Nifedipine	NC	D	I			**	30–120	See amlodipine
Nisoldipine		D	I			**	10–40	See amlodipine
Nitroglycerine	I		I			Exaggerated		Pharmacokinetics independent of age. Increased sensitivity to drug requires lower dosages
Nizatidine	NC	D	I			Exaggerated	150–300	
Nortriptyline	I	D	I	D*			10–50	Prolonged half-life; evaluation of therapeutic effect to be delayed
Olanzapine	NC	D	I		NC		2.5–10	
Olmesartan							20–40	For patients with possible depletion of intravascular volume (diuretic therapy or impaired renal function), initiate under close supervision and consider using a lower starting dose.
Omeprazole		D	I				20–40	Bioavailability slightly increased; however, no dosage adjustment required. No dosage reduction in reduced CrCl
Oxaprozin	NC	NC	D*	NC	NC		1200	Dual elimination (renal and hepatic) leads to decreased t ½ in chronic dosing; high risk for GI bleed or CNS effects

Table 5-6. (Continued)

Drug	Volume of Distribution	Clearance	Half-Life	PB (%f)	Time to Peak	Dynamics	Dose (mg/day)	Comment
Oxazepam	I	D	I	NC	I	**	10–60	
Oxybutynin	NC	NC	I	NC	NC	NC	5–15	Lower doses improve tolerability
Oxycodone	I	D	I	I	NC	I	10–20	Enhanced CNS effects and constipation noted
Pantoprazole							40	No dosage adjustment required in elderly
Paroxetine	D		I				10–40	See fluoxetine; half-life and steady-state concentration increase disproportionately to dose with single and multiple dosing
Penicillin G			I	NC			1–2 g/day	Dosage reduction in moderate to severe renal impairment
Perindopril							4–8	See benazepril
Phenobarbital		D	I	NC			30–60	Dose administration at bedtime to avoid excessive sedation; tolerance within a few weeks
Phenytoin		D	I*				200–300	Decreased serum albumin concentrations may increase clearance; monitoring of free phenytoin concentrations
Pioglitazone	*	*	*	*	*		15–15	No dosage adjustment required
Piroxicam	D	D	I	NC	D		10–20	Avoid due to long half-life (60–70 hr) and higher GI bleed risk
Pravastatin	NC	NC	NC	NC			10–40	
Prazosin	I	D	I				2–10	
Probucol	*	*	*	*	*		1000	
Propoxyphene[b]	NC	D	I	I	NC		*65 (100)	Not recommended in geriatrics
Propranolol	D	D	I	D*		**	40–480	
Quetiapine		D					25–200	Use 40% to 80% lower doses in elderly as compared to younger patients
Quinapril			I				2.5–80	See benazepril
Quinidine		D	I	NC			600–3600	Dosage reduction because of decreased clearance; dose based on side effects, therapeutic response, and concentrations (2–6 mg/L)
Rabeprazole							20	No dosage adjustment necessary
Raloxifene	NC	NC	NC				60	No dosage adjustment necessary
Ramipril							1.25–20	See benazepril

Ranitidine	D	D	I		NC		150–300	Prolonged half-life; if CrCl <50 ml/min, 150 mg every 24 hr orally or 50 mg every 18–24 hr intramuscularly or by intravenous intermittent slow infusion or direct injection
Repaglinide							1–16	Has not been studied extensively in the elderly
Risedronate							5	Not recommended for use in severe renal impairment (CrCl <30 ml/min). No dosage adjustment necessary in CrCl at least 30 ml/min or in elderly
Risperidone	NC	D	I	I	NC		0.5–2	Titrate slowly to avoid ADRs
Rivastigmine			I				3–12	Titrate dose to tolerance
Ropinirole	NC	D	I				0.75–24	Slow titration dose required; clinical significance of reduced clearance unknown
Rosiglitazone	*	*	*	*	*		4–8	No dosage adjustment
Sertraline	D	D	I	I			25–50	See fluoxetine
Simvastatin	*	*	*	NC	*		5–40	
Spironolactone			I		NC		50–100	Dosage reduction in significant renal impairment
Sulindac	No data	NC	NC	NC	NC		400	Hepatic metabolism to active metabolite; high risk for GI bleed or CNS effects
Tamoxifen	NC	D	*				20–40	Hot flashes, nausea, vomiting
Telithromycin							800	Dosage reduction in significant renal impairment and concomitant hepatic impairment
Telmisartan							40–80	See eprosartan
Temazepam	NC	NC	NC	I	NC	**	15–30	
Terazosin		D	D				1–10	Dose depends on indication; dry mouth and urinary incontinence are common
Tetracycline		I					500–2000	Rarely drug of choice
Theophylline	D	D	I	I		**	0.2–0.4 mg/kg/hr	Elderly more susceptible to side effects: CHF or liver disease decreases clearance: dose based on serum concentrations (7.5–15 mg/L)
Thioridazine		I	NC				10–400	Elderly more susceptible to side effects: prolonged half-life
Ticlopidine	I	D	I				500	Differences among brands; risk of neutropenia; only use in documented allergy to aspirin
Tigecycline							100	No significant PK differences in healthy older adults

Table 5-6. (Continued)

Drug	Volume of Distribution	Clearance	Half-Life	PB (%f)	Time to Peak	Dynamics	Dose (mg/day)	Comment
Timolol							20–80	
Tobramycin	NC	D	I				***	Dose conservatively based on weight and CrCl or measured concentrations
Tolazamide							100–1000	
Tolbutamide	D	D	I	I			500–3000	Inactive metabolite excreted via urine
Tolmetin	NC	NC	NC	NC	NC		1200	
Tolterodine	NC	D	I	NC	NC		2–4	Lower doses improve tolerability
Topiramate							50-400	Dose conservatively based on CrCl; initial dose of 25 mg daily and titrate at 25 mg daily at weekly intervals
Toremifene	I		I				60	No dosage reduction required
Tramadol		D	I	NC	NC		200–300	Max dose of 100 mg daily in CrCl < 30 ml/min
Trandolapril	I				I		0.5–4.0	Initiate at lowest dose; use lowest doses in CrCl < 30 ml/min
Trazodone			I		D		50–400	Prolonged half-life; evaluation of therapeutic effect to be delayed
Triamterene		D	I	D			50–100	More effective in combination with thiazide diuretic; avoid in patients with CrCl < 30 ml/min
Triazolam		D	I	I*	I		0.125–0.25	
Trimethoprim-sulfamethoxazole								Dosage reduction based on degree of renal impairment, severity of infection, and susceptibility of causative organisms
							CrCl (ml/min)	Dose
							15–30	One-half usual adult daily dose
							<15	Conflicting data (recommend reduced dose or no use at all)
Trospium	NC	I					20–40	Base dose on tolerability. Increased incidence of anticholinergic side effects in > 75 years of age
Valsartan							80–320	See eprosartan

Valproic acid						Individualize	When used for treatment of agitation associated with dementia, note: serum concentrations do not correlate with behavior response
Venlafaxine		D	I			50–225	Decrease dose by 25% in CrCl 10–70 ml/min. Decrease dose by 50% in hepatic impairment. Minimal side effects make this a valuable alternative in elderly
Verapamil	I	D	I		**	120–480	See amlodipine
Vinblastine	I with chronic doses	NC					
Vincristine	NC	NC					
Warfarin	I	D	I	I*	**	***	Increased age and female sex may increase risk of bleeding; 40% dosage reduction
Ziprasidone						40–200	Does not require dosage modification in the elderly. No additional benefit noted from doses above 20 mg twice daily

[a]PB (%f) = protein binding alterations (percent free fraction).
[b]Removed from the U.S. market in November 2010.
Dynamics = pharmacodynamics; dose = recommended daily dosage for geriatric patients; O = oral; P = parenteral; D = decreased; I = increased; NC = no change; * = conflicting data reported; ** = age-related alterations in sensitivity reported; and *** = dose to be individualized for particular patients.

References

1. El Desoky ES. Pharmacokinetic-pharmacodynamic crisis in the elderly. *Am J Ther*. 2007;14:488-98.
2. Klotz U. Pharmacokinetics and drug metabolism in the elderly. *Drug Metab Rev*. 2009;41(2):67-76.
3. Murray MD, Callahan JL. Improving medication use for older adults: an integrated research agenda. *Ann Intern Med*. 2003;139:425-9.
4. Hutchison LC, O'Brien CE. Changes in pharmacokinetics and pharmacodynamics in the elderly patient. *J Pharm Prac*. 2007;20(1):4-12.
5. Greenblatt JD, Harmatz JS, Shader RI. Clinical pharmacokinetics of anxiolytics and hypnotics in the elderly. Part 1. Therapeutic considerations. *Clin Pharmacokinet*. 1991;21(3):165-177.
6. Kane RL, Ouslander JG, Abrass IB, eds. Drug therapy (Chapter 14). In: *Essentials of Clinical Geriatrics*. New York: McGraw-Hill; 2004:357-88.
7. Ahmed N, Mandel R, Fain MJ. Frailty: an emerging geriatric syndrome. *Am J Med*. 2007;120:748-53.
8. Wynne HT, Cope LH, James OFW, et al. The effect of age and frailty upon acetanilide clearance in man. *Age Ageing*. 1989;18:415-6.
9. Fried PL. The epidemiology of frailty: The scope of the problem. In: Perry HM, Morley JE, Coe RM, eds. *Aging, Musculoskeletal Disorders and Care of the Frail Elderly*. New York, NY: Springer; 1993:3-16.
10. Hubbard RE, O'Mahoney MS, Calver BI, et al. Plasma esterases and inflammation in ageing and frailty. *Eur J Clin Pharmacol*. 2008;64(9):895-900.
11. Noreddin AM, Haynes V. Use of pharmacodynamic principles to optimize dosage regimens for antibacterial agents in the elderly. *Drugs Aging*. 2007;24(4):275-92.
12. Mangoni AA, Jackson SHD. Age-related changes in pharmacokinetics and pharmacodynamics: basic principles and practical applications. *Br J Clin Pharm*. 2003;57(1):6-14.
13. Muhlberg W. Pharmacokinetics of diuretics in geriatric patients. *Arch Gerontol Geriatr*. 1989;9(3):283-6.
14. Abernathy DR, Schwartz JB, Todd ED, et al. Verapamil pharmacodynamics and disposition in young and elderly hypertensive patients: Altered electrocardiographic and hypotensive responses. *Ann Intern Med*. 1986;105(3):329-36.
15. Montamat SC, Abernathy DR. Calcium antagonists in geriatric patients: Diltiazem in elderly persons with hypertension. *Clin Pharmacol Ther*. 1989;45:682-5.
16. Robertson DRC, Waller DG, Renwick AG, et al. Age-related changes in the pharmacokinetics and pharmacodynamics of nifedipine. *Br J Clin Pharmacol*. 1988;25(3):297-305.
17. Piepho RW, Fendler KJ. Antihypertensive therapy in the aged patient: Clinical pharmacokinetic considerations. *Drugs Aging*. 1991;1(3):194-211.
18. Rocci ML, Vlasses PH, Cressman MD, et al. Pharmacokinetics and pharmacodynamics of labetalol in elderly and young hypertensive patients following single and multiple doses. *Pharmacotherapy*. 1990;10(2):92-9.
19. Creasey WA, Funke PT, McKinstry DN, et al. Pharmacokinetics of captopril in elderly healthy male volunteers. *J Clin Pharmacol*. 1986;26(4):264-8.
20. Kobayashi KA, Bauer LA, Horn JR, et al. Glipizide pharmacokinetics in young and elderly volunteers. *Clin Pharm*. 1988;7(3):224-8.
21. Schwinghammer TL, Antal EJ, Kubacka RT, et al. Pharmacokinetics and pharmacodynamics of glyburide in young and elderly nondiabetic adults. *Clin Pharm*. 1991;10(7):532-8.
22. Greenblatt JD, Harmatz JS, Shader RI. Clinical pharmacokinetics of anxiolytics and hypnotics in the elderly. Part 2. Therapeutic considerations. *Clin Pharmacokinet*. 1991;21(4):262-73.
23. LeBel M, Barbeau G, Bergeron MG, et al. Pharmacokinetics of ciprofloxacin in elderly subjects. *Pharmacotherapy*. 1986;6(2):87-91.
24. Divoll M, Abernathy DR. Acetaminophen kinetics in the elderly. *Clin Pharmacol Ther*. 1981;31(2):151-6.
25. Johansson LC, Frison L, Logren U, et al. Influence of age on the pharmacokinetics and pharmacodynamics of Ximelagatran, an oral direct thrombin inhibitor. *Clin Pharmacokinet*. 2003;42(4):381-92.
26. Guay DRP. Clinical pharmacokinetics of drugs used to treat urge incontinence. *Clin Pharmacokinet*. 2003;42(14):1243-85.
27. Drover DR. Comparative pharmacokinetics and pharmacodynamics of short-acting hypnosedatives zaleplon, zolpidem, and zopiclone. *Clin Pharmacokinet*. 2004;43(4): 227-38.
28. Aronow WS, Frishman WH, Cheng-Lai A. Cardiovascular drug therapy in the elderly. *Cardiology Rev*. 2007;15(4):195-215.
29. Beyth RJ, Shorr RI. Principles of drug therapy in older patients: rational drug prescribing. *Clin Geriatr Med*. 2002;18:577-692.

30. Grandison MK, Boudinot FD. Age-related changes in protein binding of drugs: Implications for therapy. *Clin Pharmacokinet.* 2000;38:271-90.
31. Grond S, Radbruch L, Lehmann KA. Clinical pharmacokinetics of transdermal opioids. *Clin Pharmacokinet.* 2000;38(1):59-89.
32. Owen JA, Sitar DS, Berger L, et al. Age-related morphine kinetics. *Clin Pharmacol Ther.* 1983;34:364-8.
33. Hasselgren G, Hassan-Alin M, Andersson T, et al. Pharmacokinetic study of esomeprazole in the elderly. *Clin Pharmacokinet.* 2001;40(2):145-50.
34. Hatanaka T. Clinical pharmacokinetics of pravastatin, mechanisms of pharmacokinetic events. *Clin Pharmacokinet.* 2000;39(6):397-412.
35. Scripture CD, Peiper JA. Clinical pharmacokinetics of fluvastatin. *Clin Pharmacokinet.* 2001;40(4):263-81.
36. Song JC, White CM. Clinical pharmacokinetics and selective pharmacodynamics of new angiotensin converting enzyme inhibitors, an update. *Clin Pharmacokinet.* 2002;41(3);207-24.
37. Kelly JG, O'Malley K. Clinical pharmacokinetics of the newer ACE inhibitors. A review. *Clin Pharmacokinet.* 1990;19:375-84.
38. Morello KC, Wurz GT, DeGregorio MW. Pharmacokinetics of selective estrogen receptor modulators. *Clin Pharmacokinet.* 2003;42(4):361-72.
39. Oberbauer R, Kivanek P, Turnheim K. Pharmacokinetics of indomethacin in the elderly. *Clin Pharmacokinet.* 1993;24:428-34.
40. DeVane CL, Liston HL, Markowitz JS. Clinical pharmacokinetics of sertraline. *Clin Pharmacokinet.* 2002;41(15):1247-66.
41. Fischer JH, Patel TV, Fischer PA. Fosphenytoin, clinical pharmacokinetics and comparative advantages in the acute treatment of seizures. *Clin Pharmacokinet.* 2003;42(1):33-58.
42. Lenz TL, Wilson AF. Clinical pharmacokinetics of antiplatelet agents used in the secondary prevention of stroke. *Clin Pharmacokinet.* 2003;42(10):909-20.
43. Kaye CM, Nicholls B. Clinical pharmacokinetics of ropinirole. *Clin Pharmacokinet.* 2000;39(4):243-54.
44. Aminimanizani A, Beringer P, Jelliffe R. Comparative pharmacokinetics and pharmacodynamics of the newer fluoroquinolone antibacterials. *Clin Pharmacokinet.* 2001;40(3):169-87.
45. Perucca E. Clinical pharmacokinetics of new-generation antiepileptic drugs at the extremes of age. *Clin Pharmacokinet.* 2006;45(4):351-63.
46. Jann MW, Shirley KL, Small GW. Clinical pharmacokinetics and pharmacodynamics of cholinesterase inhibitors. *Clin Pharmacokinet.* 2002;41(10):719-39.
47. Harper CM, Newton PA, Walsh JR. Drug-induced illness in the elderly. *Postgrad Med.* 1989;86(2):245-56.
48. Kusserow R. Drug misuse among the older patients. Report of the Inspector General of the U.S. Department of HHS, January 1989.
49. Colt HG, Shapiro AP. Drug-induced illness as a cause for admission to a community hospital. *J Am Geriatr Soc.* 1989;37(4):323-6.
50. Geurian KL, Pitner RB, Lackland DT. Potential drug-drug interactions in an ambulatory geriatric population. *J Geriatr Drug Ther.* 1992;7(2):67-86.
51. Schneider JK. Adverse drug reactions in an elderly outpatient population. *Am J Hosp Pharm.* 1992;49:90-6.
52. Gurwitz JH, Avorn J. The ambiguous relation between aging and adverse drug reactions. *Ann Intern Med.* 1991;114(11):957-66.
53. Beyth RJ, Shorr RI. Epidemiology of adverse drug reactions in the elderly by drug class. *Drugs Aging.* 1999;14(3):231-9.
54. Budnita DS, Pollock DA, Weidenbach KN, et al. National surveillance of emergency department visits for outpatient adverse drug events. *JAMA.* 2006;296(15):1858-66.
55. Klein LE, German PS, Levine DM. Adverse drug reactions among the elderly: a reassessment. *J Am Geriatr Soc.* 1981;29:525-30.
56. Nolan L, O'Malley K. Prescribing for the elderly. Part I: sensitivity of the elderly to adverse drug reactions. *J Am Geriatr Soc.* 1988;36:142-9.
57. Terrell KM, Heard K, Miller DK. Prescribing to older ED patients. *Am J Emerg Med.* 2006;24:468-78.
58. Chutka DS, Takahashi PY, Hoel RW. Inappropriate medications for elderly patients. *Mayo Clin Proc.* 2004;79:122-39.
59. Col N, Fangle JE, Kronholm P. The role of medication noncompliance and adverse drug reaction in hospitalization of the elderly. *Arch Intern Med.* 1990;150(4):841-5.
60. Resnick NM, Marcantonio DR. How should clinical care of the aged differ? *Lancet.* 1997;350:1157-8.

61. Hammerlein A, Derendorf H, Lowenthal DT. Pharmacokinetic and pharmacodynamic changes in the elderly: clinical implications. *Clin Pharmacokinet.* 1998;35(1):49-64.

62. Dawling S, Crome P. Clinical pharmacokinetic considerations in the elderly: an update. *Clin Pharmacokinet.* 1981;17:236-63.

63. Hilmer SN, McLachlan, Le Couteur DG. Clinical pharmacology in the geriatric patient. *Fundam Clin Pharmacol.* 2007;21:217-30.

64. Cahpron DJ. Drug disposition and response. In: Delafuente JC, Stewart RB, eds. *Therapeutics in the Elderly.* Cincinnati, OH: Harvey Whitney Books; 2001:257-88.

65. Evans MA, Triggs EJ, Broe GA, et al. Systemic availability of orally administered L-dopa in the elderly Parkinsonian patient. *Eur J Clin Pharmacol.* 1980;17:215-21.

66. Bianchine JR, Calimlim LR, Morgan JP, et al. Metabolism and absorption of L-3,4 dihydroxyphenylalanine in patients with Parkinson's disease. *Ann NY Acad Sci.* 1971;179:126-40.

67. Ochs HR, Greenblatt DJ, Allen MD, et al. Effect of age and Billroth gastrectomy on absorption of desmethyldiazepam from chlorazepate. *Clin Pharmacol Ther.* 1979;26:449-56.

68. Lamy PP. *Prescribing for the Elderly.* Littleton, MA: PSG Wright;1980.

69. Kelly JG, McGarry K, O'Malley K, et al. Bioavailability of labetalol increases with age. *Br J Clin Pharmacol.* 1982;14:304-5.

70. Storstein L, Larsen A, Saevareld L. Pharmacokinetics of calcium channel blockers in patients with renal insufficiency and in geriatric patients. *Acta Med Scand.* 1984;681:25-30.

71. Ewy GA. Digoxin metabolism in the elderly. *Circulation.* 1969;39(4):449-52.

72. Rubin PC, Scott PJW, Reid JL. Prazosin disposition in young and elderly subjects. *Br J Clin Pharmacol.* 1981;12(3):401-4.

73. Cusack BJ. Pharmacokinetics in older persons. *Am J Geriatr Pharmcother.* 2004;2:274-302.

74. Miller SW, Strom JG. Drug-product selection: implications for the geriatric patient. *The Consult Pharm.* 1990;5(1):30-7.

75. Greenblatt DJ. Reduced serum albumin concentration in the elderly: a report from the Boston Collaborative Drug Surveillance Program. *J Am Geriatr Soc.* 1979;27:20-2.

76. Cooper JW, Cobb HH. Nutritional correlation and changes in a geriatric nursing home. *Nut Supp Serv.* 1988;8(8):5-7.

77. Michalets EL. Update: Clinically significant cytochrome P-450 drug interactions. *Pharmacotherapy.* 1998;18(1):84-112.

78. Schmucker DL. Aging and drug disposition: an update. *Pharmacol Rev*. 1985;37:133-48.

79. Wallace SM, Verbeek RO. Plasma protein binding of drugs in the elderly. *Clin Pharmacokinet.* 1987;12(1):41-72.

80. Somerville K, Faulkner G, Langman M. Non-steroidal anti-inflammatory drugs and bleeding peptic ulcer. *Lancet.* 1986;1:462-4.

81. Hayes MJ, Langman MJS, Short AH. Changes in drug metabolism with increasing age. *Br J Clin Pharmacol.* 1975;12(2):73-79.

82. Mather LE, Tucker GT, Pflug AE. Meperidine kinetics in man. *Clin Pharmacol Ther.* 1975;17(1):21-30.

83. Beers MH, Ouslander JG, Fingold SF, et al. Inappropriate medication prescribing in skilled-nursing facilities. *Ann Intern Med.* 1992;117:684-9.

84. Beers MH. Explicit criteria for determining potentially inappropriate medication use by the elderly, an update. *Arch Intern Med.* 1997;157:1531-6.

85. Fick DM, Cooper JW, Wade WE, et al. Updating the Beers criteria for potentially inappropriate medication use in older adults. *Arch Intern Med.* 2003;163:2716-24.

86. Greenblatt DJ, Sellers EM, Shader RI. Drug disposition in old age. *N Engl J Med.* 1982;306(18):1081-8.

87. Chapron DI. Drug disposition and response. In: Delafuente JC, Stewart RB, eds. *Therapeutics in the Elderly.* 3rd ed. Cincinnati, OH: Harvey Whitney Books Company, 2001:257-88.

88. Dawling S, Lynn K, Rosser R, et al. Nortriptyline metabolism in chronic renal failure: metabolic elimination. *Clin Pharmacol Ther.* 1982;32(3):322-9.

89. Abernathy DR, Greenblatt DJ, Shader RI. Imipramine and desipramine disposition in the elderly. *J Pharmacol Exp Ther.* 1985;232:183-8.

90. Cohen BM, Sommer BR. Metabolism of thioridazine in the elderly. *J Clin Psychopharmacol.* 1988;8(5):336-9.

91. Antal EJ, Kramer PA, Mercik SA. Theophylline pharmacokinetics in advanced age. *Br J Clin Pharmacol.* 1981;12(5):637-5.

92. Kinirons MT, O'Mahoney M. Drug metabolism and ageing. *Br J Clin Pharmacol.* 2004;57:540-4.

93. Kinirons MT, Crome P. Clinical pharmacokinetic consideration in the elderly, an update. *Clin Pharmacokinet.* 1999;33:302-12.

94. LeBlanc JM, Dasta JF, Pruchnicki MC, et al. Impact of disease states on the pharmacokinetics and pharmacodynamics of angiotensin-converting enzyme inhibitors. *J Clin Pharmacol.* 2006;46:968-80.

95. Gral T, Young M. Measured versus estimated creatinine clearance in the elderly as an index of renal function. *J Am Geriatr Soc.* 1980;28(11):492-6.

96. Smythe M, Hoffman J, Kizy K, et al. Estimating creatinine clearance in elderly patients with low serum creatinine concentrations. *Am J Hosp Pharm.* 1994;51(2):198-204.

97. Smith JM, Baldessarini RJ. Changes in prevalence, severity, and recovery in tardive dyskinesia with age. *Arch Gen Psych.* 1980;37:1368-73.

98. Feely J, Cloakley D. Altered pharmacodynamics in the elderly. *Clin Geriatr Med.* 1990;6:269-83.

99. Uchida H, Mamo DC, Mulsant BH, et al. Increased antipsychotic sensitivity in elderly patients: evidence and mechanisms. *J Clin Psych.* 2009;70(3):397-405.

100. Committee on Identifying and Preventing Medication Errors, Aspden P, Wolcott J, Bootman JL, et al., eds. *Preventing Medication Errors. Quality Chasm Series Institute of Medicine Report.* Institute of Medicine of the National Sciences; July, 2006. Available at: http://www.nap.edu/openbook.php?record_id=11623. Accessed 5/27/11.

101. Sloane PD, Zimmerman S, Brown LC, et al. Inappropriate medication prescribing in residential care/assisted living facilities. *J Am Ger Soc.* 2002;50:1001-11.

102. Spore DL, Mor V, Larrat P, et al. Inappropriate drug prescriptions for elderly residents of board and care facilities. *Am J Public Health.* 1997;87:404-9.

103. Golden AG, Preston RA, Barnett SD, et al. Inappropriate medication prescribing in homebound older adults. *J Am Ger Soc.* 1999;47:948-53.

104. Hanlon JT, Fillenbaum GG, Schmader KE, et al. Inappropriate drug use among community dwelling elderly. *Pharmacotherapy.* 2000;20:575-82.

105. Goulding MR. Inappropriate medication prescribing for elderly ambulatory patients. *Arch Intern Med.* 2004;164:305-12.

106. Aparasu RR, Fliginger SE. Inappropriate medication prescribing for the elderly by office-based physicians. *Ann Pharmacother.* 1997;31:823-9.

107. Huang B, Bachmann KA, He X, et al. Inappropriate prescriptions for the aging population of the United States: an analysis of the National Ambulatory Medical Care Survey, 1997. *Pharmacoepidemiol Drug Saf.* 2002;11:127-34.

108. Caterino JM, Emond JA, Camargo Jr CA. Inappropriate medication administration to the acutely ill elderly: a nationwide emergency department study, 1999–2000. *J Am Ger Soc.* 2004;52:1847-55.

109. Bonk ME, Krown H, Matuszewski K, et al. Potentially inappropriate medications in hospitalized senior patients. *Am J Hosp Pharm.* 2006;63:1161-65.

110. Stefanacci RG, Cavallaro E, Beers MH, et al. Developing explicit positive Beers criteria for preferred central nervous system medications in older adults. *Cons Pharm.* 2009;24(8):601-10.

111. Semla TP, Beizer JL, Higbee MD, eds. *Geriatric Dosage Handbook.* 15th ed. Hudson, OH: Lexi-Comp; 2010.

112. Aronoff GR, Bennett WM, Berns JS, et al. *Drug Prescribing in Renal Failure: Dosing Guidelines for Adults.* 5th ed. Philadelphia, PA: ACP-ASIM; 2007.

Chapter 6

Gary R. Matzke and Thomas C. Dowling

Renal Drug Dosing Concepts

Chronic kidney disease (CKD) is a progressive consequence of systemic diseases such as diabetes and hypertension as well as localized kidney injury as the result of glomerulonephritis. Over 500,000 patients in the U.S. have stage 5 CKD, which is also categorized as end-stage renal disease (ESRD). Each year, for the last several decades, up to 100,000 patients have developed ESRD and over 80,000 have died.[1] Chronic renal replacement therapy, whether peritoneal or hemodialysis, was life-sustaining for over 370,000 patients in 2007. A significant portion of the additional 170,000 who have received a kidney transplant have stage 1-4 CKD. Most stage 1-4 CKD patients are initially identified in ambulatory care clinics, while others are identified in general hospital wards and acute care environments. Population-based studies, such as NHANES III, report that the prevalence of CKD increased dramatically from 1988-1994[2] and their latest estimates suggest that approximately 25 million adults have CKD in the U.S.[3]

Renal failure can also appear abruptly, with some patients presenting with acute kidney injury (AKI) in emergency departments, clinical wards, or intensive care units.[4] The majority of AKI cases are attributed to drug therapy or renal hypoperfusion in hospitalized patients, which often requires continuous renal replacement therapies (CRRT). Regardless of the cause of acute or chronic renal impairment, these patients are at increased risk of accumulating drugs, toxic metabolites and other nephrotoxins. For any drug that relies extensively on the kidney for elimination from the body (i.e., renal clearance > 30% of total clearance) and drug concentrations in blood or plasma are clearly associated with a pharmacodynamic effect (success, failure, or toxicity), dose adjustments are necessary when renal function is considerably reduced. The aim of this chapter is to describe dosing strategies for patients with CKD, or AKI and those receiving renal replacement therapies on an intermittent and/or continuous basis.

Clinical Assessment of Renal Function

The indices of glomerular and tubular function most widely utilized clinically by nephrologists include daily urinary protein excretion rate (glomerular), urine albumin-creatinine ratio (glomerular), fractional excretion of sodium (tubular), and serum creatinine concentration (glomerular and tubular). Creatinine is excreted by glomerular filtration and tubular secretion, making creatinine clearance (CrCl) a composite index of renal function that has been strongly associated with the total and renal clearance of many drugs that are eliminated by the kidney and is the primary index of renal drug dosing in FDA product labeling.

In patients with CKD stages 1 through 5 (pre-dialysis), the Cockcroft-Gault equation (see Chapter 1) is commonly used to estimate CrCl in the presence of stable renal function. Newer equations that estimate GFR (eGFR), such as the MDRD and CKD-EPI equations, are most appropriately used for identifying CKD and staging their degree of CKD severity.[5] Although the MDRD equation was being widely employed for automated reporting of GFR by clinical laboratories, it is important to note that the CKD-EPI equation has now replaced it in many facilities. Neither of these eGFR equations has been consistently demonstrated to be equivalent to CrCl when adjusting drug doses for renal impairment.[6,7] Furthermore, recent studies in over 10,000 patients have reported that the CKD-EPI equations yield significantly higher estimates of renal function, and significantly different dose calculations, when compared to CG equation, particularly in elderly individuals and those receiving narrow therapeutic index drugs such as enoxaparin.[6,8] Thus, renal dosing practices should remain consistent with the original pharmacokinetic studies of a particular drug in CKD, which to date generally involves estimation of creatinine clearance.

Quantification of renal function in patients with AKI, where renal function and serum creatinine values are rapidly changing, is a challenging situation. Here, numerous equations for estimating CrCl based on two non-steady-state serum creatinine values have been proposed. See Chapter 1 for further discussions of appropriate use of equations to quantify renal function in various situations and patient populations. For critically ill patients with AKI receiving CRRT, estimation of both residual renal function (CrCl) and CRRT clearance are required for dose individualization (see section on dosing strategies).[9,10]

Mechanisms of Drug Clearance

Renal elimination

The process of renal drug elimination is a composite of glomerular and tubular functions, with the amount of drug cleared by the kidney (A_c) described by the following equation:

$$A_c = A_{filt} + A_{sec} - A_{reabs} \qquad \text{(Eq. 1)}$$

Initially, unbound drug is filtered through the glomerulus (A_{filt}) into the proximal tubular fluid. Once in the tubule, filtered drug may then be passively or actively reabsorbed (A_{reabs}) back into the bloodstream. This reabsorptive process is rare and occurs primarily in distal segments for unionized drugs at low urine flow rates. Drugs may also undergo active tubular secretion (A_{sec}), where unbound drug in plasma is transported into the tubular cell, and secreted into the urine, by pathways mediated by the organic anionic transporter (OAT), organic cationic transporter (OCT) or p-glycoprotein (P-GP), located along the basolateral and apical membranes of the proximal tubule.[11,12] These pathways work together to form an extremely efficient process of "detoxification," resulting in renal clearance values that can exceed GFR, and in some cases approach renal plasma flow as observed with para-aminohippurate (PAH) and several penicillins. As filtration capacity (measured as GFR) progressively diminishes in CKD, some experimental data suggest that tubular secretory mechanisms may maintain their functionality, thereby providing significant renal clearance for some drugs even in the presence of severe glomerular damage.[13]

Kidney diseases can affect both glomerular and tubular function, leading to reduced overall drug elimination. As destruction of nephrons progresses, it has traditionally been believed that the function of all segments of the remaining nephrons is affected equally.[14] Based on this assumption, the rate of drug excretion in the normal or diseased kidney can be estimated by GFR or CrCl, which are predominantly measures of glomerular function.[15] The total renal clearance of a drug from the body also depends on (1) the fraction of the drug eliminated unchanged by the normal kidney, (2) the renal mechanisms involved in drug elimination, and (3) the degree of functional impairment of each of these pathways. The fraction of unchanged drug eliminated renally (f_e) and an assessment of the relationship between renal function and the drug's parameters, such as half-life ($t½$), total clearance (CL) and renal clearance (CL_R) can be used to individualize drug therapy. Ideally, renal drug clearance is determined by quantifying the amount of drug excreted in urine relative to the AUC of drug in plasma, and renal function is measured using a GFR method such as iothalamate clearance.[16] More commonly, the relationship between CrCl and drug clearance (CL) is evaluated in a large patient population with varying renal function, as follows:

$$CL = (A \times CrCl) + B \qquad \text{(Eq. 2)}$$

$$k = (A \times CrCl) + B \qquad \text{(Eq. 3)}$$

where A is the slope of the linear relationship between CrCl and either CL or k (the elimination rate constant), and B is the non-renal CL (CL_{NR}) or non-renal k (k_{NR}), respectively. This drug-specific information can then be used to design dose adjustment strategies in patients with renal insufficiency to minimize drug toxicity and optimize therapeutic efficacy.

Role of renal drug transporters

All aspects of drug transport in the kidney may be affected by co-administration of other substances, even in patients with normal renal function. First, drugs that cause a change in GFR will alter the CL_R of other renally eliminated drugs, assuming that tubular function remains unchanged. Second, substances may alter the tubular transport of one or more secretory pathways, such P-GP, OAT or OCT, through noncompetitive inhibition or

Table 6-1. Examples of Renal Drug Transporter-Interaction Studies in Humans[18-21]

Transporter(s) (Gene)	Substrate	Inhibitor	PK Results
P-GP (ABCB1)	Fexofenadine	Probenecid	44%↓ CL/F; 70%↓ CL_R; 53%↑ AUC
	Cimetidine	Itraconazole	26%↓ CL; 30%↓ CL_R; 25%↑ AUC
	Digoxin	Itraconazole	21%↓ CL_R; 50%↑ AUC
	Digoxin	Ritonavir	42%↓ CL/F; 21%↓ CL_R; 86%↑ AUC
OAT1/4	Zidovudine	Probenecid	49%↓ CL; 56%↓ CL_R; 50%↑ $T_{1/2}$
	Ciprofloxacin	Probenecid	41%↓ CL; 64%↓ CL_R; 74%↑ AUC
OCT1 (SLC22A1)	Metformin	Cimetidine[a]	50%↓ CL/F; 50%↓ CL_R; 57%↑ AUC
			37%↓ CL/F; 17%↑ AUC
OCT2 (SLC22A2)	Amantadine	Quinidine	33%↓ CL_R

[a]Interaction observed only in patients with OCT1 GG genotype.
P-GP = p-glycoprotein; OAT1/4 = family of organic anion transporters 1–4; OCT1 = organic cation transporter 1; OCT2 = organic cation transporter 2.

degradation of transport carriers. The most common type of tubular transport interaction occurs when two substances compete for tubular secretion by the same pathway. Clinically significant drug interactions involving renal transport mechanisms have been reported for the OAT, OCT, and P-GP transporters (Table 6-1).[12] Some clinically important interactions and suspected pathways include ciprofloxacin/azlocillin (OAT), cidofovir/probenecid (OAT), oseltamivir/probenecid (OAT), itraconazole/digoxin (P-GP), itraconazole/cimetidine (P-GP), and itraconazole/quinidine (OCT/P-GP).

Although the mechanism is not well defined, an interaction between cimetidine and creatinine has been reported.[17] Cimetidine appears to block the OCT-mediated tubular secretion of creatinine, which then provides for a more accurate assessment of the GFR using a CrCl estimation method. There is increasing evidence to suggest that genetic variability of renal drug transporters, such as OCT1, may be an important determinant of urinary drug excretion. Other transporters such as the peptide transporter (PEPT) and nucleoside transporters (CNT) may also contribute to renal drug elimination of drugs such as β-lactam antibiotics and didanosine, respectively.[11,12]

Renal interactions can also be beneficial for management of toxicity, by enhancing urinary excretion of the toxin to reduce serum drug concentrations, or by inhibiting drug uptake in tubules. For example, administration of urinary acidifying agents such as ammonium chloride, reduces the renal tubular reabsorption of weak basic drugs such as xanthines, amphetamine, and phenobarbital, resulting in increased renal elimination. In contrast, urinary alkalinizing agents would reduce the renal elimination of weak basic drugs thereby enhancing systemic exposure. A known mechanism of cidofovir nephrotoxicity is intracellular localization of the drug in the proximal tubule. Use of probenecid to block cellular uptake of cidofovir provides renoprotection, thereby circumventing the development of nephrotoxicity caused by this agent.

Nonrenal Mechanisms

Metabolism

Biotransformation of drugs by Phase I (oxidative) and Phase 2 (reductive) reactions generally results in the formation of inactive metabolic products. Decreased intra-renal metabolism, decreased hepatic metabolism, and reduced renal clearance of active or toxic metabolites have all been noted in CKD and may result in significant changes in total body clearance (Table 6-2).[22-25] The kidney itself plays an important role in the metabolism of many endogenous proteins and small peptides in addition to some drugs. For example, the carbapenem antibiotic imipenem is inactivated by renal dehydrodipeptidase I (RDHP), located in high concentrations along the brush border of the nephron.[26] CKD patients have reduced RDHP activity, resulting in a prolonged elimination half life of imipenem and the need for dose adjustment in patients with CrCl < 70 ml/min. Data from animal models of CKD and evidence in patients suggests that hepatic CYP activity is reduced in the presence of renal failure.[23,25,27-29] For example, the non-renal clearance of reboxetine, which is extensively metabolized by CYP3A and minimally excreted unchanged by the kidneys, was 30% lower in ESRD patients (CKD stage 5) compared to those with mild renal impairment (CKD stage 2–3), and 67% lower than subjects with normal renal function.[29] Altered stereoselective metabolism may also occur in CKD. For example, a preferential increase in formation of metoprolol R-MAM and OHM was observed in CKD patients relative to normal controls.[30] Thus, for drugs where non-renal clearance is affected by renal disease, appropriate dose adjustments and close monitoring is needed in order to maintain steady state drug concentrations at values similar to individuals with normal renal and hepatic function.

Table 6-2. Drugs Reported to Have Reduced Non-Renal Clearance in CKD

Acyclovir[a]	Cyclophosphamide[c]	Nitrendipine[b]
Aztreonam[a]	Didanosine[a]	Nortriptyline[c]
Bufurolol[b]	Encainide[b]	Oxprenolol[b]
Bupropion[c]	Erythromycin[c]	Procainamide[c]
Captopril[c]	Felbamate[c]	Propoxyphene[c]
Carvedilol[c]	Guanadrel[b]	Propranolol[c]
Cefepime[a]	Imipenem[a]	Quinapril[a]
Cefmetazole[a]	Isoniazid[c]	Raboxetine[b]
Cefonicid[a]	Ketoprofen[a]	Raloxifene[c]
Cefotaxime[a]	Ketorolac[a]	Repaglinide[c]
Ceftibuten[a]	Lidocaine[c]	Rosuvastatin[a]
Ceftriaxone[a]	Lomefloxacin[a]	Roxithromycin[b]
Cerivastatin[b]	Losartan[c]	Simvastatin[c]
Cibenzoline[b]	Lovastatin[c]	Sparfloxacin[a]
Cilastatin[a]	Metoclopramide[a]	Telithromycin[a]
Cimetidine[a]	Minoxidil[c]	Valsartan[c]
Ciprofloxacin[a]	Morphine[c]	Vancomycin[a]
Codeine[c]	Nicardipine[c]	Verapamil[c]
	Nimodipine[c]	Zidovudine[a]

[a]Indicates that a renal dose adjustment is required; see Table 6-3 or package insert.
[b]Indicates drug not available in U.S.
[c]Indicates no FDA-approved dose adjustment in CKD provided; use with caution in CKD.

Gastrointestinal (GI) absorption

The effect of CKD on GI absorption of drugs is not well understood and the impact of AKI on GI absorption is unknown. Many patients with diabetes mellitus are known to have decreased gastric emptying and therefore delayed absorption of some drugs can be expected in the presence of diabetes. However, the extent of absorption and overall bioavailability are typically unchanged compared to patients without renal disease. While the bioavailability of a few drugs are reportedly reduced, consistent findings of impaired absorption in CKD patients is lacking. For the majority of drugs that have been evaluated, GI absorption is either unchanged or increased, suggesting that pre-systemic (or first-pass) extraction may be reduced in these patients. The absorption of some drugs such as digoxin and fluoroquinolone antibiotics may be altered due to the concomitant administration of phosphate binders.[31,32]

Volume of Distribution (V)

The V of many drugs, including aminoglycosides and cephalosporins, have been reported to be significantly increased in CKD patients.[33-35] Proposed mechanisms of increased V for various drugs include fluid overload, decreased plasma protein binding due to hypoalbuminemia or competitive binding interactions with uremic toxins, or altered tissue binding. Decreased V in patients with ESRD is rare and, if present, is due to reduced binding to tissue proteins. The two primary plasma proteins that bind acidic and basic drugs are albumin and α_1-acid glycoprotein (AAG), respectively. The protein binding for some acidic drugs such as penicillins, cephalosporins, furosemide, theophylline, and phenytoin, is reduced in patients with renal failure.[36,37] The binding of basic drugs to AAG is, however, generally unaltered in CKD patients, although increased V has been reported for some drugs such as bepridil and disopyramide.[38,39] Although changes in plasma protein binding are not usually clinically significant, close monitoring in patients receiving narrow therapeutic index drugs is warranted unless there is clinical confirmation of no associated problem.

Drug Dosing Strategies for CKD Patients

For drugs that rely to a significant degree on the kidneys for total body elimination (i.e., fe > 0.3), dose reductions may be required in patients with CKD to avoid systemic accumulation and adverse drug events. In nearly all cases, the U.S. FDA–approved drug product label (i.e., package insert) includes drug dose adjustment guidelines based on the degree of reduction in CrCl.[40]

It is important to understand the mathematical basis for dose adjustment recommendations. The following approach involves an initial estimation of the drug's CL (or k) based on either literature data or derivation of a regression equation from clinical trial data.[15,41] The next step is to use the estimates of CL or k to determine the dose adjustment factor (Q):

$$Q = k_R \div k_{norm} \qquad \text{(Eq. 4)}$$

$$Q = CL_R \div CL_{norm} \qquad \text{(Eq. 5)}$$

An assumption when using these equations is that volume of distribution does not change in the presence of renal disease and that the normal values are representative of individuals with CrCl ≥ 120 ml/min.

An alternative approach to calculating Q involves determination of the ratio (KF) of the patient's CrCl to a presumed normal CrCl of 120 ml/min, based on estimation of the fraction of drug eliminated unchanged renally in subjects with normal renal function (f_e), as:

$$Q = 1 - [fe\ (1 - KF)] \qquad \text{(Eq. 6)}$$

Use of this approach is based on the following assumptions: (1) elimination of the drug is best described by a linear, first-order process; (2) glomerular and tubular function decrease in a parallel fashion in all renal diseases; (3) other aspects of drug absorption (bioavailability), distribution (protein binding) and metabolism (non-renal clearance) remain constant; (4) metabolites of the drug are pharmacologically inactive or do not accumulate in renal disease; and (5) the pharmacodynamics (i.e., the concentration or dose response relationship) of the drug or metabolites remains unchanged by renal disease.[15,41]

Once the dosage adjustment factor (Q) for the patient has been estimated, the dosage regimen for that drug can be modified to achieve the desired serum concentration profile. If clinically significant relationships between peak and trough concentrations and efficacy or toxicity have been described then the dosage regimen should be designed to attain and maintain these target values. In all other cases, the goal of dose individualization may be to achieve similar average steady state concentrations (Css_{av}) to those typically observed in patients with normal renal function. If the goal is to maintain the same Css_{av} and the dosage form precludes modification (e.g., time-release capsule), then one must prolong the dosing interval (t). Conversely, if the standard dosing interval is desired, the dose can be reduced to maintain the desired Css_{av}. The new dosing interval (τ_R) or dose (D_R) for the patient with renal insufficiency can be calculated as follows:

$$\tau_R = \tau_{norm} \div Q \qquad \text{(Eq. 7)}$$

$$D_R = D_{norm} \times Q \qquad \text{(Eq. 8)}$$

The strategies shown in Eq. 7 and 8 are designed to achieve the same Css_{av}. However, the resultant steady state peak [Css_{max}] and trough [Css_{min}] concentrations may be markedly different in each case. The reduced dosage strategy (Eq. 8) yields lower Css_{max} and higher Css_{min} compared to the prolonged dosage interval (Eq. 7) approach, which results in values that are similar to the individual with normal renal function. If this approach yields an interval that is impractical, a new dose can be calculated using a fixed, pre-specified dose interval (τ_R), as follows:

$$D_R = [\, D_{norm} \times Q \times \tau_R] \,/\, \tau_{norm} \qquad \text{(Eq. 9)}$$

The methods of dosage individualization described above (Eq. 7–9) are applicable to clinical settings where no serum concentration data are available to guide the therapeutic decision making process. These approaches are based on data obtained from clinical pharmacokinetic studies in patients with renal impairment, and serve as the basis for making initial dosing decisions based on renal function (CrCl) as shown in Table 6-3. However, when a specific serum concentration-time profile, peak, trough or area under the concentration time curve, is required, measurement of drug concentrations and traditional therapeutic drug monitoring approaches are recommended (see the drug-specific chapters of this book).

Hemodialysis and Continuous Renal Replacement Therapy

Hemodialysis (HD) is the predominant modality of renal replacement therapy for over 350,000 individuals who reside in the U.S.[1] The medical care environment of free standing community centered dialysis units often places them outside of traditional healthcare institutions and because only a small number of pharmacists practice in this setting pharmacotherapeutic management of the patient's care is often dependent on the nursing staff. The medication burden of the typical HD-dependent patient is extensive: they often are prescribed 12 or more medications and also self select multiple over-the-counter drugs and supplements. There is thus a considerable need for community pharmacists to be cognizant of the influence of HD on the pharmacokinetics and dynamics of the medications that these patients are receiving. The establishment of consultant relationship with dialysis centers is one avenue for a pharmacist to participate in the care of these vulnerable patients, just as many pharmacists do for those who reside in skilled nursing facilities.[46] Finally, since the average age of HD patients is over 65 and they have a significant medication burden, they are prime candidates for the receipt of medication therapy management under the auspices of the MTM provisions in Medicare Part D.

This section of the chapter serves as a primer on the impact of renal replacement therapies such as hemodialysis and continuous renal replacement therapies (CRRTs) on acute and chronic drug therapy regimens and provides clinically useful dosage recommendations for many of the most commonly used medications for this patient population.

Principles of hemodialysis

The removal of a drug by dialysis is dependent on several factors, including the physiochemical and pharmacokinetic characteristics of the drug, the patient's residual renal function, volume status and acuity of their illness, a myriad of other factors mentioned in the preceding section, and finally the dialysis prescription, which consists of the selection of the dialyzer, the blood and dialysate flow rates, the degree of fluid removal, and the frequency and duration of the procedure.[47-49] Drugs that are highly protein bound have low dialysis clearances because α_1-acid glycoprotein and albumin have molecular weights in excess of 20,000 Daltons (D) and thus do not cross the dialysis membrane. Drugs that have a volume of distribution (V) greater than 2 L/kg are also poorly removed by hemodialysis. Table 6-4 outlines the key factors.

The degree of drug removal by the hemodialysis procedure, be it acute for the management of AKI or the typical three times a week regimen for the management of stage 5 chronic kidney disease (CKD), can be dramatically affected by the prescribed dialysis regimen.[47,49-51] The intensity of the hemodialysis prescription for

Table 6-3. Pharmacokinetic Parameters and Maintenance Dosages for Some Commonly Used Drugs in Patients with CKD[42–45]

			CrCl (ml/min)			
Drug	**V (L/kg)**	**fe**	**120–70**	**70–50**	**50–10**	**<10**
Acyclovir	0.7	0.40–0.70	5 mg/kg every 8 h	5 mg/kg every 8 h	5 mg/kg every 12–24 h	2.5 mg/kg every 24 h
Amantadine	4–5	0.90	100 mg every 12 h	Every 24–48 h	Every 48–72 h	Every 7 d
Amphotericin B	4	0.05–0.10	20–50 mg every 24 h	Every 24 h	Every 24 h	Every 24–36 h
Amoxicillin	0.26	0.50–0.70	250–500 mg every 8 h	Every 8 h	Every 8 h–12 h	Every 24 h
Ampicillin	0.17	0.30–0.90	250 mg–2 g every 6 h	Every 6 h	Every 6–12 h	Every 12–24 h
Atenolol	1.1	0.90	50–100 mg every 24 h	100% every 24 h	50% every 48 h	30%–50% every 96 h
Aztreonam	0.5–1	0.75	2 g every 8 h	100%	50%–75%	25%
Benazepril	0.15	0.20	10 mg every 24 h	100%	50%–75%	25%–50%
Bisoprolol	3	0.50	10 mg every 24 h	100%	75%	50%
Cefazolin	0.13–0.22	0.75–0.95	1–2 g every 8 h	Every 8 h	Every 12 h	Every 24–48 h
Cefepime	0.3	0.85	2 g every 12 h	Every 12 h	Every 16–24 h	Every 24–48 h
Cefotaxime	0.15–0.55	0.60	1 g every 6 h	Every 6 h	Every 8–12 h	Every 24 h
Cefoxitin	0.2	0.80	1–2 g every 8 h	Every 8 h	Every 8–12 h	Every 24–48 h
Ceftazidime	0.28–0.4	0.60–0.85	1–2 g every 8 h	Every 8–12 h	Every 24–48 h	Every 48 h
Ceftizoxime	0.26–0.42	0.57–1.0	1–2 g every 8–12 h	Every 8–12 h	Every 12–24 h	Every 24 h
Cefuroxime sodium	0.13–1.8	0.90	0.75–1.5 g every 8 h	Every 8 h	Every 8–12 h	Every 12 h
Cephalexin	0.35	0.98	250–500 mg every 6 h	Every 8 h	Every 12 h	Every 12 h
Cetirizine	0.4–0.6	0.60–0.70	5–20 mg every 24 h	100%	50%	25%
Cimetidine	0.8–1.3	0.50–0.70	400 mg every 12 h	100%	50%	25%
Cidofovir	0.3–0.8	0.90	5 mg/kg every 1–2wk	100%	Avoid	Avoid
Ciprofloxacin	2.5	0.50–0.70	400 mg every 12 h	100%	50%–75%	50%
Clarithromycin	2–4	0.15–0.25	0.5–1 g every 12 h	100%	75%	50%–75%
Didanosine	1	0.40–0.69	200 mg every 12 h (125 mg if < 60kg)	100%	200 mg every 24 h	50% every 24 h
Enalapril	No data	0.43	5–10 mg every 12 h	100%	75%–100%	50%
Famciclovir	1.5	0.50–0.65	500 mg every 8 h	100%	250–500 mg every 24–48 h	250 mg every 48 h
Famotidine	0.8–1.4	0.65–0.80	20–40 mg every 24 h	50%	25%	10%
Fexofenadine	5–6	0.10	60 mg every 12 h	Every 12 h	Every 12–24 h	Every 24 h
Flucytosine	0.6	0.90	37.5 mg/kg every 6 h	Every 12 h	Every 16 h	Every 24 h
Foscarnet	0.3–0.6	0.85	40 mg/kg every 8 h	28 mg/kg	15 mg/kg	6 mg/kg
Gabapentin	0.7	0.90	300–600 mg every 8 h	400 mg every 8 h	300 mg every 12–24 h	300 mg every 48 h
Ganciclovir	0.47	0.90–1.0	5 mg/kg every 12 h	Every 12 h	Every 24–48 h	Every 48–96 h
Glipizide	0.13–0.16	0.05–0.07	2.5–15 mg every 24 h	100%	50%	50%
Glyburide	0.2–0.3	0.50	1.25–20 mg every 24 h	No data	Avoid	Avoid
Insulin	0.15	None	Variable	100%	75%	50%
Insulin (Lispro)	0.26–0.36	No data	Variable	100%	75%	50%

Table 6-3. (Continued)

Drug	V (L/kg)	fe	GFR (ml/min) 120–70	70–50	50–10	<10
Itraconazole	10	0.35	100–200 mg every 12 h	100%	100%	50%
Lamivudine	0.83	0.70–0.80	150 mg every 12 h	100% every 24 h	50–150 mg every 24 h	25–50 mg
Levetiracetam	0.5–0.7	0.66	0.5–1.5 g every 12 h	0.5–1 g every 12 h	250–750 mg every 12 h	0.5–1 g every 24 h
Levofloxacin	1.1–1.5	0.67–0.87	500 mg every 24 h	100%	250 mg every 24–48 h	250 mg every 48 h
Lisinopril	0.13–0.15	0.80–0.90	5–10 mg every 24 h	100%	50%–75%	25%–50%
Meropenem	0.35	0.65	0.5–1 g every 6 h	500 mg every 6 h	250–500 mg every12 h	250–500 mg every24 h
Metformin[b]	1–4	0.90–1.0	500–850 mg every 12 h	50%	25%	Avoid
Methicillin	0.31	0.25–0.80	1–2 g every 4h	Every 4–6 h	Every 6–8 h	Every 8–12 h
Metoclopramide	2–3.4	0.10–0.22	10–15 mg every 6 h	100%	75%	50%
Metronidazole	0.3–0.9	0.20	7.5 mg/kg every 6 h	100%	100%	50%
Nizatidine	0.8–1.3	0.10–0.15	150–300 mg every 24 h	75%	50%	25%
Ofloxacin	1.5–2.5	0.68–0.80	400 mg every 12 h	100%	200–400 mg every 24 h	200 mg every 24 h
Olmesartan	0.24	0.50	20 mg every 24 h	100%	100%	50%
Oxcarbazepine[c]	0.7–0.8	0.30	300–600 mg every 12 h	100%	75%	50%
Penicillin G	0.3–0.4	0.60–0.85	0.5–4 MU every 6 h	100%	75%	20%–50%
Pentamidine	3–4	0.05	4 mg/kg every 24 h	Every 24 h	Every 24 h	Every 24–36 h
Piperacillin	0.2–0.3	0.75–0.90	3–4 g every 4h	Every 4–6 h	Every 6–8 h	Every 8 h
Quinapril	1.5	0.30	10–20 mg every 24 h	100%	75%–100%	75%
Ramipril	1.2	0.1–0.21	10–20 mg every 24 h	100%	50%–75%	25%–50%
Ranitidine	1.2–1.8	0.80	150–300 mg every 24 h	75%	50%	25%
Sotalol	1.3	0.60	160 mg every 24 h	100%	30%	15%–30%
Sparfloxacin	4.5	0.10	400 mg every 24 h	100%	50%–75%	50% every 48 h
Spironolactone	No data	0.20–0.30	25 mg every 6–8 h	Every 6–12 h	Every 12–24 h	Avoid
Stavudine	0.5	0.40	30–40 mg every 12 h	100%	50% every 12–24 h	50% every 24 h
Tetracycline	0.7	0.48–0.60	250–500 mg every 6 h	Every 8–12 h	Every 12–24 h	Every 24 h
Topiramate	0.6–0.8	0.70–0.97	200 mg every 12 h	100%	50%	25%
Trimethoprim	1–2.2	0.40–0.70	100–200 mg every 12 h	Every 12 h	Every 18 h	Every 24 h
Venlafaxine	6–7	0.05	75–375 mg every 24 h	75%	50%	50%
Vigabatrin	0.8	0.70	1–2 g every 12 h	Every 24 h	Every 48 h	Every 2–3d
Zalcitabine	0.5	0.75	0.75 mg every 8 h	Every 8 h	Every 12 h	Every 24 h

V = volume of distribution; PB = plasma protein binding; fe = fraction excreted unchanged in the urine; GFR = glomerular filtration rate (the range following GFR indicates the use of the dose that corresponds to that range of GFR in patients not on dialysis); a = seizures in end-stage renal disease; b = contraindicated when serum creatinine is >1.5 mg/dl (males) or >1.4 mg/dl (females); c = active metabolite is MHD.

patients who have stage 5 CKD has increased dramatically in the last 10 years.[51-53] This has been accomplished in part by increasing the blood and dialysate flow rates as well as the use of new high flux, large surface area, dialysis filters. Dialyzers composed of synthetic materials (e.g., polysulfone, polymethylmethacrylate, or polyacrylonitrile) readily remove drugs with molecular weights between 1,000 and 5,000 daltons (D), which in the past were likely to be considered non-dialyzable.[49,51] Thus high-molecular-weight drugs such as vancomycin are now extensively cleared by hemodialysis. In addition, significant increases in hemodialysis clearance of 50-100% have been noted for many drugs, especially antibacterial agents that have a molecular weight of less than 1,000 D.[49]

Table 6-4. Factors Affecting the Hemodialyzability of a Drug

		Impact on Dialyzability
Physicochemical and pharmacokinetic drug properties	Molecular weight < 10,000	Increases
	High water solubility	Increases
	High lipid solubility	Decreases
	Increased ionization—anionic	Decreases
	Large volume of distribution	Decreases
	High protein binding	Decreases
	Lower red blood cell partition	Decreases
Mechanical properties of the renal replacement therapy	Larger surface area of dialyzer	Increases
	Higher porosity dialysis membrane	Increases
	Higher dialysate flow rates	Increases
	Higher blood flow rate	Increases

Dosage regimen adjustment strategies for patients receiving hemodialysis

Prospective individualization of drug dosage regimens is recommended for narrow therapeutic range drugs, such as the aminoglycosides, vancomycin, and the multiple others identified in this chapter. Several factors contribute to the complexity of accomplishing this in the CKD patient who is receiving chronic hemodialysis. Of considerable importance is the long turn-around time associated with measurement and reporting of serum concentrations in the ambulatory care setting and the delay in implementing a new dosage regimen since the next dose is almost always given at the end or shortly after HD before the patient has left the dialysis center. Thus, in most ambulatory hemodialysis care situations patients will initially benefit from the recognition that a drug dosage regimen should be adjusted and the implementation of a best practical dosage regimen based on data derived from prior clinical investigations.[44] The data in the second column of Table 6-5 presents recommendations for dialysis dependent CKD patients with a residual CrCl less than 10 ml/min who are receiving intermittent hemodialysis on a thrice weekly schedule. This is the rationale for the every 48–72 hour dosage intervals for many of the agents that are included in the table since drug administration is almost always fixed to be during the last hour of or after the end of the dialysis procedure. These dosage regimens should be used with caution since there is tremendous variability in the clearance efficiency of the over 100 dialysis filters currently available.[49,54,55] Dosage recommendations for hemodialysis patients derived prior to 1995 likely provide an underestimate of patient needs because of the enhanced clearance with newer, more efficient, dialyzers and more aggressive dialysis prescriptions.

For medications that are commonly individualized on the basis of serum concentration guidance, the primary dosage regimen design issues are to avoid administration in the hours immediately before dialysis to minimize excessive removal of "standard doses" of the medication, and the use of simple consistent administration schedules that minimize the need for variable drug doses being administered on non-dialysis as well as dialysis days. For some drugs higher doses have been proposed and evaluated, to facilitate delivery during dialysis, that compensate for the enhanced removal that results from administration during dialysis.[56,57] Although this approach may increase medication cost it may enhance patient compliance and improve the efficiency of the dialysis center. The primary objective for most medications is to design a regimen for administration on dialysis days such that the dose given at the end of dialysis is sufficient to achieve the desired maximum drug concentration. In this setting, the dose to be administered after dialysis ($D_{post\text{-}HD}$) can be calculated as:

$$D_{postHD} = V \times (C_{max} - C_{postHD}) \qquad \text{(Eq. 10)}$$

$$C_{postHD} = C_{preHD} \times (e^{-kt} + e^{-kHDt}) \qquad \text{(Eq. 11)}$$

where V is the patient's estimated volume of distribution for the drug of interest, e^{-kt} is the fraction of drug remaining at the end of the dialysis procedure as a result of the patient's residual total body clearance ($k_{pt} = CL_{pt} \div V$), and e^{-kHDt} is the fraction of drug remaining as a result of elimination by the dialyzer ($k_{HD} = CL_{HD} \div V$). The duration of the dialysis procedure in hours is expressed as t. Values for CL_{pt} can be derived from the drug clearance to renal function relationships in the literature or estimated from the information in Table 6-3, while CL_{HD} values for many dialyzers and dialysis procedures will need to be acquired from reliable literature sources.[47-49]

Alternatively CL_{HD} can be measured for individual patients if a series of serum concentrations are collected using the following approach:[33]

$$CL_{HD} = \left(\frac{C_{art} - C_{ven}}{C_{art}}\right) \times (Qb\,(1 - Hct))$$

Where C_{art} is the concentration of the drug in the plasma entering the dialyzer, C_{ven} is the concentration of the drug in the plasma leaving the dialyzer, Qb is the blood flow through the dialyzer, and Hct is the patient's hematocrit. This information can be used with the measured CL_{pt} using the equation to estimate kHD described in the preceding paragraph to calculate the post HD dose (Eq. 10).

Dosage individualization strategies for patients receiving continuous renal replacement therapies

In contrast to intermittent HD, CRRTs that were developed over the past 15 years have proven to be a viable management approach for hemodynamically unstable patients with or without AKI.[10] Several variants have been developed, and there are currently two primary techniques used in many institutions around the world.[58] Drug removal by continuous venovenous hemofiltration (CVVH) occurs by convection/ultrafiltration, while continuous venovenous hemodiafiltration (CVVHDF), which is more efficient, uses convection/ultrafiltration, and diffusion as the two predominant means for drug removal.

Optimization of drug therapy for patients with AKI is often quite challenging. Interpretation of the limited literature available on drug removal by CRRT in critically ill patients is complicated by the large variation between hemofilters, the individual CRRT prescription being used, and the marked degree of interpatient variability in residual renal function and fluid volume status.[54,59,60] The essential elements that characterize each of the predominant CRRT variants are well described in two recent reviews.[61,62]

Although dosing guidelines based on data derived from *in vitro* experiments or studies in patients with stable stage 5 CKD may not reflect the clearance and volume of distribution in critically ill AKI patients, this may be the only information available for many drugs. Table 6-5 presents drug dosage recommendations for AKI patients with a creatinine clearance less than 10 ml/min who are receiving CVVH or CVVHDF compiled from many sources.[44,54,59,61,62] These recommendations differ from FDA approved product labeling in those situations where more current clinical information was available in the literature.

When there is a need to tightly control patient exposure to a given drug, be it for the enhancement of therapeutic response or the minimization of risk of adverse events, the dosage regimen for patients receiving CRRT can be individually ascertained by adding the estimated or measured drug clearance by CRRT to the patient's residual drug clearance. Once the total clearance is known, the dosage regimen can be projected using the same principles as those described for patients with stable CKD. For example the dosage regimen for

Table 6-5. Dosage Recommendations for Patients Receiving Hemodialysis, CVVH, or CVVHDF

	Dosage Recommendation		
Drug	**HD**	**CVVH**	**CVVHDF**
Acyclovir	2.5–5 mg/kg every 24 h	5–10 mg/kg every 24 h	5–10 mg/kg every 12–24 h
Amantadine	100 mg every 24–48 h	100 mg every 24–48 h	100 mg every 24–48 h
Amphotericin B	0.25–1.5 mg/kg every 24 h	0.25–1.5 mg/kg every 24 h	0.25–1.5 mg/kg every 24 h
Amoxicillin	250–500 every 24 h	ND	ND
Amikacin	IND or 5–7.5 mg/kg every 48–72 h	IND or 7.5 mg/kg every 24–48 h	IND or 7.5 mg/kg every 24–48 h
Ampicillin	1 g every 12 h	1–2 g every 8–12 h	1–2 g every 6–8 h
Ampicillin / Sulbactam	1.5–3 g every 12–24 h	1.5–3 g every 8–12 h	1.5–3 g every 6–8 h
Atenolol	25–50 mg every 48–72 h	25–50 mg every 24 h	25–50 mg every 24 h
Aztreonam	0.5 g every 12 h	1–2 g every 12 h	2 g every 12 h
Benazepril	2.5–10 mg every 12–24 h	5–20 mg every 12–24 h	5–20 mg every 12–24 h
Bisoprolol	2.5–10 mg every 24 h	5–15 mg every 24 h	5–15 mg every 24 h
Cefazolin	15–20 mg/kg every 48–72 h	1–2 g every 12 h	2 g every 12 h
Cefepime	1–2 g every 48–72 h	1–2 g every 12 h	2 g every 12 h
Ceftazidime	1 g every 24 h	1–2 g every 12 h	2 g every 12 h
Ceftriaxone	0.5–1 g every 24 h	1–2 g every 12–24 h	1–2 g every 12–24 h
Cephalexin	250–500 every 24 h	ND	ND
Cidofovir	AVOID	2 mg/kg every 7 d	2 mg/kg every 7 d
Cimetidine	300 every 8–12 h	200 every 12 h	200 every 12 h
Ciprofloxacin	0.2–0.4 g every 24 h	0.2–0.4 g every 12–24 h	0.4 g every 12 h
Clarithromycin	ND	250–500 mg every 12 h	250–500 mg every 12 h
Colistin	1.5 mg/kg every 24–48 h	2.5 mg/kg every 48 h	2.5 mg/kg every 48 h
Daptomycin	4–6 mg/kg every 48–72 h	4–6 mg/kg every 48 h	4–6 mg/kg every 48 h
Didanosine	100 mg every 24 h	200 mg every 12 h	200 mg every 12 h
Enalapril	5–10 mg every 24 h	5–10 mg every 12–24 h	5–10 mg every 12–24 h
Famciclovir	500 mg every 24 h	500 mg every 12 h	500 mg every 12 h
Famotidine	5 mg every 24 h	5–10 mg every 24 h	5–10 mg every 24 h
Fexofenadine	60 mg every 24 h	60 mg every 24 h	60 mg every 24 h
Fluconazole	0.2–0.4 g every 48–72 h	0.2–0.4 g every 24 h	0.8 g every 24 h
Foscarnet	ND	60–80 mg/kg every 48 h	60–80 mg/kg every 48 h
Gabapentin	200–300 mg every 48–72 h	300 mg every 12–24 h	300 mg every 12–24 h
Ganciclovir	0.5 mg/kg every 48–72 h	1.25 mg/kg every 24 h	2.5 mg/kg every 24 h
Gentamicin	IND or 1.5–2 mg/kg every 48–72 h	IND or 1.5–2 mg/kg every 24–48 h	IND or 1.5–2 mg/kg every 24–48 h
Glipizide	1.25–7.5 mg every 24 h	1.25–7.5 mg every 24 h	1.25–7.5 mg every 24 h
Imipenem/ cilastatin	0.25–0.5 g every 12 h	0.5 g every 8 h	0.5 g every 6 h
Lamivudine	1 mg/kg every 24 h	4 mg/kg every 24 h	4 mg/kg every 24 h
Levetiracetam	500–750 every 24 h	250–750 every 12 h	250–750 every 12 h
Levofloxacin	250–500 every 48–72 h	500 every 48 h	500 every 48 h
Meropenem	1 g every 48–72 h	0.5–1 g every 12 h	0.5–1 g every 8–12 h
Metformin	AVOID	AVOID	AVOID
Metoclopramide	5 mg every 6 h	5–10 mg every 6 h	5–10 mg every 6 h
Metronidazole	0.5 g every 8–12 h	0.5 g every 6–12 h	0.5 g every 6–12 h

Table 6-5. (Continued)

Drug	Dosage Recommendation HD	CVVH	CVVHDF
Moxifloxacin	0.4 g every 24 h	0.4 g every 24 h	0.4 g every 24 h
Ofloxacin	200 mg non HD 300 mg HD	300 mg every 24 h	300 mg every 24 h
Piperacillin	4 g every 12 h	ND	ND
Quinapril	2.5 mg every 12–24 h	2.5–5 mg every 12–24 h	2.5–5 mg every 12–24 h
Ramipril	1.25–2.5 mg every 24 h	2.5–5 mg every 24 h	2.5–5 mg every 24 h
Ranitidine	75–150 mg every 24 h	150 mg every 12–24 h	150 mg every 12–24 h
Stavudine	20 mg every 24 h	40 mg every 12 h	40 mg every 12 h
Tazobactam	2.25 g every 8–12 h	2.25–3.75 g every 6–8 h	3.75 g every 6 h
Tetracycline	250–500 every 24 h	ND	ND
Ticarcillin/ clavulanate	2 g every 12 h	2 g every 6–8 h	3.1 g every 6 h
Tobramycin	IND or 1.5–2 mg/kg every 48–72 h	IND or 1.5–2 mg/kg every 24–48 h	IND or 1.5–2 mg/kg every 24–48 h
Topiramate	50 mg every 12 h	100 mg every 12 h	100 mg every 12 h
Trimethoprim/ Sulfamethoxazole	5–15 mg/kg (TMP) every 48–72 h	2.5–7.5 mg/kg (TMP) every 12 h	2.5–7.5 mg/kg (TMP) every 12 h
Vancomycin	IND or 7.5 mg/kg every 48–72 h	IND or 10–15 mg/kg every 24–48 h	IND or 7.5–10 mg/kg every 12 h
Vigabatrin	1–2 g every 48–72 h	1–2 g every 48 h	1–2 g every 48 h
Zalcitabine	0.75 mg every 24 h	0.75 mg every 12 h	0.75 mg every 12 h

IND = individualize because desired concentrations and or pharmacodynamic endpoints may vary markedly. ND = no data available.

cefepime of a patient receiving CVVHDF will be predicated upon the sum of the patient's residual clearance and the clearance associated with CVVHDF, which can be approximated as follows:

If a patient with a CrCl of 10 ml/min is receiving CVVHDF with an AN69 filter at blood, ultrafiltrate, and dialysate flow rates of 200, 12, and 33 ml/min, respectively and is to receive cefepime while on CVVHDF, the patient's residual cefepime clearance (CL_{RES}) can be estimated using the following regression equation relating CrCl and cefepime clearance drawn from the literature.[33] The cefepime clearance of a patient with normal renal function (CrCl of 120 ml/min) would be calculated as:

$$CL_{norm}\ (\text{ml/min}) = [0.96 \times (\text{CrCl})] + 10.9$$

$$CL_{norm} = [0.96 \times 120] + 10.9$$

$$CL_{norm} = 126.1\ \text{ml/min}$$

This patient's cefepime clearance as the result of his residual CrCl value can be calculated similarly:

$$CL_{RES}\ (\text{ml/min}) = [0.96 \times (10)] + 10.9$$

$$CL_{RES} = [0.96 \times (10)] + 10.9$$

$$CL_{RES} = 20.5\ \text{ml/min}$$

The total clearance while on CVVHDF would be the sum of the patient's residual clearance and the cefepime clearance associated with CVVHDF, which can be approximated as follows:

$$CL_{CVVHDF} = [(\text{UFR} + \text{DFR}) \times f_u)] \qquad \text{(Eq. 13)}$$

(where UFR = ultrafiltrate formation rate, DFR = dialysate flow rate, and fu = fraction unbound)

$$CL_{CVVHDF} = [(12 + 33) \times 0.97] = 43.7\ \text{ml/min}$$

$$CL_T = CL_{RES} + CL_{CVVHDF} \quad \text{(Eq. 14)}$$

$$CL_T = 20.5 \text{ ml/min} + 43.7 \text{ ml/min}$$

$$CL_T = 64.2 \text{ ml/min}$$

The dosage adjustment factor would then be:

$$Q = CL_T/CL_{norm}$$

$$Q = 64.2 \div 126$$

$$Q = 0.51$$

For this patient's situation, the normal regimen of cefepime would be 2,000 mg (D_N) every 12 hours (τ_N). If one wanted to maintain D_n at 2,000 mg the extended dosing interval, τ_R would be calculated as:

$$\tau_R = \tau_N/Q$$

$$\tau_R = 12 \text{ hr}/0.51$$

$$\tau_R \approx 24 \text{ hr}$$

It is important to monitor these patients on a continual basis, as dose adjustments will be required if renal function significantly improves or worsens, or if there are prolonged interruptions in the delivery of the CRRT therapy or if it is discontinued.

Conclusion

Patients with AKI or CKD and those receiving intermittent HD or CRRT present many challenges to the clinician as they are at increased risk for adverse events due to accumulation of drugs and/or their active or toxic metabolites. Important therapeutic decisions can be made based on awareness of each patient's functional renal capacity and of the effects of renal disease on drug metabolism, metabolite formation and renal excretion. Clinicians can play a critical role in providing rational drug therapy to these patients making dose adjustments based on renal function using either traditional TDM or empiric methods, assuring avoidance of drugs with toxic metabolites, determining the optimal dose to accommodate immediate post dialysis dosing, and taking responsibility for patient outcomes.

References

1. USRDS 2010 Annual Data Report: Atlas of Chronic Kidney Disease and End-Stage Renal Disease in the United States. Bethesda, MD: National Institutes of Health, National Institutes of Diabetes and Digestive and Kidney Diseases; 2010.
2. Coresh J, Wei GL, McQuillan G, et al. Prevalence of high blood pressure and elevated serum creatinine level in the United States: Findings from the third National Health and Nutrition Examination Survey (1988–1994). *Arch Intern Med.* 2001;161:1207-16.
3. Coresh J, Selvin E, Stevens LA, et al. Prevalence of chronic kidney disease in the United States. *JAMA.* 2007;298(17):2038-47.
4. Brochard L, Abroug F, Brenner M, et al. An official ATS/ERS/ESICM/SCCM/SRLF statement: prevention and management of acute renal failure in the ICU patient. *Am J Respir Crit Care Med.* 2010;181:1128-55.
5. Stevens LA, Coresh J, Greene T, et al. Comparative performance of the CKD Epidemiology Collaboration (CKD-EPI) and the Modification of Diet in Renal Disease (MDRD) Study equations for estimating GFR levels above 60 mL/min/1.73 m^2. *Am J Kidney Dis.* 2010;56(3):486-95.
6. Spruill WJ, Wade WE, Cobb HH. Continuing the use of the Cockcroft-Gault equation for drug dosing in patients with impaired renal function. *Clin Pharmacol Ther.* 2009 Nov;86(5):468-70.
7. Gill J, Malyuk R, Djurdjev O, et al. Use of GFR equations to adjust drug doses in an elderly multi-ethnic group--a cautionary tale. *Nephrol Dial Transplant.* 2007;22(10):2894-9.

8. Melloni C, Peterson ED, Chen AY, et al. Cockcroft-Gault versus modification of diet in renal disease: importance of glomerular filtration rate formula for classification of chronic kidney disease in patients with non-ST-segment elevation acute coronary syndromes. *J Am Coll Cardiol.* 2008;51(10):991-6.
9. Bouchard J, Macedo E, Soroko S, et al. Comparison of methods for estimating glomerular filtration rate in critically ill patients with acute kidney injury. *Nephrol Dial Transplant.* 2010;25:102-7.
10. Dager W, Halilovic J. Acute kidney injury. In: Dipiro JT, Talbert RL, Yee GC, et al., eds. *Pharmacotherapy: A Pathophysiologic Approach.* New York, NY: McGraw Hill; 2011.
11. Lee W, Kim RB. Transporters and renal drug elimination. *Ann Rev Pharmacol Toxicol.* 2004;44:137-66.
12. Masereeuw R, Russel FGM. Therapeutic implications of renal anionic drug transporters. *Pharmacol Ther.* 2010;126:200-16.
13. Westenfelder C, Arevalo G, Crawford P, et al. Renal tubular function in glycerol-induced acute renal failure. *Kidney Int.* 1980;18:432-44.
14. Bricker NS, Klahr S, Lubowitz H, et al. The pathophysiology of renal insufficiency. On the functional transformations in the residual nephrons with advancing disease. *Ped Clin N Am.* 1971;18(2):595-611.
15. Tozer TN. Nomogram for modification of dosage regimens in patients with chronic renal impairment. *J Pharmacokinet Biopharm.* 1974;2:13-28.
16. Dowling TC, Frye RF, Fraley DS, et al. Comparison of iothalamate clearance methods for measuring GFR. *Pharmacother.* 1999;19(8):943-50.
17. Walser M. Assessing renal function from creatinine measurements in adults with chronic renal failure. *Am J Kidney Dis.* 1998 Jul;32(1):23-31.
18. Liu S, Beringer PM, Hidayat L, et al. Probenecid, but not cystic fibrosis, alters the total and renal clearance of fexofenadine. *J Clin Pharmacol.* 2008 Aug;48(8):957-65.
19. Wang ZJ, Yin OQ, Tomlinson B, et al. OCT2 polymorphisms and in-vivo renal functional consequence: studies with metformin and cimetidine. *Pharmacogenet Genomics.* 2008;18(7):637-45.
20. Shu Y, Brown C, Castro RA, et al. Effect of genetic variation in the organic cation transporter 1, OCT1, on metformin pharmacokinetics. *Clin Pharmacol Ther.* 2008;83(2):273-80.
21. Landersdorfer CB, Kirkpatrick CM, Kinzig M, et al. Competitive inhibition of renal tubular secretion of ciprofloxacin and metabolite by probenecid. *Br J Clin Pharmacol.* 2010;69(2):167-78.
22. Dreisbach AW. The influence of chronic renal failure on drug metabolism and transport. *Clin Pharmacol Ther.* 2009;86:553-6.
23. Vilay AM, Churchwell MD, Mueller BA. Drug metabolism and clearance in acute kidney injury. *Crit Care* 2008;12:235.
24. Flockhart DA. Cytochrome P450 Drug Interaction Table. Available at: http://medicine.iupui.edu/clinpharm/ddis/table.asp. Accessed November 11, 2010.
25. Nolin TD. Altered nonrenal drug clearance in ESRD. *Curr Opin Nephrol Hypertens.* 2008;17(6):555-9.
26. Mouton JW, Touzw DJ, Horrevorts AM, et al. Comparative pharmacokinetics of the carbapenems: clinical implications. *Clin Pharmacokinet.* 2000;39(3):185-201.
27. Guevin C, Michaud J, Naud J, et al. Down-regulation of hepatic cytochrome p450 in chronic renal failure: role of uremic mediators. *Br J Pharmacol.* 2002;137(7):1039-46.
28. Dowling TC, Briglia AE, Fink JC, et al. Characterization of hepatic cytochrome p4503A activity in patients with end-stage renal disease. *Clin Pharmacol Ther.* 2003;73(5):427-34.
29. Fleishaker JC. Clinical pharmacokinetics of reboxetine, a selective norepinephrine reuptake inhibitor for the treatment of patients with depression. *Clin Pharmacokinet.* 2000;39(6):413-27.
30. Cerqueira PM, Coelho EB, Geleilete TJ, et al. Influence of chronic renal failure on stereoselective metoprolol metabolism in hypertensive patients. *J Clin Pharmacol.* 2005;45(12):1422-33.
31. Aronson JK. Clinical pharmacokinetics of digoxin 1980. *Clin Pharmacokinet.* 1980;5(2):137-49.
32. Fish DN. Fluoroquinolone adverse effects and drug interactions. *Pharmacotherapy.* 2001;21(10: Part 2):253S-72S.
33. Matzke GR. Drug therapy individualization for patients with renal insufficiency. In: Dipiro JT, Talbert RL, Yee GC, et al., eds. *Pharmacotherapy: A Pathophysiologic Approach.* New York, NY: McGraw Hill; 2011.
34. Gilbert B, Robbins P, Livornese LL Jr. Use of antibacterial agents in renal failure. *Infect Dis Clin North Am.* 2009;23:899-924.
35. Olyaei, AJ, Bennett WM. Drug dosing in the elderly patients with chronic kidney disease. *Clin Geriatr Med.* 2009;25:459-527.
36. Grandison MK, Boudinot FD. Age-related changes in protein binding of drugs: implications for therapy. *Clin Pharmacokinet.* 2000;38(3):271-90.

37. Meijers, BKI, Bammens B, Verbeke B, et al. A review of albumin binding in CKD. *Am J Kidney Dis.* 2008;51:839-50.

38. Chan GL, Axelson JE, Price JD, et al. In vitro protein binding of propafenone in normal and uraemic human sera. *Eur J Clin Pharmacol.* 1989;36(5):495-9.

39. Pritchard JF, Matzke GR, Opsahl JA, et al. Effects of hemodialysis on plasma protein binding of bepridil. *J Clin Pharmacol.* 1995;35(2):137-41.

40. Dowling TC, Murphy JE, Matzke GR, et al. Evaluation of renal drug dosing: Prescribing information and clinical pharmacist approaches. *Pharmacotherapy.* 2010;30(8):776-86.

41. Dettli L. Elimination kinetics and dosage adjustments of drugs in patients with kidney disease. *Prog Pharmacol.* 1977;1:1-34.

42. Verbeeck RK, Musuamba FT. Pharmacokinetics and dosage adjustment in patients with renal dysfunction. *Eur J Clin Pharmacol.* 2009;65:757-73.

43. McEvoy GK, Snow EK. *American Hospital Formulary Service Drug Information.* Bethesda, MD: American Society of Health-System Pharmacists; 2010.

44. Aronoff GR, Bennett WM, Berns JS, et al. *Drug Prescribing in Renal Failure: Dosing Guidelines for Adults and Children.* 5th ed. Philadelphia, PA: American College of Physicians; 2007.

45. Thummel KE, Shen DD, Isoherranen N, et al. Appendix II. Design and optimization of dosage regimens: Pharmacokinetic data. In: Brunton LL, Lazo JS, Parker KL, eds. *Goodman and Gilman's The Pharmacological Basis of Therapeutics.* 11th ed. New York, NY: McGraw-Hill; 2005:1787-888.

46. Joy MS, DeHart RM, Gilmartin C, et al. Clinical pharmacists as multidisciplinary health care providers in the management of CKD: A joint opinion by the Nephrology and Ambulatory Care Practice and Research Networks of the American College of Clinical Pharmacy. *Am J Kidney Dis.* 2005;45(6):1105-18.

47. Secker, BS, Mueller BA, Sowinski KM. Drug dosing considerations in alternative hemodialysis. *Adv Chr Kidney Dis.* 2007;14:e17-e26.

48. Dager WE, King JH. Aminoglycosides in intermittent hemodialysis: pharmacokinetics with individual dosing. *Ann Pharmacotherapy.* 2006;40:9-14.

49. Matzke GR. Status of hemodialysis of drugs in 2002. *J Pharm Pract.* 2002;15:405-18.

50. Schulman G. Clinical application of high-efficiency hemodialysis. In: Nissenson AR, Fine RN, eds. *Handbook of Dialysis Therapy.* 4th ed. Philadelphia, PA: Saunders/Elsevier; 2008:481-97.

51. Agarwal R, Mehrotra R. End-Stage renal disease and dialysis. *NephSAP.* 2010;9:352-414.

52. Cheung AK. Hemodialysis and hemofiltration. In: Greenberg A, Cheung AK, Coffman TM, et al., eds. *Primer on Kidney Disease.* 5th ed. Philadelphia, PA: W.B. Saunders; 2008:82-99.

53. Ahmad S, Misra M, Hoenich N, et al. Hemodialysis apparatus. In: Daugirdas JT, Blake PG, Ing TS, eds. *Handbook of Dialysis.* 4th ed. Philadelphia, PA: Lippincott Williams & Wilkins; 2007:59-78.

54. Heintz BH, Matzke GR, Dager WE. Antimicrobial dosing concepts and recommendation for critically ill patients receiving continuous renal replacement therapy or intermittent hemodialysis. *Pharmacotherapy.* 2009;29:562-77.

55. Mueller BA, Pasko DA, Sowinski KM. Higher renal replacement therapy dose delivery influences on drug therapy. *Artif Organs.* 2003;27(9):808-14.

56. Scott MK, Macias WL, Kraus MA, et al. Effects of dialysis membrane on intradialytic vancomycin administration. *Pharmacotherapy.* 1997;17(2):256-62.

57. Mohamed OHK, Wahba IM, Watnick S, et al. Administration of tobramycin in the beginning of the hemodialysis session: A novel intradialytic dosing regimen. *Clin J Am Soc Nephrol.* 2007;2:694-9.

58. Li AMY, Gomersall CD, Choi G, et al. A systematic review of antibiotic dosing regimens for septic patients receiving continuous renal replacement therapy: do current studies supply sufficient data? *J Antimicrobial Chemother.* 2009;64:929-37.

59. Churchwell MD, Mueller BA. Drug dosing during continuous renal replacement therapy. *Semin Dial.* 2009;22:185-8.

60. Roberts JA, Lipman J. Pharmacokinetic issues for antibiotics in the critically ill patient. *Crit Care Med.* 2009;37(8):2941.

61. Choi G, Gomersall CD, Tian Q, et al. Principles of antibacterial dosing in continuous renal replacement therapy. *Crit Care Med.* 2009;37:2268-82.

62. Pea F, Pierluigi V, Federica P, et al. Pharmacokinetic considerations for antimicrobial therapy in patients receiving renal replacement therapy. *Clin Pharmacokinet.* 2007;46:997-1038.

Section 2: Specific Drugs and Drug Classes

7 Aminoglycosides (AHFS 8:12.02)
John E. Murphy and Kathryn R. Matthias

8 Antidepressants (AHFS 28:16.04)
Patrick R. Finley

9 Newer Antiepileptic Drugs (AHFS 28:12)
William R. Garnett, Jacquelyn L. Bainbridge, Michael D. Egeberg, and Sarah L. Johnson

10 Antirejection Agents (AHFS 92:00)
Christine Formea and Janet Karlix

11 Carbamazepine (AHFS 28:12.92)
William R. Garnett, Jacquelyn L. Bainbridge, Michael D. Egeberg, and Sarah L. Johnson

12 Digoxin (AHFS 24:04)
Robert L. Page II

13 Ethosuximide (AHFS 28:12.20)
William R. Garnett, Jacquelyn L. Bainbridge, and Sarah L. Johnson

14 Unfractionated Heparin, Low Molecular Weight Heparin (AHFS 20:12.04), and Fondaparinux (AHFS 20:12.04.92)
William E. Dager and A. Josh Roberts

15 Lidocaine (AHFS 24:04.04.08)
Paul E. Nolan, Jr. and Toby C. Trujillo

16 Lithium (AHFS 28:28)
Giulia Ghibellini and Stanley W. Carson

17 Phenobarbital (AHFS 28:12.04 and 28:24.04)
Kimberly B. Tallian and Douglas M. Anderson

18 Phenytoin and Fosphenytoin (AHFS 28:12.12)
Michael E. Winter

19 Procainamide (AHFS 24:04)
Robert L. Page II and John E. Murphy

20 Quinidine (AHFS 24:04.04)
Paul E. Nolan, Jr., Toby C. Trujillo, and Christy M. Yeaman

21 Theophylline (AHFS 86:16)
John E. Murphy and Hanna Phan

22 Valproic Acid (AHFS 28:12.92)
Barry E. Gidal

23 Vancomycin (AHFS 8:12.28)
Gary R. Matzke and Jeremiah J. Duby

24 Warfarin (AHFS 20:12.04)
Ann K. Wittkowsky

Chapter 7

John E. Murphy and Kathryn R. Matthias

Aminoglycosides (AHFS 8:12.02)

Aminoglycoside antibiotics have been available for the treatment of infections for over 60 years. They are active against a variety of aerobic Gram-negative and some aerobic Gram-positive bacteria. Agents currently available or that have been studied include amikacin, arbekacin, dibekacin, gentamicin, isepamicin, kanamycin, neomycin, netilmicin, paromomycin, sisomicin, spectinomycin, streptomycin, tobramycin, and trospectomycin. Pharmacokinetic monitoring has generally been focused on amikacin, gentamicin, and tobramycin, which will be emphasized in this chapter.

Usual Dosage Range in Absence of Clearance-Altering Factors

After adjustment to achieve desired concentrations, aminoglycoside dosing regimens vary widely because of interpatient (and to some extent intrapatient) variation in pharmacokinetics. Average adult gentamicin and tobramycin doses of 80 mg every 8 hr (smaller dose-short interval [SDSI] dosing) produce low peak concentrations in many patients.[1-3] Dosing schedules where the entire daily dose is given at one time or a larger dose is given every 24–48 hr (or even at longer intervals) are used frequently now, but these regimens are not included in current prescribing information in package inserts. These large dose-extended interval (LDEI) approaches are generally considered at least equally effective and may be less toxic when used appropriately, as compared to SDSI where smaller doses are given every 8–12 hr. LDEI approaches are generally the standard for most patients now, though certain patient types should still not be dosed in this manner. Further study of SDSI dosing should likely focus on the situations where such dosing might be more beneficial. Continuing development of consensus on who should *not be candidates* for LDEI is warranted.[4,5]

Since the kidneys eliminate aminoglycosides, decreased renal function affects the dosage interval used, but it has less effect on the size of individual doses since high peak and low trough concentrations are generally desired.

Loading dose

The following loading doses (Table 7-1) are used in SDSI approaches for gentamicin and tobramycin. Amikacin doses are approximately 2–4 times these amounts. Loading doses are not administered in the LDEI approach since it is generally expected that the concentration reaches zero or very near zero before the next dose is given. Little or no accumulation therefore occurs and high concentrations are achieved, negating the need for a loading dose with LDEI.

In neonates, a first dose of 2.5 mg/kg generally produces a peak of less than 6 mg/L.[8,10] The therapeutic implications of a low first-dose peak in this population, particularly early in life for "presumed" infections, are not clearly established.[11-14] In adults, treatment failures may occur secondary to a low first-dose peak.

There is also minimal accumulation with traditional SDSI aminoglycoside regimes due to the use of intervals of three or more times the half-life. Thus, the usual reason for loading doses, rapid achievement of concentra-

Table 7-1. Loading Doses for SDSI Approaches[6-9]

Age	SDSI Loading Dose (mg/kg)[a]
Neonates	2.5–4
Infants	2.5–3
Children	2–2.5
Adolescents, adults, geriatrics	1.5–2

[a]See dosing strategies section to determine dosing weight.

tions closer to goal steady state concentrations in situations where accumulation is extensive, does not hold. Rather, loading doses have been recommended by some to ensure achievement of a higher first-dose peak concentration. This may enhance the potential for therapeutic success due to the concentration-dependent killing of organisms by aminoglycosides, though some authors suggest that there is little evidence of a relationship of peak concentration to therapeutic outcome.[3]

Maintenance dose

LDEI and traditional SDSI maintenance doses for gentamicin and tobramycin are shown in Table 7-2. Amikacin doses are approximately 2–4 times these amounts. Arbekacin doses are similar to gentamicin and tobramycin.[10] For LDEI, amikacin doses have tended to be 15 mg/kg for adults and 20 mg/kg in neonates. Uncomplicated urinary tract infections and infections with organisms with low minimum inhibitory concentrations (MIC) may respond to lower doses in all patients.

Reduced renal function necessitates increases in the dosing interval, in some cases beyond the usual recommendation given. Some clinicians use the higher end of the dosing range for more severe infections and vice versa. However, others use target concentrations or the usual averages. The Dosing Strategies section later in the chapter provides more in-depth dosing guidelines.

Dosage Form Availability[9]

Although these drugs are distributed as the sulfate salts, the manufacturers express the doses in terms of drug equivalence; thus, $S = 1$ for calculations.

Pharmacokinetic monitoring of the aminoglycosides is generally reserved for intramuscular (IM) and intravenous (IV) dosage forms. Irrigations or implanted bone cement with aminoglycosides have resulted in nephrotoxicity and ototoxicity, however. Size of dose used, site, contact time, and degree of denuding present are all factors that affect the amount absorbed. One study found very high wound concentrations (median 304 mg/L), but peak serum concentrations tended to be quite low in comparison (median 2.1 mg/L).[29] Caution should be exercised when using high doses in localized sites and serum concentration(s) measurement may be warranted. When used specifically as an intratympanic injection in the treatment of Meniere's disease, ototoxicity may occur, though the incidence is similar to standard medical measures.[30,31] Serum concentrations are negligible.

Topical dosage forms (creams, ointments, and solutions) of gentamicin and tobramycin do not appear to require pharmacokinetic monitoring, although toxicity has been reported.

Inhalation dosing of aminoglycosides, particularly tobramycin, is used in patients with cystic fibrosis. There have also been studies on inhalation dosing of tobramycin for treatment of *Pseudomonas aeruginosa* infections in non-cystic fibrosis patients. Unfortunately, the studies were too small or of too short a duration to recommend this approach before further investigation.[32-34] Studies have shown differences in delivery and bioavailability

Table 7-2. Standard LDEI and SDSI Maintenance Doses and Dosing Intervals[9,11-22]

Age	LDEI Dosage (mg/kg)	SDSI Dosage (mg/kg)
Neonates	3.5–5 every 24–48 hr[a]	2–2.5 every 2–24 hr
Infants	4–6.5 every 24–48 hr	2–2.5 every 8–12 hr
Children	4–8 every 24–48 hr[b]	2–2.5 every 8 hr
Adolescents	4–7.5 every 24–48 hr[b]	1.5–2.5 every 8 hr
Adults	3.5–7 every 24–48 hr[b]	1–1.7 every 8 hr[c]
Younger geriatrics	4–5 every 24–48 hr[d]	1–1.7 every 8–12 hr[d]
Older geriatrics	4–5 every 24–48 hr[d]	1–1.7 every 12–24 hr[d]

[a]Data extrapolated from one study of neonates 24–42 weeks gestation given gentamicin indicated that 4 mg/kg every 24 hr resulted in 13% with troughs ≥2 mg/L [primarily (10%) those with gestational ages ≤36 weeks] and 30% with troughs of 1–<2 mg/L. A dose of 4 mg/kg/36 hr led to no troughs above 2 mg/L, only 5% with troughs ≥1 mg/L, and 75% with troughs <0.5 mg/L. With 4 mg/kg every 48 hr all but 5% had troughs <0.5 mg/L.[23]
[b]Up to 15 mg/kg of tobramycin and 35 mg/kg of amikacin have been used in patients with cystic fibrosis.[24-26]
[c]Every 8 or 12 hr initially for amikacin.
[d]Although larger doses have been used, reduced renal function with aging and the potential for therapy with other toxins should probably lead to a more conservative approach.[27,28]

depending on the devices and concentrations used.[35-40] This dosing, though generally safe in that it usually produces low serum concentrations, has been described in a case report to result in higher concentrations in the presence of renal dysfunction and positive pressure ventilation,[41] and in other cases it has been associated with acute renal failure.[42,43]

Since injectable gentamicin, tobramycin, and amikacin are available in different concentrations (i.e., pediatric and adult), care must be taken to avoid dosing confusion. Neonates have received overdoses when the dose volume for the 10-mg/ml dosage form was inadvertently used with a 40-mg/ml vial.[44] For intramuscular injection of amikacin, gentamicin, and tobramycin, the most concentrated forms are recommended. Short intravenous infusions (0.5–1 hr) and intravenous bolus injections yield pharmacokinetic profiles similar to intramuscular administration.[45] These aminoglycosides have also been administered as intrathecal and intraventricular injections, with the latter generally preferred. Table 7-3 shows the available dosage forms of amikacin, gentamicin, and tobramycin.

General Pharmacokinetic Information

Absorption

Information on the bioavailability of various dosage forms and administration methods is given in Table 7-4.

Distribution

Aminoglycosides exhibit three-compartment distribution when given by intravenous bolus.[48] The central compartment volume is quite small (approximately one-third to one-half of the volumes used for general dosing

Table 7-3. Available Dosage Forms

Drug[a]	Dosage Form
Amikacin sulfate	Injection for IV and IM use:
	50 mg/mL (pediatric) and 250 mg/mL
Gentamicin sulfate	Injection for IV and IM use:
	10 mg/mL (pediatric—available with preservative and preservative free) and 40 mg/mL
	10 mg/mL (60, 80, or 100 mg)
	Injection for IV infusion—premixed in normal saline:
	40, 60, 70, 80, and 100 mg in 50 mL
	60, 80, 90, 100, and 120 mg in 100 mL
	Premixed bone cement:
	500, 1000, and 1200 mg in 40 g acrylic cement
Tobramycin sulfate	Injection for IV and IM use:
	10 mg/mL (pediatric) and 40 mg/mL
	10 mg/mL (20 or 80 mg)
	Injection for IV infusion—premixed in normal saline:
	60 mg in 50 mL
	80 mg in 100 mL
	Injection for IV infusion—lyophilized powder:
	1200 mg in 50 mL vial
	Preservative-free solution for inhalation
	300 mg in 5-ml ampule
	Premixed bone cement:
	1000 and 1200 mg in 40 g acrylic cement

[a]Original brand names for these products (non-bone cement) were Amikin (amikacin), Garamycin (gentamicin), and Nebcin (tobramycin). All are available from multiple sources at present, but recent nationwide shortages in the United States have been reported for amikacin and tobramycin.

Table 7-4. Bioavailability of Dosage Forms (F)

Dosage Form	Bioavailability Percent and Comments
Intravenous	100% (F = 1)
Intramuscular[9,46,47]	Assumed complete (100%), although absorption rate may vary with diminished muscle mass and poor circulation; peak at 30–90 min after dosing
Oral[48,49]	≤5% with absorption usually being ≤1%; diseases of the bowel such as ulcers and inflammatory bowel disease may lead to enhanced absorption. Significant systemic exposure with use of tobramycin for selective gastrointestinal decontamination in acute renal failure patients receiving continuous renal replacement therapy (21% of patients with concentrations ≥1 mg/L)
Intraperitoneal[50,51]	55% (F = 0.55) with absorption being variable; duration of exposure and inflamed peritoneum may affect bioavailability
Intrathecal	Assumed complete (100%); passes into systemic circulation
Intratympanic[31]	Assumed complete (100%); risk of ototoxicity
Topical irrigations[9,52]	Significant with absorption dependent on site and degree of denuding present (e.g., burns, wounds, ulcers, and sinus)
Bladder irrigations[53]	Bladder irrigations in children of 14 mg of gentamicin once or twice daily did not result in detectable serum concentrations
Inhalation or nebulization[35,38-40,54-57]	Negligible, but may lead to absorption of 30% of a dose (concentrations can average 1 mg/L). Peak amikacin concentrations of 5.2–10.2 mg/L after nebulization of high dose amikacin (40–60 mg/kg) were reported in one study[57]
Polymethylmethacrylate beads[58-60] or cement[61-63] and collagen-gentamicin implants[64]	High concentration at site with variable effect on serum/plasma concentration dependent on a variety of factors of the implanted material such as drug concentration, shape, viscosity, total amount of drug, and combination of antimicrobial agents in implanted material along with patient specific factors such as renal function. Significant changes in renal function, including acute renal failure, have been reported after implantation. Intermittent higher systemic exposure can occur usually in first 72 hr post-implantation but low systemic exposure to aminoglycosides can be prolonged (>6 months post implantation)
Hypodermoclysis[65]	100% (F = 1) with time to peak approximately 1.5 hr, peak decreased compared to IM
Liposome encapsulated aminoglycosides[66-68]	Delivered inhaled, intravenously or locally; with IV, concentration in liver and spleen high; renal accumulation similar to normal dosing; persists much longer and leads to higher concentrations but does not appear to increase toxicity

with one-compartment approaches). The first distribution phase, during the first hour, is generally not detected due to its masking by the infusion time (0.5–1 hr) and peak-sampling schedule (0.5 hr after a 0.5 hr infusion, at the end of a 1 hr infusion, 1–1.5 hr after intramuscular injection, or 0.5–1 hr after intravenous bolus).

The late distribution phase involves slow distribution into and redistribution from tissues. This phase has been associated with nephrotoxicity. The final phase half-life, averaging approximately 150 hr, is generally not detected without analysis of urine collected during therapy and for a week or more after therapy is completed.

The volume of distribution (*V*) values for the aminoglycosides are based on population studies. Although some researchers have found subtle differences among the aminoglycosides, the same volume estimate is suggested for each drug. Amikacin, gentamicin, and tobramycin are generally considered to distribute into the extracellular fluid volume. Dehydration, overhydration, and ascites affect the *V*. Patients who are dehydrated may have a smaller actual *V*, while edematous patients may have a larger *V* than predicted. Seriously ill adult patients are reported to have larger *V* per body weight. The average *V* by age group is provided in Table 7-5.

Protein binding

Amikacin, gentamicin, and tobramycin are essentially not bound to plasma proteins. No adjustments in dosing or monitoring are necessary based on changes in plasma proteins.

Table 7-5. Volume of Distribution by Age Group

Age	Volume (V) (mean ± SD)[a,b]
Neonates[8,23,69-72]	0.45 ± 0.1 L/kg[c,d,e]
Infants[73]	0.40 ± 0.1 L/kg[d]
Children[74,75]	0.35 ± 0.15 L/kg[f]
Adolescents[74,75]	0.30 ± 0.1 L/kg[f]
Adults and geriatrics[28,76-78]	0.30 ± 0.13 L/kg[g]

[a]The values used for volumes approximate those in the original studies but are rounded off. Due to the variability in the ages studied, some of these age ranges and values are extrapolated or rounded off from those given in the original studies.
[b]Studies are inconsistent in the reporting of V relative to body weight. Volume may be related to actual, ideal, or an adjusted "dosing" weight; many studies have patients both above and below ideal weight. See the dosing strategies section of the chapter to estimate a patient's dosing weight and V.
[c]Premature neonates tend to have a larger V[7,8,79] (nearer 0.50–0.55 L/kg and perhaps even larger), while full-term neonates tend to have smaller values (nearer 0.40–0.45 L/kg).[6,7,23]
[d]To estimate the V for neonates and infants, actual body weight (ABW) should be used.
[e]One report indicates that the presence of sepsis increases V approximately 14%.[72]
[f]For children and adolescents, ideal body weight (IBW) is suggested for estimating V, although one study found that an adjusted body weight (BWadj) might need to be used in obese children[80] (see dosing strategies section of chapter for determining BWadj—Step 3b).
[g]For adults and geriatrics (and perhaps older children), dosing weight for use in V estimates is determined according to the instructions in the dosing strategies section of this chapter.

Elimination

The aminoglycosides are eliminated by glomerular filtration in the kidney. Studies indicating some non-renal elimination were affected by describing the pharmacokinetics assuming a one-compartment model and the occurrence of early tissue accumulation of drug. Aminoglycoside clearance correlates reasonably well with glomerular filtration rate (GFR) and creatinine clearance (CrCl).

The clearance values provided in Table 7-6 are based on approximately average renal function for each age group. Reduced renal function in any age group results in decreased clearance.

Table 7-6. Average Clearance in Patients with Normal Renal Function

Age	Clearance (Mean ± SD)[a]
Neonates[6,23,69,81,82]	0.05 ± 0.01 L/hr/kg[b,c]
Infants[83]	0.10 ± 0.05 L/hr/kg
Children[74,75,83-85]	0.13 ± 0.03 L/hr/kg
Adolescents[74,75,83,85]	0.11 ± 0.03 L/hr/kg
Adults[86]	0.08 ± 0.03 L/hr/kg
Geriatrics[86,87]	0.06 ± 0.03 L/hr/kg

[a]These values have been rounded off and approximate those found in the original studies.
[b]In newborns, renal function increases rapidly; the glomerular filtration rate tends to double during the first 14 days of life.
[c]In premature or low birth weight neonates, clearance is decreased compared to normal gestation and weight newborns. For this group, the clearance value given minus one standard deviation may be used initially. One study of extremely premature neonates (post-conception age 27.8 ± 1.8 weeks and weight 1.07 ± 0.34 kg) showed clearances of 0.007 to 0.013 L/hr/kg at 24 and 30 weeks post-conception.[79]

Half-life and time to steady state

The half-lives shown in Table 7-7 are associated with calculations that assume one-compartment distribution. The half-life of aminoglycosides may increase by 10%–20% as therapy continues, although in newborns it may decrease due to the natural rapid maturation of renal function in the first few weeks of life.

Dosing Strategies

There are several approaches to determining the initial dose and interval for treating patients with aminoglycosides. These range from use of a standard dose and interval for age (using either LDEI or SDSI approaches), to adjusting standard doses and/or intervals based on the patient's renal function, to estimating the pharmacokinetic

Table 7-7. Half-Life and Time to Steady State by Age Grouping

Age or Condition	Half-Life (Mean ± SD)	Time to Steady State[a]
Neonates[23,48,69,88]	6 ± 2 hr[b]	20–40 hr
Infants[c,73]	4 ± 1 hr	15–25 hr
Children[74,83,85,89]	1.5 ± 1 hr	3–12 hr
Adolescents[7,85,90]	1.5 ± 1 hr	3–12 hr
Adults[86,91]	2 ± 1 hr	5–15 hr
Younger geriatrics[86,91]	3.5 ± 2 hr	8–27 hr
Older geriatrics[86,91]	4 ± 2 hr	10–30 hr
Renal failure[92-94]	40–60 hr[d]	8–12 days
During peritoneal dialysis[95,96]	10–20 hr[d]	
During hemodialysis[92-94]	4.2 ± 2.3 hr	
During continuous renal replacement therapy[97]	8 hr[e]	

[a]Time to steady state assuming five half-lives using +1 SD and −1 SD of the mean t½.
[b]Premature neonates would tend to have t½ = mean +1 SD (8 hr).[23]
[c]In infants and children, half-life tends to decrease with advancing age.
[d]Approximate range.
[e]Approximate range. Arbekacin prescribed to critically ill patients receiving CVVHDF (flow rates of 0.81 L/h [filtrate] and 0.61 L/h [dialysate]).

parameters of the aminoglycoside in the specific patient using population predictors and then determining the dose and interval to produce desired peak and trough concentrations. Many studies have evaluated population values and dosage prediction techniques for the aminoglycosides. One review of SDSI concluded that individualized dosing using Sawchuk-Zaske techniques or Bayesian analysis after monitoring of drug concentrations (particularly with parameters based on the patient population being monitored) provided the best predictive performance.[98] In this section predictive approaches will be discussed.

Estimating pharmacokinetic parameters—dosing weight and volume of distribution

For *adults and geriatrics (and perhaps older children)*, the following algorithm may be followed to determine dosing weight and population volume of distribution.

To determine dosing weight:

Step 1. Patient's actual body weight (ABW) in kilograms is determined.

Step 2. Patient's ideal body weight (IBW) in kilograms is determined (see Introduction).

Step 3. ABW is compared to IBW:

(a) For a patient whose ABW/IBW ratio is 0.9 to <1.2, use of ABW is suggested for dosing weight.

(b) For a patient whose ABW/IBW ratio is ≥1.2 (classified as overweight/obese), calculate and use adjusted body weight (BW_{adj}) for dosing weight.[77,99]

BW_{adj} (kg) = IBW + 0.4 (ABW − IBW)

(c) For a patient whose ABW/IBW ratio is >0.75 to <0.9, IBW is used for dosing weight.[100]

(d) For a patient whose ABW/IBW ratio is ≤0.75 (emaciated), the patient's ABW is multiplied by 1.13 and used for the dosing weight.[77]

To estimate volume of distribution (in liters):

Step 4. The volume of distribution is determined for all patients *except* emaciated and severely ill or trauma patients using:

V = 0.3 L/kg × dosing weight (kg)

Step 5. The volume of distribution is determined for emaciated, severely ill, and trauma patients[77,101-104]:

V = 0.35 L/kg × dosing weight (kg) (emaciated patients)

V = 0.4 L/kg × dosing weight (kg) [severely ill and trauma patients (some studies show even larger V in this group)]

Estimating pharmacokinetic parameters—clearance, elimination rate constant, and half-life

Many methods for estimating the clearance and half-life of aminoglycosides have been evaluated. These methods usually relate the patient's actual or estimated CrCl to the parameter being considered [i.e., the aminoglycoside clearance (CL_{ag}) or the elimination rate constant (k)] and use one-compartment approaches to dosing.[98] Though newer methods to estimate GFR have been developed (see Chapter 1), the use of these GFR estimates to predict drug concentrations have not been studied sufficiently to recommend their use for drug dosing at this time. New methods for calibrating and standardizing serum creatinine measurements have been adopted that are expected to decrease variability in assay results among laboratories but also to decrease values 10% to 20% on average, with resulting increases in estimates of CrCl compared to when many of the studies relating CrCl to drug clearance were conducted. When CrCl estimates are used in the predictors below, it might be assumed that actual aminoglycoside clearance will be slightly less and half-life slightly longer than what is predicted and, therefore, concentrations may be slightly higher than predicted (on average). Drug dosing guidance has been provided for use of estimated CrCl by the National Institutes of Health at http://www.nkdep.nih.gov/professionals/drug-dosing-information.htm.

Estimating clearance

The following equation has been used to relate CL_{ag} to CrCl[105]:

$$CL_{ag} = CrCl$$

Estimating the elimination rate constant (k)

The elimination rate constant can be estimated using two different approaches. In the first approach, CL_{ag} is determined as above and then k is determined using the following equation:

$$k = \frac{CL_{ag}}{V}$$

where CL_{ag} and CrCl are in liters per hr (L/hr), k in hr^{-1}, and V in liters (L). CrCl is converted from milliliters per minute to liters per hour by multiplying by 0.06 [i.e., CrCl (L/hr) = CrCl (ml/min) × 0.06].

In the second approach, CrCl is related to k using the equation below[106]:

$$k = (0.0024 \times CrCl) + 0.01$$

where k is in units of hr^{-1} and CrCl in ml/min.

Estimating half-life

After determining k using either approach above, half-life (t½, in hr) is then estimated by:

$$t\,½ = \frac{0.693}{k}$$

Using estimated pharmacokinetic parameters to determine dose and interval

The parameters (k and V) estimated above are next inserted into the appropriate formula describing the dosing pattern. For example, when multiple short infusions are used for dosing, the equation in Chapter 1 describing this approach to dosing can be manipulated to solve for the dose to provide a target peak concentration after the appropriate interval has been chosen.

Standard approaches, nomograms, and algorithms—SDSI and LDEI

The average *traditional* SDSI doses frequently produce concentrations outside of the accepted traditional therapeutic range.[1,2,107-109] In adults and geriatrics, 1-mg/kg doses often result in steady state peaks of less than 6 mg/L. Use of larger doses reduces the incidence of low peaks but can also increase the incidence of elevated troughs if intervals are not simultaneously lengthened. Individualized dosing using Sawchuk-Zaske[110] or Bayesian dosing methods produce desired concentrations more reliably due to the use of measured concentrations for feedback.[98]

Traditional SDSI approaches—doses and dosing intervals

The dosing interval in all patients receiving SDSI should be approximately two to three times the half-life. The usual doses/intervals are shown in Table 7-2. Obviously, this interval value must be rounded off to a logical time (e.g., 6, 8, 12, 16, 18, 24, 36, or 48 hr). Note that the intervals can be as long as those used in LDEI approaches when patients have poor renal function. Clinicians generally do not use less than 8-hr dosing intervals for aminoglycosides, even in patients with excellent elimination, although in the past some have used 6-hr intervals in patients with very high clearance (e.g., burn patients).[110] Intervals such as 16, 18, and 36 hr should be avoided whenever possible as they can cause confusion in scheduling. The correctness of dosing times should be verified when these unusual schedules are ordered.[111]

For *newborns*, when traditional doses of 2.5 mg/kg are used dosing intervals may be based on birth weight, gestational age, or post conception age.[23] For example, one approach based on weight is as follows: 1000 g or less, interval of 24 hr; 1001–2000 g, interval of 18 hr; and over 2000 g, initial interval of 12 hr.[88] An approach using gestational age and weight suggests 2.5 mg/kg doses with intervals of 24 hr if the newborn is ≤34 weeks of gestation and <1000 g, 18 hr if ≤34 weeks of gestation and >1000 g, and 12 hr if ≥35 weeks of gestation.[8]

LDEI dosing initially was not used in certain populations (e.g., ascites, total body surface area burns >20%, pregnancy, enterococcal endocarditis, end-stage renal disease including dialysis, granulocytopenia, or cystic fibrosis).[19,112] Increasingly, studies have examined its safety and efficacy in more patient types.[18,26-28,113-121] However, several populations may require additional caution when receiving this dosing. These include enterococcal endocarditis (LDEI not recommended), pregnancy, burns, renal failure, meningitis, and osteomyelitis.[4] A simulation study suggested that many burn patients are not candidates for once-daily LDEI because of pronounced variability in the length of the aminoglycoside-free period (i.e., the time when concentrations are essentially zero). The authors suggested monitoring aminoglycoside concentrations if LDEI is used in burn patients to ensure that the aminoglycoside free period is not extensive.[122] Though efficacy studies comparing LDEI and SDSI generally show fairly similar results for many older children and adolescents, additional monitoring may also be necessary as these patients are expected to have a short aminoglycoside half-life.[6] Patients on long-term therapy with aminoglycosides are at particular risk for toxicity, whatever dosing approach is chosen, and should be monitored very carefully and appraised of the risks.

LDEI dosing—doses and dosing intervals

There are essentially four approaches to LDEI dosing found in the literature.

1. The first, and most common in studies, is to give the usual total daily dose (e.g., 80 mg or 1.5 mg/kg given every 8 hr for gentamicin and tobramycin) as a single dose once daily (e.g., 240 mg or 4.5 mg/kg every 24 hr). In some cases the dose or interval is adjusted based on measured concentrations.
2. The second approach is to give a large dose (e.g., 7 mg/kg of gentamicin or tobramycin) designed to produce a certain peak to anticipated MIC ratio (e.g., 10:1), or simply a high concentration. The initial dosing interval is based on the patient's estimated or actual renal function and $t\frac{1}{2}$ (either by using CrCl for adults and children or by gestational age in neonates) and the dose is based on estimated *V*. Intervals are usually 24, 36, or 48 hr, though some protocols may allow even longer. In some approaches it is suggested that the interval be adjusted as needed based on measured concentrations.
3. The third approach is to adjust the LDEI dose that would be used in patients with normal renal function downward based on estimated or actual CrCl, giving the dose once daily in all cases.
4. The fourth approach is individualized dosing that targets desired peak and trough concentrations. This is similar to traditional approaches except that peaks are higher and troughs usually lower.

LDEI dosing in adults

For *adults*, there are many examples in the literature of the first approach to LDEI dosing where the total daily dose is given as a single dose.[123] Studies of these methods generally show equal efficacy and in some cases reduced toxicity to multiple daily dosing. In some cases a trough concentration might be monitored and the interval extended if the concentration is not below 2 mg/L. Another suggested method simply decreases the starting dose by half if the trough is above 1 mg/L.[124]

The authors of the "Hartford" method (an example of the second approach described earlier) suggest the initial use of 7 *mg/kg* of gentamicin or tobramycin (or 15 mg/kg of amikacin) with the interval determined as follows[19]:

CrCl is ≥60 ml/min	Interval = 24 hr
CrCl is 40–59 ml/min	Interval = 36 hr
CrCl is 20–39 ml/min	Interval = 48 hr

The dosing weight is the patient's actual weight unless >20% above IBW (ABW/IBW ratio is >1.2) where the weight would be determined as in step 3b in the dosing strategies section on determining dosing weight and *V*.

In 2,184 patients treated with this method, 77% were dosed every 24 hr, 15% every 36 hr, 6% every 48 hr, and 2% >48 hr.[19] The monitoring approaches and a dosing interval adjustment nomogram for this method can be found in this chapter in the section on monitoring aminoglycoside patients.

Two examples of the third approach described earlier—keeping the dosing once daily and simply adjusting the dose downward based on renal function—are shown in Table 7-8.

An example of the fourth approach, individualized dosing, is found in a study by Rybak and colleagues.[125] Target peak concentrations in this study were 16–20 mg/L for gentamicin and tobramycin for patients with respiratory infections (60–80 mg/L for amikacin) and 10–12 mg/L for patients with other infections (40–60 mg/L for amikacin). Target trough concentrations were <1 mg/L (<4 mg/L amikacin).

A study evaluating predicted concentrations derived from the pharmacokinetic parameters of 116 patients and applied to the Hartford,[19] Example A,[20] and Example B[21] methods (the latter two shown in Table 7-8) yielded the following results.[92] Peaks were ≥10 mg/L in 100% of patients given the 7 mg/kg dose of the Hartford method, while 92% and 81% of those dosed with the Example A and B methods, respectively, achieved these peaks. Troughs were > 1 mg/L in 17%, 14%, and 13% of patients using Hartford, Example A, and Example B dosing approaches, respectfully. Thus, there appears to be a good chance of high peaks and low troughs with all the methods, but still some patients who might have benefited from concentration monitoring, particularly for lengthier regimens.

Table 7-8. Once-Daily Dosing Approaches, Dose Based on CrCl

CrCl, ml/min, Estimated or Actual	Example A[20] Dose, mg/kg[a]	Example B[21] Dose, mg/kg[b]
≥80	5.1	4.0
61–80	3.9	3.25
51–60	3.6	3.25
30–50	3.0	2.5
<30	Not used	2.0

[a]Doses are based on ABW unless ABW/IBW ratio is ≥1.35, then an adjusted body weight (BWadj) is used (see Step 3b in the dosing strategies section on determining dosing weight and *V* for determination of BWadj).
[b]Doses based on ABW.

LDEI dosing in neonates

A review by the Cochrane Neonatal Group of the National Institute for Child Health and Human development on once versus multiple daily dosing of gentamicin for suspected or proven sepsis in neonates found that there was, "insufficient evidence from the currently available RCTs (*randomized controlled trials*) to conclude whether a 'once a day' or 'multiple doses a day' regimen of gentamicin is superior in treating proven neonatal sepsis."[126] However, the authors concluded that the pharmacokinetic outcomes of LDEI were superior (higher peaks and avoidance of "toxic" trough levels) and that there is no difference in nephrotoxicity or auditory toxicity. They concluded that LDEI may be superior in treating neonatal sepsis in neonates more than 32 weeks in gestation.

For *neonates*, a variety of dosing methods have been proposed. Four are described below.

Method 1—Pharmacokinetic data generated from studies of tobramycin dosing in a large group of neonates were used to generate the LDEI dosing recommendations shown in Table 7-9.[128]

Using the recommendations in Table 7-9 and data from two studies, extrapolated predictions found that peaks greater than 5 mg/L would occur in more than 90% of the neonates. Troughs above 2 mg/L would be very rare, and troughs <1 mg/L would occur in the majority (more than 70%).[127,128]

Method 2—The authors of method 2 (shown in Table 7-10) suggest using decreasing mg/kg doses and shortening the interval based on a newborn's (first week of life) gestational age.[129] The authors of method 1 questioned the validity of certain of the modeling approaches for development of method 2.[130]

Method 3—The issue of dosing in *very low birth weight neonates* (600 g to 1500 g) was evaluated in 58 first week of life newborns.[131] The authors tested 24-hr regimens with lower doses and 48-hr regimens with larger doses and found that the optimal interval for producing desired concentrations was 48 hr. The 48-hr doses studied were *5 mg/kg in 1001–1500* g babies and *4.5 mg/kg in 600–1000* g babies. The authors cautioned that a 36-hr interval might be more appropriate for some neonates since 13% of those on 48-hr dosing had troughs <1 mg/L for over 24 hr before the next dose, suggesting the need for measuring trough concentrations in these groups.

Method 4—Another group has proposed a gentamicin dosing algorithm for *neonates* in the first 10 days of life that targets a 24-hr area under the curve ($AUC_{0\text{-}24}$) of 87.5 mg/L × hr.[132] The algorithm was based on pharmacokinetic data from 139 neonates given gentamicin. The daily dose is determined by the equation:

24-hr gentamicin dose (mg) = [0.441 + (0.0945 × gestational age)] × birth weight

where gestational age is in weeks and birth weight in kg.

Table 7-9. Method 1 Dosing Guidelines for Neonates[128]

Gestational Age (weeks)[a]	Dose (mg/kg)	Interval (hr)
<32	4	48
32–36	4	36
>36	4	24

[a]These authors had originally suggested a slightly different dosing approach (the only difference being modification of the every 36 hr dosing to be gestational age 32–37 weeks).[127]

Table 7-10. Method 2 Dosing Guidelines for Neonates[129]

Gestation Age (weeks)	Dose (mg/kg)	Interval (hr)
<30	5	48
30–34	4.5	36
>34	4	24

A study using pharmacokinetic data from 293 newborns ≤1 week of age to simulate peak and trough gentamicin concentrations from the dosing recommendations for each of the methods above concluded that all "would likely yield acceptable peak concentrations as well as trough concentrations of ≤1 mg/L for at least 50% of patients."[13] They suggested that it might be sufficient to monitor only trough concentrations when these protocols were used. Simulated peaks were ≥5 mg/L in at least 97% of patients for all the methods, while method 4 had the greatest percentage of troughs ≥2 mg/L (17%), compared to 8% or less for the others.

LDEI dosing in children

A meta-analysis of 24 eligible studies of LDEI (termed once-daily dosing or ODD) vs. SDSI use in children found consistent trends favoring LDEI in terms of lower clinical failure rate, microbiological failure rate, and combined clinical and microbiologic failure rate, though the differences were not statistically significant.[16] No significant differences were found in primary nephrotoxicity (increased serum creatinine or decreased CrCl) though LDEI was significantly better in avoiding secondary nephrotoxicity outcomes (urinary excretion of proteins or phospholipids). Finally, though reporting on ototoxicity outcomes was somewhat incomplete in the studies, the rates were very low in both arms (LDEI and SDSI) and there was no significant difference noted. These results led the authors to conclude "the available randomized evidence supports the general adoption of once-daily dosing (ODD) of aminoglycosides in pediatric clinical practice."[16] A letter to the editor discussing the previous outcomes pointed out that there are remaining gaps in knowledge that should be addressed before the authors could "confidently recommend universal change."[133] The gaps included knowledge about "(1) the incidence of ototoxicity, (2) the appropriate dose (*which varied from 4 to 7.5 mg/kg per 24 hr in included trials*), and (3) the role and appropriate mode of therapeutic drug monitoring with EIAD (*extended interval aminoglycoside dosing*)..."[133]

The authors of the meta-analysis responded that they disagreed that the evidence did not support universal change and pointed out that the original SDSI dosing approaches were developed based on no evidence as well.[134] They also noted that there was no evidence suggesting that SDSI is indicated in any subgroups (e.g., cystic fibrosis, neonates) either and that "perpetuating emphasis on spurious subgroup differences is only likely to inappropriately delay the wider adoption of single daily dosing." Finally, they noted "single daily dosing translates to lower trough values and should simplify the need for monitoring..."

In *children* there have been a number of LDEI regimens suggested and studied. One method is shown in Table 7-11 from a study of 90 patients one month to 12 years of age with urinary tract infection given once daily gentamicin.[135]

A review of 13 studies describing once daily dosing of gentamicin in infants and children found that, based on concentrations that resulted, these approaches were theoretically more efficacious with no higher toxicity than standard dosing approaches.[136] The daily dose used was 4 to 5 mg/kg in 11 of the studies and 7.5 mg/kg in one. The 13th study was the method described above and shown in Table 7-11.[135] As would be expected, peaks are higher and troughs lower in the once-daily groups.[136] Troughs exceeded 2 mg/L in 5% to 55% of the standard three times daily dosing studies as compared to 0% to 24% of the once-daily groups. The latter result of up to 24% with troughs greater than 2 mg/L in the LDEI approach is a reminder that some patients will need concentration monitoring.

LDEI dosing summary

LDEI dosing approaches may provide rapidly effective concentrations that can maximize the killing of bacteria without enhancing the risk of toxicity and may minimize or prevent the development of adaptive resistance in the bacteria. They may also reduce the need for concentration monitoring, decreasing these and other costs

Table 7-11. LDEI Once-Daily Dosing Guidelines for Children[135]

Age	Dose (mg/kg)	Interval (hr)
1 mo–<5 yr	7.5	24
5–10 yr	6	24
>10 yr (to 12 yr)	4.5	24

associated with more frequent dosing (e.g., additional administration costs).[137] Further, LDEI approaches can make treatment at home or at day treatment facilities more feasible, allowing some patients to leave hospital settings. LDEI approaches should not be used in all patient types however, until evidence supports at least equal efficacy and safety.

The variation in individual pharmacokinetic outcomes with LDEI approaches and the variation in suggestions for dosing and intervals suggest that doses may still need to be individualized using concentration monitoring, particularly for extended treatment regimes. Additional research to determine optimum LDEI regimens, therapeutic ranges, and therapeutic monitoring strategies would be helpful.

Therapeutic Ranges

SI units have been reported for several aminoglycosides but their use worldwide is rare. Thus, all drug (serum or plasma) concentrations are expressed in milligrams per liter (mg/L) in this chapter.

Though traditional SDSI approaches to dosing (i.e., 1–1.5 mg/kg every 8-hr or 12-hr) are used less frequently, there are still groups of patients where these intervals and doses are recommended. With traditional SDSI approaches for the treatment of *pneumonia,* peak concentrations of gentamicin or tobramycin—drawn approximately 0.5 hr after a 0.5-hr infusion or at the end of a 1-hr infusion—should be greater than 7 mg/L.[138] Trough concentrations—drawn approximately 0.5 hr or less before the next dose—should be 1–2 mg/L.[1,48] With amikacin, peak concentrations should be greater than 28 mg/L,[136] and trough concentrations should be 4–8 mg/L.[1,48] For *other infections*, gentamicin and tobramycin peak concentrations of greater than 5 mg/L[139] and trough concentrations between 0.5 and 2 mg/L are recommended.[122]

With LDEI *dosing* approaches, the peak concentration desired varies. Doses most often recommended in adults range from 4 to 7 mg/kg, which would produce peak concentrations of approximately 13–23 mg/L in average patients. Recommendations for children have been similar with a range of 4–8 mg/kg every 24-hr.[16,114] Patients with cystic fibrosis have received 15-mg/kg doses that produce peaks as high as 40 mg/L.[24] Though some authors advise against use of LDEI in cystic fibrosis patients,[114] a recent RCT showed equal efficacy and perhaps less nephrotoxicity (in children) with LDEI dosing.[121]

The desired trough concentration varies depending on the approach. The Hartford method assumes that the aminoglycoside concentration drops to zero 4 hr or more before the next dose.[19] Others suggest less than 1 mg/L.[125] For neonates receiving LDEI doses of 3.5–5 mg/kg of gentamicin and tobramycin every 24 hr, the trough may not go below 1 mg/L for many patients.[13,23,128,131,140,141] It is unknown whether this presents a greater risk of toxicity, although at least one study shows no apparent increase in risk.[142] However, the often brief duration of therapy for neonates and adults (5 days or less) may obscure the potential for toxicity that could occur if these doses are continued for a longer period. Greater caution should always be used in patients who will receive aminoglycosides longer than 5 days, so it is prudent to ensure the lowest possible trough concentrations. Conversely, in low birth weight newborns given 4.5–5 mg/kg every 48-hr, a small percentage of patients (13%) will be below 1 mg/L for more than 24 hr.[131] Whether this represents a higher risk of therapeutic failure or not needs to be examined as the post-antibiotic effect (PAE) seen with aminoglycosides is 6 hr or less.

In SDSI approaches, patients of very advanced age (and consequent reduced renal function) and those with diminished renal function due to other causes, may have received once daily-dosing of traditional sized aminoglycoside doses to keep peaks of 5–8 mg/L and troughs of <2 mg/L. If these same patients are given LDEI and their interval is not extended beyond 24 hr, the risk of toxicity increases.[28] This issue is critical with LDEI dosing approaches, particularly if the interval is fixed at once daily no matter what the patient's renal function might be. The advantages seen in some studies with LDEI in terms of decreased toxicity are likely due to having very low to nonexistent troughs.[143] Extrapolating the benefits of LDEI on a once-daily dosing basis to those who would have received traditional doses at extended intervals should probably not be done.

It has been suggested for traditional dosing approaches that the peak aminoglycoside concentration to MIC ratio should be greater than 4:1 and preferably greater than 8:1.[144,145] The likelihood of success appears to increase with higher values since the aminoglycosides demonstrate concentration-dependent killing. This characteristic of aminoglycosides is exploited in LDEI dosing approaches. When a favorable peak to MIC ratio cannot be attained, synergistic agents or another antibiotic with good organism sensitivity should be used.

The Hartford LDEI dosing approach using 7 mg/kg for gentamicin and tobramycin was based on the assumption of need for a 10:1 peak to MIC ratio for best results and assumes an MIC of 2 mg/L for organisms.[19]

Others have made similar dosing suggestions.[114] The success of other LDEI approaches using lower doses and the fact that some organisms have lower MICs should lead clinicians and researchers to consider regimens that take advantage of knowledge of the actual MIC to adjust dose size. Since organisms sometimes demonstrate different levels of susceptibility to the various aminoglycosides, it is also conceivable that using the aminoglycoside to which the organism is most susceptible could allow for use of lower doses. Since total dose exposure appears to relate to toxicity, use of the lowest effective dose is desirable.

Therapeutic Monitoring

Suggested sampling times and effect on therapeutic range

Peak aminoglycoside concentrations usually should be drawn 0.5 hr after a 0.5-hr infusion or less than 15 min after a 1-hr infusion for consistency of evaluation among patients, sites, and studies. The true peak occurs precisely at the end of the infusion. However, to avoid possible pre-distribution values and unrelated problems in blood drawing times, these recommendations have been generally adopted. If doses are given as bolus injections, *peak* concentrations should be drawn 1 hr after the injection.

The true *trough* aminoglycoside concentration occurs precisely before the next infusion or bolus begins (i.e., if dosage interval 12 hr the trough concentration would occur at 12 hr after start of previous dose but prior to next dose). Trough aminoglycoside concentrations are usually scheduled for 30 min or less before a dose assuming that previous dose and next dose are administered per prescribed dosing interval (i.e., if the next dose is administered 3 hr late a concentration measured at 30 minutes prior to that dose would be lower than the trough concentration on the regular schedule). Again, unrelated delays in sample collection and the need for consistency in the evaluation of efficacy and toxicity lead to the recommendation to check the trough approximately 30 min before the next dose.

When peak and trough concentrations are not measured at the correct time, the concentrations at the correct times should be estimated using the measured concentrations to determine whether the dosing regimen is meeting desired concentration goals.

Serial collection refers to multiple sampling within a dosage interval, along with a sample pre-dose if the sampling interval is not after the first dose. Drug concentration measurements should be collected approximately one half-life apart for improved accuracy (to reduce the impact of assay error). A number of studies have examined the accuracy of using four versus three versus two versus one concentration measurement.[146-148] Recommendations vary (three versus two versus one) and cost considerations as well as patient discomfort are obviously important. For traditional SDSI dosing, two concentrations continue to predominate monitoring suggestions, while for LDEI many recommendations are for one measurement. Others suggest more traditional approaches for LDEI where a "peak" is drawn at some point in the hour or so after a dose (fairly similar to traditional "peak" measurements) with a second concentration measured approximately two estimated half-lives later (usually 6–12 hr). Doses and intervals may then be individualized to ensure achievement of a trough concentration of zero or near zero. Others recommend that no concentration measurements are needed when LDEI is used in patients with normal renal function who do not have confounding factors.[127,149]

Bayesian approaches tend to enhance the accuracy of subsequent dose adjustments when fewer concentrations are measured. However, inaccurate information about dose and sample collection timing can make any concentration report problematic. Varying the definition of when peak concentrations are to be drawn will affect the desired concentrations. These times must be standardized to ensure appropriate and consistent dosing within and among various institutions.

Concentration measurement frequency

Monitoring of aminoglycoside concentrations helps to ensure therapeutic peak concentrations (though of reduced necessity when large doses are used), which enhances the likelihood of clinical response, and to reduce the possibility of toxicity. When SDSI approaches were the norm, it was argued that aminoglycoside concentrations were monitored too soon and too often based on the number of patients who have short-term therapy (4 days or less), who do not exhibit toxicity despite elevated aminoglycoside concentrations, and who survive despite "subtherapeutic" concentrations.[150] Many authors still support the value of measurements, while some deny the value, and others suggest reducing the number of measurements around a dose or the total frequency of measurement.[19,151-153] A study published in 2005 found an association between pharmacist-managed aminoglycoside therapy and improvements in health care and economic outcomes for Medicare patients receiving these drugs.[154] This suggests that monitoring concentrations and adjusting doses to achieve desired concentrations improves these outcomes.

Certain patients may not derive benefit from having aminoglycoside concentrations measured, and clinicians should evaluate the cost to benefit for each patient.[152,155,156] In a patient whose risk of death from infection is significant or the risk of toxicity high, the assurance of adequate concentrations would appear to be worthwhile.

Initial concentration measurement

If a course of SDSI aminoglycoside therapy is planned (3 or more days), peak and trough concentration determinations can enhance the potential for adequate therapy. These measurements should be obtained early in treatment (first or second day) to ensure adequate peak concentrations or to allow for early dosage adjustment to achieve target concentrations. A study of burn patients demonstrated rapid achievement of therapeutic steady state concentrations when first dose measurements were used to guide therapy.[157] Patients also had fewer dosing changes than with conventional dosing where concentrations were not measured early in therapy. Thus, early assessment has utility if it is known that a full course of therapy is fairly certain. Unless a patient has considerably reduced renal function or their intervals are shorter than 8 hr, steady state conditions are usually in place by the second dose. A study in neonates showed that early measurements after a loading dose led to fewer dose adjustments, fewer concentration measurements, and more rapid attainment of desired concentrations than with standard dosing protocols where concentrations were measured later.[158] In neonates it has also been shown that pharmacokinetic parameters do not change sufficiently between day 2 of life compared to days 3 or 4, so early monitoring in a course of therapy for these patients is acceptable when a full course of therapy is planned.[82] Whether other approaches to monitoring would lead to similar therapeutic outcomes and fewer measurements of concentrations is unknown.

Recommendations for initial monitoring of LDEI dosing generally suggest measurements on the first or second day of treatment. As mentioned previously, it has also been suggested that no monitoring is necessary if the patient has normal renal function, no confounding factors, and therapy will be for 5 days or less.[149] A study evaluating the utility of TDM in neonates given LDEI in the first week of life demonstrated no improvement in prediction of final dosing interval over model-based predictions, leading the authors to suggest that there is little value in monitoring concentrations.[132] Conversely, another study with a fairly small sample size showed that patients on LDEI who were monitored and had doses adjusted had decreased nephrotoxicity.[159]

Follow-up concentration measurements

The need to recheck aminoglycoside concentrations depends on several factors.

- *The duration of therapy is extended.*
- *Serum creatinine (or other measure of significant change in renal function) rises or falls considerably.*
- *More aggressive dosing (e.g., shorter intervals with higher troughs or very high peaks) is used or initial troughs do not reach target concentrations on* LDEI. Rechecking of the trough (at least) would be necessitated by a small rise in serum creatinine (e.g., ~ 20%) in these cases. However, if the targeted trough based on initial serum concentrations were approximately 1 mg/L or less for traditional dosing, small changes in serum creatinine would not usually indicate significant increases in the trough concentration so the need for dosage adjustment would not be as likely.
- *Unexpected values result.* In health systems without well-developed procedures for ensuring the correct timing of concentration measurements, the potential for error is high, particularly if the dose times and collection times are not reported to the clinician. Peaks that are drawn late will be lower than anticipated, and troughs drawn early will be higher. The times of dose administration and blood sampling are important. When unexpected results are obtained and the need to know the concentrations is considered to be high, concentrations should be redrawn with strict instructions as to the time of dose, duration of infusion, and sampling times for both the peak and trough. If only one concentration appears inaccurate, it should be the one to be repeated. As a rule, all orders for aminoglycoside concentration measurements should be written with strict timing instructions unless a scheduling service is provided for ordered drug concentrations.

Other approaches to monitoring

After initiating therapy using the Hartford method (explained in dosing strategies section in this chapter), a single concentration measured between 6 and 14 hr after a dose is plotted on Figure 7-1.[19] The concentration result suggests adjustments to therapy if the place it falls does not represent the current dosing interval.

In a follow-up report, the authors suggested discontinuation of monitoring concentrations in their institution for "patients: (a) receiving 24-hr dosing regimens, (b) without concurrently administered nephrotoxic agents (e.g., amphotericin, cyclosporine, vancomycin), (c) without exposure to contrast media, (d) not quadriplegic or amputee, (e) not in the intensive care unit, and (f) <60 years old."[149] Adoption of these suggestions at their institution yielded extrapolated savings of >$100,000/year (value in 1995 dollars) for their 600-bed, tertiary-care hospital and did not demonstrate an increase in nephrotoxicity (ototoxicity was not evaluated).[149]

In one evaluation of monitoring of once-daily aminoglycoside dosing, the author suggested that there is little evidence that can stand up to critical appraisal for differences in outcomes or toxicity between LDEI and SDSI and that extrapolation of need for peak concentration monitoring from SDSI to LDEI is not valid based on evidence.[160] The author further suggested that there is little evidence to suggest a need for a peak of 10 times the MIC and concluded with the following recommendations. First, monitor the patient for efficacy (e.g., temperature, white blood cell count, how the patient feels, etc.) and toxicity outcomes, particularly auditory and vestibular as they are the most life altering for patients. Second, tell patients who are to receive the drugs for more than a couple of days about the ototoxicity risks and explain the early symptoms such as "tinnitus, loss of hearing, a sense of fullness in the ears, headache, nausea and vomiting, giddiness, lightheadedness, vertigo, nystagmus and ataxia." Clinicians should then ask the patient about these daily and discontinue the aminoglycoside if at all possible if the symptoms occur and cannot be attributed to another cause. Third, serum creatinine can be monitored to assess whether renal toxicity is occurring, and finally, "every attempt should be made to minimize the duration of aminoglycoside therapy."[160]

Assay issues

Although assay quality for aminoglycosides is good, some variation exists between methods and laboratory quality should be evaluated.[161] Assay errors may be more important when the trough (i.e., low) concentration is used to adjust doses, leading some to suggest sampling earlier in the interval.[162] Other factors can affect assay

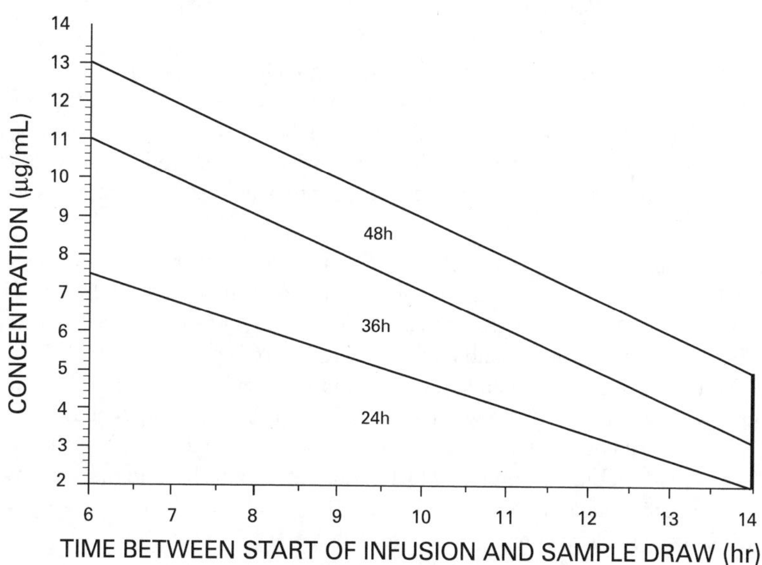

Figure 7-1. Nomogram for concentration monitoring and interval adjustment of gentamicin and tobramycin at 7 mg/kg.

Source: *Reproduced with permission from the American Society of Microbiology.*

results. One study showed differences in peak (but not trough) concentrations of gentamicin and tobramycin when serum concentrations were compared to samples collected with sodium citrate (12% decrease primarily due to dilution), EDTA (5% decrease), and heparin (17%–22% depending on heparin concentration).[163] These interactions might be more important in LDEI situations. Though not an assay issue per se, one report documented the potential for erroneously high tobramycin concentrations when samples were taken by finger stick in a patient whose hands were contaminated with drug after inhalation of nebulized tobramycin.[164]

Summary of aminoglycoside concentration monitoring

It seems reasonable to assume that patients treated appropriately using either larger traditional doses or LDEI approaches with adjustment of dosing interval based on renal function will have sufficiently high aminoglycoside peak concentrations to improve the chance of therapeutic success, unless the organism is resistant. This assumption should reduce the need to monitor peak concentrations. Thus, suggestions to avoid measuring concentrations early in therapy for such patients who have normal renal function seem reasonable. However, serum creatinine should be followed in such a setting. For therapy that will be extended beyond a few days an aminoglycoside concentration measurement is suggested. Furthermore, confounding factors such as concomitant nephrotoxins, impaired physiology (e.g., ascites, burns, advanced age, or early age), or changing serum creatinine should signal the need for more aggressive monitoring.

Pharmacodynamic Monitoring

Concentration-related efficacy

Much of the work on concentration related efficacy occurred when the aminoglycosides were given using SDSI approaches (i.e., every 8 hr or 12 hr). Moore and colleagues determined that patients with bacteremia responded better when peak gentamicin or tobramycin concentrations were above 5 mg/L and when peak amikacin concentrations were above 20 mg/L.[139] They also found that peaks of all three agents needed to be higher for patients with Gram-negative pneumonia (7 mg/L for gentamicin and tobramycin and 28 mg/L for amikacin).[138] Binder and colleagues found a 71% response rate in febrile immunocompromised patients with hematologic malignancies whose gentamicin or tobramycin peak was >4.8 mg/L but only 30% response if the peak was ≤4.8 mg/L.[165]

Deziel-Evans and colleagues showed that peak concentration to MIC ratios might be a better predictor of success.[144] Ratios of 4:1 or more improved survival rate. Others have shown improvement if the ratio is at least 3:1 for infections with Gram-negative organisms.[166]

Moore and colleagues also observed a graded dose-response effect with peak to MIC ratios and showed that the likelihood of success increased as the peak to MIC ratio increased.[145] With a ratio of less than 2:1 as unity, the relative odds of clinical response were 4.35 times higher at a peak to MIC ratio of 6–8:1 and 8.41 times higher at a ratio of 10:1 or more. These results were supported by a study of patients with nosocomial pneumonia where a 10:1 ratio in the first 2 days of treatment predicted a 90% probability of temperature and leukocyte reduction.[167]

Per the Clinical and Laboratory Standards Institute recommendations for antimicrobial susceptibility testing, MIC values of 16 mg/L or higher for gentamicin and tobramycin and 64 mg/L or higher for amikacin are considered resistant.[168] It has been suggested that organisms should be considered resistant at gentamicin and tobramycin MICs of 4 mg/L or higher and amikacin MICs of 16 mg/L or higher.[145,146] However, if a peak to MIC ratio of at least 4:1 is desired, gentamicin and tobramycin peak concentrations of 16 mg/L would be required for an organism with an MIC of 4 mg/L. Prior to LDEI dosing, clinicians would have been hesitant to use aminoglycoside doses that could produce such concentrations. Since the goal of some LDEI methods is a 10:1 ratio, a peak of 40 mg/L would be required, which represents a value beyond the majority of LDEI dosing approaches. The use of additional antibiotics with synergistic effect may enhance the potential for successful outcome when organisms are relatively resistant to aminoglycosides.

Concentration- or exposure-related toxicity

Aminoglycosides cause nephrotoxicity, ototoxicity (vestibular and cochlear), and neuromuscular toxicity. It is possible that LDEI is less toxic than SDSI due to saturable uptake of aminoglycosides in the proximal renal tubule cells and the inner ear. One study showed that enzyme markers of nephrotoxicity were lower with once daily vs. multiple daily dosing despite higher daily doses.[169] It is not clear however, whether LDEI is less ototoxic than SDSI.[170]

Nephrotoxicity has been related to a number of factors, including excessive trough concentrations, daily area-under-the curve (AUC_{0-24}) exposure, prolonged drug exposure (including low-dose), and co-administration with other nephrotoxic agents.[41,125,171-173] The exact relationship has been vigorously debated, but it is generally accepted that in SDSI approaches, troughs of gentamicin and tobramycin should be as low as possible (<2 mg/L) and that troughs of amikacin should be <8 mg/L, if possible. With a number of LDEI dosing approaches, the goal is to have the trough reach <0.1 mg/L for several hours before the next dose is given.

Increased rates of nephrotoxicity were reported in one study with LDEI twice daily dosing versus once daily dosing (15.4% versus 0%, respectively) potentially due to the increased AUC_{0-24}.[125] The predicted probability of nephrotoxicity was 50% if LDEI twice-daily and once-daily dosing prescribed with an AUC_{0-24} of approximately 130 and 750 mg•hr/L, respectively (60 and 675 mg•hr/L if concurrent vancomycin therapy).[125]

Renal function must be monitored in patients receiving aminoglycosides. Factors such as decreased renal function and concomitant treatment with other nephrotoxins increase the incidence of nephrotoxicity. Fortunately, most nephrotoxicity resolves after therapy is discontinued due to the ability of the kidneys to regenerate tubules.[174] Serum creatinine should be monitored at the beginning of therapy and routinely throughout treatment. The frequency of monitoring varies according to the patient's stability.

Though not generally considered an appropriate reason to recommend TDM, litigation associated with aminoglycoside therapy may be prevented or at least reduced by monitoring serum creatinine and aminoglycoside concentrations and by dosage adjustment to provide target concentrations in the generally accepted therapeutic range. More important of course, patients may have a greater likelihood of successful treatment without toxicity.

In general, serum creatinine should be monitored daily in any aminoglycoside patient whose serum creatinine varies by about 25% or more between measurements. For patients with stable measurements, serum creatinine may be monitored approximately every 3 days. Renal dysfunction associated with aminoglycosides can take several days to manifest as rising serum creatinine; therefore, it may be useful to check serum creatinine 2–3 days after treatment is completed in some cases. Since reductions in renal function tend to improve however, this is unnecessary for most patients. In the presence of other factors that may affect renal function (e.g., treatment with other nephrotoxins or hypotensive episodes), it is suggested that serum creatinine should be monitored more frequently (daily to every other day).

Various urine tests and BUN also can be used to monitor renal function. Though not suggested for routine monitoring, urine can be tested for, among other things, decreasing specific gravity (indicating reduced ability to concentrate urine), excretion of protein, cells, and casts and fractional excretion of sodium, potassium, magnesium, and uric acid.[174] Although an increase in BUN may indicate decreasing renal function, it can also be caused by other factors. Diminished urine output over time relative to intake of fluid may also be a sign of decreasing renal function.

One study of LDEI dosing showed timing of dosing as an independent risk factor for nephrotoxicity.[112] Patients receiving their dose during midnight to 7:30 a.m. had a higher incidence of nephrotoxicity. These findings have led some authors to suggest that after the first dose, which must be given as soon as possible in sick individuals even if it must be given during the night (or resting period), further LDEI doses should be switched to administration in the morning or early afternoon (active period).[175] There is evidence that liver disease and biliary obstruction are associated with increased potential for nephrotoxicity.[176,177]

Ototoxicity has been related to prolonged drug exposure and can be monitored by vestibular and auditory tests.[178,179] These tests are, however, notoriously difficult to use in many settings. Symptoms of ototoxicity include dizziness, vertigo, tinnitus, roaring in the ears, and hearing loss. When practical, patients should be questioned regarding such symptoms periodically. Deafness is usually irreversible and may evolve after therapy is concluded. One study found that 33 of 33 subjects with permanent ototoxicity complained of symptoms of vestibular toxicity within 1 to 3 weeks of initiation of gentamicin, yet vestibular toxicity was not recognized prior to discharge by clinicians in 32 of 33.[179] Peak and trough concentrations did not correlate with ototoxicity nor did observance of safe dosage ranges, though all but one of the patients received long term therapy. The authors of this study recommended frequent monitoring and paying attention to signs and symptoms of ototoxicity since early identification may reduce risk, informing all patients about the risks of ototoxicity, and using other agents whenever feasible.[179]

It has been suggested that the choice of aminoglycoside can play an important role in the risk of ototoxicity, though prolonged duration of therapy is probably the most frequently cited factor. Older age, bacteremia, poor physical condition, fever, liver and renal impairment, and the combination with another ototoxic agent are also often reported.[27,115,180] Genetic predisposition may also play a role.[181] Iron chelators and radical scavengers have been reported to prevent ototoxicity in guinea pigs but these have not been adopted for human use.[182]

Neuromuscular toxicity also has occurred with the aminoglycosides; they should be used with caution in patients receiving neuromuscular blocking agents and in patients with muscular disorders such as myasthenia gravis and Parkinsonism. The risk of neuromuscular blocking problems is likely enhanced with use of LDEI approaches in these patients.[183]

Other symptoms of toxicity that occur to a minor extent (less than 3% incidence) include hypersensitivity, headache, nausea and vomiting, and abnormal liver function tests. Some brands of aminoglycosides may contain sodium bisulfite, which can cause allergic reactions including anaphylaxis in certain individuals. A syndrome of endotoxin-like reactions has been reported with the use of gentamicin for LDEI dosing.[184,185] One product apparently contained enough endotoxin that the large dose led to pyrogenic adverse consequence for patients. Products of two companies, American Pharmaceutical Partners (40-mg/ml dosage forms) and ESI Lederle (20 lots only), were voluntarily withdrawn after these reports due to possible association with this adverse event, but clinicians should watch for similar reactions when LDEI approaches are used.

In a study of 61 metabolic and respiratory stable preterm neonates who received gentamicin for suspected infection, higher peak serum gentamicin concentrations were associated with an increased incidence of microalbuminuria, natriuresis, and calciuria.[186] Due to these potential complications in neonates, it is recommended that urine albumin/urine creatinine, urine calcium/urine creatinine, and fractional excretion of sodium and potassium be monitored if monitoring gentamicin concentrations are not feasible.[186]

Drug-Drug Interactions[9,48,138]

In vitro sensitivity studies have found that the administration of *beta-lactams, extended-spectrum penicillins,* or *vancomycin* with an aminoglycoside can have a synergistic effect, improving the response to therapy. However, *in vitro* studies also have shown that concomitant administration of *carbenicillin, mezlocillin,* and *ticarcillin* decreases aminoglycoside concentrations. The time between collection of blood and concentration determination should be as short as possible when the agents are used to treat patients receiving aminoglycosides. Samples should be refrigerated until analyzed.

In vitro studies have indicated that a precipitate may form when aminoglycosides are administered concomitantly with *cefoperazone* and *cephalothin* or *in vitro* inactivation may occur with various *beta-lactams.* These agents should not be mixed together for infusion. A study of *piperacillin-tazobactam* and gentamicin showed no interaction.[187]

In vivo studies indicated that concomitant administration of *beta-lactams* or *extended-spectrum penicillins* might decrease the half-life and increase clearance of the aminoglycosides, especially in patients with renal failure. Although an interaction has been suggested to be more likely in patients with reduced renal function, it appears that there is no need to consider separating gentamicin and ampicillin dosing times.[188] *In vivo* studies also have found an increase in aminoglycoside toxicity when administered concomitantly with other nephrotoxic agents or potent diuretics like *acyclovir, amphotericin B, carboplatin, bacitracin, capreomycin, cisplatin, colistin, furosemide, ethacrynic acid, mannitol, vancomycin, urea, other aminoglycosides,* and possibly some *cephalosporins.*

Drug–Disease State or Condition Interactions

The following disease states or conditions influence certain aspects of aminoglycoside pharmacokinetics.

- *Ascites*[189,190]—The volume of distribution may increase by as much as 25%.
- *Burns*[191-194]—Clearance and volume of distribution may increase while half-life may increase or decrease.
- *Cirrhosis*[195]—Critically ill patients with cirrhosis and sepsis may have 40% larger volume (L/kg) and 38% lower clearance than similar patients without cirrhosis.
- *Cystic fibrosis*[24,25,196-201]—The volume of distribution or clearance may increase. Larger doses have been recommended for both LDEI and SDSI approaches. Once daily dosing is as effective in patients with cystic fibrosis as SDSI and may be less toxic in children.[201]

- *Dialysis—hemodialysis, peritoneal dialysis*[99,170,202-208]—Clearance increases and half-life decreases compared to values obtained when patient is not on dialysis. Studies of the use of a once-daily dose of aminoglycosides intraperitoneally differ on whether it provides appropriate coverage.[51,207,208] During peritoneal dialysis, efficiency of removal can be affected by various solutes in the dialysis solution and by the integrity of the peritoneal membrane. During hemodialysis, drug removal is affected by numerous variables including dialysate and blood flow rates, efficiency of dialyzer, positive and negative pressures, and length of dialysis. Aminoglycoside concentrations demonstrate a rebound phenomenon after hemodialysis, where the concentration increase may be due to redistribution from tissue. Therefore, sampling should be delayed approximately 2 hr after dialysis to avoid the possibility of dosing errors based on this phenomenon.[95] Several pharmacokinetic studies have been published evaluating different hemodialysis dosing methods (pre-dialysis, during dialysis, and post-dialysis). While most studies have evaluated the use of post-dialysis aminoglycoside dosing, this dosing strategy can lead to higher aminoglycoside AUC_{0-24} exposure between hemodialysis sessions since a patient's aminoglycoside concentrations remains fairly stable between sessions if there is no renal function. To decrease AUC_{0-24} exposure between sessions, lower aminoglycoside doses are administered that are potentially sub-therapeutic. Another strategy is to either administer a dose during the beginning of a hemodialysis session or 2-6 hr prior to a scheduled hemodialysis session in order to mimic renal clearance with dialysis.[204-206] This strategy may allow for higher doses to be administered, increasing the probability of achieving goal peak concentration while minimizing AUC_{0-24} between hemodialysis sessions. Concern for use of this dosing strategy relates to the potentially high aminoglycoside exposure if the hemodialysis session was not completed as scheduled.[204-206]
- *Febrile neutropenia*[209]—The use of SDSI versus LDEI dosing methods has been evaluated in a few studies. There are potential concerns about LDEI monotherapy if extended periods of time are allowed with low aminoglycoside concentrations.
- *Intensive care setting/severely ill patients*[101,102,104,210,211]—Patients may have a volume of distribution 25%–50% higher than normal and increased clearance.
- *Hepatic dysfunction*[212]—Serum cystatin C may be a better predictor of GFR for aminoglycoside dosing due to potential for overestimating GFR with the Cockcroft and Gault equation in hepatic dysfunction.
- *Hypothermia (therapeutic)*[213,214]—Patients may have a larger volume of distribution and longer half-life.
- *Malnutrition or underweight (<90% IBW)*[215]—For underweight patients with serum creatinine <1 mg/dl, estimated creatinine clearance may overestimate aminoglycoside clearance. An adjustment factor of 0.69 has been proposed.
- *Meningitis*[216]—Minimal concentrations of aminoglycosides have been reported in cerebrospinal fluid after intravenous administration but may be increased slightly in patients with meningitis.
- *Obesity*[99]—See dosing strategies section on dosing weight and volume of distribution determination, Step 3b—The volume of distribution does not increase proportionally with increasing weight.
- *Pancreatitis*[217]—The volume of distribution may increase by as much as 25%.
- *Patent ductus arteriosus*[218]—Clearance may decrease by ~11% and volume of distribution may increase by ~13%.
- *Postoperative, mechanical ventilation*[219]—The volume of distribution increases.
- *Postpartum*[220]—The volume of distribution is increased over normal; 1.5 times the IBW for dosing weight should be used in estimations of volume of distribution. A study showed that use of BW_{adj} (similar to use in obese patients) provided good prediction of volume.[221] The first approach is slightly more aggressive.
- *Pregnancy*—Certain aminoglycosides are known to cause fetal harm (e.g., streptomycin- and kanamycin induced ototoxicity) when administered during pregnancy.[9,48] It is not known whether amikacin, gentamicin, and tobramycin cause fetal harm or whether LDEI approaches would increase risk. One study of LDEI vs. SDSI dosing in 38 laboring women found peak concentrations of 13 to 25 mg/L after a 5.1 mg/kg dose in the mothers and extrapolated mean peak cord blood concentrations of 6.9 mg/L in the newborns (compared to 2.9 mg/L for SDSI) and no noted adverse effects.[48] As always, the benefits should outweigh the risks, and patients should be warned of potential hazard to the fetus, particularly with longer duration therapy.
- *Prematurity*[222-225]—Decreases in renal tubular function after administration of aminoglycosides may be more pronounced in premature neonates.

Summary

- LDEI dosing approaches are now often considered the standard for all but a few patient categories. Continuing development of consensus on the types of patients who should not be given this type of dosing is warranted. Generally, LDEI is not recommended in patients who are pregnant or those with renal failure, osteomyelitis, meningitis, enterococcal endocarditis, or extensive burns.
- All patients must have their renal function monitored.
- All patients in whom it is feasible should be queried about signs and symptoms of ototoxicity or have audiometric testing conducted if therapy is to be continued beyond a few days.
- All patients should be informed of the risks of aminoglycoside ototoxicity if long-term therapy is considered.
- The duration of dosing should be kept as limited as possible because total exposure seems to be an important factor in toxicity, although some patients may become toxic from limited doses.[29] Use of larger doses with LDEI could theoretically allow for a shorter duration of treatment due to more rapid elimination of organisms.
- It appears that less monitoring (i.e., no monitoring at all to one concentration versus two) is possible with LDEI approaches as long as the interval is adjusted appropriately, the patient has normal renal function, there are no contraindicating factors, and treatment will not be extended.
- Extrapolation of results from SDSI studies to LDEI and vice versa should be avoided.

References

1. Murphy JE. Aminoglycosides: another look at current and future roles in antimicrobial therapy. *Pharmacotherapy*. 1990;10:217-23.
2. Hurley SC, Hegman G. Attainment of adequate serum aminoglycoside concentrations. Proceedings of the American Society of Hospital Pharmacists 45th Annual Meeting. San Francisco, CA; June 1988.
3. McCormack JP, Jesesson PJ. A critical reevaluation of the therapeutic range of aminoglycosides. *Clin Infect Dis*. 1992;14:320-39.
4. Rodvold KA, Danziger LH, Quinn JP. Single daily doses of aminoglycosides. *Lancet*. 1997;350:1412.
5. McDade E, Wagner J, Moffett B, et al. Once-daily gentamicin dosing in pediatric patients without cystic fibrosis. *Pharmacotherapy*. 2010;30(3):248-53.
6. Waterberg KL, Kelly HW, Angelus P, et al. The need for a loading dose of gentamicin in neonates. *Ther Drug Monit*. 1989;11:16-20.
7. Semchuk W, Borgmann J, Bowman L. Determination of a gentamicin loading dose in neonates and infants. *Ther Drug Monit*. 1993;15:47-51.
8. Isemann BT, Kotagal UR, Mashni SM, et al. Optimal gentamicin therapy in preterm neonates includes loading doses and early monitoring. *Ther Drug Monit*. 1996;18:549-55.
9. Aminoglycosides. In McEvoy GK, ed. *AHFS Drug Information*. Bethesda, MD, American Society of Health-System Pharmacists, Inc.; 2011:8:12.02.
10. Suzuki K, Tanikawa K, Matsuzaki T. Pharmacokinetics and dosing of arbekacin in preterm and term newborns. *Ped Internatl*. 2003;45:175-9.
11. Hale LS, Durham CR. A simple, weight-based, extended-interval gentamicin dosage protocol for neonates. *Am J Health-Syst Pharm*. 2005;62:1613-6.
12. Murphy JE, Roether AM. Two nomograms for determining extended-dosing intervals for gentamicin in neonates. *Am J Health-Syst Pharm*. 2008;65(7):624-30.
13. Murphy JE. Prediction of gentamicin peak and trough concentrations from six extended-interval dosing protocols for neonates. *Am J Health-Syst Pharm*. 2005;62:823-7.
14. Hoff D, Wilcox R, Tollefson L, et al. Pharmacokinetic outcomes of a simplified, weight-based, extended-interval gentamicin dosing protocol in critically ill neonates. *Pharmacotherapy*. 2009;29(11):1297-1305.
15. Nestaas E, Bangstad H-J, Sandvik L, et al. Aminoglycoside extended interval dosing in neonates is safe and effective: a meta-analysis. *Arch Dis Child Fetal Neonatal Ed*. 2005;90:F294-F300.
16. Contopoulos-Ioannidis DG, Giotis ND, Baliatsa DV, et al. Extended-interval aminoglycoside administration for children: A meta-analysis. *Pediatrics*. 2004;114:e111-e118.
17. Vigano A, Principi N, Brivio L, et al. Comparison of 5 milligrams of netilmicin per kilogram of body weight once daily

versus 2 milligrams per kilogram thrice daily for treatment of gram-negative pyelonephritis in children. *Antimicrob Agents Chemother*. 1992;36:1499-1503.

18. Uijtendal EV, Rademaker CMA, Schobben A, et al. Once-daily versus multiple-daily gentamicin in infants and children. *Ther Drug Monit*. 2001;23:506-13.
19. Nicolau DP, Freeman CD, Belliveau PP, et al. Experience with a once-daily aminoglycoside program administered to 2,184 adult patients. *Antimicrob Agents Chemother*. 1995;39:650-5.
20. Gilbert DN, Lee BL, Dworkin RJ, et al. A randomized comparison of the safety and efficacy of once-daily gentamicin or thrice-daily gentamicin in combination with ticarcillin-clavulanate. *Am J Med*. 1998;105:182-91.
21. Prins JM, Weverling GJ, de Blok K, et al. Validation and nephrotoxicity of a simplified once-daily aminoglycoside dosing schedule and guidelines for monitoring therapy. *J Antimicrob Chemother*. 1996;40:2494-9.
22. Begg E, Vella-Brincat J, Robertshawe B, et al. Eight years' experience of an extended-interval dosing protocol for gentamicin in neonates. *J Antimicrob Chemother*. 2009;63:1043-9.
23. Murphy JE, Austin ML, Frye RF. Evaluation of gentamicin pharmacokinetics and dosing protocols in 195 neonates. *Am J Health-Syst Pharm*. 1998;55:2280-8.
24. Bragonier R, Brown NM. The pharmacokinetics and toxicity of once-daily tobramycin therapy in children with cystic fibrosis. *J Antimicrob Chemother*. 1998;42:103-6.
25. Bates RD, Nahata MC, Jones JW, et al. Pharmacokinetics and safety of tobramycin after once-daily administration in patients with cystic fibrosis. *Chest*. 1997;112:1208-13.
26. Canis F, Huson MO, Turck D, et al. Pharmacokinetics and bronchial diffusion of single daily dose amikacin in cystic fibrosis patients. *J Antimicrob Chemother*. 1997;39:431-3.
27. Paterson DL, Robson JMB, Wagener MM. Risk factors for toxicity in elderly patients given aminoglycosides once daily. *J Ger Intern Med*. 1998;13:735-9.
28. Koo J, Tight R, Rajkumar V, et al. Comparison of once-daily versus pharmacokinetic dosing of aminoglycosides in elderly patients. *Am J Med*. 1996;101:177-83.
29. Fridberg O, Jones I, Sjoberg L, et al. Antibiotic concentrations in serum and wound fluid after local gentamicin or intravenous dicloxacillin prophylaxis in cardiac surgery. *Scan J Infect Dis*. 2003;35:251-4.
30. Chia SH, Gamst AC, Anderson JP, et al. Intratympanic gentamicin therapy for Meniere's disease: A meta-analysis. *Otol Neurotol*. 2004;25:544-52.
31. De Beer L, Stokroos R, Kingma H. Intratympanic gentamicin for Meniere's disease. *Acta Otolaryngol*. 2007;127(6):605-12.
32. LoBue PA. Inhaled tobramycin: Not just for cystic fibrosis anymore? *Chest*. 2005;127:1098-1100. (Editorial)
33. Rubin BK. Aerosolized antibiotics for non-cystic fibrosis bronchiectasis. *J Aerosol Med Pulm Drug Deliv*. 2008;21(1):71-6.
34. Bilton D, Henig N, Morrissey B, et al. Addition of inhaled tobramycin to ciprofloxacin for acute exacerbations of *Pseudomonas aeruginosa* infection in adult bronchiectasis. *Chest*. 2006;130(5):1503-10.
35. Touw DJ, Jacobs FAH, Brimicombe RW, et al. Pharmacokinetics of aerosolized tobramycin in adult patients with cystic fibrosis. *Antimicrob Agents Chemother*. 1997;41:184-7.
36. Coates AL, MacNeish CF, Lands LC, et al. A comparison of the availability of tobramycin for inhalation from vented vs. unvented nebulizers. *Chest*. 1998;113:951-6.
37. Touw DJ, Vinks ATMM, Mouton JW, et al. Pharmacokinetic optimization of antibacterial treatment in patients with cystic fibrosis. *Clin Pharmacokinet*. 1998;35:437-59.
38. Geller DE, Rosenfeld M, Waltz DA, et al. Efficiency of pulmonary administration of tobramycin solution for inhalation in cystic fibrosis using an improved drug delivery system. *Chest*. 2003;123:28-36.
39. Gibson RL, Emerson J, McNamara S, et al. Significant microbiological effect of inhaled tobramycin in young children with cystic fibrosis. *Am J Resp Crit Care Med*. 2003;167:841-9.
40. Hubert D, Leroy, S, Nove-Josserand R, et al. Pharmacokinetics and safety of tobramycin administered by the PARI eFlow rapid nebulizer in cystic fibrosis. *J Cyst Fibrosis*. 2009;8(5):332-7.
41. Kahler DA, Schowenderdt KO, Fricker FJ, et al. Toxic serum trough concentrations after administration of nebulized tobramycin. *Pharmacotherapy*. 2003;23:543-5.
42. Cannella CA, Wilkinson ST. Acute renal failure associated with inhaled tobramycin. *Am J Health-Syst Pharm*. 2006;63:1858-61.
43. Izquierdo MJ, Gomez-Alamillo C, Ortiz F, et al. Acute renal failure associated with use of inhaled tobramycin for treatment of chronic airway colonization with *Pseudomonas aeruginosa*. *Clin Nephrol*. 2006;66(6):464-7.
44. Murphy JE, Job ML, Ward ES. Dosing error due to use of adult concentration of gentamicin injection rather than the pediatric concentration. *Hosp Pharm*. 1996;31:219-20, 230.
45. Meunier F, Van der Auwera P, Schmit H, et al. Pharmacokinetics of gentamicin after iv infusion or iv bolus. *J Antimicrob*

Chemother. 1987;19:225-31.

46. Pechere JC, Dugal R. Clinical pharmacokinetics of aminoglycoside antibiotics. *Clin Pharmacokinet*. 1979;4:170-99.
47. Mayer PR, Brown CH, Carter RA, et al. Intramuscular tobramycin pharmacokinetics in geriatric patients. *Drug Intell Clin Pharm*. 1986;20:611-5.
48. Zaske DE. Aminoglycosides. In: Evans WE, Schentag JJ, Jusko WJ, eds. *Applied Pharmacokinetics: Principles of Therapeutic Drug Monitoring*. 3rd ed. Vancouver, WA: Applied Therapeutics; 1992:14-1-14-47.
49. Mol M, van Kan HJM, Schultz MJ, et al. Systemic tobramycin concentrations during selective decontamination of the digestive tract in intensive care unit patients on continuous venovenous hemofiltration. *Intensive Care Med*. 2008;34:903-6.
50. Smeltzer BD, Schwartzman MS, Bertino JS. Amikacin pharmacokinetics during continuous ambulatory peritoneal dialysis. *Antimicrob Agents Chemother*. 1988;32:236-40.
51. Low CL, Bailie GR, Evans A. Pharmacokinetics of once-daily IP gentamicin in CAPD patients. *Peritoneal Dialysis Int*. 1996;16:379-84.
52. Wong KK, Marglani O, Westerberg BD, et al. Systemic absorption of topical gentamicin sinus irrigation. *J Otolaryngol Head Neck Surg*. 2008;37(3):395-8.
53. Defoor W, Ferguson D, Mashni S, et al. Safety of gentamicin bladder irrigations in complex urological cases. *J Urology*. 2006;175:1861-4.
54. Crosby SS, Edwards WAD, Brennan C, et al. Systemic absorption of aminoglycosides instilled through the endotracheal tubes of ten hospitalized patients. *Drug Intell Clin Pharm* 1987;21:19A.
55. McCall CY, Spruill WJ, Wade WE. The use of aerosolized tobramycin in the treatment of a resistant pseudomonal pneumonitis. *Ther Drug Monit*. 1989;11:692-5.
56. Ramsey BW, Pepe MS, Quan JM, et al. Intermittent administration of inhaled tobramycin in patients with cystic fibrosis. *N Engl J Med*. 1999;340:23-30.
57. Davis KK, Kao PN, Jacobs SS, et al. Aerosolized amikacin for treatment of pulmonary *Mycobacterium avium* infections: an observational case series. *BMC Pulm Med*. 2007;7:2.
58. Walenkamp GHIM, Vree TB, Van Rens TJG. Gentamicin-PMMA beads: pharmacokinetic and nephrotoxicological study. *Clin Orthop*. 1986;205:171-83.
59. Anagnostakos K, Wilmes P, Schmitt E, et al. Elution of gentamicin and vancomycin from polymethylmeth-acrylate beads and hip spacers in vivo. *Acta Orthopaedica*. 2009;80(2):193-7.
60. Rasyid H, van der Mei H, Frijlink H, et al. Concepts for increasing gentamicin release from handmade bone cement beads. *Acta Orthopaedica*. 2009;80(5):508-13.
61. Dune NJ, Hill J, McAfee P, et al. Incorporation of large amounts of gentamicin sulphate into acrylic bone cement: effect on handling and mechanical properties, antibiotic release, and biofilm formation. *Proc Inst Mech Eng H*. 2008;222(3):255-65.
62. Patrick BN, Rivey MP, Allington DR. Acute renal failure associated with vancomycin- and tobramycin-laden cement in total hip arthroplasty. *Ann Pharmacotherapy*. 2006;40(11):2037-42.
63. McLaren RL, McLaren AC, Veron BL. Generic tobramycin elutes from bone cement faster than proprietary tobramycin. *Clin Orthop Relat Res*. 2008;466:1372-6.
64. Gomez GGV, Guerrero TS, Llack MC, et al. Effectiveness of collagen-gentamicin implant for treatment of "dirty" abdominal wounds. *World J Surg*. 1999;23:123-7.
65. Champoux N, DuSouch P, Ravaoarinoro M, et al. Single-dose pharmacokinetics of ampicillin and tobramycin administered by hypodermoclysis in young and older healthy volunteers. *Br J Clin Pharmacol*. 1996;42:325-31.
66. Schiffelers R, Storm G, Bakker-Woudenberg I. Liposome-encapsulated aminoglycosides in preclinical and clinical studies. *J Antimic Chemother*. 2001;48:333-44.
67. Mugabe C, Azghani AO, Omri A. Liposome-mediated gentamicin delivery: development and activity against resistant strains of *Pseudomonas aeruginosa* isolated from cystic fibrosis patients. *J Antimicrob Chemother*. 2005;55:269-71.
68. Okusanya O, Bhavnani S, Hammel J, et al. Pharmacokinetic and pharmacodynamics evaluation of liposomal amikacin for inhalation in cystic fibrosis patients with chronic pseudomonal infection. *Antimicrob Agents Chemother*. 2009;53(9):3847-54.
69. Botha JH, du Preez MJ, Miller R, et al. Determination of population pharmacokinetic parameters for amikacin in neonates using mixed-effect models. *Eur J Clin Pharmacol*. 1998;53:337-41.
70. Carlstedt BC, Uaamnulchal M, Day RB, et al. Aminoglycoside dosing in pediatric patients. *Ther Drug Monit*. 1989;11:38-43.
71. Bloome MR, Warren AJ, Ringer I, et al. Evaluation of an empirical dosing schedule for gentamicin in neonates. *Drug Intell Clin Pharm*. 1988;22:618-22.
72. Lingvall M, Reith D, Broadbent R. The effect of sepsis upon gentamicin pharmacokinetics in neonates. *Br J Clin*

Pharmacol. 2005;59:54-61.

73. Gennrich JL, Nitake M. Devising an aminoglycoside dosage regimen for neonates seven to ninety days chronological age. *Neonatal Pharmacol Q*. 1992;1:45-50.
74. Shevchuk YM, Taylor DM. Aminoglycoside volume of distribution in pediatric patients. *DICP Ann Pharmacotherapy*. 1990;24:273-6.
75. Jacobson PA, West NJ, Price J, et al. Gentamicin and tobramycin pharmacokinetics in pediatric bone marrow transplant patients. *Ann Pharmacotherapy*. 1997;31:1127-31.
76. Ristuccia AM, Cunha BA. The aminoglycosides. *Med Clin North Am*. 1982;66:303-12.
77. Traynor AM, Nafziger AN, Bertino JS. Aminoglycoside dosing weight correction factors for patients of various body sizes. *Antimicrob Agents Chemother*. 1995;39:545-8.
78. Debord J, Charmes JP, Marquet P, et al. Population pharmacokinetics of amikacin in geriatric patient studies with the NPEM-2 algorithm. *Int J Clin Pharmacol Ther*. 1997;35:24-7.
79. Allegaert K, Anderson BJ, Cossey V, et al. Limited predictability of amikacin clearance in extreme premature neonates at birth. *Br J Clin Pharmacol*. 2005;61:39-48.
80. Koshida R, Nakashima E, Taniguchi N, et al. Prediction of the distribution volumes of cefazolin and tobramycin in obese children based on physiological pharmacokinetic concepts. *Pharm Res*. 1989;6:486-91.
81. Faura CC, Feret MA, Horga JF. Monitoring serum levels of gentamicin to develop a new regimen for gentamicin dosage in newborns. *Ther Drug Monit*. 1991;13:268-76.
82. Knight JA, Davis EM, Manouilov K, et al. The effect of postnatal age on gentamicin pharmacokinetics in neonates. *Pharmacotherapy*. 2003;23:992-6.
83. Bass KD, Larkin SE, Paap C, et al. Pharmacokinetics of once-daily gentamicin dosing in pediatric patients. *J Pediatric Surg*. 1998;33:1104-7.
84. Kelman AW, Thomson AH, Whiting B, et al. Estimation of gentamicin clearance and volume of distribution in neonates and young children. *Br J Clin Pharmacol*. 1984;18:685-92.
85. Ho KK, Bryson SM, Thiessen JJ, et al. The effects of age and chemotherapy on gentamicin pharmacokinetics and dosing in pediatric oncology patients. *Pharmacotherapy*. 1995;15:754-64.
86. Zaske DE, Cipolle RJ, Rotschafer JC, et al. Gentamicin pharmacokinetics in 1,640 patients: method of control of serum concentrations. *Antimicrob Agents Chemother*. 1982;21:407-11.
87. Zaske DE, Irvine P, Strand LM, et al. Wide interpatient variations in gentamicin dose requirements for geriatric patients. *JAMA*. 1982;248:3122-6.
88. Charlton CK, Needelman H, Thomas RW, et al. Gentamicin dosage recommendations for neonates based on half-life predictions from birth-weight. *Am J Perinatol*. 1986;3:28-32.
89. Lanao JM, Dominguez-Gil A, Malaga S, et al. Modification in the pharmacokinetics of amikacin during development. *Eur J Clin Pharmacol*. 1982;23:155-60.
90. Hoecker JL, Pickering LK, Swaney J, et al. Clinical pharmacology of tobramycin in children. *J Infect Dis*. 1978;137:592-6.
91. Murphy JE, Barzanjy S, Nguyen Y, et al. Aminoglycoside pharmacokinetics and evaluation of predicted concentrations from large dose, extended interval dosing protocols. *Eur J Hosp Pharm Science*. 2006;12:67-71.
92. Halstenson CE, Berkseth RO, Mann HJ, et al. Aminoglycoside redistribution phenomenon after hemodialysis: netilmicin and tobramycin. *Int J Clin Pharmacol Ther Toxicol*. 1987;25:50-5.
93. Sowinski K, Magner S, Lucksiri A, et al. Influence of hemodialysis on gentamicin pharmacokinetics, removal during hemodialysis, and recommended dosing. *Clin J Am Soc Nephrol*. 2008;3:355-61.
94. Dager W, King J. Aminoglycosides in intermittent hemodialysis: pharmacokinetics with individual dosing. *Ann Pharmacotherapy*. 2006;40:9-14.
95. Reguer L, Colding H, Jensen H, et al. Pharmacokinetics of amikacin during hemodialysis and peritoneal dialysis. *Antimicrob Agents Chemother*. 1977;11:214-8.
96. Kaojarern S, Arkaravichien W, Indraprasit S, et al. Dosing regimen of gentamicin during intermittent peritoneal dialysis. *J Clin Pharmacol*. 1989;29:140-3.
97. Ikawa K, Morikawa N, Suyama H, et al. Pharmacokinetics and pharmacodynamics of once-daily arbekacin during continuous venovenous hemodiafiltration in critically ill patients. *J Infect Chemother*. 2009;15:420-3.
98. Erdman SM, Rodvold KA, Pryka RD. An updated comparison of drug dosing methods, part III: aminoglycoside antibiotics. *Clin Pharmacokinet*. 1991;20:374-88.
99. Bauer LA, Blouin RA, Griffen WO, et al. Amikacin pharmacokinetics in morbidly obese patients. *Am J Hosp Pharm*. 1980;37:519-22.
100. Tointon MM, Job ML, Peltier TT, et al. Alterations in aminoglycoside volume of distribution in patients below ideal

body weight. *Clin Pharm*. 1987;6:160-2.

101. Hassan E, Ober JD. Predicted and measured aminoglycoside pharmacokinetic parameters in critically ill patients. *Antimicrob Agents Chemother*. 1987;11:1855-8.
102. Townsend PL, Fink MP, Stein KL, et al. Aminoglycoside pharmacokinetics: dosage requirements and nephrotoxicity in trauma patients. *Crit Care Med*. 1989;17:154-7.
103. Romano S, Gonzalez P, Tejada P, et al. Influence of diagnostic and treatment factors in the population pharmacokinetics of gentamicin. *J Clin Pharm Ther*. 1998;23:141-8.
104. Lugo G, Castaneda-Hernandez G. Relationship between hemodynamic and vital support measures and pharmacokinetic variability of amikacin in critically ill patients with sepsis. *Crit Care Med*. 1997;25:806-11.
105. Beringer PB, Winter ME. Aminoglycosides. In: Winter ME. *Basic Clinical Pharmacokinetics*. 5th ed. Baltimore, MD: Wolters Kluwer: Lippincott, Williams & Wilkins; 2010.
106. Sarubbi FA, Hull HH. Amikacin serum concentrations: prediction of levels and dosage guidelines. *Ann Intern Med*. 1978;89:612-8.
107. Ismail R, Haw AHSM, Azman M, et al. Therapeutic drug monitoring of gentamicin: a 6-year follow-up audit. *J Clin Pharm Ther*. 1997;22:21-5.
108. Eltahawy AT, Bahnassy AA. Aminoglycoside prescription, therapeutic monitoring and nephrotoxicity at a university hospital in Saudi Arabia. *J Chemother*. 1996;8:278-83.
109. Saunders NJ, Adams DJ, Lynn WA. Antimicrobial practice: a prospective laboratory-based audit of gentamicin use and therapeutic monitoring. *J Antimicrob Chemother*. 1995;36:729-36.
110. Sawchuk RJ, Zaske DE. Pharmacokinetics of dosing regimens which utilize multiple intravenous infusions: gentamicin in burn patients. *J Pharmacokinet Biopharm*. 1976;4:183-95.
111. Murphy JE, Job ML, Ward ES. Rectifying incorrect dosage schedules. *Am J Hosp Pharm*. 1990;47:2235-6.
112. Prins JM, Weverling GJ, van Ketel RJ, et al. Circadian variations in serum levels and the renal toxicity of aminoglycosides in patients. *Clin Pharmacol Ther*. 1997;62:106-11.
113. Livingston JC, Llata E, Rinehart E, et al. Gentamicin and clindamycin therapy in postpartum endometritis: The efficacy of daily dosing versus dosing every 8 hr. *Am J Obstet Gyn*. 2003;188:149-52.
114. Knoderer CA, Everett JA, Buss WF. Clinical issues surrounding once-daily aminoglycoside dosing in children. *Pharmacotherapy*. 2003;23:44-56.
115. El Bakri F, Pallett A, Smith AG, et al. Ototoxicity induced by once-daily gentamicin. *Lancet*. 1998;351:1407-8.
116. Postovsky S, Ben Arush MW, Kassis E, et al. Pharmacokinetic analysis of gentamicin thrice and single daily dosage in pediatric cancer patients. *Pediatr Hematology Oncol*. 1997;14:547-54.
117. Mitra AG, Whitten MK, Laurent SL, et al. A randomized, prospective study comparing once-daily gentamicin versus thrice-daily gentamicin in the treatment of puerperal infection. *Am J Obstet Gynecol*. 1997;177:786-92.
118. Tod M, Lortholary O, Seytre D, et al. Population pharmacokinetic study of amikacin administered once or twice daily to febrile, severely neutropenic adults. *Antimicrob Agents Chemother*. 1998;42:849-56.
119. Pession A, Prete A, Paolucci G. Cost-effectiveness of ceftriaxone and amikacin as single daily dose for the empirical management of febrile granulocytopenic children with cancer. *Chemotherapy*. 1997;43:358-66.
120. Finnell DL, Davis GA, Cropp CD, et al. Validation of the Hartford nomogram in trauma surgery patients. *Ann Pharmacotherapy*. 1998;32:417-21.
121. Smyth A, Tan KH, Hyman-Taylor P, et al. Once versus three-times daily regimes of tobramycin treatment for pulmonary exacerbations of cystic fibrosis—The TOPIC study: a randomized controlled trial. *Lancet*. 2005;365:573-8.
122. Loey LL, Tschida SJ, Rotschafer JC, et al. Wide variation in single, daily-dose aminoglycoside pharmacokinetics in patients with burn injuries. *J Burn Care Rehabil*. 1997;18:116-24.
123. Preston S, Briceland L. Single daily dosing of aminoglycosides. *Pharmacotherapy*. 1995;15(3):297-316.
124. Cooke RPD, Grace RJ, Gover PA. Audit of once-daily dosing gentamicin therapy in neutropenic fever. *Int J Clin Pract*. 1997;51:229-31.
125. Rybak MJ, Abate BJ, Kang SL, et al. Prospective evaluation of the effect of an aminoglycoside dosing regimen on rates of observed nephrotoxicity and ototoxicity. *Antimicrob Agents Chemother*. 1999;43:1549-55.
126. Rao SC, Srinivasjois R, Hagan R, et al. One dose per day compared to multiple doses per day of gentamicin for treatment of suspected or proven sepsis in neonates. *Cochrane Database of Systematic Reviews*. 2006, Issue 1. Art. No.: CD005091. DOI: 10.1002/14651858.CD005091.pub2. Last assessed as up to date March 10, 2010. http://www2.cochrane.org/reviews/en/ab005091.html. Accessed January 2, 2011.
127. de Hoog M, Schoemaker RC, Mouton JW, et al. Tobramycin population pharmacokinetics in neonates. *Clin Pharmacol Ther*. 1997;62:392-9.

128. de Hoog M, Mouton JW, Schoemaker RC, et al. Extended-interval dosing of tobramycin in neonates: Implications for therapeutic drug monitoring. *Clin Pharmacol Ther*. 2002;71:349-58.

129. Stolk LML, Degraeuwe PLJ, Nieman FHM, et al. Population pharmacokinetics and relationship between demographic and clinical variables and pharmacokinetics of gentamicin in neonates. *Ther Drug Monit*. 2002;24:527-31.

130. de Hoog MMD, Mouton JW, van den Anker JN. Letters to the editor. *Ther Drug Monit*. 2003;25:256-7.

131. Rastogi A, Agarwal G, Pyati S, et al. Comparison of two gentamicin schedules in very low birth weight infants. *Pediatr Infect Dis J*. 2002;21:234-40.

132. DiCenzo, R, Forrest A, Slish JC, et al. A gentamicin pharmacokinetic population model and once-daily dosing algorithm for neonates. *Pharmacotherapy*. 2003;23:585-91.

133. Best EJ, Gazarian M. Extended-interval aminoglycosides in children: More guidance is needed. *Pediatrics*. 2005;115:827-8. (Letter)

134. Contopoulos-Ioannidis DG, Ioannidis JPA. In reply. *Pediatrics*. 2005;115:828. (Letter)

135. Carapetis JR, Jaquiery AL, Buttery JP, et al. Randomized, controlled trial comparing once daily and three times daily gentamicin in children with urinary tract infections. *Pediatr Infect Dis J*. 2001;20:240-6.

136. Miron D. Once daily dosing of gentamicin in infants and children. *Pediatr Infect Dis J*. 2001;20:1169-73.

137. Hitt CM, Klepser ME, Nightingale CH, et al. Pharmacoeconomic impact of once-daily aminoglycoside administration. *Pharmacotherapy*. 1997;17:810-4.

138. Moore RD, Smith CR, Lietman PS. Association of aminoglycoside plasma levels with therapeutic outcome in gram-negative pneumonia. *Am J Med*. 1984;77:657-62.

139. Moore RD, Smith CR, Leitman PS. The association of aminoglycoside plasma levels with mortality in gram-negative bacteremia. *J Infect Dis*. 1984;149:443-8.

140. Hayani KC, Hatzopoulos FK, Frank AL, et al. Pharmacokinetics of once-daily dosing of gentamicin in neonates. *J Pediatr*. 1997;131:76-80.

141. Ettlinger JJ, Bedford KA, Lovering AM, et al. Pharmacokinetics of once-a-day netilmicin (6 mg/kg) in neonates. *J Antimicrob Chemother*. 1996;38:499-505.

142. Langhendries JP, Battisti O, Bertrand JM, et al. Adaptation in neonatology of the once-daily concept of aminoglycoside administration: evaluation of a dosing chart for amikacin in an intensive care unit. *Biol Neonate*. 1998;74:351-62.

143. Barclay ML, Kirkpatrick CMJ, Begg EJ. Once daily aminoglycoside therapy. Is it less toxic than multiple daily doses and how should it be monitored? *Clin Pharmacokinet*. 1999;36:89-98.

144. Deziel-Evans LM, Murphy JE, Job ML. Correlation of pharmacokinetic indices with therapeutic outcome in patients receiving aminoglycosides. *Clin Pharm*. 1986;5:319-24.

145. Moore RD, Lietman PS, Smith CR. Clinical response to aminoglycoside therapy: Importance of the ratio of peak concentration to minimal inhibitory concentration. *J Infect Dis*. 1987;155:93-9.

146. Mann HJ, Wittgrodt ET, Baghaie AA, et al. Effect of pharmacokinetic sampling methods on aminoglycoside dosing in critically ill surgery patients. *Pharmacotherapy*. 1998;18:371-8.

147. Jameson JP, Lewis JA. Three-point versus two-point method for early individualization of aminoglycoside doses. *DICP*. 1991;25:635-7.

148. Matthews J, Chow MSS. Simpler approaches to aminoglycoside monitoring. *Am J Hosp Pharm*. 1994;51:2847-8.

149. Nicolau DP, Wu AHB, Finocchiaro S, et al. Once-daily aminoglycoside dosing: Impact on requests and costs for therapeutic drug monitoring. *Ther Drug Monit*. 1996;18:263-6.

150. Averbuch M, Weintraub M, Nolte F. Gentamicin blood levels: ordered too soon and too often. *Hosp Form*. 1989;24:598-612.

151. Begg EJ, Barclay ML, Kirkpatrick CJM. The therapeutic monitoring of antimicrobial agents. *Clin Pharmacol*. 1999;47:23-30.

152. Logsdon BA, Phelps SJ. Routine monitoring of gentamicin serum concentrations in pediatric patients with normal renal function is unnecessary. *Ann Pharmacotherapy*. 1997;31:1514-8.

153. MacGowan A, Reeves D. Serum aminoglycoside concentrations: The case for routine monitoring. *J Antimicrob Chemother*. 1994;34:829-37.

154. Bond CA, Raehl CL. Clinical and economic outcomes of pharmacist-managed aminoglycoside or vancomycin therapy. *Am J Health-Syst Pharm*. 2005;62:1596-605.

155. Massey KL, Hendeles L, Neims A. Identification of children for whom routine monitoring of aminoglycoside serum concentrations is not cost-effective. *J Pediatr*. 1986;109:897-901.

156. Robinson D. Gentamicin monitoring in pediatric patients. *Ann Pharmacotherapy*. 1997;31:1539-40.

157. Hollingsed TC, Harper DF, Jennings JP, et al. Aminoglycoside dosing in burn patients using first dose pharmacokinetics.

J Trauma. 1993;35:394-8.

158. Glover ML, Shaffer CL, Rubino CM, et al. A multicenter evaluation of gentamicin therapy in the neonatal intensive care unit. *Pharmacotherapy*. 2001;21:7-10.
159. Bartal C, Schlaeffer F, Reisenberg K, et al. Pharmacokinetic dosing of aminoglycosides: a controlled trial. *Am J Med*. 2003;114:194-8.
160. McCormack JP. An emotional-based medicine approach to monitoring once-daily aminoglycosides. *Pharmacotherapy*. 2000;20:1524-7.
161. Blaser J, Konig C, Fatio R, et al. Multicenter quality control study of amikacin assay for monitoring once-daily dosing regimens. *Ther Drug Monit*. 1995;17:133-6.
162. Zaera S, Hermida J, Tutor JC. Effect of analytical inaccuracy on dose adjustment for vancomycin, amikacin, and tobramycin using the Abbottbase Pharmacokinetic Systems. *Ther Drug Monit*. 2002;24:696-700.
163. Rodriguez-Mendizabal M, Lucena MI, Cabello MR, et al. Variations in blood levels of aminoglycosides related to in vitro anticoagulant usage. *Ther Drug Monit*. 1998;20:88-91.
164. Redmann S, Wainwright C, Stacey S, et al. Misleading high tobramycin plasma concentrations can be caused by skin contamination of fingerprick blood following inhalation of nebulized tobramycin (TOBI®). *Ther Drug Monit*. 2005;27:205-7.
165. Binder L, Schiel X, Binder C, et al. Clinical outcome and economic impact of aminoglycoside peak concentrations in febrile immunocompromised patients with hematologic malignancies. *Clin Chem*. 1998;44:408-14.
166. Bezirtzoglou E, Golegou S, Savvaidis I. A relationship between serum gentamicin concentrations and minimal inhibitory concentration. *Drugs Expt Clin Res*. 1996;2:57-60.
167. Kashuba ADM, Nafziger AN, Drusano GL, et al. Optimizing aminoglycoside therapy for nosocomial pneumonia caused by gram-negative bacteria. *Antimicrob Agents Chemother*. 1999;43:623-9.
168. M100-S19 Performance Standards for Antimicrobial Susceptibility Testing; Nineteenth Information Supplement. Clinical and Laboratory Standards Institute. January 2009.
169. Olsen KM, Rudis MI, Rebuck JA, et al. Effect of once-daily dosing vs. multiple daily dosing of tobramycin on enzyme markers of nephrotoxicity. *Crit Care Med*. 2004;32:1678-82.
170. Kirkpatrick CMJ, Duffull SB, Begg EJ. Once-daily aminoglycoside therapy: potential ototoxicity. *Antimicrob Agents Chemother*. 1997;41:879. (Letter)
171. Cosgrove S, Vigliani G, Campion M, et al. Initial low-dose gentamicin for *staphylococcus aureus* bacteremia and endocarditis is nephrotoxic. *Clin Infect Dis*. 2009;48(6):713-21.
172. Buchholtz K, Larsen C, Hassager C, et al. Severity of gentamicin's nephrotoxic effect on patients with infective endocarditis: a prospective observational cohort study of 373 patients. *Clin Infect Dis*. 2009;48(1):65-71.
173. Rougier F, Ducher M, Maurin M, et al. Aminoglycoside dosages and nephrotoxicity: quantitative relationships. *Clin Pharmacokinet*. 2003;42(5):493-500.
174. Mingeot-Leclercq M, Tulkens PM. Aminoglycosides: Nephrotoxicity. *Antimicrob Agents Chemother*. 1999;43:1003-12.
175. Beauchamp D, Labrecque G. Aminoglycoside nephrotoxicity: Do time and frequency of administration matter? *Curr Opinion Crit Care*. 2001;7:401-8.
176. Sawyers CL, Moore RD, Lerner SA, et al. A model for predicting nephrotoxicity in patients treated with aminoglycosides. *J Infect Dis*. 1986;153:1062-8.
177. Desai TK, Tsang TK. Aminoglycoside nephrotoxicity in obstructive jaundice. *Am J Med*. 1998;85:47-50.
178. Beaubien AR, Desjardins S, Ormsby E, et al. Incidence of amikacin ototoxicity: A sigmoid function of total drug exposure independent of plasma levels. *Am J Otolaryngol*. 1989;10:234-43.
179. Black FO, Pesznecker S, Stallings V. Permanent gentamicin vestibulotoxicity. *Otol Neurotol*. 2004;25:559-69.
180. Barclay ML, Begg EJ. Aminoglycoside toxicity and relation to dose regimen. *Adverse Drug React Toxicol Rev*. 1994;13:207-34.
181. Hamasaki K, Rando RR. Specific binding of aminoglycosides to a human rRNA construct based on a DNA polymorphism which causes aminoglycoside-induced deafness. *Biochem*. 1997;36(40):12323-8.
182. Schacht J. Aminoglycoside ototoxicity: prevention in sight? *Otolaryngol Head Neck Surg*. 1998;118:674-7.
183. Dotan ZA, Hana R, Simon D, et al. The effect of vecuronium is enhanced by a large rather than a modest dose of gentamicin as compared to no preoperative gentamicin. *Anesth Analg*. 2003;96:750-4.
184. Anonymous. Endotoxin-like reactions associated with intravenous gentamicin—California, 1998. *Morbidity Mortality Weekly Rep*. 1998;47:877-80.
185. Lucas KH, Schliesser SH, O'Neill MG. Shaking, chills, and rigors with once-daily gentamicin. *Pharmacotherapy*. 1999;19:1102-4.

186. Tugay S, Bircan Z, Caglayan C, et al. Acute effects of gentamicin on glomerular and tubular functions in preterm neonates. *Pediatr Nephrol*. 2006;21:1389-92.

187. Hitt CM, Patel KB, Nicolau DP, et al. Influence of piperacillin-tazobactam on pharmacokinetics of gentamicin given once daily. *Am J Health-Syst Pharm*. 1997;54:2704-8.

188. Daly JS, Dodge RA, Glew RH, et al. Effect of time and temperature on inactivation of aminoglycosides by ampicillin at neonatal dosages. *J Perinatol*. 1997;17:42-5.

189. Sampliner R, Perrier D, Powell R, et al. Influence of ascites on tobramycin pharmacokinetics. *J Clin Pharmacol*. 1984;24:43-6.

190. Gill MA, Kern JW. Altered gentamicin distribution in ascitic patients. *Am J Hosp Pharm*. 1979;36:1704-6.

191. Zaske DE, Sawchuk RJ, Gerding DN, et al. Increased dosage requirements of gentamicin in burn patients. *J Trauma*. 1976;16:824-8.

192. Loirat P, Rohan J, Baillet A, et al. Increased glomerular filtration rate in patients with major burns and its effect on the pharmacokinetics of tobramycin. *N Engl J Med*. 1978;299:915-9.

193. Conil JM, Georges B, Breden A, et al. Increased amikacin dosage requirements in burn patients receiving a once-daily regimen. *Int J Antimicrob Agents*. 2006;28:226-30.

194. Bracco D, Landry C, Dubois M, et al. Pharmacokinetic variability of extended interval tobramycin in burn patients. *Burns*. 2008;34:791-6.

195. Lugo G, Castaneda-Hernandez G. Amikacin Bayesian forecasting in critically ill patients with sepsis and cirrhosis. *Ther Drug Monit*. 1997;19:271-6.

196. Delage G. Desautels L, Legault S, et al. Individualized aminoglycoside dosage regimens in patients with cystic fibrosis. *Drug Intell Clin Pharm*. 1988;22:386-9.

197. Massie J, Cranswick N. Pharmacokinetic profile of once daily intravenous tobramycin in children with cystic fibrosis. *J Paediatr Child Health*. 2006;42:601-5.

198. Smyth AR, Bhatt J. Once-daily versus multiple-daily dosing with intravenous aminoglycosides for cystic fibrosis. Cochrane Database of Systematic Reviews 2010, Issue 1. Art. No.: CD002009. DOI: 10.1002/14651858.CD002009.pub3. http://www2.cochrane.org/reviews/en/ab002009.html. Last assessed as up-to-date: April 14. 2009. Accessed January 2, 2011.

199. Lam W, Tjon J, Seto W, et al. Pharmacokinetic modeling of a once-daily dosing regimen for intravenous tobramycin in paediatric cystic fibrosis patients. *J Antimicrob Chemother*. 2007;59:1135-40.

200. Touw DJ, Knox AJ, Smyth A. Population pharmacokinetics of tobramycin administered thrice daily and once daily in children and adults with cystic fibrosis. *J Cyst Fibros*. 2007;6:327-33.

201. Beringer PM, Vinks AATMM, Jelliffe RW, et al. Pharmacokinetics of tobramycin in adults with cystic fibrosis: implications for once-daily administration. *Antimicrob Agents Chemother*. 2000;44(4):809-13.

202. Indraprasit S, Ukaravichien V, Pummangura C, et al. Gentamicin removal during intermittent peritoneal dialysis. *Nephron*. 1986;44:18-21.

203. Goetz DR, Pancorbo S, Hosg S, et al. Prediction of serum gentamicin concentrations in patients undergoing hemodialysis. *Am J Hosp Pharm*. 1980;37:1077-83.

204. Mohamed O, Wahba I, Watnick S, et al. Administration of tobramycin in the beginning of the hemodialysis session: a novel intradialytic dosing regimen. *Clin J Am Soc Nephrol*. 2007;2:694-9.

205. Matsuo H, Hayashi J, Ono K, et al. Administration of aminoglycosides to hemodialysis patients immediately before dialysis: a new dosing modality. *Antimicrob Agents Chemother*. 1997;41(12):2597-601.

206. Teigen M, Duffull S, Dang L, et al. Dosing of gentamicin in patients with end-stage renal disease receiving hemodialysis. *J Clin Pharmacol*. 2006;46:1259-67.

207. Lai, M, Kao M, Chen C, et al. Intraperitoneal once-daily dose of cefazolin and gentamicin for treating CAPD peritonitis. *Perit Dial Int*. 1997;17:87-9.

208. Anding K, Krume B, Pelz K, et al. Pharmacokinetics and bactericidal activity of a single daily dose of netilmicin in the treatment of CAPD-associated peritonitis. *Int J Clin Pharm Ther*. 1996;34:465-9.

209. Inparajah M, Wong C, Sibbald C, et al. Once-daily gentamicin dosing in children with febrile neutropenia resulting from antineoplastic therapy. *Pharmacotherapy*. 2010;30(1):43-51.

210. Mann HJ, Fuhs DW, Awang R, et al. Altered aminoglycoside pharmacokinetics in critically ill patients with sepsis. *Clin Pharm*. 1987;6:148-53.

211. Arenas Lopez S, Mulla H, Durward A, et al. Extended-interval gentamicin: population pharmacokinetics in pediatric critical illness. *Pediatr Crit Care Med*. 2010;11(2):267-74.

212. Hermida J, Tutor JC. Serum cystatin C for the prediction of glomerular filtration rate with regard to the dose adjustment of amikacin, gentamicin, tobramycin, and vancomycin. *Ther Drug Monit*. 2006;28:326-31.

213. Mercer J, Neyens R. Aminoglycoside pharmacokinetic parameters in neurocritical care patients undergoing induced

hypothermia. *Pharmacotherapy.* 2010;30(7):654-60.

214. Liu X, Borooah M, Stone J, et al. Serum gentamicin concentrations in encephalopathic infants are not affected by therapeutic hypothermia. *Pediatrics.* 2009;124:310-5.

215. Khuu T, Bagdasarian G, Leung J, et al. Estimating aminoglycoside clearance and creatinine clearance in underweight patients. *Am J Health-Syst Pharm.* 2010;67(5):274-9.

216. Allegaert K, Scheers I, Brajanoski G, et al. Cerebrospinal fluid compartmental pharmacokinetics of amikacin in neonates. *Antimicrob Agents Chemother.* 2008;52(6):1934-9.

217. Carr MR, Dick SP, Bordley J, et al. Gentamicin dosing requirement in patients with acute pancreatitis. *Surgery.* 1988;103:533-7.

218. Williams BS, Ransom JL, Gal P, et al. Gentamicin pharmacokinetics in neonates with patent ductus arteriosus. *Crit Care Med.* 1997;25:273-5.

219. Triginer C, Fernandez R, Izquirdo I, et al. Gentamicin pharmacokinetic changes related to mechanical ventilation. *DICP Ann Pharmacotherapy.* 1989;23:923-4.

220. Briggs GG, Ambrose P, Nageotte MP. Gentamicin dosing in post-partum women with endometritis. *Am J Obstet Gynecol.* 1989;160:309-13.

221. Cropp CD, Davis GA, Ensom MHH. Evaluation of aminoglycoside pharmacokinetics in postpartum patients using Bayesian forecasting. *Ther Drug Monit.* 1998;20:68-72.

222. Locksmith GJ, Chin A, Vu T, et al. High compared with standard gentamicin dosing for chorioamnionitis: A comparison of maternal and fetal serum drug levels. *Obstet Gynecol.* 2005;105:473-9.

223. Giapros VI, Andronikou SK, Cholevas VI, et al. Renal function and effect of aminoglycoside therapy during the first ten days of life. *Ped Nephrology.* 2003;18:46-52.

224. Thingvoll E, Guillet R, Caserta M, et al. Observational trial of a 48-hour gentamicin dosing regimen derived from Monte Carlo simulations in infants born at less than 28 weeks gestation. *J Pediatr.* 2008;153(4):530-4.

225. Garcia B, Barcia E, Perez F, et al. Population pharmacokinetics of gentamicin in premature newborns. *J Antimicrob Chemother.* 2006;58(2):372-9.

Chapter 8

Patrick R. Finley

Antidepressants (AHFS 28:16.04)

Antidepressants have been prescribed for the treatment of mood disorders for over 50 years. However, it has only been within the past decade that the popularity of this class of medications has increased dramatically.[1] Recent data suggests that antidepressants have joined opioid analgesics and lipid-lowering agents as the three medication classes most commonly prescribed in contemporary practice. The popularity of antidepressant medications can be attributed to an enhanced awareness of the prevalence of depression, as well as the discovery and release of newer agents perceived to be safer than tricyclic alternatives. An additional benefit of prescription antidepressants is their clinical utility and effectiveness in the treatment of a wide range of illnesses, ranging from FDA-approved indications such as major depression, anxiety disorders, and smoking cessation, to unapproved uses such as insomnia, premature ejaculation, and weight management.[2]

Given the popularity of the antidepressant drug class, concerns about their collective potential for causing drug interactions and potentially serious side effects are well founded. As depression has been strongly associated with a wide variety of common medical conditions that are chronically treated with medications (e.g., heart disease, diabetes, Parkinson's disease), concerns about drug-drug and drug-disease interactions are particularly salient.[3]

While the practice of therapeutic drug monitoring (TDM) has been well described for tricyclic antidepressants, their use has been steadily declining in favor of selective serotonin reuptake inhibitors (SSRI), serotonin norepinephrine reuptake inhibitors (SNRI), and norepinephrine reuptake inhibitors (NRI).[4] The benefits of TDM are not as apparent for these newer agents. However, an appreciation for the pharmacokinetic disposition of *all* antidepressants is vital in order to ensure the safe and efficacious use of these medications across a broad and diverse patient population.

In general, the successful incorporation of pharmacokinetic principles into the clinical use of antidepressants requires slightly different considerations than with many other drug classes. For instance, many patients who receive adequate or optimal antidepressant therapy may have drug concentrations that are considerably different than values considered normal or therapeutic. When a patient is responding well, the dosage should not be altered simply to bring the concentration into a previously defined range unless toxicity is a concern. Dosing is usually based on observed efficacy and tolerability rather than measured drug concentrations.[5–7] Also, it should be kept in mind that assumptions about the pharmacokinetics and pharmacodynamics of these drugs are based on concentrations achieved in the plasma rather than concentrations determined from the actual site of action in the central nervous system, where sampling is impractical. Nonetheless, the pharmacokinetic parameters of the antidepressants will often be a factor in determining safe and appropriate therapy.

In this chapter, the population parameters, metabolic fate, and monitoring concerns for all antidepressants currently marketed in the United States are summarized. It should be noted that, although there are other psychotropic compounds prescribed for the treatment of depression (e.g., lithium, buspirone, lamotrigine and second generation antipsychotics), a complete discussion of the wide variety of medications is beyond the scope of this chapter, The disposition of most antidepressants has not been well studied in certain patient populations such as children and adolescents. Thus, the primary focus of this chapter will be on adult pharmacokinetic parameters. Similarly, the impact of other medical conditions and impairments has not been well described for most antidepressants. At the end of the chapter a brief but largely theoretical discussion of conditions that may influence antidepressant disposition is provided as well as specific recommendations about drug dosing and therapeutic monitoring.

Usual Dosage Range in Absence of Clearance-Altering Factors[7–9]

The respective dosage ranges for all antidepressants in the treatment of major depression are summarized in Table 8-1. Antidepressant dosing practices for other indications may vary considerably from these ranges. For example, the use of SSRI for obsessive-compulsive disorder (OCD) or panic disorder requires small initial doses to avoid excessive activation (e.g., fluoxetine 5–10 mg daily). Maintenance doses, however, are often greater for the treatment of these anxiety disorders than for major depression, where 40–80 mg daily of fluoxetine is more commonly used for treatment.[2,10]

The typical daily doses listed in Table 8-1 are generally consistent with those approved for adults by the FDA. Since steady state concentrations can vary more than ten-fold with empiric dosing recommendations and there are substantial inherent differences in pharmacodynamic sensitivity, some patients may require doses greater or less than those listed in the table. For example, daily doses of venlafaxine often exceed the FDA-recommended maximum of 225 mg. Although higher doses are associated with an increased risk of hypertension and tachycardia, clinicians often find that doses greater than 225 mg daily are necessary to achieve complete remission of symptoms. Ultimately, the therapeutic effects and toxicities observed will effectively determine prescribed maintenance doses, so routine and thorough patient monitoring is vital.

Table 8-1. Oral Dosage Ranges

Drug	Initial Dosage[a]	Usual Daily Dosage
Amitriptyline	25 mg daily	100–300 mg
Amoxapine	50 mg daily	100–600 mg
Bupropion	100 mg twice daily	200–450 mg
Bupropion sustained release	150 mg daily	300–400 mg
Bupropion extended release	150 mg daily	300–450 mg
Citalopram	10–20 mg daily	20–40 mg
Clomipramine[b]	25–100 mg daily	75–250 mg
Desipramine	25 mg daily	100–300 mg
Desvenlafaxine	50 mg daily	50-100 mg
Doxepin	25 mg daily	100–300 mg
Duloxetine	20–30 mg daily	60–120 mg
Escitalopram	5–10 mg daily	10–20 mg
Fluoxetine	10–20 mg daily	10–40 mg
Fluvoxamine[b]	50 mg daily	100–300 mg
Imipramine	25 mg daily	100–300 mg
Maprotiline	25 mg daily	75–225 mg
Mirtazapine	15 mg daily	15–45 mg
Nortriptyline	25 mg daily	50–150 mg
Paroxetine	10–20 mg daily	10–40 mg
Phenelzine	15 mg daily	30–60 mg
Protriptyline	15 mg daily	15–60 mg
Selegiline (transdermal patch)	6 mg daily	6–12 mg
Sertraline	25–50 mg daily	50–100 mg
Trazodone	50 mg daily	150–600 mg
Tranylcypromine	10 mg daily	20–40 mg
Trimipramine	25 mg daily	50–300 mg
Venlafaxine	37.5 daily	150–375 mg

[a]In geriatric patients the starting dose is generally less than for younger adults.
[b]The dosage given is for obsessive-compulsive disorder. Labeling for treatment of depression has not been approved in the United States.

Dosage Form Availability

Antidepressant medications are currently available in a wide variety of oral dosing formulations (e.g., tablets, capsules, and solution). An injectable preparation of amitriptyline is suitable for intramuscular administration and a transdermal patch of a monoamine oxidase inhibitor (MAOI; selegiline) is available. Table 8-2 provides the available dosage forms.

Table 8-2. Dosage Form Availability

Drug	Dosage Form	Brand Name
Amitriptyline	Tablets: 10, 25, 50, 75, 100, and 150 mg	Elavil
	Parenteral injection: 10 mg/ml	Elavil
Amoxapine	Tablets: 25, 50, 100, and 150 mg	Asendin
Bupropion	Tablets: 75 and 100 mg	Wellbutrin
	Tablets (sustained release): 100, 150, and 200 mg	Wellbutrin SR, Zyban
	Tablets (extended release): 150 and 300 mg	Wellbutrin XL
Citalopram	Tablets: 10, 20, and 40 mg	Celexa
	Oral solution: 10 mg/5 ml	
Clomipramine	Capsules: 25, 50, and 75 mg	Anafranil
Desipramine	Tablets: 10, 25, 50, 75, 100, and 150 mg	Norpramin
	Capsules: 25 and 50 mg	Pertofrane
Desvenlafaxine	Tablets (extended release): 50 and 100 mg	Pristiq
Doxepin	Capsules: 10, 25, 50, 75, 100, and 150 mg	Adapin
		Sinequan
	Oral solution: 10 mg/ml	Sinequan
Duloxetine	Capsules: 20, 30, and 60 mg	Cymbalta
Escitalopram	Tablets: 5, 10, 20 mg	Lexapro
	Oral solution: 5 mg/5 ml	
Fluoxetine	Tablets: 10, 20 mg	Prozac
	Capsules: 10, 20, and 40 mg	Prozac, Sarafem
	Capsules (delayed-release): 90 mg	Prozac Weekly
	Oral solution: 20 mg/5 ml	Prozac
Fluvoxamine	Tablets: 25, 50, and 100 mg	Luvox
Imipramine	Tablets: 10, 25, and 50 mg	Tofranil
	Capsules: 75, 100, 125, and 150 mg	Tofranil-PM
Maprotiline	Tablets: 25, 50, and 75 mg	Ludiomil
Mirtazapine	Tablets: 15, 30, and 45 mg	Remeron
	Tablets (orally disintegrating tablet) 15, 30, and 45 mg	
Nortriptyline	Capsules: 10, 25, 50, and 75 mg	Aventyl, Pamelor
	Oral solution: 10 mg/5 ml	Aventyl, Pamelor
Paroxetine	Tablets: 10, 20, 30, and 40 mg	Paxil
	Oral solution: 10 mg/5 ml	Paxil
	Controlled release: 12.5, 25, 37.5 mg	Paxil CR
Phenelzine	Tablets: 15 mg	Nardil
Protriptyline	Tablets: 5 and 10 mg	Vivactil

Table 8-2. (Continued)

Drug	Dosage Form	Brand Name
Selegiline	Transdermal patch: 6, 9, 12 mg	Emsam
Sertraline	Tablets: 25, 50, and 100 mg	Zoloft
	Oral solution: 20 mg/ml	
Tranylcypromine	Tablets: 10 mg	Parnate
Trazodone	Capsules: 50, 100, 150, and 300 mg	Desyrel
Trimipramine	Capsules: 25, 50, and 100 mg	Surmontil
Venlafaxine	Tablets: 25, 37.5, 50, 75, and 100 mg	Effexor
	Capsules (sustained-release): 37.5, 75, and 150 mg	Effexor XR

General Pharmacokinetic Information

The major pharmacokinetic parameters for commercially available antidepressants in healthy adults are summarized in Table 8-3.[9] Antidepressants tend to be highly lipophilic compounds, permitting their passage across the blood brain barrier into the central nervous system. They are usually basic amines with pK as ranging from 7–10. Most antidepressants are rapidly and completely absorbed in the small intestine but undergo extensive presystemic elimination in the liver (i.e., high first pass effect). This characteristic makes plasma concentrations highly variable among patients receiving identical doses. The extent of extraction by the liver classifies these drugs as moderate to high clearance, with extraction ratios of 0.5–0.8.

The presence of food in the gastrointestinal tract does not alter the extent or rate of absorption for most antidepressants, which is important because patients are generally instructed to ingest their antidepressants during or shortly after meals to minimize nausea. One exception to this pattern can be found with sertraline, where the presence of food in the GI tract has been demonstrated to increase the AUC by 65%. The clinical significance of this finding is unclear.

Most antidepressants are highly bound to plasma proteins (>80%), with the notable exceptions of venlafaxine (27%) and escitalopram (56%). Volumes of distribution greatly exceed body weight, implying that antidepressants accumulate in tissues, and concentrations are much higher in this compartment than in the plasma. Since as little as 3% of the total body burden of some antidepressants resides in the circulating plasma, extracorporeal methods of drug elimination (hemodialysis and hemoperfusion) have little benefit in the treatment of overdosage.[11] Fortunately, the most popular class of antidepressants (SSRI) appears to be less toxic in overdose than the older tricyclic antidepressants.[9,12–14]

All FDA-approved antidepressants undergo hepatic transformation prior to excretion. For the most part this is a Phase 1 reaction and with many of the antidepressants the primary metabolic pathway produces an active metabolite.[9,16] Examples include amitriptyline (nortriptyline), imipramine (desipramine), fluoxetine (norfluoxetine), sertraline (desmethylsertraline), venlafaxine (o-desmethylvenlafaxine), and bupropion (hydroxybupropion). The clinical importance of these metabolites can be quite profound. For instance, demethylation of fluoxetine produces a moiety with comparable activity (relative to the parent compound) but it has a much longer half-life (7–15 days vs. 1–4 days) and concentrations exceed those of fluoxetine once steady state is achieved. Similarly, the activity of hydroxybupropion is roughly half that of the parent compound but concentrations at steady state are 7–10 times higher.[17]

Generally, the terminal half-lives of most antidepressants are approximately 24 hours. Therefore, steady state concentrations would be achieved within roughly 4 days. The pharmacologic half-life of these medications is probably much longer, as evidenced by the delayed onset of therapeutic effects commonly observed (e.g., 1–2 weeks). Similarly, the pharmacologic actions of these medications may persist for weeks after discontinuation. For example, the effects of irreversible MAO inhibitors (such as phenelzine, selegiline, and tranylcypromine) may be evident for as long as 2 weeks, necessitating a relatively long washout period before the risk of drug and dietary interactions has diminished.

Table 8-3. Pharmacokinetic Parameters for Antidepressants in Healthy Adults[5,6,12,15]

Drug	Bioavailability (%)[a]	Clearance (L/h)[b]	Volume of Distribution (L/kg)	Half-Life (hr)
Amitriptyline	30–60	19–72	6–36	9–46
Amoxapine	46–82	42–73[c]	8–14	
Bupropion	>90	126–140	27–63	9–21
Citalopram	95	23–38	14	23–45
Clomipramine	36–62	23–122	9–25	15–62
Desipramine	33–51	78–168	24–60	12–28
Desvenlafaxine	80	210	3.4	9–15
Doxepin	13–45	41–61	9–33	8–25
Duloxetine	[c]	114	11–50	9–19
Escitalopram	80	36	12–26	27–32
Fluoxetine	>70	5–42	12–42	26–220
Fluvoxamine	>90	33–320	>5	9–28
Imipramine	30–70	32–102	9–23	6–28
Maprotiline	70–90	17–34	16–32	27–50
Mirtazapine	50	[c]	4.5	13–34
Nefazodone	>20	[c]	0.2–1.0	2–8
Nortriptyline	46–70	17–79	15–32	18–56
Paroxetine	>90	15–92	3–28	7–37
Phenelzine	[c]	[c]	[c]	1.5–4.0
Protriptyline	75–90	8–23	15–31	54–198
Selegiline	25–30	16	[c]	18–25
Sertraline	>44	96	>20	22–36
Tranylcypromine	[c]	[c]	1.1–5.7	1.5–3.5
Trazodone	70–90	7–12	1–2	3–14
Trimipramine	18–63	40–105	17–48	16–40
Venlafaxine	92	40–129	2–23	2–11

[a]Values are generally low for many of these drugs due to extensive presystemic elimination.
[b]Values approach or exceed hepatic blood flow due to an inherent artifact in calculating clearance from oral dose data.
[c]Reliable values are not available in the literature.

The metabolic fate of the various antidepressants is shown in Table 8-4. The primary isoenzymes metabolizing the parent drug and the primary metabolite(s) are listed.

Dosing Strategies

Dosing and titration methods for antidepressants vary considerably from patient to patient and medication to medication. With the SSRI, for instance, there is no mention made of titration methods in the manufacturers' package inserts (PI) yet many clinicians find it a worthwhile practice to initiate treatment at lower doses (e.g., 5 mg fluoxetine daily) in the interest of improving adherence and treatment outcomes.[18] With SNRI, NRI, and TCA, there are more specific recommendations found in the PI, which are designed to minimize the risk of adverse effects while the clinician advances treatment toward a therapeutic dose. The rationale and recommendations associated with these respective approaches can be found below.

As a rule, loading doses are generally not practical or useful for antidepressants available at the present time. Side effects are quite common with the initiation of most antidepressants, and higher initial doses would

Table 8-4. Metabolic Fate of Antidepressants[72,73]

Drug	CYP450 Isoenzyme	Primary Metabolite(s)[a]
Amitriptyline	1A2, 2C19, 3A4	Nortriptyline (2D6), Hydroxy amitriptyline
Amoxapine	2C19 > 1A2, 2D6, 3A4	7-Hydroxy amoxapine, 8-hydroxy amoxapine
Bupropion	2B6	Hydroxy-bupropion (2D6)
Citalopram	2C19, 3A4 > 2D6	Desmethyl-citalopram (2D6), Didesmethyl-citalopram (2D6)
Clomipramine	2C19, 1A2	*N*-Desmethyl-clomipramine (2D6)
Desipramine	2D6	Hydroxy-desipramine
Desvenlafaxine	UGT > 3A4	Desvenlafaxine-glucuronide
Doxepin	2D6 > 1A2, 2C9, 2C19, 3A4	Desmethyl-doxepin
Duloxetine	2D6, 1A2	Hydroxy-duloxetine
Escitalopram	3A4 > 2C19, 2D6	Desmethyl-escitalopram (2D6), Didesmethyl-escitalopram (2D6)
Fluoxetine	2C9, 2D6 > 3A4	Norfluoxetine (2D6)
Fluvoxamine	1A2, 2D6	None
Imipramine	1A2 > 2C19, 3A4	Desipramine (2D6), 2-hydroxy-imipramine
Maprotiline	2D6	Desmethyl-maprotiline
Mirtazapine	3A4 > 2D6 > 1A2	Desmethyl-mirtazapine
Nefazodone	3A4	Hydroxy-nefazodone, *m*-Chlorophenylpiperazine (2D6)
Nortriptyline	2D6	10-Hydroxy-nortriptyline
Paroxetine	2D6	None
Protriptyline	2D6	Desmethyl-protriptyline
Selegiline	2B6	Desmethyl-selegiline, L-methamphetamine, L-amphetamine
Sertraline	2C9, 3A4	Desmethyl-sertraline
Trazodone	3A4	*m*-Chlorophenylpiperazine (2D6)
Trimipramine	2D6	Desmethyl-trimipramine
Venlafaxine	2D6 > 3A4	*o*-Desmethyl-venlafaxine (2D6)

[a]Isoenzyme responsible for the metabolism of primary metabolite is indicated in parentheses.

be poorly tolerated. Fortunately, most of these side effects are transient and less severe with lower doses (e.g., gastrointestinal distress and insomnia associated with SSRI and SNRI) and will abate with continued treatment.

Since the onset of therapeutic benefit is usually not evident for 1–2 weeks after initiation, and maximum benefit may require 3–4 weeks, the rate of titration is most strongly influenced early on by tolerability rather than efficacy. Recommended titration methods for bupropion are more specific in order to account for the risk of seizures that have been linked to total daily doses as well as aggressive initiation. For most antidepressants titration is designed to improve general tolerability and is left to the prescriber's discretion.

Other factors that may influence titration include the severity of target symptoms and the treatment setting (inpatient vs. outpatient). As most patients are prescribed antidepressants for mild to moderate symptoms and are seen in an ambulatory care setting, slow titration is often preferred and is usually associated with increased medication adherence. It should be noted that the elderly often respond more slowly to the pharmacological effects of antidepressants and therapeutic trials may be considerably longer in this population (6–8 weeks vs. 3–4 weeks in the general population).[19]

When an effective dose is identified, it may be advisable to assess drug concentrations for certain antidepressants that possess experimental evidence of an effective therapeutic range (i.e., certain of the tricyclics). With antidepressants such as the SSRI and SNRI, efficacy and toxicity have not been closely correlated with drug concentrations and therapeutic drug monitoring is only recommended under uncommon circumstances such as hepatic or renal insufficiency, supra-therapeutic doses, or history of poor compliance. While a recommended therapeutic range for bupropion has not been determined, concerns about the accumulation of the active metabolite (hydroxybupropion) and subsequent seizures may warrant plasma concentration monitoring in patients with hepatic or renal impairment.

For tricyclic antidepressants, a variety of dosing strategies have been proposed. For instance, several methods use a concentration determined shortly after the initial dose to select a constant dosage for reaching a targeted concentration at steady state. These methods, which have been thoroughly reviewed elsewhere, have acceptable accuracy and probably have been underutilized.[20] They require use of a previously established mathematical relationship between the drug concentration determined one or more times after a single dose and the concentration produced at steady state following constant dosing. The use of this type of predictive approach with a new patient assumes that the patient's drug disposition pattern will be similar to that of the previously tested population.

Several concentrations determined after the first dose can be used to estimate clearance and to predict a dosage for a targeted steady state with simple mathematical relationships. Nomograms are also available for this purpose. The most applicable drug for prospective dosing methods is nortriptyline with its widely accepted therapeutic range.[20]

For most patients, linearity can be assumed in drug disposition with most antidepressants, and dosage can be adjusted according to the principles outlined elsewhere in this book. Dosage changes made to achieve a new concentration should always be guided by feedback from acute and chronic pharmacological effects (presence or lack of side effects and therapeutic effects). Nonlinearity may be encountered occasionally and can be manifested by an exaggerated pharmacologic response to a dosage increase.[21] This is attributed to a disproportional increase in the concentration of a drug and/or metabolites. For example, a doubling of the daily dose of paroxetine has been shown to increase steady state plasma concentrations five-fold in some patients.[22] Non-linearity in the dose-concentration relationship has also been described for fluoxetine. While the clinical significance of nonlinearity is debatable, this pharmacokinetic anomaly may suggest that smaller dose increments should be used during titration.[9]

Therapeutic Range

The effective and appropriate dosing recommendations for many psychotropic medications are often different than those found in the manufacturers' package insert. With antidepressants, the effective maintenance doses are often *lower* than the FDA-approved package insert for several reasons. For instance, dose-ranging or fixed-dose studies are usually conducted among study subjects with moderate-severe symptoms and little if any medical comorbidity (and corresponding potential for drug interactions). However, most patients treated with antidepressants have mild-moderate symptoms and are concurrently suffering from several other medical illnesses and receiving other medications that may interact with antidepressants or alter patients' sensitivity to their effects.

An additional reason that the manufacturers often endorse a higher dosing range has to do with preclinical study designs. By including higher doses in clinical trials, researchers may be able to enroll a smaller study population and still demonstrate relatively superior treatment effects (in comparison to placebo) while minimizing the possibility of Type II study error. Effective therapeutic doses may also contrast with published recommendations for pharmacokinetic reasons. For instance, huge interindividual variations in clearance values have been reported for many of the antidepressants. Steady state concentrations can vary 10-fold with fluoxetine at fixed dosages, and 40-fold variations have been reported with tricyclic agents. Much of this variability can be attributed to differences in the genetic expression of liver enzymes (e.g., genetic polymorphism of the CYP 2D6 isoenzyme). Genetic variability may also influence the activity of transport proteins, such as p-glycoprotein, which regulate CNS concentrations, leading to further variability and patient response.

The antidepressants with the best established therapeutic ranges are nortriptyline, imipramine, desipramine, and amitriptyline.[23] The SSRI and other antidepressants have not been reported to have a concentration range correlated with clinical response or adverse events.[24] Average steady state concentrations from usual doses have been reported, which may be useful in assessing medication adherence or the presence of drug-drug interactions, but are not necessarily predictive of response.

The use of drug concentrations to determine adequate dosages for antidepressants is complicated by the lack of rigorously defined therapeutic ranges. Furthermore, the use of average dosage ranges with the cyclic antidepressants is complicated by the variability of patient response to various concentrations (i.e., pharmacodynamic variations). Due to the vast differences in pharmacokinetic parameters among various patient populations, clinical response continues to be the best indicator of adequate dosage.

Tricyclic antidepressants

Several studies confirmed that a curvilinear therapeutic window exists for nortriptyline and the best antidepressant response is frequently obtained with a concentration of 50–150 mcg/L.[5,25,26] The recommended therapeutic range for nortriptyline (or other TCAs) in children has not been determined, but clinical experience suggests that safe and effective concentrations are comparable to or slightly lower than those achieved by adults.[27] It should be noted, however, that the effects of tricyclics on cardiac conduction and blood pressure parameters can be considerably different in children than mature adults and EKG monitoring is always advised.

The combined plasma concentration of imipramine and its demethylated metabolite, desipramine, is frequently 180–350 mcg/L when optimal antidepressant response is observed.[23] However, the dose–response curve is thought to be more linear compared to that of nortriptyline and the upper limit of the range is less distinct. Desipramine concentrations of 115–250 mcg/L are frequently therapeutic.

It is rarely justified for imipramine plus desipramine concentrations to exceed 350 mcg/L. However, an occasional patient will have excessive concentrations from usual doses, probably due to genetically determined poor hepatic hydroxylation ability. A combined concentration >500 mcg/L should prompt great concern as TCAs can slow cardiac conduction in a concentration-dependent manner. Concentrations approaching 500 mcg/L may result in serious EKG abnormalities such as QT prolongation or asystole. A concentration of 1000 mcg/L for any tricyclic antidepressant may herald extreme toxicity (seizures, arrhythmias, coma) and is sometimes used to define an overdose. Unfortunately, some side effects of TCAs can occur at any concentration and cannot be used to reflect the drug concentration.[27]

Evidence for amitriptyline's therapeutic range is not as strong.[28] On the lower end, combined concentrations of amitriptyline plus nortriptyline that are less than 100–200 mcg/L tend not to be therapeutic except in a small number of patients. Concentrations greatly exceeding this range (e.g., >450 mcg/L) have been associated with anticholinergic delirium.[29]

Other antidepressants

Efforts to predict therapeutic response from drug concentrations with newer agents have not been quite as fruitful. Research investigations in recent years have begun to focus more intently upon genetic differences in metabolic capacity than traditional clinical pharmacokinetic domains. The therapeutic ranges listed in Table 8-4 reflect the steady state concentrations observed in pooled populations of responsive patients, as opposed to genuine therapeutic ranges identified from rigorous controlled trial conditions. Responders may exist outside of the ranges listed, and some nonresponders may have steady state concentrations within the desired ranges. Nonetheless, drug concentration measures may be useful in verifying adherence, documenting drug interactions, and monitoring safety in special populations such as the elderly, children, or patients with renal or hepatic impairment.

Several studies examined whether a therapeutic range exists for fluoxetine.[30,31] Multiple reports found no relationship between drug concentrations and clinical effects. However, other data suggest the existence of a possible therapeutic window where high concentrations of the metabolite, norfluoxetine, are associated with nonresponse. Overall, the best response appears when the combined fluoxetine plus norfluoxetine concentration is less than 500 mcg/L.

A small flexible dose study with sertraline reported a significant correlation between drug concentrations and effectiveness as maintenance treatment.[32] A relatively low concentration of 25–50 mcg/L was adequate for maintaining therapeutic effects, but this association has not been replicated in a larger study population. Naturalistic studies with citalopram, fluoxetine, and sertraline reported large differences in inter-individual concentrations with therapeutic doses and lower apparent clearance values for women and the elderly.[24,33] Correlations between drug concentrations and response or toxicity were not found.

Three reports examined the value of monitoring bupropion concentrations.[34–36] Data suggested that hydroxymetabolite concentrations greater than 1200 mcg/L may undermine response. For bupropion alone, concentrations associated with clinical response appear to be in the 20–50 mcg/L range and are usually <100 mcg/L.

There have also been attempts to demonstrate an association with venlafaxine concentrations and clinical response.[37,38] Unfortunately, authors have reported a very wide range of concentrations relative to dose and little evidence of a true therapeutic range. More recently, researchers have employed positron emission tomography (PET) to study the correlation between the occupancy of serotonin reuptake sites by SSRI/SNRI in the brain and daily dosages, drug concentrations, and patient response.[39] They reported a nonlinear relationship, with occupancy rates greater 80%, correlated with positive outcomes and that there was little gained from further dosage increases (i.e. a therapeutic plateau). Interestingly, the researchers confirmed that doses generally prescribed for treatment response were also associated with achievement of this 80% threshold (fluoxetine 20 mg daily; sertraline 25 mg daily; paroxetine 20–40 mg daily; citalopram 20–40 mg daily; and venlafaxine 75 mg daily) Two published reports have linked trazodone concentrations with observed clinical effects.[40,41] A therapeutic threshold concentration of 650 mcg/L was reported but, as this medication is only rarely used for its antidepressant properties due to potent sedating effects, the clinical utility of this association is limited.

Table 8-5 summarizes the available information on therapeutic ranges of the various antidepressants.

Table 8-5. Potential Therapeutic Concentrations of Antidepressants

Drug	Concentrations Associated with Therapeutic Doses (mcg/L)[a]
Amitriptyline[43–45]	120–250[b,c]
Amoxapine[46]	200–600[d]
Bupropion[34,47]	20–50, <100[e]
Citalopram[8]	40–300
Clomipramine[48–50]	100–250[b,f]
Desipramine[27]	>115–250
Desvenlafaxine	N/A
Doxepin[51]	>110–250[b,d]
Duloxetine	N/A
Escitalopram	N/A
Fluoxetine[33]	75–450[g]
Fluvoxamine[8]	20–500
Imipramine[52,53]	180–350[b,c]
Maprotiline[56]	200–600[b,d]
Mirtazapine[8]	20–40
Nefazodone[8]	150–1000
Nortriptyline[23,55]	50–150[h]
Paroxetine	10–600
Phenelzine	N/A
Protriptyline[56,57]	75–250[d]
Selegiline	N/A
Sertraline	20–200
Tranylcypromine	N/A
Trazodone[58,59]	500–1500
Trimipramine[60]	100–300[d]
Venlafaxine[8]	50–150

[a]Applies to treatment of major depression. Concentration monitoring may be particularly helpful in situations of overdosage, inadequate response, diagnosis of noncompliance, and investigation of drug interactions.
[b]Parent drug plus desmethyl metabolite.
[c]Therapeutic range is less established than for nortriptyline. Concentrations >450 mcg/L frequently correlate with delirium and anticholinergic toxicity. Some responders occur below this range.
[d]No established therapeutic range; responders are frequently in this range.
[e]Limited data are available but suggest that high parent drug concentrations (>100 mcg/L) may be disadvantageous; one small study suggested that high hydroxylated metabolite concentrations correlated with the lack of antidepressant response.
[f]Parent drug concentrations. Metabolite concentrations may be somewhat higher. Therapeutic range is not well established.
[g]Sparse data are available. Metabolite concentrations may fall in the same range as for the parent drug but persist longer after discontinuance of dosing due to a prolonged half-life.
[h]Clear therapeutic window with curvilinear response. Many patients with concentrations greater than 150 mcg/L show a poor response; a better response occurs if the dose is decreased to produce concentrations within the range.
NA = data not available.

Therapeutic Monitoring

Suggested sampling times

Accurate interpretation of drug concentrations requires the achievement of steady state conditions. For most of these drugs, the minimum time to steady state is 3–4 days. Exceptions are protriptyline and fluoxetine. Because of the long half-life of the drug or metabolite, at least 2 weeks of constant dosing with protriptyline and up to 4 weeks for fluoxetine may be required before steady state conditions occur. For antidepressants with relatively short half-lives such as venlafaxine and duloxetine, steady state concentrations of the parent drugs may be reached in 2 days. When concentration monitoring is indicated, an accepted standardized time for drawing blood is approximately 12 hours after the previous dose, usually in the morning. Trough concentration measurements are acceptable. If therapeutic monitoring of antidepressants is indicated for a given patient, no established frequency has been recommended. Concentration monitoring may be advisable when: (1) a significant dosage change occurs, (2) a patient is exhibiting serious symptoms of toxicity at doses within the therapeutic range, (3) a medication is ineffective and/or noncompliance is suspected, (4) a potential drug interaction may be present, or (5) renal or hepatic function significantly changes.

Further Considerations for Sampling

Analytical methods used to quantify antidepressant concentrations in plasma vary in their expense, sensitivity, reliability, and ease of operations. Currently employed methods include radioimmunoassay, high performance liquid chromatography, gas chromatography, and enzyme and fluorescence immunoassay methods (EMIT and TDX). All are sensitive enough to provide reliable data for routine monitoring purposes, but the laboratory must maintain an internal and external quality control program. Recently, NMR spectroscopy has been employed to estimate antidepressant concentrations in the brain. With fluoxetine and norfluoxetine, researchers reported that CNS concentrations were roughly 10 times those reported in the periphery. It is hoped that these efforts to quantify antidepressant concentrations in the effective compartment (the brain) will inspire future efforts to explore correlations with efficacy and/or toxicity.[42]

Pharmacodynamic Monitoring

Drug-drug interactions

The CYP450 isoenzyme inhibitory potential of the various antidepressants is summarized in Table 8-6. The capacity for some newer drugs to inhibit isoforms of the cytochrome P450 (CYP450) system in recent years has stimulated much research in this field. While much can be learned about the inhibitory effects of these medications from in vitro investigations, the potential for and severity of observed drug interactions remains largely unpredictable. This may be due to phenotypic variations among the liver enzymes, as well as differences in study design (single dose versus steady state, dosing strength, sampling methods, etc.). More in-depth discussions of this phenomenon have been published elsewhere.[61–65]

Among the SSRIs, fluoxetine and paroxetine strongly inhibit CYP2D6 in vitro. Fluoxetine also has been shown to be a mild inhibitor of CYP2C9; its metabolite, norfluoxetine, is a potent inhibitor of CYP3A4, which may be of clinical relevance as steady state concentrations of the metabolite usually exceed the parent compound. Fluvoxamine is unique among the SSRIs in its potent inhibition of CYP1A2. It also inhibits CYP2C9 and CYP3A4. Sertraline is a mild inhibitor of CYP2D6 and CYP2C9. Citalopram and escitalopram are also mild inhibitors of CYP2D6.

While bupropion has only a mild affinity for the CYP2D6 isoenzyme in vitro, subsequent in vivo studies have revealed a potent inhibitory effects on this enzyme and clinically significant drug interactions have been reported.[66,67] Duloxetine has also demonstrated potent inhibitory effects on the metabolism of CYP2D6 substrates.[68] Venlafaxine and mirtazapine do not appear to have a significant potential for inhibiting CYP450 isoenzymes.

Select drug-drug interactions are shown in Table 8-7. Many other interactions may exist and new ones are postulated or demonstrated frequently so these should only be considered as a limited set of examples.

Table 8-6. Inhibitory Potential of Selected Antidepressants

Medication	CYP 1A2	CYP 2C9	CYP 2C19	CYP2D6	CYP3A4
Bupropion	---	---	---	+++	---
Citalopram	---	---	---	+	---
Desvenlafaxine	---	---	---	---	---
Duloxetine	---	---	---	+++	---
Escitalopram	---	---	---	+	---
Fluoxetine	+	+	+	+++	++
Fluvoxamine	+++	+++	+++	---	+++
Paroxetine	---	---	---	+++	---
Sertraline	+	---	+	+	+
Venlafaxine	---	---	---	+	---

--- = minimal; + = mild; ++ = moderate; +++ = strong.

Drug–Disease State or Condition Interactions

Adolescence

Milligram per kilogram dose requirements may be higher in adolescents compared with adults due to more efficient hepatic elimination and differences in body composition (e.g., lower percentage of body fat). Chronic therapy may require relatively higher doses to maintain the same concentration.[69] Divided doses may be necessitated by shorter half-life as well.

Advanced age

Geriatric patients (age > 65 years) have decreased ability to metabolize many medications, including antidepressants. Drug concentrations are often higher at steady state due to lower clearance, though some elderly will show no apparent impairment in clearance compared to younger patients because the activity of CYP450 enzymes does not decrease uniformly with age.[19,70] CYP2D6 is still preserved in the elderly while total P450 content decreases markedly after age 70 years.[68] Plasma half-lives are considerably longer in the elderly due to decreased clearance as well as larger volumes of distribution secondary to higher body fat composition. The pharmacodynamic action of psychotropic medications may also be inherently different in the elderly and they may consequently be more sensitive to cognitive or sedating effects. This sensitivity may be attributed, in part, to changes in the integrity of the blood-brain barrier that occur with age and ultimately permit increased CNS penetration of lipophilic agents.[71] As a result of these physiological distinctions, the elderly should empirically receive smaller initial doses of all antidepressants (e.g., one-third to one-half reduction).

Alcoholism, alcoholic liver disease

The usual result of alcoholic liver disease is impairment of drug metabolism accompanied by a longer half-life and higher steady state concentrations. An increase in the severity of adverse drug reactions is possible.[74] Further, patients commonly report an increased sensitivity to the subjective effects of alcohol when antidepressants are concurrently administered with subsequent impairment in motor and cognitive function. Alcohol dependence or abuse may also dampen or reverse the therapeutic benefits of antidepressants.

Cardiac disease

Little data exist on alterations of pharmacokinetic parameters in cardiac disease. Orthostatic hypotension may become worse, especially with tricyclic antidepressants and trazodone. Caution is also required due to tachycardia and anticholinergic effects of tricyclics. Tricyclic antidepressants may be relatively contraindicated in severe conduction defects, while the SSRIs and bupropion appear to be relatively safe in patients with cardiac disease and there is evidence that SSRIs may improve cardiac outcomes in the depressed population.[75,76]

Table 8-7. Selected Antidepressant Drug Interactions

Drug	Combined Therapy	Interaction	Suggested Action
Bupropion	Carbamazepine, phenobarbital, phenytoin	Reduce antidepressant concentration	Monitor effects closely
	Monoamine oxidase inhibitors[b]	Potential toxicity	Contraindicated
	Drugs with seizure activity	Combined increased risk	Use with caution
	Venlafaxine	Increased venlafaxine concentration	Monitor effects closely
Duloxetine	Type 1C antiarrhythmics	Increased antiarrhythmic concentration	Caution advised
	Beta-blockers (propranolol, metoprolol)	Increased beta-blocker concentrations	Caution advised
	Tricyclic antidepressants	Increased TCA concentrations	Decrease TCA dose
	Benzodiazepines	Increased sedation, other side effects	Avoid or lower doses and monitor
Mirtazapine	Monoamine oxidase inhibitors[b]	Potential serotonin syndrome	Contraindicated
SSRIs[a]	Benzodiazepines (alprazolam, midazolam, triazolam)	Increased anxiolytic concentration with fluvoxamine	Monitor effects, may require reduced dosage
	Antiarrhythmics (Type IC)	Increased antiarrhythmic concentration	Caution advised
	Beta-blockers (propranolol, metoprolol)	Increased beta-blocker concentration	Caution advised
	Carbamazepine	Increased concentration in some patients	Monitor carbamazepine concentration
	Cimetidine	Increased SSRI concentration	Usually no action required
	Clozapine	Increased concentration from fluvoxamine and fluoxetine	Monitor clozapine concentration
	Codeine	Inhibited metabolism to morphine by CYP2D6 inhibitors	Use non-interacting SSRI or other antidepressant
	Estrogens	Increased concentration	Use with caution
	Monoamine oxidase inhibitors[b]	Possible serotonin syndrome	Contraindicated combination
	Phenytoin	Increased concentration with fluoxetine, possible with fluvoxamine and sertraline	Monitor phenytoin concentration
	Sumatriptan	Possible serotonin syndrome	Avoid combination if possible
	Theophylline	Increased concentration with fluvoxamine	Monitor theophylline concentration, use lower doses as needed
	Tramadol	Possible serotonin syndrome	Avoid combination if possible
	Tricyclic antidepressants	Reciprocal inhibition	Monitor, use lower doses as needed
	Warfarin	Increased warfarin effects	Monitor prothrombin time
Tricyclic antidepressants	Anticholinergics	Increased adverse effects	Use lower initial doses
	Antipsychotics	Mutual inhibition with some increased concentration	Use lower initial doses
	Carbamazepine, barbiturates	Decreased tricyclic antidepressant concentration	Monitor effects and concentrations as needed
	Cimetidine, disulfiram, methadone, quinidine, SSRIs[a] bupropion, duloxetine	Increased concentration of some drugs or metabolites	Monitor concentrations when appropriate
	Monoamine oxidase inhibitors[b]	Fatal reaction possible	Contraindicated combination
	Valproate	Tricyclic antidepressants can increase	Monitor concentration and effects

Table 8-7. (Continued)

Drug	Combined Therapy	Interaction	Suggested Action
Venlafaxine	Bupropion	Increased venlafaxine concentrations	Monitor effects closely
	Cimetidine	Increased venlafaxine concentration	No action usually required, monitor
	Haloperidol	Increased haloperidol concentration	Monitor and adjust doses as needed
	Monoamine oxidase inhibitors	Toxicity	Contraindicated

[a]SSRIs = selective serotonin reuptake inhibitors.
[b]Severe reactions, including death, have occurred when monoamine oxidase inhibitors have been combined with antidepressants. Symptoms that suggest a serotonin syndrome include tremors, myoclonus, diaphoresis, nausea, vomiting, dizziness, and hyperthermia.

SNRIs and bupropion have been associated with small but statistically significant elevations in blood pressure and/or heart rate, and routine monitoring is advisable when these medications are prescribed.

Hepatic insufficiency

As the liver metabolizes virtually all antidepressants, significant hepatic compromise may lead to accumulation of the parent compound(s) and some metabolites. Similarly, liver dysfunction may lead to a decrease in first pass metabolism and an increase in apparent bioavailability. In general, hepatic compromise will affect drugs undergoing phase I reactions (such as oxidative metabolism) to a greater extent than phase II reactions (conjugation).[77] Most psychotropic medications undergo phase I metabolic processes. For example, the disposition of duloxetine is dramatically affected by even moderate liver impairment (e.g., 5-fold increase reported in AUC). As a result, empiric dosage reduction and/or increases in dosing intervals are encouraged for all antidepressants whenever significant liver damage is evident. Antidepressants with narrow therapeutic indices or those that possess potentially toxic metabolites (e.g., bupropion) should be avoided.

Inflammatory disease states

Protein binding may be altered due to increases in alpha-1-acid glycoprotein. In theory, increases in plasma protein binding may decrease the free concentration of antidepressant in the plasma, leading to a decrease in CSF concentrations (as the blood brain barrier is relatively impermeable to bound drug). However, the clinical importance of protein binding changes has not been demonstrated.

Nutritional status

Severe malnutrition may alter protein binding and potentially impact therapeutic outcomes. Although literature documentation is limited, caution is warranted.

Renal insufficiency

Parent drug concentrations of most cyclic antidepressants are not greatly affected, but conjugated water-soluble metabolites can show excessive accumulation in renal insufficiency. In moderate to severe renal failure (i.e., CrCl = 10–50 ml/min), adverse consequences may be more likely to occur with normal doses so initial doses should be decreased by 50%–75% for antidepressants such as bupropion, mirtazapine, paroxetine, and venlafaxine.[77]

Smoking status

Smoking has an inductive effect on hepatic microsomal enzymes responsible for metabolizing cyclic antidepressants. More rapid drug elimination and decreased steady state concentrations may result. This effect is best described for medications metabolized via the CYP 1A2 isoenzyme, but other pathways may be affected. Due to the high interindividual variability in clearance values, empiric changes in dosing recommendations for smokers are not endorsed at this time.

Thyroid disease

Documentation of effects of thyroid disease on the pharmacokinetics of antidepressants is lacking. Hypothyroidism may mimic depression and result in a lack of antidepressant response until the underlying problem is treated. l-Triiodothyronine (T3) is sometimes used as an adjunct to antidepressant therapy in relative nonresponders.[78]

References

1. Olfson M, Marcus SC, Druss B, et al. National trends in the outpatient treatment of depression. *JAMA*. 2002;287:203-9.
2. Lee KC, Feldman MD, Finley PR. Beyond depression: evaluation of newer indications and offlabel uses for SSRIs (Part 1 of 2). *Formulary*. 2002;37:40-51.
3. Ranga K, Krishnan R. Comorbidity and depression treatment. *Biol Psychiatry*. 2003;53:701-6.
4. Hirschfeld RMA. Efficacy of SSRI's and newer antidepressants in severe depression: comparison with TCAs. *J Clin Psychiatry*. 1999;60:326-35.
5. DeVane CL, Jarecke R. Cyclic antidepressants. In: Evans WE, Schentag JJ, Jusko WJ, eds. *Applied Pharmacokinetics, Principles of Therapeutic Drug Monitoring*. 3rd ed. Vancouver, WA: Applied Therapeutics; 1992.
6. Preskorn SH, Dorey RC, Jerkovich GS. Therapeutic drug monitoring of tricyclic antidepressants. *Clin Chem*. 1988;34:822-8.
7. DeVane CL. *Fundamentals of Monitoring Psychoactive Drug Therapy*. Baltimore, MD: Williams & Wilkins; 1990.
8. Medlewicz J. Optimizing antidepressant use in clinical practice: towards criteria for antidepressant selection. *Br J Psychiatry*. 2001;179 (suppl 42):1-3.
9. DeVane CL. Differential pharmacology of newer antidepressants. *J Clin Psychiatry*. 1998;59 (suppl 20):85-93.
10. Ballenger JC, Davidson JR, Lecrubier Y, et al. Consensus statement on panic disorder from the International Consensus Group on Depression and Anxiety. *J Clin Psychiatry*. 1998;59 (suppl 8):47-54.
11. Pentel PR, Bullock ML, DeVane CL. Hemoperfusion for imipramine overdose: elimination of active metabolites. *J Toxicol Clin Toxicol*. 1982;19:239-48.
12. DeVane CL. Metabolism and pharmacokinetics of selective serotonin reuptake inhibitors. *Cell Mol Neurobiol*. 1999;19:443-66.
13. Borys DJ, Setzer SC, Ling LJ, et al. The effect of fluoxetine in the overdose patient. *J Toxicol Clin Toxicol*. 1990;28:331-40.
14. Barbey JT, Roose SP. SSRI safety in overdose. *J Clin Psychiatry*. 1998;59:42-8.
15. Rudorfer MV, Potter WZ. Metabolism of tricyclic antidepressants. *Cell Mol Neurobiol*. 1999;19:373-409.
16. Sharma A, Goldberg MJ, Cerimele BJ. Pharmacokinetics and safety of duloxetine, a dual-serotonin and norepinephrine reuptake inhibitor. *J Clin Pharmacol*. 2000;40:161-7.
17. Jefferson JW, Pradko JF, Muir KT. Bupropion for major depressive disorder: pharmacokinetic and formulation considerations. *Clinical Therapeutics* 2005;27:1685-95.
18. Finley PR. Depression and coexisting medical illness: treatment considerations. *The Rx Consultant*. 2004;13:1-8.
19. DeVane CL, Pollock BG. Pharmacokinetic considerations of antidepressant use in the elderly. *J Clin Psychiatry*. 1999;60(suppl 20):38-44.
20. DeVane CL, Rudorfer MV, Potter WZ. Dosage regimen design for cyclic antidepressants: a review of pharmacokinetic methods. *Psychopharmacol Bull*. 1991;27:619-31.
21. Nelson JC, Jatlow PI. Nonlinear desipramine kinetics: prevalence and importance. *Clin Pharmacol Ther*. 1987;41:666-70.
22. Kaye CM, Haddock RE, Langley PF, et al. A review of the metabolism and pharmacokinetics of paroxetine in man. *Acta Psychiatr Scand*. 1989;80 (suppl 35):60-75.
23. Glassman AH, Schildkraut JJ, Orsulak PJ, et al. Tricyclic antidepressant blood level measurements and clinical outcome. *Am J Psychiatry*. 1985;142:155-63.
24. Mitchell PB. Therapeutic drug monitoring of non-tricyclic antidepressant drugs. *Clin Chem Lab Med*. 2004;42:1212-8.
25. Kragh-Sorensen P, Hansen CE, Baastrup PC, et al. Self-inhibiting action of nortriptyline's antidepressant effect at high plasma levels. *Psychopharmacology*. 1976;45:305-14.
26. Perry PJ, Browne JL, Alexander B, et al. Two prospective dosing methods for nortriptyline. *Clin Pharmacokinet*. 1984;9:555-63.
27. Nelson JC, Jatlow PI, Bock J, et al. Major adverse reactions during desipramine treatment. *Arch Gen Psychiatry*. 1982;39:1055-61.

28. Breyer-Pfaff U, Giedke H, Gaertner HJ, et al. Validation of a therapeutic plasma level range in amitriptyline treatment of depression. *J Clin Psychopharmacol*. 1989;9:116-21.

29. Preskorn SH, Irwin HA. Toxicity of tricyclic antidepressants—kinetics, mechanism, intervention: a review. *J Clin Psychiatry*. 1982;43:151-6.

30. Goodnick PJ. Pharmacokinetics of second generation antidepressants: fluoxetine. *Psychopharmacol Bull*. 1991;27:503-12.

31. Amsterdam JD, Fawcett J, Quitkin FM, et al. Fluoxetine and norfluoxetine plasma concentrations in major depression: a multicenter study. *Am J Psychiatry*. 1997;154:963-9.

32. Mauri MC, Fiorentini A, Cerveri G, et al. Long-term efficacy and therapeutic drug monitoring of sertraline in major depression. *Hum Psychopharmacol*. 2003;18:385-8.

33. Lundmark J, Reis M, Bengtsson F. Therapeutic drug monitoring of sertraline: variability factors as displayed in a clinical setting. *Ther Drug Monit*. 2000;22:446-54.

34. Golden RN, DeVane CL, Laizure SC, et al. Bupropion in depression. II. The role of metabolites in clinical outcome. *Arch Gen Psychiatry*. 1988;45:145-9.

35. Goodnick PJ. Blood levels and acute response to bupropion. *Am J Psychiatry*. 1992;149:399-400.

36. Preskorn SH. Antidepressant response and plasma concentrations of bupropion. *J Clin Psychiatry*. 1983;44(suppl 5):137-9.

37. Reis M, Lundmark J, Bjork H, et al. Therapeutic drug monitoring of racemic venlafaxine and its main metabolites in an everyday clinical setting. *Ther Drug Monit*. 2002:24:545-53.

38. Veefkind AH, Haffmans PMJ, Hoencamp E. Venlafaxine serum levels and CYP2D6 genotype. *Ther Drug Monit*. 2000;22:202-8.

39. Meyer JH, Wilson AA, Sagrati S, et al. Serotonin transporter occupancy of five selective serotonin reuptake inhibitors at different doses: an [11C]DASB positron emission tomography study. *Am J Psychiatry*. 2004;161:826-35.

40. Monteleone P, Gnocchi G, Delrio G. Plasma trazodone concentrations and clinical response in elderly depressed patients: a preliminary study. *J Clin Psychopharmacol*. 1989;9:284-7.

41. Mihara K, Yasui-Furukori N, Kondo T, et al. Relationship between plasma concentrations of trazodone and its active metabolite, m-chlorophenylpiperazine, and its clinical effect in depressed patients. *Ther Drug Monit*. 2002;24:563-6.

42. Bolo NR, Hode Y, Nedelec JF, et al. Brain pharmacokinetics and tissue distribution in vivo of fluvoxamine and fluoxetine by fluorine magnetic resonance spectroscopy. *Neuropsychopharmacology*. 2000;23:428-38.

43. Young RC. Hydroxylated metabolites of antidepressants. *Psychopharmacol Bull*. 1991;27:521-32.

44. Ziegler VE, Co BT, Taylor JR, et al. Amitriptyline plasma levels and therapeutic response. *Clin Pharmacol Ther*. 1976;19:795-801.

45. Kupfer DJ, Hanin I, Spiker DG, et al. Amitriptyline plasma levels and clinical response in primary depression. *Clin Pharmacol Ther*. 1977;22:904-11.

46. Boutelle WE. Clinical response and blood levels in the treatment of depression with a new antidepressant drug, amoxapine. *Neuropharmacology*. 1980;19:1229-31.

47. Preskorn SH. Should bupropion dosage be adjusted based upon therapeutic drug monitoring? *Psychopharmacol Bull*. 1991;27:637-43.

48. Reisby N, Gram LF, Beck P, et al. Clomipramine: plasma levels and clinical effects. *Commun Psychopharmacol*. 1979;5:341-51.

49. Traskman L, Asberg M, Bertilsson L, et al. Plasma levels of clomipramine and its desmethyl metabolite during treatment of depression. Differential biochemical and clinical effects of the two compounds. *Clin Pharmacol Ther*. 1979;26:600-10.

50. Stern RS, Marks IM, Mawson D, et al. Clomipramine and exposure for compulsive rituals II: plasma levels, side effects and outcome. *Br J Psychiatry*. 1980;136:161-6.

51. Linnoila M, Seppala T, Mattila MJ, et al. Clomipramine and doxepin in depressive neurosis: plasma levels and therapeutic response. *Arch Gen Psychiatry*. 1980;37:1295-9.

52. Reisby N, Gram LF, Beck P, et al. Imipramine: clinical effects and pharmacokinetic variability. *Psychopharmacology*. 1977;54:263-72.

53. Glassman AH, Perel JM, Shostak M, et al. Clinical implications of imipramine plasma levels for depressive illness. *Arch Gen Psychiatry*. 1977;34:197-204.

54. Gwirtsman HE, Ahles S, Halaris A, et al. Therapeutic superiority of maprotiline versus doxepin in geriatric depression. *J Clin Psychiatry*. 1983;44:449-53.

55. Montgomery S, Braithwaite R, Dawling S, et al. High plasma nortriptyline levels in the treatment of depression. *Clin Pharmacol Ther*. 1978;23:309-14.

56. Biggs JT, Holland WH, Sherman WR. Steady-state protriptyline levels in an outpatient population. *Am J Psychiatry*. 1975;132:960-2.

57. Moody JP, Whyte SF, MacDonald AJ, et al. Pharmacokinetic aspects of protriptyline plasma levels. *Eur J Clin Pharmacol*. 1977;11:51-6.

58. Putzolu S, Pecknold JC, Baiocchi L. Trazodone: clinical and biochemical studies II. Blood levels and therapeutic responsiveness. *Psychopharmacol Bull*. 1976;12:40-1.

59. Mann JJ, Georgotas A, Newton R, et al. A controlled study of trazodone, imipramine, and placebo in outpatients with endogenous depression. *J Clin Psychopharmacol*. 1981;1:75-80.

60. Suckow RF, Cooper TB. Determination of trimipramine and metabolites in plasma by liquid chromatography with electrochemical detection. *J Pharm Sci*. 1984;73:1745-8.

61. Nemeroff CB, DeVane CL, Pollock BG. Antidepressants and the cytochrome P450 system. *Am J Psychiatry*. 1996;153:311-20.

62. Ereshefsky L, Riesenman C, Lam YW. Antidepressant drug interactions and the cytochrome P450 system: the role of cytochrome P450 2D6. *Clin Pharmacokinet*. 1995;29(suppl 1):10-9.

63. Preskorn S, Werder S. Detrimental antidepressant drug-drug interactions: are they clinically relevant? *Neuropsychopharmacology*. 2006;31:1605-12.

64. Spina E, Santoro V, D'Arrigo C. Clinically relevant pharmacokinetic drug interactions with second-generation antidepressants: an update. *Clin Ther.* 2008; 30:1206-27.

65. Finley PR.Drug interactions with psychotropic medications. *Rx Consultant*. 2009; 7:1-10.

66. Kennedy SH, McCann SM, Masellis M, et al. Combining bupropion SR with venlafaxine, paroxetine, or fluoxetine: a preliminary report on pharmacokinetic, therapeutic, and sexual dysfunction effects. *J Clin Psychiatry*. 2002;63:181-6.

67. Kotlyar M, Brauer LH, Tracy TS, et al. Inhibition of CYP2D6 activity by bupropion. *J Clin Psychopharmacol*. 2005;25:226-9.

68. Preskorn SH, Greenblatt DJ, Flockhart D, et al. Comparison of duloxetine, escitalopram, and sertraline effects on CYP 2D6 function in healthy volunteers. *J Clin Psychopharmacol*. 2007;27:28-34.

69. Geller B. Psychopharmacology of children and adolescents: pharmacokinetics and relationships of plasma/serum levels to response. *Psychopharmacol Bull*. 1991;27:401-10.

70. DeVane CL, Pollock BG. Pharmacokinetic considerations of antidepressant use in the elderly. *J Clin Psychiatry*. 1999;60(suppl 20):38-44.

71. Grinberg LT, Thal DR. Vascular pathology in the aged brain. *Acta Neuropathol*. 2010; 119:277-90.

72. Greenblatt DJ, von Moltke LL, Harmatz JS, et al. Human cytochromes and some newer antidepressants: kinetics, metabolism, and drug interactions. *J Clin Psychopharmacol*. 1999;19(suppl 1):23S-35S.

73. Caccia S. Metabolism of newer antidepressants: an overview of the pharmacological and pharmacokinetic implications. *Clin Pharmacokinet*. 1998;34:281-302.

74. Shoaf SE, Linnoila M. Interaction of ethanol and smoking on the pharmacokinetics and pharmacodynamics of psychotropic medications. *Psychopharmacol Bull*. 1991;27:577-94.

75. Roose SR, Glassman AH. Cardiovascular effects of tricyclic antidepressants in depressed patients with and without heart disease. *J Clin Psychiatry Monograph*. 1989;7:1-18.

76. Glassman GH, O'Connor CM, Califf RM, et al. Sertraline treatment of major depression in patients with acute MI or unstable angina. *JAMA*. 2002;288:701-9.

77. Lane EA. Renal function and the disposition of antidepressants and their metabolites. *Psychopharmacol Bull*. 1991;27:533-40.

78. Goodwin FK, Prange A, Post R, et al. Potentiation of antidepressant effects by L-triiodothyronine in tricyclic nonresponders. *Am J Psychiatry*. 1982;139:34-8.

Chapter 9

*William R. Garnett, Jacquelyn L. Bainbridge, Michael D. Egeberg, and Sarah L. Johnson**

Newer Antiepileptic Drugs (AHFS 28:12)

Twelve antiepileptic drugs (AEDs) have been approved by the FDA since 1993 with several more in development. These drugs differ in structure and mechanism of action from the older AEDs (phenytoin, carbamazepine, phenobarbital, and valproic acid). The pharmacokinetic profiles of the newer AEDs are generally more predictable.

In the International League Against Epilepsy's "Guidelines for therapeutic monitoring of antiepileptic drugs," the League stated: "Use of blood levels to adjust dosage so that numbers fall within the "therapeutic range" is a waste of time and money and may even be dangerous if effective and well-tolerated therapy is changed simply because levels are not in the published ranges. It is better to develop a target range for each patient based on severity of epilepsy and tolerance of side effects."[1] In this scenario, the patient would act as his or her own historic control. In addition to this guidance, clinical studies have not been carried out specifically to determine target concentration ranges for any new antiepileptic drug. Thus, the need for therapeutic monitoring of drug concentrations with these agents is limited, but pharmacokinetic approaches to dosing may still have value in many cases. Therapy with these agents is, however, generally started at a low dose and titrated to patient response. High initial doses and rapid dose escalation have been shown to significantly increase the incidence of side effects with lamotrigine, tiagabine, topiramate, zonisamide, lacosamide, and vigabatrin. Table 9-1 provides the dosage forms of the twelve drugs in order of their approval by the FDA.

Felbamate (Felbatol)

Felbamate blocks the glycine receptor on the *N*-methyl-d-aspartate (NMDA) complex, thereby inhibiting the response to NMDA neuronal excitation. Felbamate may also prevent seizure propagation by blocking voltage-dependent sodium channels, calcium channels and bursting from kainic acid, as well as affecting the gamma-aminobutyric acid (GABA) system. It is structurally related to meprobamate, but dependency does not develop and there are no withdrawal effects.[2] Felbamate is approved for use in patients with refractory partial or generalized seizures and in patients with Lennox-Gastaut syndrome at doses of up to 3.6 g/day in adults and up to 45 mg/kg/day in children. Due to an increased risk of aplastic anemia and liver failure, the FDA currently limits the use of felbamate to patients who are refractory to other antiepileptic agents and places the following restrictions on its use: (1) Full hematological evaluations should be performed before therapy, frequently during therapy, and for a significant time after discontinuing therapy, and (2) liver function tests (AST, ALT, and bilirubin) should be done before therapy is started and at frequent intervals while the patient is taking felbamate, though the exact monitoring schedule is left to the clinical judgment of the prescriber.

Table 9-2 provides various pharmacokinetic parameters and general dosing guidelines for felbamate. The drug displays linear pharmacokinetics, and available oral products are rapidly absorbed. Food does not affect the absorption of the tablet dosage form, and the apparent bioavailability is estimated to be complete. Felbamate is distributed to a variety of organs including the liver, kidney, heart, lung, spleen, muscle, gonads, eyes, and brain and protein binding (mainly albumin) is limited.[3] Approximately 40%–50% of a given dose will be excreted unchanged in the urine with the rest undergoing liver metabolism. Felbamate is a substrate for CYP3A4, CYP2E1, and uridine-diphospho-glucuronyltransferase (UDPGT). The half-life is decreased in patients taking enzyme-inducing drugs such as carbamazepine and phenytoin as compared to drug-naïve patients. Felbamate concentrations in children are less than the concentrations in adults receiving comparable mg/kg doses, suggesting a more rapid elimination in the pediatric population.[3,4] Elderly subjects require a lower initial dose and slower rates of titration.[5] Gender does not affect the pharmacokinetics of felbamate, nor does race, renal function, or liver function.[4,6] The effects of pregnancy on the pharmacokinetics of felbamate are unknown at this time.[7]

*The authors would like to thank Holly Cooper for her contributions to this chapter.

Table 9-1. Dosage Forms of Newer Antiepileptic Drugs

Felbamate (Felbatol)	400- and 600-mg tablets
	600 mg/5 ml suspension
Gabapentin (Neurontin)	100-, 300-, and 400-mg capsules
	600- and 800-mg tablets
	250 mg/5 ml oral solution
Lamotrigine (Lamictal)	25-, 100-, 150-, and 200-mg tablets
	5-, and 25-mg chewable, dispersible tablets[a]
	25-, 50-, 100-, and 200-mg extended-release tablets
	25-, 50-, 100-, and 200-mg orally-disintegrating tablets
Tiagabine (Gabitril)	2-, 4-, 12-, and 16- mg tablets
Topiramate (Topamax)	25-, 50-, 100-, and 200-mg tablets
	15- and 25-mg sprinkle capsules[b]
Levetiracetam (Keppra)	250-, 500-, 750-, and 1000-mg tablets
	100 mg/ml oral suspension
	500 mg/5 ml IV injection
	500- and 750-mg extended-release tablets
Oxcarbazepine (Trileptal)	150-, 300-, and 600-mg tablets
	300 mg/5 ml oral suspension
Zonisamide (Zonegran)	25-, 50-, and 100-mg capsules
Pregabalin (Lyrica)	25-, 50-, 75-, 100-, 150-, 200-, 225-, and 300-mg capsules
Lacosamide (Vimpat)	50-, 100-, 150-, 200-mg tablets
	10-mg/ml oral solution
	200-mg/20 ml IV injection
Rufinamide (Banzel)	200- and 400-mg tablets
Vigabatrin (Sabril)	500-mg tablet
	500-mg powder for solution[c]

[a]May be swallowed, chewed, or diluted with 5 ml of water or fruit juice and taken immediately.
[b]May be swallowed whole but not chewed.
[c]Must be mixed with water before dose is given.

Felbamate inhibits CYP2C19, increases the half-life and decreases the clearance of phenobarbital, phenytoin, and valproic acid, and probably affects the pharmacokinetics of other drugs extensively metabolized by this enzyme. Interestingly, felbamate decreases the concentration of carbamazepine but increases the concentration of the active 10, 11-di-epoxide metabolite. The doses of phenobarbital, phenytoin, carbamazepine, and valproic acid should be decreased by 30%–50% when felbamate is added.[8,9]

In contrast to other antiepileptic drugs, felbamate is associated with CNS stimulation. Side effects include insomnia, decreased appetite, and weight loss.[4] At least 32 cases of aplastic anemia and 16 cases of hepatic failure have been reported. Aplastic anemia may be the result of the formation of an uncommon but toxic metabolite.[4] The incidence of aplastic anemia is higher in women with a history of autoimmune disease. Patients taking felbamate should have frequent CBCs and liver function tests.[10]

Table 9-2. Pharmacokinetic and Dosing Summary for Felbamate

Bioavailability (F)	100% (F = 1)
*t*max	1–4 hr
*t*½	16–23 hr (drug naive patients)
	11–16 hr (when receiving enzyme-inducing antiepileptics)
V	0.7–1.0 L/kg
Clearance	26 ± 3 ml/hr/kg
Protein binding	20%–35%
Elimination	50% renal, 50% hepatic
Therapeutic range	30–60 mg/L[7,11]
Usual dose	Adults: Initiate at 1200 mg/day (in three to four divided doses) then increase by 1200 mg/day weekly to a max dose of 3600 mg/day
Pediatrics	Initiate at 15 mg/kg/day (in three to four divided doses) then increase by 15 mg/kg/day weekly to 45 mg/kg/day
	Max dose: 3600 mg/day
Pregnancy	Unknown

Gabapentin (Neurontin)

Although gabapentin was designed to potentiate GABA at neuronal receptor sites, it does not work at either GABA A or GABA B receptors. It interacts with a specific high-affinity binding site that is an auxiliary protein subunit of voltage-gated calcium channels. It also causes a dose-proportional non-synaptic release of GABA, which increases the concentration of GABA in the brain. Gabapentin may also slightly increase GABA by enhancing its rate of synthesis from glutamate. It may decrease the concentration of glutamate, and it inhibits sodium channels by mechanisms different than phenytoin and carbamazepine. Gabapentin readily crosses the blood-brain barrier and concentrates in brain tissue by an active transport process that may saturate at higher plasma concentrations.[12]

Gabapentin is indicated as adjunctive therapy for patients with partial seizures with or without secondary generalization.[13] It is widely used in the treatment of pain and also for anxiety, panic attacks, migraine headaches, and other CNS disorders. The initial dose is 900 mg/day, given in 3–4 divided doses that are usually titrated upward over 3 days; the dose is then titrated to the patient's response.[14] The initially approved dose of up to 3.6 g is inadequate for many patients, and doses up to 10 g have been reported. Because the CNS side effects do not seem to be dose-dependent, gabapentin can be rapidly titrated to response.

Following oral administration, gabapentin binds to a sodium-independent L-like amino acid transport system that facilitates transport across the gut into the bloodstream and across the blood-brain barrier to the site of activity in the brain.[15] However, binding to the L-amino acid transport system becomes saturated, and the bioavailability of gabapentin decreases with increasing dose (see Table 9-3 for pharmacokinetic parameters and general dosing guidelines).[16] Gabapentin exhibits dose-dependent bioavailability where bioavailability decreases with increasing dose and, therefore, achieved concentrations are not proportional to dose. Bioavailability may be increased by giving the drug more frequently (i.e., four times a day rather than three).[17] Absorption is somewhat delayed with peak concentrations occurring 2–4 hours after an oral dose. Food does not affect the absorption rate, but a high-protein meal will increase absorption.[18,19] Absorption appears to vary more between subjects than within a single subject.[20] The bioavailability of gabapentin given orally in a capsule and in a solution is comparable, though it is not well absorbed after rectal administration.[21] Gabapentin has a bitter taste when put into solution.

Gabapentin does not undergo liver metabolism and is excreted unchanged in the urine with a half-life of 5–9 hours.[22] Its clearance is proportional to creatinine clearance, and young children (< 5 years) have higher and more variable clearances than older children. On a mg/kg dose basis, 33% larger doses would be required in children < 5 years of age compared to older children.[23,24] Age-related decreases in renal function decrease

Table 9-3. Pharmacokinetic and Dosing Summary for Gabapentin

Bioavailability (F)	Decreases with an increase in dose (F = 0.6 at low doses, 0.35 at high doses)	
*t*max	2–4 hr	
V	0.65–1.4 L/kg	
*t*½	5–7 hr	
Clearance	150 ml/min	
Protein binding	<10%	
Elimination	Almost 100% renal	
Therapeutic range	12–20 mg/L[7,11]	
Usual dose	Adults: Initiate at 900 mg/day and increase up to 3600 mg/day. Doses of 5–10 g have been well tolerated.	
Pediatrics	10–15 mg/kg/day	
Dosing in renal dysfunction[a]	CrCl (ml/min)	Dose (mg)
	> 60	400 three times a day
	30–60	300 twice a day
	15–30	300 every day
	< 15	300 every other day
Anephric[b]	200–300 mg after each 4 hr hemodialysis	
Pregnancy	Unknown	

[a]These guidelines were established before there was significant experience with large doses of gabapentin (i.e., 5–10 g). The ultimate guide to dosing is a patient's response, so the dose may be increased in patients with renal dysfunction if clinical benefit based on the guidelines was limited and no side effects are noted.
[b]If the patient is anephric and on dialysis, give 200 to 300 mg after each 4-hr hemodialysis session.

gabapentin clearance, and the dose should be decreased in patients with renal impairment.[25] Gabapentin is removed by hemodialysis, and a replacement dose of 200 to 300 mg for each 4 hours of dialysis has been suggested.[26] Gender, race, and hepatic function do not affect the pharmacokinetics. The effects of pregnancy on the pharmacokinetics of gabapentin are unknown at this time.

Gabapentin does not undergo liver metabolism and is poorly protein bound, so it is not associated with many significant pharmacokinetic drug interactions. Concurrent administration with antacids may decrease absorption by 20%, therefore it is recommended that gabapentin be taken at least 2 hours after an antacid.[27] Cimetidine may decrease clearance by 10%.[26] Dosage adjustments are usually not necessary.

Gabapentin is generally well tolerated, with central nervous system (CNS) effects such as fatigue, somnolence, dizziness, ataxia, nystagmus, tremor, and diplopia noted at the onset of therapy. As tolerance develops, the CNS side effects seem to plateau.[28] Other side effects include weight gain, edema, and behavioral abnormalities.[29–32] Rash is uncommon. The consequences of overdose appear to be minimal.[33] Withdrawal symptoms have been reported.

Lamotrigine (Lamictal)

Lamotrigine was originally synthesized as a folate antagonist, though it has very weak activity in that regard. It is a member of the phenyltriazine class and is believed to work by blockade of voltage-sensitive sodium currents, slow binding of inactivated sodium channels, blockade of voltage-activated calcium currents, inhibition of presynaptic N-type calcium channels, and inhibition of glutamate and aspartate release.[34] It inhibits the sodium channel in a manner that is different from other sodium channel inhibiting drugs such as phenytoin and carbamazepine.

Lamotrigine is approved as adjunctive therapy for patients 2 years or older with partial seizures, primary generalized tonic-clonic seizures, and Lennox-Gastaut syndrome. It is also indicated as monotherapy in patients 16 years or older being converted from carbamazepine, phenytoin, phenobarbital, primidone, or valproate monotherapy and is effective in a wide range of seizures, including partial, primary generalized tonic-clonic, myoclonic, and absence. Lamotrigine is indicated for the treatment of bipolar disorder as well.

The pharmacokinetics of lamotrigine appear to be linear. Table 9-4 provides a summary of the pharmacokinetics and general dosing guidelines. Bioavailability is believed to be complete. Administration with food may reduce the maximum peak concentration but does not alter the total amount of drug absorbed. While the amount absorbed from the dispersible tablet given rectally is not the same as the amount following oral administration, there is adequate absorption to make this an alternative route of administration.[35,36] Absorption also occurs when the compressed tablet is given rectally. Lamotrigine is metabolized predominately by glucuronidation catalyzed by UDPGT in the liver to inactive metabolites that are excreted renally.[37,38] A 25% decrease in elimination half-life at steady state has been reported, suggesting that lamotrigine induces its own metabolism.[39] Half-life is significantly affected by enzyme inducers and inhibitors.[39,40]

Clearance is unaffected by age, gender, or dose, though some studies have shown an increase in children and decrease in the elderly.[39-43] Clearance is influenced by body weight and concurrent therapy with other antiepileptic drugs, and has been reported to be 25% lower in non-Caucasians.[40] Metabolic clearance is reduced in patients with hepatic impairment, and patients with renal disease should also be monitored closely and may require a decrease in dose.[44] During hemodialysis, ~20% of lamotrigine is removed. Patients with Gilbert's syndrome may show reduced clearance.[45] Clearance during monotherapy increases markedly during pregnancy; >300% from pre-pregnancy baseline.[46] This increase begins in the first trimester and continues through the third.[46-48] After delivery, concentrations increase rapidly to pre-pregnancy levels, occurring as early as 1–2 weeks post-partum.[46] The half-life in patients taking enzyme inducers (e.g., carbamazepine, phenytoin, phenobarbital, primidone, and rifampin) is 12–14 hours and the half-life in patients taking enzyme inhibitors (e.g., valproic acid) can exceed 59 hours. The interaction between lamotrigine and valproate is believed to result from competition during glucuronidation.[38] Acetaminophen, in doses of 900 mg in healthy volunteers, increased the total body clearance of lamotrigine by 15%.[49]

Lamotrigine does not typically affect the metabolism of other drugs and does not affect the concentration of carbamazepine or its active 10, 11-di-epoxide metabolite.[40,50,51] Side effects may be increased in patients taking carbamazepine when lamotrigine is added, suggesting a potential pharmacodynamic interaction.[52] Lamotrigine may slightly decrease concentrations of ethinyl estradiol, thus caution should be advised in patients taking concomitant oral contraceptives. Conversely, concurrent use of oral contraceptives in patients on lamotrigine has resulted in a decrease in lamotrigine concentrations and breakthrough seizures.[53,54] There have been reports of lamotrigine side effects occurring during the oral contraceptive placebo week in some patients. Possible solutions to this issue include decreasing the lamotrigine dose during the placebo week or switching the patient to an oral contraceptive without a placebo week.

Table 9-4. Pharmacokinetic and Dosing Summary for Lamotrigine

Bioavailability (F)	100% (F = 1)
*t*max	1.4–4.8 hr
*t*½	22 hr
	15 hr (with enzyme-inducing antiepileptics)
	> 59 hr (with valproic acid)
V	0.9–1.3 L/kg[57]
Clearance	0.076 L/hr/kg[57]
Protein binding	55%
Elimination	Hepatic via glucuronidation
Therapeutic range	2.5–15 mg/L[7,11]
Usual dose	Maintenance dose: 300–500 mg/day in patients taking enzyme-inducing antiepileptics; doses up to 700 mg/day have been well tolerated. 100–200 mg/day in patients taking valproic acid
Pregnancy	Marked decrease in serum concentrations beginning in first trimester and further decreasing until late pregnancy. After delivery, serum concentrations rapidly increase to pre-pregnancy levels within a few weeks.

The most common side effects of lamotrigine are headache, nausea, vomiting, ataxia, somnolence, dizziness, sedation, blurred vision, diplopia, and other visual disturbances. The incidence of CNS effects is increased in patients taking carbamazepine concurrently. A generalized, morbilliform skin rash has been reported in up to 10% of patients taking lamotrigine; however, this is considered to be benign and resolves without treatment. Rarely, serious rashes may develop including Stevens-Johnson syndrome and toxic epidermal necrolysis, which have systemic involvement and can be life-threatening.[55] It occurs more frequently in children than in adults and high starting doses, rapid dosage titration, and concurrent valproic acid therapy (due to increased lamotrigine half-life) increase the incidence of rash. Therefore, the dose of lamotrigine should be started low and gradually titrated to the patient's response (commonly over several months). Doses up to 700 mg/day have been well tolerated in patients not taking enzyme inhibitors concurrently.[56] Drug Reaction with Eosinophilia and Systemic Syndrome (DRESS) has also been reported with lamotrigine.

Tiagabine (Gabitril)

Tiagabine was specifically designed to block the reuptake of GABA into presynaptic terminals. It selectively inhibits the neuronal and glial reuptake of GABA and enhances GABA-mediated inhibition at both GABA A and GABA B receptors.[58] It is approved as adjunctive therapy for patients 12 years or older with partial seizures.

The pharmacokinetics and general dosing guidelines for tiagabine are shown in Table 9-5. Tiagabine exhibits linear absorption and the tmax, dose-adjusted Cmax, and AUC are independent of the administered dose, indicating linear pharmacokinetics.[59,60] A one-compartment model with first-order absorption and elimination adequately describe the tiagabine concentration-time profile.[61] Food delays absorption, but does not alter the extent. Tiagabine is highly protein bound, and valproic acid can dramatically increase the percentage unbound. Tiagabine is extensively metabolized by CYP3A4 and by glucuronidation, with only 2% excreted as the parent drug.[62] Half-life is short and is reduced in patients taking enzyme-inducing drugs such as phenytoin and carbamazepine and prolonged in patients taking enzyme-inhibiting drugs such as valproic acid.[63,64] However, tiagabine does not interact with drug-metabolizing enzymes to any clinically significant extent.[65-68] The pharmacokinetics are not affected by increasing age, smoking, race, or renal impairment.[69-71] Impaired liver function has been shown to decrease tiagabine elimination.[72] The effects of pregnancy on the pharmacokinetics of tiagabine are unknown at this time.

The primary side effects of tiagabine are CNS related. Adverse reactions reported include nausea, irritability, abdominal pain, asthenia, amblyopia, incoordination, tremors, speech disorders, nervousness, paresthesia, abnormal thinking, somnolence, and dizziness.[73] The incidence of CNS side effects may be reduced by slow dosage titration and may decrease over time.[74,75] Tiagabine has not been associated with weight gain or visual field defects.[76,77]

Table 9-5. Pharmacokinetic and Dosing Summary for Tiagabine (Gabitril)

Bioavailability (F)	90% (F = 0.9)
*t*max	45 min fasting, 2.5 hr non-fasting
*t*½	5–13 hr
	3.2 hr (enzyme-inducing antiepileptics)
	5.7 hr (valproic acid)
V	1.1–1.3 L/kg
Clearance	109 ml/min
Protein binding	96% (valproic acid decreases the bound percentage to 60%)
Elimination	Extensively hepatic (CYP 3A4 and glucuronidation)
Therapeutic range	20–100 mcg/L[7,11]
Usual dose	Initiate at 4 mg/day and titrate at weekly intervals up to 56 mg/day, if needed. Give in 2–4 divided doses
Pregnancy	Unknown

Topiramate (Topamax)

Topiramate blocks voltage-dependent sodium channels and inhibits the d-amino-3-hydroxy-5-methyl isoxazole-4-propionic acid (AMPA) subtype of the glutamate receptor and the release of glutamate. It also potentiates GABA-mediated inhibitory neurotransmission (at GABA A receptors) and modulates voltage-gated calcium ion channels.[78] It is a weak inhibitor of carbonic anhydrase.[79] Topiramate is approved as monotherapy for patients 10 years or older with partial onset or primary generalized tonic-clonic seizures. It is also approved as adjunctive therapy in patients with partial onset seizures or primary generalized tonic-clonic seizures and in the treatment of Lennox-Gastaut syndrome in patients 2 years or older. Further, it is indicated for the prophylaxis of migraine headaches in adults and may be useful in pediatric patients with a variety of seizure types, including myoclonic seizures and possibly infantile spasms.[80]

Table 9-6 provides the pharmacokinetics and general dosing guidelines for topiramate. Dose proportionality studies of the drug show that the Cmax increases linearly but is not dose proportional.[81] It is fairly rapidly absorbed, and administration with food delays the rate but not the extent of absorption.[82,83] The volume of distribution may change depending on dose. It was reported to be 58 L after a 100 mg dose and 38.5 L after a 1.2 g dose.[84] This change may reflect saturation of low-capacity binding sites on erythrocytes. A small amount of topiramate is excreted in the milk of nursing mothers.[85] There does not seem to be a saturable carrier mechanism restricting transport across the blood-brain barrier and the concentration in CSF is equal to the unbound proportion of topiramate in plasma, implying that the delivery to the brain occurs via transfer from the unbound plasma pool.[86] Plasma protein binding is low and variable and a high-affinity, low-capacity binding of topiramate to erythrocytes has been reported.

About 70% of an administered dose of topiramate is excreted unchanged in the urine and the remainder may be metabolized by hydroxylation, hydrolysis, or glucuronidation. There is no change in half-life after multiple dosing. Clearance appears to change with dose and was reported to be 36 ml/min following a 100 mg dose and 22.5 ml/min following a 1.2 g dose.[86] Weight-adjusted clearance appears to be higher in children than adults. For the same mg/kg dose, the resulting concentrations are 33% lower in children. No age effect per se has been reported in older patients. If older patients have decreased renal function as a function of age, they will have decreased clearance. Clearance is decreased by 42% in patients with moderate renal impairment (CrCl 30–69 ml/min) and by 54% in patients with severe impairment (CrCl < 30 ml/min). It is recommended that half of the usual dose be used to initiate titrating therapy and that the time between dosage adjustments be increased in patients with reduced renal function. It is also recommended that a dosage reduction of 50% be employed for patients with moderate to severe renal impairment. Hemodialysis increases the clearance of topiramate four- to six-fold. After dialysis, a supplemental dose may be required, taking into account the duration of dialysis, the clearance rate of the dialysis system, and the patient's effective renal clearance. In general, a supplemental dose equivalent to half of the daily dose of topiramate may be given. About half of this should be given before dialysis and the other half after dialysis. Clearance may also be decreased in patients with hepatic impairment.[87,88]

Table 9-6. Pharmacokinetic and Dosing Summary for Topiramate

Bioavailability (F)	80% (F = 0.8)
*t*max	2 hr
$t^{1/2}$	18–23 hr
V	0.6–0.8 L/kg
Clearance	20–30 ml/min
Protein binding	13%–41%
Elimination	Renal, unchanged (70%)
Therapeutic range	5–20 mg/L[7,11]
Usual dose	Initiate at 12.5–50 mg/day and increase at weekly intervals up to 400 mg/day (two divided doses)
Dosing in renal dysfunction	Use half the usual dose and increase the interval between dosing adjustments.
Pregnancy	Unknown

Metabolism of topiramate is increased by enzyme-inducing drugs. For example, phenytoin and carbamazepine induce topiramate metabolism and decrease concentrations by 48% and 40%, respectively, while valproic acid causes a 14% decrease in clearance, leading to increased concentrations.[89-91] Topiramate is a moderate enzyme inhibitor and has been reported to cause a 0%–25% increase in phenytoin concentrations.[92] Two patients taking carbamazepine were reported to develop toxicity after topiramate was added to their regimen.[93] Topiramate may increase concentrations of the 4-ene valproic acid metabolite, which has been shown to be hepatotoxic. These interactions are especially important if concurrent antiepileptic drugs are withdrawn after dosage stabilization with topiramate, as the concentrations will rebound.[94,95] At doses of approximately 200 mg/day and higher, topiramate is a moderate enzyme inducer. It may increase the clearance of oral contraceptives in a dose-dependent manner (e.g., doses >100 mg/day), and patients should report changes in menstrual patterns.[96] Women on oral contraceptives should be cautioned about breakthrough bleeding and the potential need for supplementary contraception. A 12% decrease in digoxin concentration has been reported when given concomitantly with topiramate. Because topiramate depresses CNS function, it may have an additive effect with other CNS depressants. There is a 1.5% increase in incidence of kidney stones in patients taking topiramate; the incidence is higher in men. Both kidney stones and paresthesia have been reported with other carbonic anhydrase inhibitors (e.g., zonisamide) as well.[80] Patients taking topiramate should be encouraged to maintain adequate fluid intake to reduce the incidence of kidney stones.

The most common side effects seen with topiramate are CNS related.[97] These side effects include dizziness, psychomotor slowing, difficulty concentrating, speech and language problems, somnolence, paresthesia, cognitive slowing, and fatigue. Cognitive complaints are the most common reason for discontinuing the drug. Word finding difficulties associated with topiramate were found to be independent of the dosage titration schedule and were related to a subgroup of patients with a specific biologic vulnerability.[98] Anorexia, nausea, and weight loss have been reported. Glaucoma, metabolic acidosis, and oligohidrosis (decreased sweating) have also been reported.[99–102]

The incidence of CNS side effects with topiramate increases with high initial doses and high maintenance doses. Therefore, the dose should be low initially and escalated to the patient's response.[84] The package insert suggests an initial starting dose of 50 mg/day in divided doses with dosage increments of 50 mg/day each week in adults to improve tolerability.[103] Some clinicians start at an even lower dose and escalate more slowly (i.e., 12.5 to 25 mg per week).

Levetiracetam (Keppra)

Levetiracetam is the S-enantiomer of the ethyl analog of piracetam. It is ineffective in the classic screening models for acute seizures and does not appear to interact with any known inhibitory or excitatory neurotransmitters. It inhibits burst firing without affecting normal excitatory neurotransmitters or normal neuronal excitability. Therefore, levetiracetam inhibits seizures by a unique mechanism of action that may involve a reduction in high-voltage activated calcium currents and delayed-rectifier potassium currents as well as a unique action on GABA currents.[104] It is hypothesized that levetiracetam may bind to the synaptic vesicle glycoprotein 2A (SV2A) region in the central nervous system, which appears to be important in neurotransmitter release. Levetiracetam is approved for use in patients 4 years or older as adjunctive therapy for the treatment of partial onset seizures, in patients 12 years or older for the treatment of myoclonic seizures, and in patients 6 years or older with primary generalized tonic-clonic seizures.

The pharmacokinetics and general dosing approaches for levetiracetam are shown in Table 9-7. Levetiracetam is rapidly and completely absorbed following oral administration with peak concentrations occurring in about 1 hour.[105,106] Bioavailability of all dosage forms is complete and absorption is linear and independent of dose. Food decreases the rate but not the extent of absorption. Protein binding is low. In animal models, levetiracetam concentrations in the brain increase linearly with dose increases.

About 66% of a dose is excreted unchanged in the urine, and the remaining portion is metabolized by hydrolysis of the acetamide group to three inactive metabolites. Neither the CYP nor the UGT isoenzyme systems are involved in the metabolism. The clearance is decreased and half-life prolonged in patients with renal dysfunction, necessitating a dose reduction.[107,108] The pharmacokinetics of levetiracetam are not affected by mild to moderate liver dysfunction. Clearance in children is relative to body weight and about 130%–140% that of an adult, reflecting better renal elimination.[109] Preliminary data indicate that concentrations of levetiracetam decline by as much as 50% during pregnancy.[46]

Pharmacokinetic drug interactions with levetiracetam are unlikely because metabolism is neither induced nor inhibited, and there is negligible protein binding.[110] It does not affect the metabolism of other drugs.[111,112]

Table 9-7. Pharmacokinetic and Dosing Summary for Levetiracetam

Bioavailability (F)	100% (F = 1) (all dosage forms)		
*t*max	1 hr		
*t*½	6–8 hr		
	Increased in patients with renal dysfunction		
V	0.5–0.7 L/kg		
Clearance	0.96 ml/min/kg		
Protein binding	< 10%		
Elimination	66% renal with the remaining drug being metabolized by hydrolysis that is independent of CYP450		
Therapeutic range	8–26 mg/L[7,11]		
Usual dose	Adult: Initiate at 1000 mg daily (in two divided doses) then increase by 1000 mg/day every 2 weeks to maximum of 3000 mg daily		
Pediatrics	Initiate therapy at 20 mg/kg/day (in two divided doses) then increase by 20 mg/kg/day every 2 weeks to a maximum of 60 mg/kg/day		
Dosing in renal impairment	CrCl (ml/min)	Dosage (mg)	Frequency
	> 80	500–1500	every 12 hr
	50–80	500–1000	every 12 hr
	30–50	250–750	every 12 hr
	< 30	250–500	every 12 hr
ESRD patients using dialysis	—	500–1000	every 12 hr
Pregnancy	Increased clearance		

A pharmacodynamic interaction has been reported between levetiracetam and carbamazepine. When added to patients taking carbamazepine, there is an increased incidence of CNS side effects that is not related to a change in the concentrations of carbamazepine or its active metabolite.[113]

Levetiracetam has generally been well tolerated with the most common side effects involving the CNS such as somnolence, asthenia, dizziness, vertigo, and headaches.[114] Psychiatric events and behavioral symptoms such as depression, nervousness, emotional lability, and hostility have been reported. A significantly higher incidence of upper respiratory tract infections has been reported in children and adults. These infections were not associated with any signs of immune impairment and did not disrupt therapy.[115,116]

Oxcarbazepine (Trileptal)

Oxcarbazepine is the 10-keto analogue of carbamazepine. Functionally, oxcarbazepine is a prodrug because it undergoes presystemic reduction in the liver to 10, 11-dihydro-10-hydroxy-carbamazepine.[117] This monohydroxylated derivative (MHD) is the active form of oxcarbazepine and exists as a racemic mixture. The two enantiomers of MHD showed similar median effective dose values in animal models of antiepileptic drug activity. The mechanism of action of oxcarbazepine is similar to carbamazepine in that it (as the MHD) blocks voltage-sensitive sodium channels, modulates the voltage-activated calcium currents, and increases potassium conductance. The spectrum of anti-seizure activity is similar for the two drugs.[118] Oxcarbazepine is indicated as monotherapy in patients 4 years or older for the treatment of partial seizures and as adjunctive therapy for patients 2 years or older with partial seizures.

Table 9-8 provides the pharmacokinetics and general dosing guidelines for oxcarbazepine. Oxcarbazepine is rapidly and almost completely absorbed following oral administration with peak concentrations occurring within 1–3 hours and peak concentrations of MHD occurring within 4–6 hours.[119] Administration with a high-fat or high-protein meal increases the area under the concentration curve of MHD by 16% and 23%, respectively. The accumulation of MHD following chronic dosing of oxcarbazepine is reported to be more than

Table 9-8. Pharmacokinetic and Dosing Summary for Oxcarbazepine

Bioavailability (F)	90% (F = 0.9)
t_{max}	1–3 hours oxcarbazepine, 4–6 hr MHD
$t_{½}$	2 hr (oxcarbazepine)
	9 hr (MHD)
V	12.5 ± 12.9 L/kg (oxcarbazepine)
	11.7 L (R-isomer of MHD)
	13.8 L (S-isomer of MHD)
Protein binding	60% (oxcarbazepine)
	40% (MHD)
Elimination	Oxcarbazepine is extensively metabolized to MHD by non-inducible cytosolic ketoreductases, which is then eliminated unchanged in the urine and as glucuronides of MHD
Therapeutic range	12.6–35 mg/L (MHD)[7,11]
Usual dose	Adult: Initiate at 600 mg/day (in divided doses). Increase by 600 mg/day at weekly intervals to a recommended maintenance dose of 1200 mg/day. Doses above 1200 mg have been used effectively but side effects are dose limiting
	If carbamazepine is replaced by oxcarbazepine, the dose of oxcarbazepine is 1.5 times the dose of carbamazepine
Pediatrics	Initiate at 16–20 mg/kg/day (in two divided doses). Maximum dose is 600 mg/day
Pregnancy	Significant increase in drug clearance of the active MHD metabolite

would be expected based on linear pharmacokinetics. Oxcarbazepine and MHD pass rapidly through biologic membranes including the blood-brain barrier and both cross the placenta and are excreted into breast milk, though breast feeding is not discouraged because of this (the infant should be monitored for clinical changes). Oxcarbazepine is rapidly and extensively metabolized to MHD by a stereoselective biotransformation mediated by a cytosolic, nonmicrosomal, and noninducible arlketone reductase. MHD is excreted unchanged in the urine or undergoes further metabolism by glucuronide conjugation.[120] CYP450 isoenzymes are minimally involved in the metabolism of either oxcarbazepine or MHD. The clearance of MHD is decreased in patients with impaired renal function but is not affected by liver disease. Limited data indicate that pregnancy increases the clearance of MHD.[46] The clearance in children is 2–5 times faster than in adults relative to body weight.[121]

Drug interactions may occur with both oxcarbazepine and MHD.[122] Oxcarbazepine reduces the bioavailability of ethinylestradiol and levonorgestrel by 48% and 32%, respectively, and breakthrough bleeding has been reported.[123] When given in doses of approximately 1200 mg/day or higher, oxcarbazepine has been reported to increase the concentrations of phenytoin by ~40% and phenobarbital by ~15%, consistent with inhibition of CYP2C19. At doses of approximately 1200 mg/day or higher, it decreases the concentrations of carbamazepine, lamotrigine, and felodipine via induction of CYP3A4.[124,125] Oxcarbazepine may induce UGT. Unlike carbamazepine, oxcarbazepine does not induce its own metabolism. The clearance of MHD is increased in patients taking enzyme-inducing drugs. Neither cimetidine nor erythromycin, both potent inhibitors of CYP isoenzymes, affect the pharmacokinetics of MHD.[122] Verapamil may decrease the plasma concentration of MHD by 20%.[126]

The side effect profile of oxcarbazepine is similar to carbamazepine with the most frequently reported side effects being somnolence or sedation, headache, dizziness, vertigo, ataxia, nausea, vomiting, fatigue, abdominal pain, tremor, dyspepsia, abnormal gait, abnormal vision, and diplopia.[127-128] The reported incidence of hyponatremia, defined as a serum sodium < 125 mmol/L, is higher than with carbamazepine and has been reported in up to 25% of patients. The incidence may be higher in older patients and in patients taking sodium-depleting diuretics.[129-131] There is a cross reactivity of 25% to 31% for rash between carbamazepine and oxcarbazepine.[132] While oxcarbazepine has been reported to be better tolerated than carbamazepine, this has only been studied in patients taking immediate-release carbamazepine. The tolerability of oxcarbazepine has not been compared to extended-release carbamazepine formulations (i.e., Carbatrol, Tegretol-XR), which have been reported to be better tolerated than immediate-release carbamazepine, as these formulations lead to lower peaks.

Zonisamide (Zonegran)

Zonisamide is a sulfonamide derivative that was initially approved for use in Japan and Korea, where it was used for 10 years prior to approval in the United States. It inhibits seizures by multiple mechanisms of action, including blocking voltage-dependent sodium channels, T-type calcium channels and actively inhibiting the release of excitatory neurotransmitters such as glutamate.[133] Zonisamide is a weak inhibitor of carbonic anhydrase activity and also affects dopamine and serotonin release. It has been approved for use in the United States as adjunctive therapy in adults with partial seizures. However, based on its use in Japan and Korea, it appears to be effective in a variety of seizure types including generalized tonic-clonic seizures, absence seizures, and myoclonic seizures.[134]

Table 9-9 provides the pharmacokinetics and general dosing guidelines for zonisamide. Zonisamide is completely absorbed.[135] Absorption is independent of dose, and the AUC is dose proportional. Administration with food reduces the rate but not the extent of absorption.

Following administration, zonisamide is distributed throughout the body. The drug rapidly crosses the blood brain barrier, and in animals the concentration in the CSF is comparable to the concentration in the plasma. Zonisamide crosses the placenta and enters into breast milk. It is about 40% bound to albumin, and erythrocytes have a higher binding affinity than plasma proteins. The binding to erythrocytes is saturable at low doses, but does not affect the pharmacokinetics. Zonisamide has mixed hepatic (70%) and renal (30%) elimination and CYP3A4 is the main isoenzyme involved in its metabolism, but CYP2D6, CYP2C19, and CYP3A5 are also involved.[136] Larger doses relative to body weight are needed in children to achieve concentrations comparable to adults, suggesting a faster clearance.[137] Pharmacokinetic parameters in the elderly are reported to be comparable to younger adults. The effects of pregnancy on the pharmacokinetics of zonisamide have not been well studied, but one case report suggests that clearance may increase at the end of the second trimester.[138]

Zonisamide does not induce or inhibit the metabolism of other drugs and is reported to not interact with other drugs, including oral contraceptives.[139] However, enzyme-inducing drugs such as phenytoin and carbamazepine will increase the clearance and decrease the half-life of zonisamide. Enzyme inhibiting drugs like valproic acid decrease the clearance and increase the half-life of zonisamide.[140]

The most commonly reported side effects of zonisamide are headache, nausea, agitation, irritability, fatigue, dizziness, somnolence, anorexia, psychomotor slowing, ataxia, abdominal pain, and confusion.[141] These are

Table 9-9. Pharmacokinetic and Dosing Summary for Zonisamide

Bioavailability (F)	Presumed complete (F = 1)
t_{max}	2–6 hr
$t_{1/2}$	63 hr (105 hr in red blood cells)
V	1.45 L/kg
Clearance	0.30–0.35 ml/min/kg (no concurrent enzyme-inducing AEDs)
	0.5 ml/min/kg (concurrent enzyme-inducing AEDs)
Protein binding	40% to albumin
Elimination	Hepatic (70%) and renal (30%)
Therapeutic range	10–38 mg/L[7,11]
Usual dose[a]	Initiate at 100 mg/day and increase by 100 mg/day every 2 weeks up to 400 to 600 mg/day in adults. Doses may be given once a day.[b]
Pregnancy	Unknown, but clearance may be increased beginning at the end of the second trimester.[138]

[a]The contents of the capsule may be opened and mixed with water, apple juice, apple sauce, or pudding for patients who have trouble taking an oral solid. The mixture is stable for 48 hours.

[b]There is approximately a 28% variability around the mean concentration with once-daily dosing and 14% variability with twice-daily dosing. If the drug is given once a day, it should be given at night.

increased with rapid dose escalation and reduced with a slower rate of titration. Zonisamide has been associated with a slight increase in incidence of renal calculi (3.3% with zonisamide and 2.4% with placebo).[142] It is a sulfonamide and should be used very cautiously in a person with a history of allergy to sulfas. However, the incidence of rash has been very low. It has also been associated with oligohidrosis and hyperthermia in pediatric patients, resulting in heat stroke and hospitalization.[143]

Pregabalin (Lyrica)

Pregabalin is a GABA analogue. It is the pharmacologically active S-enantiomer of gabapentin and is similar in structure and action. Pregabalin binds with high affinity to an auxiliary subunit of the voltage-gated calcium channels in CNS tissues. It may decrease the release of several neurotransmitters through modulation of calcium channel function and may increase the density of GABA transporter protein and the rate of functional GABA transport.

Pregabalin is indicated as adjunctive therapy for adult patients with partial onset seizures. It is also indicated for the treatment of diabetic peripheral neuropathy, post-herpetic neuralgia, and fibromyalgia. The typical starting dose is 150 mg/day in two to three divided doses. This can be increased at weekly intervals up to a maximum of 600 mg/day. Pregabalin is approximately 2.5 times more potent than gabapentin.

Pharmacokinetic and dosing summaries are provided for pregabalin in Table 9-10. The oral bioavailability is high and not dependent on dose.[144] The rate of absorption is decreased if administered with food, which decreases Cmax by 25% to 30% and increases tmax from 1.5 to 3 hours. However, the administration of pregabalin with food has no clinically relevant effect on total absorption and, unlike gabapentin, its absorption from the gut is not saturable.[144]

Table 9-10. Pharmacokinetic and Dosing Summary for Pregabalin

Bioavailability (F)	90% (F = 0.9)	
t_{max}	1–1.5 hr	
$t_{1/2}$	5–6.5 hr	
V	0.5 L/kg	
Clearance	67–81 ml/min (proportional to creatinine clearance)	
Protein binding	None	
Elimination	90%–99% renal	
Therapeutic range	2.8–8.2 mg/L[144]	
Usual dose	Initiate at 150 mg/day (in two to three divided doses) then increase by 150 mg/day at weekly intervals	
	Maximum 600 mg/day	
Dosing in renal dysfunction[a]	CrCl (ml/min)	Dose (mg)
	> 60	150–600/day
	30–60	75–300/day
	15–30	25–150/day
	< 15	25–75/day
Anephric[b]	Dose (mg)	Supplemental dose (mg)
	25	25 or 50
	25–50	50 or 75
	50–75	75 or 100
	75	100 or 150
Pregnancy	Unknown	

[a]Total daily dose (mg/day) should be divided into 2–3 doses for CrCl >30 ml/min, 1–2 doses for CrCl 15–30 ml/min, and as a single daily dose for CrCl <15 ml/min.
[b]Supplementary dose is a single additional dose given immediately after each 4-hour hemodialysis session and is based on the normal daily dose for patient.

Protein binding is negligible, and the drug undergoes little metabolism (< 2%) with most of a dose excreted unchanged in urine.[144] The half-life is approximately 6 hours. Since pregabalin does not undergo liver metabolism, it has not been shown to induce or inhibit hepatic enzymes. Clearance is proportional to creatinine clearance and age or disease related decreases in renal function decrease its clearance, necessitating dosage decreases in patients with renal impairment. Pregabalin is removed by hemodialysis, and a supplementary dose given after each 4-hour dialysis session has been suggested.[144] No differences in pharmacokinetics due to race or gender have been observed, and the effects of pregnancy on pharmacokinetics are unknown at this time.[144] Adequate pharmacokinetic studies in pediatrics have not been performed.

Pregabalin does not undergo liver metabolism and is poorly protein bound, so it is not associated with significant drug interactions.[144,145] It may impair cognition and motor function, and these effects may be additive with other agents such as oxycodone, ethanol, or lorazepam.[144]

Pregabalin has a similar side effect profile to gabapentin. It is generally well tolerated with central nervous system (CNS) effects such as somnolence, dizziness, ataxia, and diplopia noted at the onset of therapy. As tolerance develops, the CNS side effects seem to plateau.[144] Other side effects include weight gain, edema, and behavioral abnormalities.

Lacosamide (Vimpat)

Lacosamide is a functionalized amino acid that is an optical antipode of L-serine.[146] Unlike traditional sodium channel blocking AEDs, which primarily target the fast inactivation of these channels, lacosamide works by a novel mechanism to enhance slow inactivation without affecting fast inactivation.[147] Lacosamide is indicated for adjunct treatment of partial-onset seizures in patients 17 years or older. Dosing is initiated at 50 mg twice daily and increased by 100 mg/day at weekly intervals to a maintenance dose of 200–400 mg/day.

The pharmacokinetics and general dosing guidelines of lacosamide are summarized in Table 9-11. After oral administration, lacosamide is rapidly and completely absorbed from the GI tract and has linear, dose-proportional pharmacokinetcs.[146,148] Lacosamide has complete oral bioavailability, and food does not affect the rate or extent of absorption.[149] Peak serum concentrations occur 1-4 hours after oral administration.[147] When infused over 30 or 60 minutes, IV administration produces concentrations similar to oral administration and Cmax is reached at the end of infusion.[150] Lacosamide has limited protein binding.[149] Elimination of lacosamide is primarily renal with approximately 40% of the dose being excreted unchanged in the urine.[149] Up to 30% of an administered dose is converted to the inactive O-desmethyl metabolite by CYP2C19, though this is considered to be of minor relevance.[149] No dose adjustments are necessary in patients with mild to moderate renal dysfunction, though, a maximum dose of 300 mg/day is recommended for patients with severe renal dysfunction (creatinine clearance < 30 ml/min).[148] Lacosamide is removed by hemodialysis so a supplemental dose of up to 50% of the patient's normal maintenance dose is recommended following hemodialysis.[149] In patients with mild to moderate hepatic impairment, cautious titration and a maximum dose of 300 mg/day are recommended.[148] Lacosamide has not been studied in patients with severe hepatic impairment, and its use is

Table 9-11. Pharmacokinetic and Dosing Summary for Lacosamide

Bioavailability	100% (F = 1)
t_{max}	1–4 hr
$t_{½}$	13 hr
V	0.6 L/kg
Protein binding	<15%
Elimination	Partially metabolized by CYP2C19, eliminated renally
Therapeutic range	10–20 mg/L,[151] though some clinical trials have reported mean serum concentrations less than 10 mg/L when the maximum recommended dose of 400 mg/day is used.[147]
Usual dose	Initiate therapy at 100 mg/day (in two divided doses) and increase by 100 mg/day weekly up to 200 to 400 mg/day
Pregnancy	Unknown

not recommended in this population.[149] The effects of pregnancy on the pharmacokinetics of lacosamide are unknown at this time.

Due to its low protein binding, minimal interaction with the CYP450 enzyme system, and primarily renal elimination, lacosamide has a low propensity for clinically significant drug interactions.[148] Clinical trials have shown it to have no effect on other AEDs, metformin, digoxin, or oral contraceptives.[146] However, carbamazepine, phenytoin, and phenobarbital have been shown to decrease concentrations of lacosamide by 15%–25%.[149] At therapeutic concentrations, lacosamide was shown to not induce or inhibit any CYP450 enzymes,[149] although at supratherapeutic concentrations, it can inhibit CYP2C19.[146]

Lacosamide is generally well tolerated with a majority of adverse events affecting the CNS and GI tract.[147] Dizziness is the most commonly reported adverse event and appears to be dose-related.[148] Other dose-related adverse effects include nausea, vomiting, diplopia, headache, and blurred vision.[147-149] In some patients, liver function tests were slightly elevated and returned to baseline levels once lacosamide was discontinued.[149-152] A small prolongation of the PR interval has been noted, but not deemed to be of clinical significance; however, caution should be exercised when administering lacosamide to patients with known cardiac conduction problems or in combination with other drugs known to increase the PR interval.[147,149,152] When using lacosamide in combination with traditional sodium channel blocking agents (e.g. phenytoin, carbamazepine, oxcarbazepine, lamotrigine), a small increase in some typical adverse events, including dizziness, nausea, vomiting, diplopia, blurred vision, fatigue, coordination abnormalities, tremor, nystagmus, and somnolence, has been reported.[153] These effects may be attenuated by decreasing the dose of the traditional sodium channel blocking agent.

Rufinamide (Banzel)

Rufinamide is a triazole derivative that acts to prolong the inactive state of neuronal sodium channels.[154] At high concentrations, rufinamide has also been shown to inhibit the mGluR5 glutamate receptor.[154] Rufinamide is indicated for the adjunctive treatment of seizures associated with Lennox-Gastaut syndrome in adults and children 4 years or older. In adults, dosing is initiated at 400–800 mg/day (in two divided doses) and increased by 400–800 mg/day every 2 days up to a target and maximum dose of 3200 mg/day. In children and adolescents, dosing is weight based and initiated at 10 mg/kg/day (in two divided doses) and increased by ~10 mg/kg/day every 2 days up to a target and maximum dose of 45 mg/kg/day or 3200 mg/day (whichever is lower).

The pharmacokinetic parameters and general dosing guidelines of rufinamide are summarized in Table 9-12. After oral administration, rufinamide is slowly absorbed.[155] This is due to the fact that it does not dissolve in water and it poorly dissolves in the fluids of the GI tract.[156] Peak concentrations are achieved 4–6 hours after administration.[154] The oral bioavailability of rufinamide is considered to be 85%; however, this is based on a study consisting of a single 600 mg dose given to healthy volunteers. It has been established that as the dose increases, the bioavailability of rufinamide decreases. Therapeutic doses are typically higher than 600 mg, so

Table 9-12. Pharmacokinetic and Dosing Summary for Rufinamide

Bioavailability	85% (F = 0.85) (decreases with higher doses)
t_{max}	4–6 hr
$t_{½}$	6–10 hr
V	~50 L
Protein binding	34%
Elimination	Hepatic metabolism (hydrolysis of carboxamide group via carboxylesterases – not P450 dependent); primarily renal elimination
Therapeutic range	Not established[155]
Usual dose	Adult: Initiate therapy at 400–800 mg/day (in two divided doses) and increase by 400–800 mg/day every 2 days up to 3200 mg/day
Pediatrics	Initiate therapy at 10 mg/kg/day (in two divided doses) and increase by ~10 mg/kg/day every 2 days up to 45 mg/kg/day or 3200 mg/day (whichever is lower)
Pregnancy	Unknown

bioavailability is expected to be less than 85% in most patients.[155] It is recommended that rufinamide be given with food, as extent of absorption increases and time to peak concentration decreases in the fed state.[154] Rufinamide exhibits low protein binding.[156] Its volume of distribution is dependent on the dose and body surface area (BSA) of the patient, but at the recommended maintenance dose and average adult BSA, the volume of distribution is approximately 50 L.[154]

The major pathway for rufinamide metabolism is hydrolysis of its carboxamide group to inactive metabolites via hepatic carboxylesterases, which is a non-CYP450 system.[155] Despite this non-CYP450 metabolic pathway, rufinamide is a weak inducer of CYP3A4 and a weak inhibitor of CYP2E1.[154] Elimination of rufinamide and its metabolites is primarily renal. Renal impairment does not significantly affect the pharmacokinetics of rufinamide so no dose adjustments are necessary in this population.[154,155] No data have been published regarding the use of rufinamide in patients with hepatic impairment.[153,155] The effects of pregnancy on the pharmacokinetics of rufinamide are unknown at this time.

Despite not being metabolized by the CYP450 system, drug interactions are a concern with rufinamide, especially in children. In adults, valproate causes a small increase in rufinamide concentrations, but in children this increase can be as much as 70%, necessitating a decrease in rufinamide dose of approximately 50%.[146,154,155] Lamotrigine has been shown to increase concentrations of rufinamide as well.[144] Drugs that have been shown to decrease rufinamide concentrations include phenytoin, phenobarbital, primidone, carbamazepine, and vigabatrin.[146,155,156] Rufinamide has been shown to increase concentrations of phenytoin and phenobarbital and to decrease concentrations of carbamazepine, lamotrigine, triazolam, and oral contraceptives.[146,154-156]

Rufinamide is generally well tolerated. The most common side effects include headache, dizziness, diplopia, fatigue, somnolence, nausea, and vomiting.[154-157] It can shorten the QT interval and is consequently contraindicated in patients with familial short QT syndrome.[154,156] It should also be used with caution in patients taking other medications that can decrease the QT interval.

Vigabatrin (Sabril)

Vigabatrin is a GABA analog that acts as an irreversible inhibitor of GABA transaminase, the enzyme responsible for the breakdown of GABA.[158,159] Vigabatrin is indicated for the treatment of infantile spasms in children 1 month to 2 years of age and for the treatment of refractory complex partial seizures in adults. In adults, dosing is initiated at 1000 mg/day (in two divided doses) and increased by 500 mg/day weekly to a target dose of 3,000 mg/day. Pediatric dosing is weight based and should be initiated at 50 mg/kg/day (in two divided doses). The dose should then be escalated by 25-50 mg/kg/day every three days up to a maximum of 150 mg/kg/day.

The pharmacokinetics and general dosing guidelines of vigabatrin are summarized in Table 9-13. After oral administration, vigabatrin is rapidly absorbed.[158,159] Its oral bioavailability is somewhat low, and food does not appear to significantly affect absorption.[158,159] Vigabatrin is not expected to have any interactions with drugs that are highly protein bound, as it does not bind to plasma proteins.[158-160] Vigabatrin is widely distributed throughout the body.[161] It is possible to measure vigabatrin concentrations doing so may provide some clinical benefit. As vigabatrin acts to irreversibly inhibit GABA transaminase, its activity persists for far longer than it is detectable in the serum.[158,159] For the effects of vigabatrin to diminish, the body must synthesize new GABA transaminase which takes approximately five to seven days.[158]

Hepatic metabolism of vigabatrin is negligible with nearly 100% of the dose being excreted unchanged in the urine.[158,159] Clearance is higher in children than in adults, which necessitates higher doses on a mg/kg basis in the younger population.[159,162] Furthermore, in children less than 22 months old, clearance is up to 40% higher than in older children.[162] The elimination half-life of vigabatrin is short, but the actions of the drug are apparent long after drug concentrations become undetectable.[159,160,162] Lower doses are necessary in patients with renal dysfunction (CrCl < 80 ml/min). Hepatic dysfunction has no impact on vigabatrin dosing.[159] The effects of pregnancy on the pharmacokinetics of vigabatrin are unknown at this time.

Vigabatrin has a very low potential for interactions with other drugs because of its renal elimination and lack of metabolism. However, there is a clinically significant interaction between vigabatrin and phenytoin. Specifically, when vigabatrin therapy is initiated in a patient taking phenytoin, phenytoin concentrations may decrease by up to 40%.[158] No other clinically significant interactions appear to occur with vigabatrin.[158,159] The package insert for vigabatrin states that it is an inducer of CYP2C9, but this has not been described in primary literature.

Table 9-13. Pharmacokinetic and Dosing Summary for Vigabatrin

Bioavailability (F)	60% –70% (F = 0.6–0.7)	
t_{max}	1–2 hr	
$t_{½}$	5–8 hr	
V	1.1 L/kg	
Protein binding	Negligible	
Elimination	Primarily eliminated unchanged in urine	
Usual dose	Adults: Initiate therapy at 1000 mg per day (in two divided doses) and increase by 500 mg/day weekly to a target dose of 3000 mg/day	
Pediatrics	Initiate therapy at 50 mg/kg/day (in two divided doses) and increase by 25–50 mg/kg/day every three days to a maximum of 150 mg/kg/day	
Dosage in renal dysfunction	CrCl (ml/min)	Dose adjustment
	51–80	Decrease dose by 25%
	31–50	Decrease dose by 50%
	10–30	Decrease dose by 75%
Pregnancy	Unknown	

Vigabatrin is generally well tolerated, but reports of irreversible visual field defects have significantly limited its use. Visual field defects appear in approximately one third of all patients treated with vigabatrin, and these defects are often not recognized early on by patients.[163] To prevent significant visual field defects from developing, adults should have a visual field test at baseline and every six months while on vigabatrin therapy. Infants should have the test performed at baseline, every three months for the first 18 months of therapy, and every six months thereafter.[163] Other common adverse effects of vigabatrin include fatigue, dizziness, somnolence, and weight gain.[158,163] Depression has been reported to occur in approximately 12% of patients, so caution should be exercised when using vigabatrin in patients with a history of psychiatric disorders.[158,163]

Use of the Newer Antiepileptic Drugs

The availability of newer drugs with different mechanisms of action has increased the options for treating patients with epilepsy. No patient with epilepsy should be considered refractory until several different single agents or combinations of antiepileptic drugs have been tried; however, therapy should begin with the antiepileptic drug considered the most effective for the patient's seizure type. Doses of the drug of first choice should be increased gradually until the patient becomes seizure free or to the maximum dose tolerated by the patient. A second drug with a different mechanism of action that is appropriate for the seizure type should then be added. This approach is referred to as "rational polytherapy." In selecting the second drug, consideration should also be given to avoiding potential drug interactions and to overlapping drug side effects, if possible. It is not always possible to avoid drug interactions and drug interactions do not necessarily contraindicate the use of interacting drugs, though they do mandate closer patient monitoring. It should be mentioned that although sophisticated technologies exist, not all mechanisms of action may have been identified for many of the AEDs. This may explain the efficacy of a different drug of the same class when a patient has failed therapy with a drug in that class.

When combination therapy is employed, the two drugs should be given in adequate doses and for an adequate period of time to assess the frequency of seizures. One estimate is that the trial period at full dosage should encompass the period normally encompassing five seizures. Thus, the less frequent the seizures, the more difficult it is to determine if the therapy is effective. If the patient has a positive response to the second drug or becomes seizure free, consideration should be given to withdrawing the first drug. The ultimate goal of antiepileptic drug therapy is to make the patient seizure free with minimal or no side effects.

The Therapeutics and Technology Assessment Subcommittee and Quality Standards Subcommittee of the American Academy of Neurology and the American Epilepsy Society reviewed the newer AEDs for the treatment of new-onset and refractory epilepsy.[164,165] These reports identify seizure types and syndromes where the use of the newer AEDs are appropriate either as initial monotherapy or as off-label use for situations that have not been approved by the FDA. These guidelines use an evidence-based approach to ensure the concept that the selection of an AED should be based on the seizure type or syndrome, the patient's age, concomitant medications, AED tolerability, safety, and efficacy and not just on the package insert and FDA-approved indications.

Generic Substitution of AEDs

In recent years there has been much controversy regarding the safety and efficacy of generic formulations of AEDs. Many patients and practitioners have noted increased side effects or loss of seizure control in some individuals switched from brand-name drug to a generic equivalent. This effect has, perhaps, been more pronounced in patients switching between multiple generic formulations (i.e., generic to generic substitution). It has been postulated that pharmacokinetic differences between formulations or batch to batch variations may be the culprit in these cases. Several studies have been published recently showing increased incidence of epilepsy-related emergency department utilization following an A-rated switch in AED.[166-168] Further, one study showed increased incidence of medical utilization and increased risk of epilepsy-related medical events when a generic AED was used compared to use of brand-name formulations.[169]

Contrary to the previously mentioned studies, a group from the FDA published a paper showing, on average, a difference in Cmax between generic and innovator products of 4.35% and a difference in AUC of 3.56%.[170] These data covered a variety of drug classes and encompassed generics approved between 1996 and 2007. The major limitation of this study, however, was the stipulation that, when submitting a new formulation for FDA approval, generic drug manufacturers were not required to submit data from all bioequivalence studies conducted, but rather can choose to submit only favorable data. This loophole was not closed until mid-2009. Data presented at the 2009 American Academy of Neurology (AAN) Annual Meeting showed that variations in AUC and Cmax can be as high as 21% and 40%, respectively, when switching between generic formulations of carbamazepine.[171] The same group presented data for other AEDs at the 2010 AAN Annual Meeting, but concluded that, in most cases, generic formulations of AEDs are accurate copies of the innovator product.[172] As the data set is limited and no consensus has been reached in the medical community, this continues to be a topic of much contention.

References

1. Commission on Antiepileptic Drugs, International League Against Epilepsy. Guidelines for therapeutic monitoring of antiepileptic drugs. *Epilepsia*. 1993;34:585-7.
2. Sofia RD. Felbamate: mechanism of action. In: Levy RH, Mattson RH, Meldrum BS, eds. *Antiepileptic Drugs*. 5th ed. New York, NY: Raven Press; 2002:791-7.
3. Sachdeo R, Narang-Sachdeo SK, Shumaker RC, et al. Tolerability and pharmacokinetics of monotherapy felbamate doses of 1,200-6,000 mg/day in subjects with epilepsy. *Epilepsia*. 1997;38:887-92.
4. Pellock JM, Perhach JL. Felbamate: In: Levy RH, Mattson RH, Meldrum BS, eds. *Antiepileptic Drugs*, 5th ed. Philadelphia, PA: Lippincott Williams & Wilkins; 2002:302-17.
5. Richens A, Banfield CR, Salfi M, et al. Single and multiple dose pharmacokinetics of felbamate in the elderly. *Br J Clin Pharmacol*. 1997;44:129-34.
6. Chang SI, McAuley JW. Pharmacotherapeutic issues for women of childbearing age with epilepsy. *Ann Pharmacother*. 1998;32:794-801.
7. Johannessen SI, Tomson T. Pharmacokinetic variability of newer antiepileptic drugs. *Clin Pharmacokinet*. 2006;45(11):1061-75.
8. Glue P, Banfield CR, Perhach JL, et al. Pharmacokinetic interactions with felbamate. In vitro-in vivo correlation. *Clin Pharmacokinet*. 1997;33:214-24.
9. Riva R, Albani F, Contin M, et al. Pharmacokinetic interactions between antiepileptic drugs. Clinical considerations. *Clin Pharmacokinet*. 1996;6:470-93.
10. Natsch S, Hekster YA, Keyser A, et al. Newer anticonvulsant drugs: role of pharmacology, drug interactions and adverse reactions in drug choice. *Drug Safety*. 1997;17:228-40.
11. Johannessen SI, Battino D, Berry DJ, et al. Therapeutic drug monitoring of the newer antiepileptic drugs. *Ther Drug Monit*. 2003;25:347-63.
12. Luer MS, Hamani C, Dujovny M, et al. Saturable transport of gabapentin at the blood-brain barrier. *Neurol Res*. 1999;21:559-62.
13. LaRoche SM, Helmers SL. The new antiepileptics. *JAMA*. 2004;291:605-14.

14. Beydoun A, Uthman BM, Sachellares JC. Gabapentin: pharmacokinetics, efficacy, and safety. *Clin Neuropharmacol.* 1995;18:469-81.
15. Vajda FJE. Gabapentin: Chemistry, biotransformation, pharmacokinetics, and interactions. In: Levy RH, Mattson RH, Meldrum BS, et al., eds. *Antiepileptic Drugs*. 5th ed. Philadelphia, PA: Lippincott Williams & Wilkins; 2002:334-9.
16. Stewart BH, Kugler AR, Thomson RR, et al. A saturable transport mechanism in the intestinal absorption of gabapentin is the underlying cause of the lack of proportionality between increasing dose and drug levels in plasma. *Pharm Res.* 1993;10:276-81.
17. Gidal BE, DeCerce J, Bockbrader HN, et al. Gabapentin bioavailability: effect of dose and frequency of administration in adult patients with epilepsy. *Epilepsy Res.* 1998;31:91-9.
18. Gidal BE, Maly MM, Kowalski JW, et al. Gabapentin absorption: effect of mixing with foods of varying macronutrient composition. *Ann Pharmacother.* 1998;32:405-9.
19. Gidal BE, Maly MM, Budde J, et al. Effect of a high protein meal on gabapentin pharmacokinetics. *Epilepsy Res.* 1996;23:71-6.
20. Gidal BE, Radulovic LL, Kruger S, et al. Inter- and intra-subject variability in gabapentin absorption and absolute bioavailability. *Epilepsy Res.* 2000;40:123-7.
21. Kriel RL, Birnbaum AK, Cloyd JC, et al. Failure of absorption of gabapentin after rectal administration. *Epilepsia.* 1997;38:1242-4.
22. McLean MJ. Clinical pharmacokinetics of gabapentin. *Neurology*. 1994;44(Suppl 5):S17-22
23. Ouellet D, Bockbrader HN, Wesche DL, et al. Population pharmacokinetics of gabapentin in infants and children. *Epilepsy Res.* 2001;47:229-41.
24. Haig GM. Bockbrader HN, Wesche DL, et al. Single-dose gabapentin pharmacokinetics and safety in healthy infants and children. *J Clin Pharmacol.* 2001;41:507-14.
25. Blum RA, Comstock TJ, Sica DA, et al. Pharmacokinetics of gabapentin in subjects with various degrees of renal function. *Clin Pharmacol Ther.* 1994;56:154-9.
26. Andrews CO, Fischer JH. Gabapentin: a new agent for the management of epilepsy. *Ann Pharmacother.* 1994;28:1188-96.
27. Bruni J. Gabapentin as adjunctive therapy for partial seizures. *Epilepsia.* 1999;40(suppl. 6):S27-S28.
28. Ramsay RE, Pryor FM. Gabapentin: Adverse effects. In: Levy RH, Mattson RH, Meldrum BS, et al., eds. *Antiepileptic Drugs*. 5th ed. Philadelphia, PA: Lippincott Williams & Wilkins; 2002:354-9.
29. Gueguen A, Guy C, Caarty O, et al. Edematous syndrome and alithiasic cholecystitis induced by gabapentin. *Presse Med.* 2002;31:1559.
30. Drabkin R, Calhoun L. Anorgasmia and withdrawal syndrome in a woman taking gabapentin. *Can J Psychiatry.* 2003;48:125-6.
31. Jablonowski K, Margolesse HC, Chouinard G. Gabapentin-induced paradoxical exacerbation of psychosis in a patient with schizophrenia. *Can J Psychiatry* 2002;47:975-6.
32. Pinninti NR, Mahajan DS. Gabapentin-associated aggression. *J Neuropsychiatry Clin Neurosci.* 2001;13:424.
33. Klein-Schwartz W, Shepherd JG, Gorman S, et al. Characterization of gabapentin overdose using a poison center case series. *J Toxicol Clin Toxicol.* 2003;41:11-5.
34. Leach MJ, Randall AD, Stefani A, et al. Lamotrigine: mechanisms of action. In: Levy RH, Mattson RH, Meldrum BS, et al., eds. *Antiepileptic Drugs*. 5th ed. Philadelphia, PA: Lippincott Williams & Wilkins; 2002:363-9.
35. Dickins M, Chen C. Lamotrigine: Chemistry, biotransformation, and pharmacokinetics. In: Levy RH, Mattson RH, Meldrum BS, et al., eds. *Antiepileptic Drugs*. 5th ed. Philadelphia, PA: Lippincott Williams & Wilkins; 2002:370-9.
36. Birnbaum AK, Kriel RL, Im Y, et al. Relative bioavailability of lamotrigine chewable dispersible tablets administered rectally. *Pharmacotherapy*. 2001;21:158-62.
37. Rambeck B, Wolf P. Lamotrigine clinical pharmacokinetics. *Clin Pharmacokinet.* 1993;25:433-43.
38. Garnett WR. Lamotrigine: Interaction with other drugs. In: Levy RH, Mattson RH, Meldrum BS, et al., eds. *Antiepileptic Drugs*. 5th ed. Philadelphia, PA: Lippincott Williams & Wilkins; 2002:380-8.
39. Hussein Z, Posner J. Population pharmacokinetics of lamotrigine monotherapy in patients with epilepsy: retrospective analysis of routine monitoring data. *Br J Clin Pharmacol.* 1997;43:457-65.
40. Grasela TH, Fiedler KJ, Cox E, et al. Population pharmacokinetics of lamotrigine adjunctive therapy in adults with epilepsy. *J Clin Pharmacol.* 1999;39:373-84.
41. Mikati MA, Fayuad M, Koleilat M, et al. Efficacy, tolerability, and kinetics of lamotrigine in infants. *J Pediatr.* 2002;141:31-5.
42. Andersson GD. Children versus adults: pharmacokinetics and adverse-effect differences. *Epilepsia.* 2002;43(Suppl 3):53-9.

43. Battino D, Croci D, Granata T, et al. Single-dose pharmacokinetics of lamotrigine in children: influence of age and antiepileptic co-medication. *Ther Drug Monit.* 2001;23:217-22.

44. Marcelin P, de Bony F, Garret C, et al. Influence of cirrhosis on lamotrigine pharmacokinetics. *Br J Clin Pharmacol.* 2001;51:410-4.

45. Posner J, Cohen AF, Land G, et al. The pharmacokinetics of lamotrigine (BW430C) in healthy subjects with unconjugated hyperbilirubinemia (Gilbert's syndrome). *Br J Clin Pharmacol.* 1989;28(1):117-20.

46. Tomson T, Battino D. Pharmacokinetic and therapeutic drug monitoring of newer antiepileptic drugs during pregnancy and the puerperium. *Clin Pharmacokinet.* 2007;46(3):209-19.

47. Ohman I, Vitols S, Tomson T. Lamotrigine in pregnancy: pharmacokinetics during delivery, in the neonate, and during lactation. *Epilepsia.* 2000;41:709-13.

48. Tran TA, Leppik IE, Elesi K, et al. Lamotrigine clearance during pregnancy. *Neurology.* 2002;59:251-5.

49. Garnett WR. Lamotrigine: pharmacokinetics. *J Child Neurol.* 1997;12(Supp 1):S10-S15.

50. Eriksson AS, Boreus LO. No increase in carbamazepine-10, 11-epoxide during addition of lamotrigine treatment in children. *Ther Drug Monit.* 1997;19:499-501.

51. Gidal BE, Rutecki P, Shaw R, et al. Effect of lamotrigine on carbamazepine epoxide/carbamazepine serum concentration ratios in adult patients with epilepsy. *Epilepsy Res.* 1997;28:207-11.

52. Besag FM, Berry DJ, Pool F, et al. Carbamazepine toxicity with lamotrigine: pharmacokinetic or pharmacodynamic interaction? *Epilepsia.* 1998;39:183-7.

53. Sabers A, Buchholt JM, Uldall P, et al. Lamotrigine plasma levels reduced by oral contraceptives. *Epilepsy Res.* 2001;47:151-4.

54. Holdich T, Whiteman P, Orme M, et al. Effect of lamotrigine on the pharmacology of the combined oral contraceptive pill. *Epilepsia.* 1991;32(Suppl 1):96.

55. Biton V. Pharmacokinetics, toxicology and safety of lamotrigine in epilepsy. *Expert Opin Drug Metab Toxicol.* 2006 Dec;2(6):1009-18.

56. Matsuo F, Gay P, Madsen J, et al. Lamotrigine high-dose tolerability and safety in patients with epilepsy: a double-blind, placebo-controlled, eleven-week study. *Epilepsia.* 1996;37:857-62.

57. Ramsay RE, Pellock JM, Garnett WR, et al. Pharmacokinetics and safety of lamotrigine (Lamictal) in patients with epilepsy. *Epilepsy Res.* 1991;10:191-200.

58. Giardina WJ. Tiagabine: Mechanisms of action. In: Levy RH, Mattson RH, Meldrum BS, et al., eds. *Antiepileptic Drugs.* 5th ed. Philadelphia, PA: Lippincott Williams & Wilkins; 2002:675-80.

59. Sommerville KW, Collins SD. Tiagabine: Chemistry, biotransformation, and pharmacokinetics. In: Levy RH, Mattson RH, Meldrum BS, et al., eds. *Antiepileptic Drugs.* 5th ed. Philadelphia, PA: Lippincott Williams & Wilkins; 2002:681-90.

60. Samara EE, Gustavson LE, El-Shourbagy T, et al. Population analysis of the pharmacokinetics of tiagabine in patients with epilepsy. *Epilepsia.* 1998;39:868-77.

61. Ingwersen SH, Pedersen PC, Groes L, et al. Population pharmacokinetics of tiagabine in epileptic patients on monotherapy. *Eur J Pharm Sci.* 2000;11:247-54.

62. Schachter SC. Pharmacology and clinical experience with tiagabine. *Expert Opin Pharmacother.* 2001;2:179-87.

63. Gustavson LE, Mengel HB. Pharmacokinetics of tiagabine, a gamma-aminobutyric acid-uptake inhibitor, in healthy subjects after single and multiple doses. *Epilepsia.* 1995;36:605-11.

64. So EL, Wolff D, Graves NM, et al. Pharmacokinetics of tiagabine as add on therapy in patients taking enzyme inducing anti-epilepsy drugs. *Epilepsy Res.* 1995;22:221-6.

65. Sommerville KW. Tiagabine: drug interactions. In: Levy RH, Mattson RH, Meldrum BS, et al., eds. *Antiepileptic Drugs.* 5th ed. Philadelphia, PA: Lippincott Williams & Wilkins; 2002:692-97.

66. Richens A, Marshall RW, Dirach J, et al. Absence of interaction between tiagabine, a new antiepileptic drug, and the benzodiazepine triazolam. *Drug Metabol Drug Interact.* 1998;14:159-77.

67. Thomsen MS, Groes L, Agerso H, et al. Lack of pharmacokinetic interaction between tiagabine and erythromycin. *J Clin Pharmacol.* 1998;38:1051-6.

68. Snel S, Jansen JA, Pedersen PC, et al. Tiagabine, a novel antiepileptic agent: lack of pharmacokinetic interaction with digoxin. *Eur J Clin Pharmacol.* 1998;54:355-7.

69. Snel S, Jansen JA, Mengel HB, et al. The pharmacokinetics of tiagabine in healthy elderly volunteers and elderly patients with epilepsy. *J Clin Pharmacol.* 1997;37:1015-20.

70. Walker MC, Patsalow PN. Clinical pharmacokinetics of new antiepileptic drugs. *Pharmacol Ther.* 1995;67:351-84.

71. Cato A, Gustavson LE, Qian J, et al. Effect of renal impairment of the pharmacokinetics and tolerability to tiagabine. *Epilepsia.* 1998;39:43-7.

72. Lau AH, Gustavson LE, Sperelakis R, et al. Pharmacokinetics and safety of tiagabine in subjects with various degrees of hepatic function. *Epilepsia.* 1997;38:445-51.

73. Adkins JC, Noble S. Tiagabine. A review of its pharmacodynamic and pharmacokinetic properties and therapeutic potential in the management of epilepsy. *Drugs*. 1998;55:437-60.

74. Schacter SC. Tiagabine: adverse effects. In: Levy RH, Mattson RH, Meldrum BS, et al., eds. *Antiepileptic Drugs*. 5th ed. Philadelphia, PA: Lippincott Williams & Wilkins; 2002:710-5.

75. Pellock JM. Tiagabine (gabitril) experience in children. *Epilepsia.* 2001;42 (Suppl 3):49-51.

76. Kalviainen R. Long-term safety of tiagabine. *Epilepsia.* 2001;42(Suppl 3):46-8.

77. Krauss GL, Johnson MA, Sheth S, et al. A controlled study comparing visual function in patients treated with vigabatrin and tiagabine. *J Neurol Neurosurg Psychiatry*. 2003;74:339-43.

78. White HS. Topiramate: Mechanisms of action. In: Levy RH, Mattson RH, Meldrum BS, et al., eds. *Antiepileptic Drugs*. 5th ed. Philadelphia, PA: Lippincott Williams & Wilkins; 2002:719-26.

79. Rosenfeld WE. Topiramate: A review of preclinical, pharmacokinetic, and clinical data. *Clin Ther*. 1997;19:1294-308.

80. Langtry HD, Gillis JC, Davis R. Topiramate. A review of its pharmacodynamic and pharmacokinetic properties and clinical efficacy in the management of epilepsy. *Drugs*. 1997;54:752-73.

81. Doose DR, Streeter AJ. Topiramate: chemistry, biotransformation, and pharmacokinetics. In: Levy RH, Mattson RH, Meldrum BS, et al., eds. *Antiepileptic Drugs*. 5th ed. Philadelphia, PA: Lippincott Williams & Wilkins; 2002:727-34.

82. Perucca E. Pharmacokinetic profile of topiramate in comparison with other new antiepileptic drugs. *Epilepsia.* 1996;37(Suppl 2):S8-13.

83. Doose DR, Walker SA, Gisclon LG, et al. Single-dose pharmacokinetics and effect of food on the bioavailability of topiramate, a novel antiepileptic drug. *J Clin Pharmacol.* 1996;36:884-91.

84. Garnett WR Clinical pharmacology of topiramate: a review. *Epilepsia.* 2000;41 (Suppl 1):S61-S65.

85. Ohman I, Vitols S, Luef G, et al. Topiramate kinetics during delivery, lactation, and in the neonate: preliminary observations. *Epilepsia.* 2002;43:1157-60.

86. Christensen J, Hojskov CS, Dam M, et al. Plasma concentration of topiramate correlates with cerebrospinal fluid concentration. *Ther Drug Monit.* 2001;23:529-35.

87. Sachdeo RC. Topiramate: Clinical profile in epilepsy. *Clin Pharmacokinet*. 1998;34:335-46.

88. Schneiderman JH. Topiramate: pharmacokinetics and pharmacodynamics. *Can J Neurol Sci.* 1998;25:S3-5.

89. Bourgeois BF. Drug interaction profile of topiramate. *Epilepsia.* 1996;37 (Suppl 2):S14-17.

90. Johannessen SI. Pharmacokinetics and interaction profile of topiramate: review and comparison with other newer antiepileptic drugs. *Epilepsia.* 1997;38(Suppl 1):S18-23.

91. Rosenfeld WE, Liao S, Kramer LD, et al. Comparison of the steady-state pharmacokinetics of topiramate and valproate in patients with epilepsy during monotherapy and concomitant therapy. *Epilepsia.* 1997;38:324-33.

92. Sachdeo RC, Sachdeo SK, Levy RH, et al. Topiramate and phenytoin pharmacokinetics during repetitive monotherapy and combination therapy to epileptic patients. *Epilepsia.* 2002;43:691-6.

93. Mack CJ, Kuc S, Mulcrone SA, et al. Interaction of topiramate with carbamazepine: two case reports and a review of clinical experience. *Seizure*. 2002;11:464-7.

94. May TW, Rambseck B, Jurgens U. Serum concentrations of topiramate in patients with epilepsy: influence of dose, age, and co-medication. *Ther Drug Monit*. 2002;24:366-74.

95. Contin M, Riva R, Albani F, et al. Topiramate therapeutic monitoring in patients with epilepsy: effect of concomitant antiepileptic drugs. *Ther Drug Monit.* 2002;24:332-7.

96. Rosenfeld WE, Doose DR, Walker SA, et al. Effect of topiramate on the pharmacokinetics of an oral contraceptive containing norethindrone and ethinyl estradiol in patients with epilepsy. *Epilepsia.* 1997;38:317-23.

97. Sachdeo RC, Karia RM. Topiramate: adverse effects. In: Levy RH, Mattson RH, Meldrum BS, et al., eds. *Antiepileptic Drugs*. 5th ed. Philadelphia, PA: Lippincott Williams & Wilkins; 2002:760-64.

98. Mula M, Trimlbe MR, Thompson P, et al. Topiramate and word-finding difficulties in patients with epilepsy. *Neurology*. 2003;60:1104-7.

99. Medeiros FA, Zhang XY, Bernd AS, et al. Angle-closure glaucoma associated with ciliary body detachment in patients using topiramate. *Arch Ophthalmol*. 2003;121:282-5.

100. Thambi L, Kapcala LP, Chambers W, et al. Topiramate-associated secondary angle-closure glaucoma: a case series. *Arch Ophthalmol*. 2002;120:1108.

101. Nieto-Barrera M, Nieto-Jimenez M, Candau R, et al. Anhidrosis and hyperthermia associated with treatment with topiramate. *Rev Neurol*. 2002;34:114-6.

102. Arcas J, Ferrer T. Roche MC, et al. Hypohidrosis related to the administration of topiramate to children. *Epilepsia.*

2001;42:1363-5.

103. Biton V, Edwards KR, Montouris GD, et al. Topiramate titration and tolerability. *Ann Pharmacother*. 2001;35:173-9.

104. Margineanu DG, Klitgaard H. Levetiracetam: mechanisms of action. In: Levy RH, Mattson RH, Meldrum BS, et al., eds. *Antiepileptic Drugs*. 5th ed. Philadelphia, PA: Lippincott Williams & Wilkins; 2002:419-27.

105. Patsalos PN. Levetiracetam: chemistry, biotransformation, pharmacokinetics, and drug interactions. In: Levy RH, Mattson RH, Meldrum BS, et al., eds. *Antiepileptic Drugs*. 5th ed. Philadelphia, PA: Lippincott Williams & Wilkins; 2002:428-32.

106. Patsalos PN. Pharmacokinetic profile of levetiracetam: toward ideal characteristics. *Pharmacol Ther*. 2000;85:77-85.

107. Radtke RA. Pharmacokinetics of levetiracetam. *Epilepsia*. 2001;42 (Suppl 4):24-7.

108. Welty TE, Gidal BE, Ficker DM, et al. Levetiracetam: a different approach to the pharmacotherapy of epilepsy. *Ann Pharmacother*. 2002;36:296-304.

109. Pellock JM, Glauser TA, Bebin EM, et al. Pharmacokinetic study of levetiracetam in children. *Epilepsia*. 2001;42:1574-9.

110. Nicolas JM, Clollart P, Gerin B, et al. In vitro evaluation of potential drug interactions with levetiracetam, a new antiepileptic agent. *Drug Metab Dispos*. 1999;27:250-4.

111. Benedetti MS. Enzyme induction and inhibition by new antiepileptic drugs: a review of human studies. *Fundam Clin Pharmacol*. 2000;14:301-19.

112. Perucca E, Gidal BE, Baltes E. Effects of antiepileptic co-medication on levetiracetam pharmacokinetics: a pooled analysis of data from randomized adjunctive therapy trials. *Epilepsy Res*. 2003;53:47-56.

113. Sisodiya SM, Sander JW, Patsalos PN. Carbamazepine toxicity during combination therapy with levetiracetam: a pharmacodynamic interaction. *Epilepsy Res*. 2002;48:217-9.

114. Biton V. Levetiracetam: Adverse experiences. In: Levy RH, Mattson RH, Meldrum BS, et al., eds. *Antiepileptic Drugs*. 5th ed. Philadelphia, PA: Lippincott Williams & Wilkins; 2002:442-7.

115. Harden C. Safety profile of levetiracetam. *Epilepsia*. 2001;42(Suppl 4):36-9.

116. Ben-Menachem E, Gilland E. Efficacy and tolerability of levetiracetam during 1-year follow-up in patients with refractory epilepsy. *Seizure*. 2002;12:131-5.

117. McLean MJ. Oxcarbazepine: Mechanisms of action. In: Levy RH, Mattson RH, Meldrum BS, et al., eds. *Antiepileptic Drugs*. 5th ed. Philadelphia, PA: Lippincott Williams & Wilkins; 2002:451-8.

118. Beydoun A, Kutlay E. Oxcarbazepine. *Expert Opin Pharmacother*. 2002;3:59-71.

119. Degen PH, Flesch G, Cardot JM, et al. The influence of food on the disposition of the antiepileptic oxcarbazepine and its major metabolites in healthy volunteers. *Biopharm Drug Dispos*. 1994;15:519-26.

120. Lloyd P, Flesch G, Dieterle W. Clinical pharmacology and pharmacokinetics of oxcarbazepine. *Epilepsia*. 1994;35(Suppl 3):S10-S13.

121. Van Heiningen PN, Eve MD, Oosteruis B, et al. The influence of age on the pharmacokinetics of the antiepileptic agent oxcarbazepine. *Clin Pharmacol Ther*. 1991;50:410-9.

122. Albani F, Riva R, Baruzzi A. Oxcarbazepine: interactions with other drugs. In: Levy RH, Mattson RH, Meldrum BS, et al., eds. *Antiepileptic Drugs*. 5th ed. Philadelphia, PA: Lippincott Williams & Wilkins; 2002:466-9.

123. Klosterskkov JP, Saano V, Haring P, et al. Possible interaction between oxcarbazepine and an oral contraceptive. *Epilepsia* 1992;33:1149-52.

124. Lakehal F, Wurden CJ, Kalhorn TF, et al. Carbamazepine and oxcarbazepine decrease phenytoin metabolism through inhibition of CYP2C19. *Epilepsy Res*. 2002;52:79-83.

125. May TW, Rambeck B, Jurgens U. Influence of oxcarbazepine and methsuximide on lamotrigine concentrations in epileptic patients with and without valproic acid co-medication: results of a retrospective study. *Ther Drug Monit*. 1999;21:175-81.

126. Flesch G. Overview of the clinical pharmacokinetics of oxcarbazepine. *Clinical drug investigation*. 2004;24 (4):185-203.

127. Kramer G. Oxcarbazepine: adverse effects. In: Levy RH, Mattson RH, Meldrum BS, et al., eds. *Antiepileptic Drugs*. 5th ed. Philadelphia, PA: Lippincott Williams & Wilkins; 2002:479-86.

128. Beydoun A. Safety and efficacy of oxcarbazepine: results of randomized, double-blind trials. *Pharmacotherapy*. 2000;20:152S-158S.

129. Holtmann M, Krause M, Opp J, et al. Oxcarbazepine-induced hyponatremia and the regulation of serum sodium after replacing carbamazepine with oxcarbazepine in children. *Neuropediatrics*. 2002;33:298-300.

130. Sachdeo RC, Wasserstein A, Mesenbrink PJ, et al. Effects of oxcarbazepine on sodium concentration and water handling. *Ann Neurol*. 2002;51:613-20.

131. Isojarvi JI, Huuskonen Ue, Pakarinen AJ, et al. The regulation of serum sodium after replacing carbamazepine with oxcarbazepine. *Epilepsia*. 2001;42:741-5.

132. Beran RG. Cross-reactive skin eruption with both carbamazepine and oxcarbazepine. *Epilepsia.* 1993;34:163-5.

133. MacDonald RL. Zonisamide: mechanisms of action. In: Levy RH, Mattson RH, Meldrum BS, et al., eds. *Antiepileptic Drugs.* 5th ed. Philadelphia, PA: Lippincott Williams & Wilkins; 2002:867-72.

134. Seino M, Fujitani B. Zonisamide: clinical efficacy and use in epilepsy. In: Levy RH, Mattson RH, Meldrum BS, et al., eds. *Antiepileptic Drugs.* 5th ed. Philadelphia, PA: Lippincott Williams & Wilkins; 2002:885-91.

135. Shah J, Shellenberger K, Canafax DM. Zonisamide: chemistry, biotransformation, and pharmacokinetics. In: Levy RH, Mattson RH, Meldrum BS, et al., eds. *Antiepileptic Drugs.* 5th ed. Philadelphia, PA: Lippincott Williams & Wilkins; 2002:873-9.

136. Kochak GM, Page JG, Buchanan RA, et al. Steady-state pharmacokinetics of zonisamide, an antiepileptic agent for treatment of refractory complex partial seizures. *J Clin Pharmacol.* 1998;38:166-71.

137. Hashimoto Y, Odani A, Tanigawara Y, et al. Population analysis of the dose-dependent pharmacokinetics of zonisamide in epileptic patients. *Biol Pharm Bull.* 1994;17:323-6.

138. Oles KS, Bell WL. Zonisamide concentrations during pregnancy. *Ann Pharmacother.* 2008;42(7):1139-41.

139. Mather GG, Shah J. Zonisamide: drug interactions. In: Levy RH, Mattson RH, Meldrum BS, et al., eds. *Antiepileptic Drugs.* 5th ed. Philadelphia, PA: Lippincott Williams & Wilkins; 2002:880-4.

140. Riva R, Albani F, Contin M, et al. Pharmacokinetic interactions between antiepileptic drugs. *Clin Pharmacokinet.* 1996;31:470-93.

141. Lee IB. Zonisamide: adverse effects. In: Levy RH, Mattson RH, Meldrum BS, et al., eds. *Antiepileptic Drugs.* 5th ed. Philadelphia, PA: Lippincott Williams & Wilkins; 2002:892-8.

142. Kubota M, Nishi-Nagase M, Sakakihara Y, et al. Zonisamide-induced urinary lithiasis in patients with intractable epilepsy. *Brain Dev.* 2000;22:230-3.

143. Shimizu T, Yamashita Y, Satoi M, et al. Heat stroke-like episode in a child caused by zonisamide. *Brain Dev.* 1997;19:366-8.

144. Ben-Menachem E. Pregabalin pharmacology and its relevance to clinical practice. *Epilepsia.* 2004;45(suppl. 6):13-18.

145. Brodie MJ, Wilson EA, Wesche DL, et al. Pregabalin drug interaction studies: Lack of effect on the pharmacokinetics of carbamazepine, phenytoin, lamotrigine, and valproate in patients with partial epilepsy. *Epilepsia.* 2005;46(9):1407-13.

146. Luszcki JJ. Third-generation antiepileptic drugs: mechanisms of action, pharmacokinetics and interactions. *Pharmacol Rep.* 2009;61(2):197-216.

147. Halász P, Kälviäinen R, Mazurkiewicz-Beldzińska M, et al. Adjunctive lacosamide for partial-onset seizures: Efficacy and safety results from a randomized controlled trial. *Epilepsia.* 2009;50(3):443-53. Epub 2009 Jan 17.

148. Chung SS. Lacosamide: new adjunctive treatment option for partial-onset seizures. *Expert Opin Pharmacother.* 2010;11(9):1595-602.

149. Cross SA, Curran MP. Lacosamide: in partial-onset seizures. *Drugs.* 2009;69(4):449-59.

150. Biton V, Rosenfeld WE, Whitesides J, et al. Intravenous lacosamide as replacement for oral lacosamide in patients with partial-onset seizures. *Epilepsia.* 2008;49(3):418-24.

151. Greenaway C, Ratnaraj N, Sander JW, et al. A high-performance liquid chromatography assay to monitor the new antiepileptic drug lacosamide in patients with epilepsy. *Ther Drug Monit.* 2010;32(4):448-52.

152. Harris JA, Murphy JA. Lacosamide: an adjunctive agent for partial-onset seizures and potential therapy for neuropathic pain. *Ann Pharmacother.* 2009;43(11):1809-17.

153. Davies K, Doty P, Eggert-Formella A, et al. Evaluation of lacosamide efficacy and safety as adjunctive therapy in patients receiving traditional sodium channel blocking AEDs. Poster presented at: 63rd Annual Meeting of the American Epilepsy Society (AES); December 4–8, 2009; Boston, MA.

154. Wisniewski CS. Rufinamide: a new antiepileptic medication for the treatment of seizures associated with Lennox-Gastaut syndrome. *Ann Pharmacother.* 2010;44(4):658-67.

155. Perucca E, Cloyd J, Critchley D, et al. Rufinamide: clinical pharmacokinetics and concentration-response relationships in patients with epilepsy. *Epilepsia.* 2008;49(7):1123-41.

156. Hakimian S, Cheng-Hakimian A, Anderson GD, et al. Rufinamide: a new anti-epileptic medication. *Expert Opin Pharmacother.* 2007;8(12):1931-40.

157. Elger CE, Stefan H, Mann A, et al. A 24-week multicenter, randomized, double-blind, parallel-group, dose-ranging study of rufinamide in adults and adolescents with inadequately controlled partial seizures. *Epilepsy Res.* 2010;88(2-3):255-63.

158. Gidal BE, Privitera MD, Sheth RD, et al. Vigabatrin: a novel therapy for seizure disorders. *Ann Pharmacother.* 1999;33(12):1277-86.

159. Johannessen SI, Tomson T. Pharmacokinetic variability of newer antiepileptic drugs: When is monitoring needed? *Clin Pharmacokinet.* 2006;45(11):1061-75.

160. Perucca E. Clinical pharmacokinetics of new-generation antiepileptic drugs at the extremes of age. *Clin Pharmacokinet*. 2006;45(4):351-63.

161. Durham SL, Hoke JF, Chen TM. Pharmacokinetics and metabolism of vigabatrin following a single oral dose of [14C] vigabatrin in healthy male volunteers. *Drug Metab Dispos*. 1993;21(3):480-4.

162. Perucca E. Pharmacokinetic variability of new antiepileptic drugs at different ages. *Ther Drug Monit*. 2005;27(6):714-7.

163. Waterhouse EJ, Mims KN, Gowda SN. Treatment of refractory complex partial seizures: role of vigabatrin. *Neuropsychiatr Dis Treat*. 2009;5:505-15.

164. French JA, Kanner AM, Bautista J, et al. Efficacy and tolerability of the new antiepileptic drugs II: treatment of refractory epilepsy: report of the Therapeutics and Technology Assessment Subcommittee and Quality Standards Subcommittee of the American Academy of Neurology and the American Epilepsy Society. *Neurology*. 2004;62(8):1261-73.

165. French JA, Kanner AM, Bautista J, et al. Efficacy and tolerability of the new antiepileptic drugs I: treatment of new onset epilepsy: report of the Therapeutics and Technology Assessment Subcommittee and Quality Standards Subcommittee of the American Academy of Neurology and the American Epilepsy Society. *Neurology*. 2004;62(8):1252-60.

166. Zachry WM III, Doan QD, Clewell JD, et al. Case-control analysis of ambulance, emergency room, or inpatient hospital events for epilepsy and antiepileptic drug formulation changes. *Epilepsia*. 2009;50(3):493-500.

167. Rascati KL, Richards KM, Johnsrud MT, et al. Effects of antiepileptic drug substitutions on epileptic events requiring acute care. *Pharmacotherapy*. 2009;29(7):769-74.

168. Hansen RN, Campbell JD, Sullivan SD. Association between antiepileptic drug switching and epilepsy-related events. *Epilepsy Behav*. 2009;15(4):481-5.

169. Labiner DM, Paradis PE, Manjunath R, et al. Generic antiepileptic drugs and associated medical resource utilization in the United States. *Neurology*. 2010;74(20):1566-74.

170. Davit BM, Nwakama PE, Buehler GJ, et al. Comparing generic and innovator drugs: a review of 12 years of bioequivalence data from the United States Food and Drug Administration. *Ann Pharmacother*. 2009;43(10):1583-97.

171. Chuang K, Krauss GL, CAO YJ. Evaluating FDA Bioequivalence standards for generic carbamazepine formulations. Poster presented at: 61st Annual Meeting of the American Academy of Neurology (AAN); April 25–May 2, 2009; Seattle, WA.

172. Krauss GL, Davit BM, Caffo BS, et al. Comparing bioequivalence of generic antiepilepsy drugs (AEDs). Poster presented at: 62nd Annual Meeting of the American Academy of Neurology (AAN); April 10–17, 2010; Toronto, Ontario.

Chapter 10

Christine M. Formea and Janet L. Karlix

Antirejection Agents (AHFS 92:00)

Cyclosporine is a large lipophilic polypeptide that has been a cornerstone of transplant immunosuppression. It inhibits T-lymphocytes and also inhibits production and release of lymphokines, including interleukin-2.[1,2] Cyclosporine is indicated for the prevention of rejection in kidney, liver, and heart transplantation as well as for selected other disorders.[1,2]

Three oral cyclosporine products are available: Sandimmune (the original formulation), Neoral, and AB rated generic cyclosporine microemulsions. The gastrointestinal absorption of Sandimmune is variable and incomplete and displays significant intra- and interpatient variability in bioavailability.[1] Neoral is an oral cyclosporine formulation that becomes a microemulsion in aqueous environment and demonstrates increased bioavailability when compared to Sandimmune.[2] The AB rated generic cyclosporine microemulsions have similar bioavailability to Neoral and Sandimmune.

Tacrolimus (Prograf) is a macrolide immunosuppressant with its properties attributed to potent inhibition of T-lymphocytes.[3] It is indicated for the prevention of rejection following kidney, liver, and heart transplantation.[3]

Sirolimus (Rapamune) is a macrocyclic lactone with potent immunosuppressive activity that results from inhibition of T-lymphocyte proliferation and antibody production.[4] It is indicated for the prevention of rejection in kidney transplant recipients older than 13 years of age.[4]

Usual Dosage Range in Absence of Clearance-Altering Factors

The following dosing recommendations for the antirejection agents are based on average pharmacokinetic parameters (see Tables 10-1 to 10-3). However, due to the wide inter- and intrapatient pharmacokinetic variability, individual monitoring is absolutely necessary. Initial and maintenance doses may differ between transplant centers, transplantation type, and patient population. Doses are generally adjusted to achieve center-defined blood trough concentrations. Long-term administration is required to prevent rejection. All of these products should be taken on a consistent schedule relative to meals and time of day.

Dosage Form Availability

A variety of dosage forms are available for the three agents (see Table 10-4). Cyclosporine and tacrolimus have intravenous dosage forms that should only be used when patients are unable to take medications orally since additional side effects may occur with the intravenous forms.

Table 10-1. Dosing Recommendations for Cyclosporine[1,2,5-8]

Dosage Form	Initial Dosage[a-c]	Maintenance Dosage[a-c]
Intravenous	5–6 mg/kg as a single IV dose given 4-12 hours before transplant	5–6 mg/kg once daily IV dose
Oral capsules and solutions	10–15 mg/kg single dose given 4–12 hours before transplant	4–15 mg/kg/day given in two divided doses

[a]Cyclosporine is most commonly administered orally every 12 hr. However, pediatric patients may require every 8-hr dosing. Pediatric patients may require and tolerate higher mg/kg doses.
[b]Due to anaphylactic risk, intravenous cyclosporine should only be used until patients are able to take oral cyclosporine products. The IV dosage of cyclosporine is one third the recommended oral dosage.
[c]Patients with renal or hepatic impairment should receive doses at the lowest value of the recommended IV and oral dosing ranges.

Table 10-2. Dosing Recommendations for Tacrolimus[3,9]

Dosage Form	Initial Dosage[a-e]
Intravenous	For heart (adult): 0.01 mg/kg/day continuous infusion For kidney/liver (adult): 0.03–0.05 mg/kg/day continuous infusion For liver (child): 0.03-0.05 mg/kg/day continuous infusion
Oral capsule	For liver (child): 0.15–0.2 mg/kg/day (divided every 12 hr) For heart (adult): 0.075 mg/kg/day (divided every 12 hr) For kidney (adult): 0.1-0.2 mg/kg/day (divided every 12 hr) For liver (adult): 0.1–0.15 mg/kg/day (divided every 12 hr)

[a]In general, children require and tolerate higher mg/kg tacrolimus doses than adults.
[b]Initiation with oral therapy is recommended. If IV therapy is necessary, conversion to capsules is recommended as soon as oral therapy is tolerated. The first oral dose of tacrolimus should be administered 8–12 hours after discontinuation of the continuous IV infusion.
[c]Patients with renal or hepatic impairment should receive doses at the lowest value of the recommended IV and oral dosing ranges.
[d]Tacrolimus and cyclosporine should not be used simultaneously. Tacrolimus or cyclosporine should be discontinued for at least 24 hours before initiating the other agent.
[e]Begin daily tacrolimus continuous infusions no sooner than 6 hours after transplant.

Table 10-3. Dosing Recommendations for Sirolimus[4,10,11]

Dosage Form	Loading Dose[a-d]	Maintenance Dose[b-f]
Oral (tablet and solution)		
Low to moderate immunologic risk:	6 mg once on Day 1	2 mg once daily
High immunologic risk[g]:	15 mg once on Day 1	5 mg once daily

[a]The sirolimus loading doseshould be given as soon as possible after transplantation.
[b]No sirolimus dosage adjustment is needed for renal impairment.
[c]In mild to moderate hepatic impairment, the sirolimus maintenance dose should be reduced by one third. In severe hepatic impairment the maintenance dose should be reduced by one-half. The loading dose does not need to be modified.
[d]For patients 13 years of age or older weighing less than 40 kg, the loading dose should be adjusted to 3 mg/m^2 and the maintenance dose should be adjusted to 1 mg/m^2/day.
[e]Sirolimus should be administered 4 hours after cyclosporine solution or capsule dosage.
[f]Due to the long half-life of sirolimus, avoid frequent dose adjustments of sirolimus based on non-steady state sirolimus blood concentrations. Interpretation of non-steady state sirolimus concentrations may result in sirolimus underdosing or overdosing.
[g]High immunologic risk includes African Americans, recipients of another transplant after a failure and/or high reactive panel antibodies (PRA >80%).

Table 10-4. Cyclosporine,[1,2,5,12,13] Tacrolimus,[3,9] and Sirolimus[4,11] Dosage Forms

Drug	Dosage Form	Product
Cyclosporine	Intravenous solution 50 mg/mL (5-mL ampule)	Sandimmune injection; multi-source availability
	Oral capsules Liquid-filled capsule 25 and 100 mg	Sandimmune; Neoral; multi-source availability
	Oral solutions 100 mg/mL	Sandimmune; Neoral; multi-source availability
Tacrolimus	Intravenous solution 5 mg/mL (1-mL ampule)	Prograf
	Oral capsules 0.5, 1, and 5 mg	Prograf, multi-source availability
Sirolimus	Oral tablets 0.5, 1, and 2 mg	Rapamune
	Oral solution 1 mg/mL	Rapamune

General Pharmacokinetic Information

Absorption[14]

The absorption of antirejection agents may be impacted by drug-food, drug-herb, or drug-drug interactions. Transport and metabolism of the antirejection agents is affected by activity of the cytochrome P450 3A enzyme system and P-glycoprotein, which may be under the control of genetic and environmental factors. Absorption of oral antirejection agents is variable, making therapeutic drug monitoring essential and particularly critical in the first 2 weeks post transplantation. Cyclosporine, tacrolimus, and sirolimus should be taken consistently with regard to time and food in order to reduce variability in drug exposure.

Cyclosporine has widely variable pharmacokinetics depending upon the formulation (Sandimmune versus Neoral).[15-19] Oral Sandimmune formulations demonstrate lower bioavailability than oral Neoral formulations and more erratic absorption. This results in Sandimmune's larger intra- and interpatient variability than other forms of cyclosporine. Conversely, absorption of Neoral is more consistent over time, with less intrapatient variability. In addition to type of cyclosporine formulation, absorption may be impacted by first-pass metabolism, gastric motility, mode of administration, drug-drug, drug-herb, and drug–food interactions. Time to peak concentration is different with Neoral (1–2 hr) compared to Sandimmune (2–3 hr).

Tacrolimus.[3,14] The oral absorption of tacrolimus is variable and incomplete. Oral bioavailability ranges from 9% to 43%. Intestinal CYP3A4 metabolism, gastric motility, and P-glycoprotein activity all affect its absorption. Although the manufacturer makes no recommendation for tacrolimus to be taken on an empty stomach, food alters tacrolimus absorption in terms of rate and reduced extent. Unlike cyclosporine, the bioavailability of tacrolimus is not affected by the presence of bile salts.

Sirolimus.[4,14] Since high fat food increases drug absorption, patients should take sirolimus tablets and oral solution in a consistent manner, with or without food. Oral bioavailability is approximately 14% for sirolimus oral solution; however, the mean bioavailability of sirolimus tablets increases by about 27% relative to the oral solution in healthy persons, thus sirolimus oral solution and oral tablets are not bioequivalent, though the 2 mg dose of the two formulations has been shown to result in clinically equivalent outcomes.

Table 10-5 provides the bioavailability of the various dosage forms of *cyclosporine, tacrolimus, and sirolimus.*

Distribution

Cyclosporine distributes widely into body fluids and tissues. In solid organ transplant recipients, the cyclosporine volume of distribution at steady state after intravenous dosing is between 3-5 L/kg.[2,5] Cyclosporine distributes in a concentration-dependent manner in blood: 41%–58% in erythrocytes, 4%–9% in lymphocytes, 5%–12% in granulocytes, and 33%–47% in plasma. Cyclosporine crosses the placenta and is detected in breast milk.

Tacrolimus. The partitioning of tacrolimus between plasma and whole blood is dependent on hematocrit, tacrolimus concentration, plasma protein concentration, and temperature of the sample.[3,9] Tacrolimus crosses the placenta and is detected in breast milk.

Sirolimus has a large volume of distribution.[4,11,21,22] In human whole blood, sirolimus is extensively distributed into cellular components: red blood cells (95%), plasma (3%), lymphocytes (1%), and granulocytes (1%). Women are advised to use effective contraception before sirolimus initiation, during sirolimus treatment, and 12 weeks after conclusion of sirolimus treatment. Although trace amounts of sirolimus can be detected in the milk of rats, it is unknown whether sirolimus distributes into human breast milk.

Table 10-5. The Bioavailability of Dosage Forms of Cyclosporine, Tacrolimus, and Sirolimus[1-7,9-12,20,21]

Dosage Form	Bioavailability Comments
Cyclosporine oral capsules and solution	30% (range = 10%–89%)[a]
Tacrolimus oral capsules	Variable (mean 25%, range 9%–43%)
Sirolimus oral solution and tablets	15%[b]

[a]Sandimmune is not bioequivalent to Neoral and cannot be used interchangeably without the supervision of a physician.
[b]Concomitant administration of cyclosporine promotes sirolimus absorption and increases sirolimus bioavailability.

Table 10-6 provides the volume of distribution information for *cyclosporine, tacrolimus, and sirolimus.*

Table 10-6. Volume of Distribution (V)

Drug[2-4,12]	V (range or mean ± SD; L/kg)
Cyclosporine	3–5
Tacrolimus[a]	0.85–1.94
Sirolimus	12 ± 8

[a]Whole blood.

Protein binding

Cyclosporine is 90% bound to proteins (primarily lipoproteins), and approximately 50% of the drug in the blood is bound to erythrocytes.[1-3,5-8,23]

Tacrolimus is highly bound in the plasma (99%) to albumin and alpha-1-acid glycoprotein.[3]

Sirolimus is approximately 92% bound to human plasma proteins.[4] Its binding has been shown to be associated with serum albumin (97%), alpha 1-acid glycoprotein, and lipoproteins.

Elimination

Metabolism and excretion

Cyclosporine, *tacrolimus*, and *sirolimus* are extensively metabolized by the hepatic and gut cytochrome P-450 3A enzyme systems (CYP3A) and counter-transported by P-glycoprotein. Patients receiving potent CYP3A and P-glycoprotein inhibitors may require a decreased dose or increased dosing interval. Patients receiving potent CYP3A and P-glycoprotein inducers may require an increased dosage and a reduced interval dosing. Careful monitoring of blood concentrations is warranted with concomitant administration of antirejection agents and CYP3A inhibitors or inducers. Dosing adjustments may be needed in hepatic failure for *cyclosporine*, *tacrolimus*, and *sirolimus*.

Cyclosporine is highly metabolized by hepatic biotransformation into more than 25 metabolites.[5-7] Cyclosporine and its metabolites are eliminated principally through the bile, while 0.1% is excreted unchanged in the urine.

Tacrolimus is extensively metabolized via CYP3A. Hydroxylation and demethylation are primary in vitro biotransformation pathways.[3] Tacrolimus is primarily eliminated in feces, with less than 1% of an intravenous dose excreted unchanged in the urine.

Sirolimus is metabolized by hydroxylation and/or O-demethylation into seven major metabolites.[4] Its excretion is primarily fecal with 2% excreted in the urine.

Table 10-7 summarizes the clearance values for *cyclosporine, tacrolimus,* and *sirolimus.*

Half-life and time to steady state

Cyclosporine.[1,2,5,12] The half-life of cyclosporine varies between products. Sandimmune ranges from 10 to 27 hours with an average of approximately 19 hours. Neoral ranges from 5 to 18 hours with an average of 8.4 hours. The wide variation in half-life may be due to enterohepatic recycling of the drug, drug interactions, and age. Pediatric patients have a shorter half-life, often requiring every 8-hour dosing rather than the usual 12-hour interval.

Tacrolimus.[25] The elimination half-life of tacrolimus is variable with a mean of 12 hours (range of 4–41 hours). Due to a long half-life with extensive distribution, dosage changes may take several days to reach steady state.

Sirolimus.[21] The observed elimination half-life of sirolimus in stable renal transplant patients on a 14-day regimen including sirolimus, cyclosporine, and prednisone was 62 ± 12 hours. Administration of an appropriate loading dose will provide near steady state drug concentrations within 1 day in most patients. Hepatic impairment will increase half-life.

Table 10-7. Terminal Elimination Half-Life ($t_{1/2}$)

Drug[3,4,12]	$t_{1/2}$ (mean ± SD or range; hours)
Cyclosporine	
Oral	19 (10–27)
Tacrolimus	
Oral[a]	34.8 ± 11.4
IV[a]	34.2 ± 7.7
Sirolimus	
Oral[b]	62 ± 16

[a]Healthy volunteers.
[b]Renal transplant patients.

Therapeutic Range

Due to the difficulty of correlating antirejection agent concentrations with the immediate clinical outcome of immunosuppression, many transplant centers have established their own specific guidelines for immunosuppressive regimens.[26] Table 10-8 gives approximate therapeutic ranges for cyclosporine, tacrolimus, and sirolimus.

Cyclosporine. Generally, approximate desired values for cyclosporine trough concentrations on every 12-hour intervals is 100–500 mcg/L. In solid organ transplantation, patients are maintained at the higher end of the therapeutic range initially and then the desired concentration is often lowered over time to minimize nephrotoxicity and over-immunosuppression. Patients at high risk for rejection may have better outcomes with higher trough blood concentrations.

Table 10-8. Suggested Therapeutic Ranges for Blood Trough Measurements

Drug	Range (mcg/L)
Cyclosporine	
Kidney	100–350
Kidney/pancreas	250–350
Liver	200–500
Bone marrow	250–500
Heart	300–500
Small bowel	300–500
Tacrolimus	5–20
Sirolimus	5–15

There are several different assays available; though the consensus is that assays specific for the parent compound correlate best with clinical events. Such assays include high performance liquid chromatography (HPLC), fluorescence polarization immunoassay, and monoclonal radioimmunoassays.[27,28]

Tacrolimus.[29-31] The therapeutic range for a tacrolimus blood trough concentration is 5–20 mcg/L as measured in whole blood.[29] Most transplant centers strive to maintain concentrations at the higher end of this range during the initial period after transplantation (< 3 months). After that time, most patients have successful outcomes and avoid toxicity with trough concentrations at the lower end of this range.[30]

Tacrolimus concentrations can be measured in plasma (processed at 37°C) or whole blood. Whole blood concentrations are generally 10–30 times higher than the corresponding plasma concentrations.[31] A consensus conference recommended whole blood as the preferred method of tacrolimus monitoring, because it requires less lab time and a less sensitive assay due to higher concentrations.[29]

Sirolimus.[21] When used with cyclosporine and corticosteroids, a sirolimus whole blood trough concentration range of 5–15 mcg/L has been associated with prevention of acute rejection and adverse effects; however, various transplant centers may have developed their own specific guidelines.

Therapeutic Monitoring

Suggested sampling times

Therapeutic efficacy and toxicity have been associated with cyclosporine, tacrolimus, and sirolimus trough concentrations. More frequent monitoring should be performed in patients who are likely to demonstrate altered pharmacokinetic parameters. These patients include hepatically impaired, children, African Americans, or those with concomitant use of potent CYP3A inducers or inhibitors. Therapeutic drug monitoring should be performed more frequently in the early post-transplantation period and less frequently in stable transplant recipients.

Cyclosporine.[5-7,32,33] Therapeutic efficacy has been established according to trough concentrations. Sampling times should be consistent and are usually obtained at hour 12 after a dose (trough). To document acceptable steady state values, cyclosporine blood concentrations should be assessed 3–5 days after initiation of therapy, a dosage adjustment, or initiation or discontinuation of known CYP3A inducers or inhibitors. Some centers monitor area under the curve (AUC) with limited sampling strategies at time 0, 2, and 4 hours past the dose to establish therapeutic efficacy and toxicity.

Tacrolimus.[25,32] Therapeutic efficacy and toxicity have been established according to trough concentrations. Sampling times should be consistent and are usually obtained at hour 12 after a dose (trough). Tacrolimus trough concentrations should be assessed 3–5 days after initiation of therapy, after a dosage adjustment, or after initiation or discontinuation of known CYP3A inducers or inhibitors.

Sirolimus.[4] Therapeutic efficacy has been established according to trough concentrations. Sampling times should be consistent and obtained just before the daily dose (trough). The first sirolimus trough level should be checked at least 3 to 4 days after the loading dose. Frequent sirolimus dose adjustments before reaching steady state may result in under-dosing or over-dosing of sirolimus due to the drug's long half-life. After maintenance dose adjustment, patients should remain on the new maintenance dose for 7 to 14 days before adjusting the dose based on trough concentrations. Blood concentrations should be carefully monitored when initiating or discontinuing a low-dose cyclosporine regimen.

Pharmacodynamic Monitoring

Concentration-related efficacy

The establishment of concentration-efficacy (rejection) relationships for cyclosporine,[34-37] tacrolimus,[30,38,39] and sirolimus[4,21] are difficult for many reasons. There is a lack of direct evidence of a correlation between specific trough concentrations and efficacy; however, in a dose-concentration relationship, higher blood concentrations result in greater immunosuppression and increased side effects. Long-term therapeutic goals include prevention of graft rejection, graft survival, and patient survival. Many transplant centers use retrospective analyses to determine appropriate concentration-related efficacy parameters at their centers.

Concentration-related toxicity

Cyclosporine demonstrates many concentration-related toxicities.[7,37] The most common are nephrotoxicity and neurotoxicity, and these usually respond to dosage reductions. Other toxicities include dermatologic, hepatic, gastrointestinal, and hematological effects. Most of these effects resolve with dose reduction or discontinuation.

Most tacrolimus toxicities are dose and concentration dependent and include nephrotoxicity and neurotoxicity.[3]

Sirolimus demonstrates dose and concentration-related toxicities including nephrotoxicity, elevations in triglycerides and cholesterol, and decreases in platelets and hemoglobin.[4]

Table 10-9 lists the common toxicities for *cyclosporine, tacrolimus, and sirolimus.*

Non-concentration-related toxicity

Cyclosporine, tacrolimus, and sirolimus are associated with development of malignancies, and post-transplant lymphoproliferative disorders (PTLD) and latent virus reactivation.

Cyclosporine. The intravenous formulation is associated with sensitivity reactions due to the solubilizing agent Cremophor EL. Intravenous cyclosporine should only be used when oral therapy is not possible.

Table 10-9. Common Toxicities and Monitoring Approaches for Cyclosporine (C), Tacrolimus (T), and Sirolimus (S)[3,7,9,20,37]

Adverse Effect	Monitoring Parameter
Nephrotoxicity (C/S/T)	Serum creatinine, blood urea nitrogen, urine output, biopsy, proteinuria, cyclosporine or tacrolimus trough concentrations, concomitant nephrotoxic drugs
Hypertension (C/T)	Blood pressure
Electrolyte abnormalities (C/T)	Potassium, magnesium, phosphate, uric acid, bicarbonate concentrations
Neurotoxicity (C/T)	Tremors, seizures, headache, altered mental status and motor function, psychiatric changes, encephalopathy, parasthesia, insomnia
Hepatotoxicity (C/T/S)	Bilirubin and liver function tests
Infections (C/T/S)	White blood cell count, temperature
Hyperlipidemia (C/T/S)	Serum cholesterol and triglycerides
Gingival hyperplasia (C)	Check gums routinely
Hirsutism (C)	Evaluate for hair growth
Gastrointestinal (C/T)	Diarrhea, nausea, vomiting, constipation, anorexia
Dermatologic (C/T)	Pruritus, rash, acne, dry skin, alopecia
Bone marrow suppression (C/T/S)	Red and white blood cells, platelets
Delayed wound healing (S)	Impaired healing and dehiscence
Malignancy/lymphoma (C/T/S)	Routine checks for development of malignancy
Post-transplant diabetes mellitus (T)	Blood glucose, frequent urination, frequent hunger or thirst

Tacrolimus.[3,9,20] There is an increased risk of anaphylaxis as well as cardiac arrhythmias with intravenous tacrolimus due to castor oil derivatives in the formulation. Intravenous tacrolimus should only be used when oral therapy is not possible. Patients should be closely monitored for the first 30 minutes and frequently thereafter during the tacrolimus intravenous infusion. Epinephrine and oxygen should be at the bedside in case anaphylaxis occurs. Additional toxicities include myocardial hypertrophy and post-transplant diabetes mellitus (PTDM).

Sirolimus.[4] Hypersensitivity reactions may occur including anaphylaxis, exfoliative dermatitis, angioedema, and hypersensitivity vasculitis. Additional toxicities include interstitial lung disease, peripheral edema, abdominal pain, and arthralgia.

Drug-Drug Interactions

Cyclosporine, Tacrolimus, and Sirolimus. Due to their CYP3A hepatic metabolism and P-glycoprotein gastrointestinal transport characteristics, other agents may alter disposition of cyclosporine, tacrolimus, and sirolimus. P-glycoprotein, a membrane-bound protein that acts as an active transport drug efflux pump, is found in many tissues including those of the intestinal lumen. Drugs, herbal supplements, and foods that affect CYP3A and P-glycoprotein have the potential to significantly interact with these drugs resulting in subtherapeutic immunosuppressant concentrations leading to graft failure or supratherapeutic concentrations leading to concentration-dependent toxicities.[40] Cyclosporine and tacrolimus are both inhibitors and substrates of CYP3A and P-glycoprotein. Sirolimus is a substrate for both CYP3A and P-glycoprotein.

Patients taking these drugs concomitantly with HMG-CoA reductase inhibitors (statins) including lovastatin, atorvastatin, simvastatin, pravastatin, and fluvastatin should be monitored closely for signs of myopathy or rhabdomyolysis; if signs and symptoms of myopathy occur then statin therapy should be temporarily withheld or discontinued.[1,2] Like many drugs, immunosuppressant drug absorption is reduced when co-administered with aluminum or magnesium hydroxide containing antacids; therefore, separating aluminum/magnesium hydroxide antacid doses is recommended.[25] There is the possibility of reduced immune response after vaccination. Attenuated live vaccines (e.g., MMR, oral polio, BCG, yellow fever, typhoid) should be avoided during treatment with antirejection agents.[1-4] Severe hyperkalemia may result from concomitant use of cyclosporine or tacrolimus with potassium-sparing diuretics or potassium supplements.[1-3]

Cyclosporine blood concentrations decrease when administered concomitantly with orlistat due to reduced absorption.[1,2] Cyclosporine may decrease clearance of colchicine, digoxin, HMG-CoA reductase inhibitors (statins), and prednisolone resulting in toxicity.[1,2] Cyclosporine increases sirolimus blood concentrations; therefore, if used together, sirolimus should be administered 4 hours after cyclosporine.[1,2]

Tacrolimus and mycophenolate mofetil co-administration results in higher mycophenolic acid (MPA) exposure than cyclosporine and mycophenolate mofetil co-administration.[3]

Sirolimus can be coadministered with acyclovir, atorvastatin, digoxin, glyburide, nifedipine, norgestrel/ethinyl estradiol, prednisolone, and sulfamethoxazole/trimethoprim without dosage adjustments.[4]

Table 10-10 lists the common drug interactions for cyclosporine, tacrolimus, and sirolimus.

Table 10-10. Drug Interactions with Cyclosporine (C), Tacrolimus (T), and Sirolimus (S)[a,1-7,9,11,20,25,41]

Potentiate Renal Dysfunction	Decrease CL[b]	Increase CL[c]
ACE[d] inhibitors (C/T)	Antibiotics[e] (C/T/S)	Anticonvulsants[f] (C/T/S)
Aminoglycosides (C/T)	Antifungals[g] (C/T/S)	Rifampin (C/T/S)
Amphotericin B (lipid also) (C/T)	Ca channel blockers[h] (C/T/S)	Octreotide (C)
Cotrimoxazole (SMX–TMP) (C)	Aluminum/Mag Hydroxide (T)	Ticlopidine (C)
Melphalan (C)	Grapefruit juice (C/T/S)	St. John's Wort (C/T/S)
Non-steroidal anti-inflammatory drugs (NSAIDs) (C/T)	Allopurinol (C)	Nafcillin (C)
	Bromocriptine (C/T/S)	Rifabutin (T/S)
Tacrolimus (C)	Danazol (C/T/S)	Rifapentine (S)
Cyclosporine (T)	Metoclopramide (C/T/S)	Caspofungin (T)
Ganciclovir (C/T)	Chloramphenicol (T)	*Sirolimus* (T)
Cisplatin (T)	Cimetidine (T/S)	Terbinafine (C)
Ketoconazole (C)	Nefazadone (T)	
Cimetidine (C)	Protease inhibitors[i] (T/S)	
Ranitidine (C)	Oral contraceptives (C/T)	
Vancomycin (C)	Methylprednisolone (C/T)	
Ciprofloxacin (C)	Omeprazole (T)	
Fiber acid derivatives (C)	Cyclosporine[j] (T/S)	
	Imatinib (C)	
	Amiodarone (C)	
	Colchicine (C)	
	Quinupristin/dalfopristin (C)	

[a]Though not all interactions are reported for each agent, there is a possibility that some occur in the other agents as well. Some interactions are well documented, while others "may" occur. C = reported for cyclosporine, T = reported for tacrolimus, S = reported for sirolimus.
[b]Enzyme inhibitors that decrease antirejection drug metabolism in liver and/or gut.
[c]Hepatic and/or gut enzyme inducers that increase antirejection drug metabolism in liver and/or gut.
[d]Angiotensin converting enzyme inhibitors.
[e]Antibiotics: clarithromycin, erythromycin, telithromycin, and troleandomycin.
[f]Anticonvulsants: carbamazepine, phenobarbital, phenytoin.
[g]Antifungals: fluconazole, voriconazole, itraconazole, clotrimazole, and ketoconazole.
[h]Calcium channel blockers: diltiazem, nicardipine, nifedipine, and verapamil.
[i]Protease inhibitors: indinavir, nelfinavir, ritonivir, and saquinivir.
[j]Concomitant administration of cyclosporine and sirolimus results in elevated sirolimus blood concentrations; therefore, it is recommended that the daily sirolimus dose be taken 4 hours after administration of cyclosporine.

Drug–Disease State or Condition Interactions

Gastroparesis decreases the absorption and affects the disposition of all three antirejection agents when given orally. Table 10-11 shows the important disease state and condition interactions for these agents.

Table 10-11. Effects of Disease State and Condition Interactions[5-7,21,25]

Condition	Effect on Clearance	Effect on Half-Life
Hemodialysis	No change (C/T/S)	No change (C/T/S)
Peritoneal dialysis	No change (C/T/S)	No change (C/T/S)
Hepatic dysfunction	Decreased (C/T/S)	Extended (C/T/S)

References

1. Sandimmune (cyclosporine) [package insert]. Novartis Pharmaceuticals Corp., East Hanover, NJ; October 2009. http://www.pharma.us.novartis.com/product/pi/pdf/sandimmune.pdf. Accessed: January 10, 2011.
2. *Micromedex® Health Care Series* [intranet database]. Version 5.1. Greenwood Village, CO: Thomson Reuters (Healthcare) Inc. Neoral (cyclosporine). http://www.thomsonhc.com/hcs/librarian. Accessed: January 10, 2011.
3. *Micromedex®* Health Care Series [intranet database]. Version 5.1. Greenwood Village, CO: Thomson Reuters (Healthcare) Inc. Prograf (tacrolimus). http://www.thomsonhc.com/hcs/librarian. Accessed: January 10, 2011.
4. *Micromedex®* Health Care Series [intranet database]. Version 5.1. Greenwood Village, CO: Thomson Reuters (Healthcare) Inc. Rapamune (sirolimus). http://www.thomsonhc.com/hcs/librarian. Accessed: January 10, 2011.
5. Cyclosporine. In: McEvoy GK, ed. AHFS Drug Information 2010. Bethesda, MD: American Society of Health-System Pharmacists, Inc.; 2010:3758-72.
6. Noble S, Markham A. Cyclosporine. A review of the pharmacokinetic properties, clinical efficacy, and tolerability of a microemulsion-based formulation (Neoral). *Drugs*. 1995;50(5):924-41.
7. Fahr A. Cyclosporine clinical pharmacokinetics. *Clin Pharmacokinet*. 1993;24(6):472-95.
8. Mochon M, Cooney G, Lum B, et al. Pharmacokinetics of cyclosporine after renal transplant in children. *J Clin Pharmacol*. 1996;36(7):580-6.
9. Tacrolimus. In: McEvoy GK, ed. AHFS Drug Information 2010. Bethesda, MD: American Society of Health-System Pharmacists, Inc.; 2010:3785-90.
10. Vasquez EM. Sirolimus: a new agent for prevention of renal allograft rejection. *Am J Health-Syst Pharm*. 2000;57:437-51.
11. Sirolimus. In: McEvoy GK, ed. AHFS Drug Information 2010. Bethesda, MD: American Society of Health-System Pharmacists, Inc.; 2010:3780-5.
12. *Micromedex®* Health Care Series [intranet database]. Version 5.1. Greenwood Village, CO: Thomson Reuters (Healthcare) Inc. Cyclosporine. http://www.thomsonhc.com/hcs/librarian. Accessed January 10, 2011.
13. Cyclosporine. In: Orange Book Online 2010. U.S. Department of Health and Human Services, Food and Drug Administration, Center for Drug Evaluation and Research, Office of Pharmaceutical Science, Office of Generic Drugs. Rockville, MD; 2010. http://www.accessdata.fda.gov/scripts/cder/ob/default.cfm. Accessed July 12, 2011.
14. Christians U, Strom T, Zhang YL, et al. Active drug transport of immunosuppressants: new insights for pharmacokinetics and pharmacodynamics. *Ther Drug Monit*. 2006;28(1):39-44.
15. Kaplan B, Lown K, Craig R, et al. Low bioavailability of cyclosporine microemulsion and tacrolimus in a small bowel transplant recipient: possible relationship to intestinal P-glycoprotein activity. *Transplantation*. 1999;67(2):333-5.
16. Cupta SK, Manfro RC, Tomlanovich SJ, et al. Effect of food on the pharmacokinetics of cyclosporine in healthy subjects following oral and intravenous administration. *J Clin Pharmacol*. 1990;30(7):643-53.
17. Ducharme MP, Warbasse LH, Edwards DJ. Disposition of intravenous and oral cyclosporine after administration with grapefruit juice. *Clin Pharmacol Ther*. 1995;57(5):485-91.
18. Brunner LJ, Munar MY, Vallian J, et al. Interaction between cyclosporine and grapefruit juice requires long-term ingestion in stable renal transplant recipients. *Pharmacotherapy*. 1998;18(1):23-9.
19. Lown KS, Mayo RR, Leichtman AB, et al. Role of intestinal P-glycoprotein (mdrl) in interpatient variation in the oral bioavailability of cyclosporine. *Clin Pharmacol Ther*. 1997;62(3):248-60.
20. Spencer CM, Goa KL, Gillis JC. Tacrolimus: an update of its pharmacology and clinical efficacy in the management of organ transplantation. *Drugs*. 1997;54(6):925-75.
21. Mahalati K, Kahan BD. Clinical pharmacokinetics of sirolimus. *Clin Pharmacokinet*. 2001;40(8):573-85.
22. Kahan BD. Sirolimus: a comprehensive review. *Expert Opin Pharmacother*. 2001;2(11):1903-17.
23. Shibata N, Minouchi T, Yamaji A, et al. Relationship between apparent total body clearance of cyclosporine A and its erythrocyte-to-plasma distribution ratio in renal transplant patients. *Biol Pharm Bull*. 1995;18(1):115-21.

24. Zimmerman JJ, Kahan BD. Pharmacokinetics of sirolimus in stable renal transplant patients after multiple oral dose administration. *J Clin Pharmacol*. 1997;37:405-15.

25. Venkataramanan R, Swaminathan A, Prasad T, et al. Clinical pharmacokinetics of tacrolimus. *Clin Pharmacokinet*. 1995;29(6):404-30.

26. Meier-Kriesche HU, Li S, Gruessner RWG, et al. Immunosuppression: evolution in practice and trends, 1994-2004. *Am J Transplant*. 2006;6(2):1111-31.

27. Shaw LM, Kaplan B, Brayman KL. Prospective investigations of concentration-clinical response for immunosuppressive drugs provide the scientific basis for therapeutic drug monitoring. *Clin Chem*. 1998;44(2):381-7.

28. Kahan BD, Welsh M, Schoenberg L, et al. Variable oral absorption of cyclosporine. A biopharmaceutical risk factor for chronic renal allograft rejection. *Transplantation*. 1996;62(5):599-606.

29. Jusko WJ, Thompson AW, Fung J, et al. Consensus document: therapeutic monitoring of tacrolimus (FK-506). *Ther Drug Monit*. 1995;17:606-14.

30. Oellerich M, Armstrong VW, Schultz E, et al. Therapeutic drug monitoring of cyclosporine and tacrolimus. *Clin Biochem*. 1998;31(5):309-16.

31. Kelly PA, Burkhart GJ, Venkataramanan R. Tacrolimus: a new immunosuppressive agent. *Am J Health-System Pharm*. 1995;52:1521-35.

32. Qazi YA, Forrest A, Tornatore K, et al. The clinical impact of 1:1 conversion from Neoral to a generic cyclosporine (Gengraf) in renal transplant recipients with stable graft function. *Clin Transplant*. 2006;20:313-17.

33. Masuda S, Inui K. An up-date review on individualized dosage adjustment of calcineurin inhibitors in organ transplant patients. *Pharmacol Ther*. 2006;112:184-98.

34. Kahan BD. Pharmacokinetic considerations in the therapeutic application of cyclosporine in renal transplantation. *Transplant Proc*. 1996;28(4):2143-6.

35. Awni W, Heim-Duthoy K, Kasiske BL. Monitoring of cyclosporine by serial posttransplant pharmacokinetic studies in renal transplant patients. *Transplant Proc*. 1990;22(3):1343-4.

36. Dunn J, Grevel J, Mapoli K, et al. The impact of steady state cyclosporine concentrations on renal allograft outcome. *Transplantation*. 1990;49(1):30-4.

37. Lindholm A, Welsh M, Rutzky L, et al. The adverse impact of high cyclosporine clearance rates on the incidences of acute rejection and graft loss. *Transplantation*. 1993;55(5):985-93.

38. Undre NA, Stevenson P, Schafer A. Pharmacokinetics of tacrolimus: clinically relevant aspects. *Transplant Proc*. 1999;31(suppl 7A):21S-24S.

39. Ringe B, Braun F, Lorf T, et al. FK and MMF in clinical liver transplantation: experience with a steroid sparing concept. *Transplant Proc*. 1998;30(4):1415-6.

40. Lo A, Burkhart GJ. P-glycoprotein and drug therapy in organ transplantation. *J Clin Pharmacol*. 1999;39:995-1005.

41. *Micromedex®* Health Care Series [intranet database]. Version 5.1. Greenwood Village, CO: Thomson Reuters (Healthcare) Inc. Vfend (voriconazole). http://www.thomsonhc.com/hcs/librarian. Accessed January 10, 2011.

Chapter 11

William R. Garnett, Jacquelyn L. Bainbridge, Michael D. Egeberg, and Sarah L. Johnson

Carbamazepine (AHFS 28:12.92)

Carbamazepine is approved by the FDA for the treatment of partial seizures with complex symptomology, generalized tonic-clonic seizures, and mixed seizure patterns in adults and children. It is also approved for the treatment of trigeminal and glossopharyngeal neuralgia in adults and may be useful in the treatment of other types of neuropathy. The extended-release formulation is approved for the treatment of bipolar I disorder in adults. Originally, carbamazepine was marketed for the treatment of trigeminal neuralgia and was later found to be effective for the treatment of seizures.[1] It is ineffective in absence or myoclonic seizures and can worsen or precipitate absence seizures.[2] Target concentrations (4–12 mg/L) have only been evaluated for the treatment of seizures, though this range has also been suggested for other conditions.

Usual Dosage Range in the Absence of Clearance-Altering Factors

Carbamazepine is unique in that it induces its own metabolism (autoinduction), which complicates dosing. Autoinduction takes approximately 3–5 weeks on a fixed dosing regimen.

Generally, doses are started at one fourth to one third of the expected maintenance dose and gradually increased to allow for development of tolerance to side effects, especially central nervous system (CNS) related side effects. For adults (≥15 yr), dosing may be initiated with 400 mg/day in divided doses and increased by 200 mg daily at weekly intervals, up to 1600 mg/day. For children 12–15 yr the initial dosing is the same as for adults, though the maximum recommended dose is 1000 mg/day. For patients 6–12 yr of age, the initial starting dose is 200 mg/day (100 mg twice daily), which can then be increased by 100 mg daily at weekly intervals up to 1000 mg/day. For patients less than 6 yr of age, the initial dose is 10–20 mg/kg/day, given in 3–4 divided doses, and may be increased at weekly intervals up to 35 mg/kg/day. Children less than 12 yr old may be converted to extended-release preparations if they receive 400 mg/day or more. The same total daily dose is used and given in 2 equally divided doses. Elderly patients may be started at 100 to 200 mg daily and increased in weekly intervals by 100 mg daily up to 1000 mg/day.[3] Table 11-1 summarizes the initial and maximum daily dosing recommendations for carbamazepine.

The dose is titrated based on the patient's clinical response and tolerability of side effects,[4] especially CNS side effects.[5] Methods for rapid loading in critically ill patients using carbamazepine suspension and tablets have been described.[6–8] One rapid switch-over technique using the pharmacokinetics derived from a single 10 mg/kg dose has been used to convert patients from other AEDs to carbamazepine.[8] Using this approach, the conversion to carbamazepine with the removal of other AEDs was achieved in 6 days, with no adverse effects.

Since the metabolism of carbamazepine is subject to enzyme induction and inhibition, the maintenance dosage will depend in part on the presence or absence of other drugs that may induce or inhibit hepatic enzymes (see Drug-Drug Interactions section).

There is significant intersubject variability in the pharmacokinetics of carbamazepine, which can impact the frequency of daily dosing. Some patients may be dosed twice a day, while others may require dosing as often as four times a day with immediate-release tablets. The dosage form can also affect the frequency of daily dosing. Controlled- and sustained-release dosage forms are designed for every 12-hour dosing, while the suspension is usually administered four times daily. However, the total daily dose is the same, no matter which formulation is being used, since bioavailability is fairly uniform. Table 11-2 summarizes the available dosage forms of carbamazepine products.

There has been much discussion regarding whether generic versions of carbamazepine are truly equivalent to the brand name products. While there are numerous case reports of patients experiencing break-through seizures or side effects after a switch from one formulation to another, controlled trials have demonstrated bioequivalency of the generic formulations compared to the brand formulation. The argument against generic

Table 11-1. Initial and Maximum Maintenance Dosing and Dosage Forms

Dosage Form and Age Groups	Initial Dose	Maximum Maintenance Doses
Intravenous	Not available	
Oral (tablets or suspension):		
Slow titration generally indicated		
Children <6 years	10–20 mg/kg/day	35 mg/kg/day
Children 6–12 years	100 mg twice daily	1000 mg/day
Children 12–15 years	200 mg twice daily	800–1000 mg/day
Adults >15 years	200 mg twice daily	1200 mg/day
Elderly	100 mg once or twice daily	1000 mg/day
Oral (tablets or suspension):		
Rapid loading for critically ill patients[a]		
Children (≤12 years)	10 mg/kg	
Children (>12 years) and Adults	8 mg/kg	

[a]This rapid loading procedure should result in peak concentrations of around 10 mg/L. A routine maintenance dose should be started 6–8 hr after the loading dose.

Table 11-2. Dosage Form Availability

Dosage Form	Product
Intravenous	None available (in development)
Oral immediate-release tablets	
100 mg chewable	Tegretol
200 mg	Tegretol, Epitol, Carbamazepine (multiple sources)
Oral suspension: 100 mg/5 ml	Tegretol
Extended-release tablets	
100 mg, 200 mg, 400 mg	Tegretol-XR
Extended-release capsules[a]	
100 mg, 200 mg, 300 mg	Carbatrol
Rectal enema	Use suspension diluted 1:1 with water

[a]May be used as a sprinkle.

products is that there is a potential that clinically important variations might occur with frequent switches of immediate-release dosage forms. Also, individual patients may have a narrow therapeutic range for seizure control and incidence of side effects. Therefore, it is prudent to initiate patients on one formulation and maintain them on that formulation unless they are converted to a sustained- or controlled-release dosage form.

General Pharmacokinetic Information

Absorption

The oral bioavailability of all formulations is considered equivalent, however, the rate of absorption can vary between formulations. Since no intravenous form of carbamazepine is currently available for human use, the absolute bioavailability is unknown. A 2% oral solution has been suggested to be 100% bioavailable and may be used for comparisons.[9] The gastrointestinal (GI) absorption of immediate-release carbamazepine is slow, erratic, and unpredictable, due to carbamazepine's slow rate of dissolution and/or anticholinergic properties.[10] Secondary peaks in drug concentration may occur due to a slow but constant rate of absorption and absorption occurring in the upper and lower intestine.[10,11] There is no first pass metabolism. There is significant inter- and intraindividual variability in the absorption rate for immediate-release tablets and circadian variation in the rate of absorption may be observed, with an evening dose being absorbed more slowly than a morning dose.[12] Table 11-3 summarizes the bioavailability of the different formulations of carbamazepine.

Concurrent administration with food affects the rate but not the extent of absorption. Immediate-release tablets, extended-release tablets, and the suspension should be administered with a meal, while the extended-release capsules (Carbatrol) can be taken without regard to food.[17] Food may increase the rate of carbamazepine absorption from the extended-release tablets. In one report the administration of a single dose of immediate-release carbamazepine with an acidic beverage (cola) resulted in an enhanced rate and extent of carbamazepine absorption.[18]

A linear relationship between dose and concentration has been shown at doses between 600 and 1400 mg/day; however, at higher doses the increases in the steady state concentration tend to be less than proportional. Carbamazepine may exhibit saturable absorption; doses higher than 20 mg/kg of the immediate-release tablet may be less absorbed. Carbamazepine undergoes a simultaneous first-order and zero-order absorption with about 35% of the available dose being absorbed at a zero-order rate.[19]

Carbatrol is the extended-release capsule formulation that contains immediate-release, intermediate-release, and extended-release beads of carbamazepine. Tegretol-XR, the extended-release tablet, utilizes the OROS system, which is a matrix system with a semipermeable membrane for drug delivery. These formulations can be given twice a day, preferably at 12-hr intervals. When immediate-release carbamazepine administered every 6 hr was compared with either extended-release carbamazepine capsules or tablets given every 12 hr, they were bioequivalent.[13,14]

Results from a 5-day study of normal volunteers indicate that Carbatrol is bioequivalent to Tegretol-XR, but there was less variability in the rate of absorption with Carbatrol.[15] Variability in GI transit time may affect the absorption of Tegretol-XR.[11]

The FDA reported that moisture might decrease the potency of carbamazepine immediate-release tablets by up to one-third or more; therefore, these tablets must be stored in a cool, dry place.[20] Tablets that are continuously exposed to 97% relative humidity at room temperature for 2 weeks become hardened and dissolve poorly.[21]

Distribution

Animal studies indicate that carbamazepine distributes rapidly and uniformly to various organs and tissues, achieving higher concentrations in organs of high blood flow (e.g., liver, kidney, and brain).[10] The drug has been detected in the cerebral spinal fluid (CSF), brain, duodenal fluids, bile, and saliva.[16] The 10, 11-epoxide metabolite has also been detected in the CSF. Carbamazepine rapidly crosses the placenta, and accumulates in fetal tissue with higher concentrations in the liver and kidney than the brain and lungs.[16] The placenta does not participate in the metabolism of carbamazepine.[22]

Table 11-3. Bioavailability of Dosage Forms

Dosage Form	Bioavailability/Comments
Intravenous	Not available
Immediate-release tablets	85%–90% (F = 0.85–0.9)[8,9]
Chewable tablets	85%–90% (F = 0.85–0.9)[10,11]
Oral suspension	85%–90%, (F = 0.85–0.9) but at a faster rate compared to immediate-release tablets.[13]
Extended-release capsules and tablets	85%–90%, (F = 0.85–0.9) capsules may provide less variation in the concentration-time curve than extended-release tablets.[14,15]
Rectal enema (extemporaneous compounding required)	80%–100% *as compared to immediate-release tablets* (F = 0.7 to 0.9) in total amount absorbed but with longer time to peak.[16]

The carbamazepine concentration in breast milk is about 25%–60% of the concentration in the mother's plasma.[10] Strong and highly significant correlations between saliva and plasma concentrations have been found over a wide range of carbamazepine concentrations following citric acid stimulation of saliva.[23] The utility of salivary sampling is limited however, and should be restricted to those occasions when a blood sample cannot be obtained.

The volume of distribution of carbamazepine varies by age (Table 11-4).[3] Carbamazepine binds to albumin and to alpha-1-acid glycoprotein (AAG).[5] The concentration of AAG and the free (unbound) fraction of carbamazepine may vary with the presence of inflammation, trauma, concurrent antiepileptic drug therapy, and age (Table 11-4).[24] Binding is slightly less in neonates than in other age groups,[10] though it has recently been reported that carbamazepine binds to nonglycated albumin, which decreases with age.[25] There was a higher free fraction in elderly patients that was attributed to the decrease in nonglycated albumin. The study suggested that this might explain the increased sensitivity to carbamazepine that has been reported in the elderly.

Monitoring of the unbound concentration may be indicated when the patient's clinical presentation does not coincide with the plasma concentration (e.g., presence of side effects or lack of response).[26] However, there is no defined target concentration range for unbound carbamazepine and unbound concentrations are not routinely measured. Poorly controlled diabetic patients may have an increased unbound fraction of carbamazepine due to a decrease in nonglycosylated albumin concentrations, which may make measurement of unbound concentrations useful in some diabetic patients.[27]

Elimination

Though carbamazepine does not appear to undergo first-pass metabolism, it is about 99% metabolized by oxidation, hydroxylation, direct conjugation with glucuronic acid, and sulfur conjugation pathways. Oxidation and hydroxylation pathways account for about 65% of its metabolism.[28] The most important carbamazepine metabolite is 10, 11-epoxide, which appears to be active and may contribute to the efficacy and toxicity of carbamazepine.[29,30] The isoenzymes responsible for catalyzing 10, 11-oxidation of carbamazepine in the human liver are CYP3A4, CYP2C8, and CYP1A1. CYP3A4 is the most important of the three.[31] While there is some polymorphic distribution of CYP2C8, it does not seem to have a major effect on the pharmacokinetics of carbamazepine. CYP1A2 and uridine diphospho-glucuronosyltransferase (UGT) are involved in forming the inactive metabolites of carbamazepine.[32,33]

The 10, 11-epoxide metabolite is further metabolized to a diol metabolite by a xenobiotic epoxide hydrolase.[33] Clearance of the 10, 11-epoxide metabolite is higher than that of the parent drug.[34] The metabolites and a small percentage of unchanged drug are excreted in the urine (72%) and feces (28%), (with 1%–3% excreted unchanged).[3] Drug interactions may alter the formation of the 10, 11-epoxide metabolite without altering the carbamazepine concentration.[35]

The metabolism of carbamazepine may be altered by other drugs and by itself (autoinduction), with clearance increasing on continued dosing.[36] Autoinduction begins 3–5 days after the initiation of therapy and takes 3–5 weeks to complete.[36,37] The 10, 11-epoxide diol pathway is the pathway primarily affected. Autoinduction occurs with each dosage increase in children and adults.[37,38] Because of autoinduction, concentrations achieved initially can be expected to fall over time on a fixed dose. This should be considered early in therapy and during dosage titration since a drop in carbamazepine concentration on a fixed dose may reflect autoinduction rather than patient nonadherence. The potential for other drugs to enhance or inhibit the metabolism of carbamazepine makes drug-drug interactions likely and potentially significant.[1]

Table 11-4. Volume of Distribution and Percent Bound to Protein[24]

Age Category	Volume (L/kg)[a]	Protein Binding (%)
Neonates	1.5	65–70
Children	1.9	75
Adults (>15 years)	0.6–2	75

[a]Based on actual body weight.

Since there is no intravenous form of carbamazepine, all reported clearance values are relative to bioavailability (CL/F), which is assumed to be nearly complete. Table 11-5 shows clearance values relative to patient age. Carbamazepine clearance increases with continued dosing and can be altered by enzyme-inducing or inhibiting drugs.[39] It decreases with increasing age and as weight increases in children 2–16 years old.[40] In children 1–14 years old, clearance has been shown to increase linearly with total body weight and nonlinearly with age; thus, older children have a lower clearance with respect to total body weight than do younger ones.[38] One study showed no effect for older patients, though others have shown that older patients may have altered pharmacokinetics.[41–43] Carbamazepine is metabolized by oxidative metabolism, which does decrease with age.[44] One population pharmacokinetic analysis demonstrated an age-related decrease in CL/F.[45]

Clearance relative to mass has been shown to decrease with increasing body mass. It has also been shown to increase with surface area and dose,[46] though the relationship of clearance to dose remains controversial.[47] Carbamazepine concentrations were significantly higher in lean subjects (BMI < 20) than those with a normal body mass index (BMI 20 to 25); the degree of obesity may affect carbamazepine concentrations.[48] Weight reduction in one patient did not affect carbamazepine clearance.[49]

A study done in patients aged 6–17 years to test for the associations of carbamazepine clearance with physical measurements, age, and plasma hormonal levels found urinary clearance of carbamazepine and its metabolites was proportional to the size of the liver, which was larger compared to adults, relative to total body weight.[50]

Table 11-5. Clearance Based on Age

Age (yr)	Clearance (L/hr/kg)[a]
Children: initial dosing	
0–3 years	0.32
4–9 years	0.19
10–15 years	0.12
Children (≤15 years): chronic dosing	0.05–0.4[b]
Adults (>15 years)	
Initial dosing	0.01–0.03
Chronic dosing	0.05–0.1

[a]Clearance relative to bioavailability (CL/F)

[b]Though the clearance range includes a lower value than what are reported as the means for initial dosing, it should be assumed that all patients will undergo autoinduction to some degree, with initial clearance lower than the clearance observed after autoinduction is complete.

Half-life and time to steady state

The half-life ($t_{1/2}$) of carbamazepine changes with continued dosing and is affected by other drugs. The time to steady state depends on the completion of autoinduction.[39] A true half-life is difficult to ascertain from measured concentrations because of the variability of absorption, as it may continue throughout the dosing interval. Table 11-6 summarizes the half-life and time to steady state. The 10, 11-epoxide metabolite of carbamazepine has a half-life of 25–43 hours with single doses and 6.1 hours with chronic fixed dosing.[3,51]

Table 11-6. Half-Life and Time to Steady State[2,3]

Dosing	Half-Life (hr)	Time to Steady State
Single dose	25–65	N/A[a]
Chronic dose	12–17	N/A[a]
Concurrent antiepileptic drug	5–14	N/A[a]

[a]Time to steady state is not applicable (N/A) to single doses and, due to autoinduction, is based more realistically not on the half-life, but rather on the time for full autoinduction to occur when dosing chronically (3–5 weeks).

Dosing Strategies

The variability in the pharmacokinetics of carbamazepine makes dosage prediction difficult. Statistical models and population methods are generally not clinically useful,[52,53] though a Bayesian nonlinear method that used three to four data points was shown to be clinically acceptable.[54] In a study of 829 adult patients with 1834 concentration measurements, clearance relative to bioavailability (CL/F) predictors were developed using NONMEM analysis and the following regression equations resulted for carbamazepine used alone or in combination with several other antiepileptic agents[45]:

1. CL/F (L/hr) = [(0.0134 X ABW) + 3.58], *where ABW = actual body weight*
2. If the patient is also receiving phenytoin, the CL/F determined in (1) is multiplied by 1.42.
3. If the patient is receiving phenobarbital or felbamate in addition to carbamazepine, the CL/F determined in (1) is multiplied by 1.17.
4. If the patient is receiving phenytoin and phenobarbital or felbamate, the CL/F determined in (1) is multiplied by 1.62.
5. If the patient is ≥70 years of age, the CL/F determined in (1 to 4) is multiplied by 0.749.

The predicted clearance values can be used to estimate the post-induction dose of carbamazepine. An additional 50 patients were used to test the predictors developed in the study and the mean prediction error was 0.6 mg/L and the median absolute error 2.4 mg/L.[45]

Tegretol XR should not be crushed or chewed. Patients taking this product should be warned that the casing will be excreted in the feces and will increase in size. Carbatrol capsules may be opened and the contents used as a sprinkle. Both formulations have reduced peak to trough fluctuation and may be associated with fewer of the side effects related to higher peak concentrations. The twice a day dosing of both formulations may also improve patient adherence.

The sustained-release carbamazepine capsules (Carbatrol) may be opened and mixed with a diluent and quickly administered through a feeding tube if the tube is larger than 12 French. In an ex vivo study, the contents of the 200 and 300 mg capsules were mixed with 30 ml of either sterile water, D5W, normal saline, or apple juice. The suspension was aspirated into a 60 ml syringe and administered down a 12 French pediatric tube, a 16 French Levine tube, and a 20 French gastrostomy tube. The tubes were flushed with two additional washings of diluent. All fluid coming through the tubes was collected and assayed. Sporadic clogging was noted with the pediatric and Levine tubing when sterile water or D5W was used, but a reproducible recovery was found for all three types of tubing when the fluid was normal saline or apple juice.[55] The ability to administer the contents of Carbatrol via feeding tubes was evaluated in six children. The contents of one capsule was added to 15 ml of liquid and flushed with 10 ml of water. Four children had 152 of 154 doses administered without difficulty. Two patients had tube occlusions, but these children had a history of frequent tube occlusions.[56] If this technique is used, the dose should be administered immediately after the suspension is made.

Therapeutic Range

The reported therapeutic range of carbamazepine is 4–12 mg/L for the treatment of seizures and the range for psychiatric disorders and trigeminal neuralgia is assumed to be the same.[4] The therapeutic range for a given patient must be individually determined with the goal of therapy as cessation of seizures while minimizing side effects.

The 10, 11-epoxide metabolite of carbamazepine is active and may contribute to efficacy as well as toxicity. Drug interactions may increase the concentration of the metabolite without changing the carbamazepine concentration. Ideally, the clinician should measure both the parent drug and the metabolite, but an assay for 10, 11-epoxide is not commercially available. Nevertheless, the contribution of this metabolite should be considered when the response to carbamazepine is evaluated.

Patients in the therapeutic range may still show limited response. One study compared the pharmacokinetics of carbamazepine in 16 controlled and 15 uncontrolled adult patients with epilepsy. The uncontrolled patients were taking higher doses of carbamazepine and had higher serum concentrations. There were no pharmacokinetic differences between the two groups. The lack of efficacy in the uncontrolled group was felt to be pharmacodynamic resistance and not related to any pharmacokinetic factor.[57]

Therapeutic Monitoring

Suggested sampling times and effect on therapeutic range

Patients should have baseline measurements that include a CBC with platelet count, reticulocytes, serum iron, lipid panel, liver function tests, urinalysis, BUN, thyroid function tests, serum sodium and ophthalmic exams. Follow-up measurements, including carbamazepine concentration determinations, can be done at the clinician's judgment, but should be considered when there is a change in therapy, change in seizure status or when unacceptable side effects occur.

The sampling time for carbamazepine depends on the duration of treatment and whether the clinician is evaluating efficacy or side effects. A blood sample is not needed for carbamazepine concentration determination after the first dose unless a rapid loading dose was given in an emergency situation and there is a desire to ensure concentrations are as desired by a clinician. While concentrations should be determined during dosage titration to evaluate end-points, they may be expected to fall due to autoinduction. Autoinduction must also be considered when doses are changed during chronic therapy. A trough concentration measurement drawn just before the morning dose is most appropriate for the evaluation of efficacy.

The dose of carbamazepine should be started low and titrated to patient response. The rate of titration will determine sample collection. If the dose is being increased weekly or every 2 weeks, autoinduction will occur for some time and the concentration will change, even with good adherence. Samples may be obtained during this period to correlate dose with side effects or with seizure control, but sampling will be more meaningful after autoinduction is complete.

Many side effects associated with carbamazepine are concentration related, and each patient has a threshold for the occurrence of side effects.[58] Therefore, for some patients the sample may be appropriately obtained when side effects are occurring. Given the variability of absorption from immediate- and controlled-release products, it is difficult to predict when the peak carbamazepine concentration will occur.

Pharmacodynamic Monitoring

Concentration-related efficacy

The effectiveness of carbamazepine as an antiepileptic drug is associated with concentrations of 4–12 mg/L.[4] This range is intended as a guide—not as an absolute—because of the variable amount of free drug, the contribution of the 10, 11-epoxide metabolite, and the intersubject variability in response. The target concentration for a given patient should be determined by patient response and occurrence of side effects. A concentration should be obtained and documented along with the dose and concomitant drugs when the patient is doing well in terms of seizure management and side effects. This provides some ability for patients to be their own control when evaluating concentrations in the future.

Concentration-related toxicity

A concentration of >15 mg/L is associated with a higher frequency of side effects. Symptoms of toxicity include dizziness, ataxia, drowsiness, nausea, vomiting, tremor, agitation, nystagmus, urinary retention, headache, blurred vision, diplopia, dysrhythmias, coma, seizures, twitches, respiratory disorders, and neuromuscular disturbances.[2,3,20] Patients on monotherapy have fewer side effects and tolerate higher concentrations of carbamazepine than do patients on polytherapy.[59] The occurrence of side effects can be reduced or minimized by slow titration, decreasing the dose, giving smaller doses more frequently, or switching to a sustained- or controlled-release product.

Slow dosage titration allows a patient time to develop tolerance to certain side effects associated with carbamazepine. The use of sustained-release or controlled-release dosage forms reduces the peak to trough fluctuations and may reduce associated side effects. A dose reduction may decrease side effects in some patients without loss of seizure control.

Other possible concentration-related side effects include hyponatremia, syndrome of inappropriate antidiuretic hormone secretion (SIADH), and osteomalacia.[5] An exact dose and concentration effect for these side effects has not been established, but they occur more frequently at higher doses or after prolonged exposure. Carbamazepine has been associated with atrioventricular block, especially in older women, and it is suggested that careful monitoring of the ECG and drug concentration be done in elderly patients.[60,61] Carbamazepine is associated with skin rash and rarely with a Stevens-Johnson reaction. The mechanism may involve reactive metabolites in the epidermis.[62] One case of skin rash was associated with an increased concentration of nicotinamide and vitamin B6.[63] Other case reports of adverse reactions include hearing loss, alopecia, hypogammaglobulinemia, tubulointerstitial nephritis, an auditory disturbance (flat A tone), abnormal pitch perception, and pemphigus.[64–70]

Idiosyncratic reactions also include bone marrow suppression, aplastic anemia, and agranulocytosis, which are all very rare. Carbamazepine can cause a leukopenia that is not considered dangerous or a harbinger of agranulocytosis or aplastic anemia, so a decrease in the white blood cell (WBC) count is not an automatic requirement for stopping carbamazepine. Many patients taking carbamazepine routinely have low WBCs without being immunosuppressed. Carbamazepine appears to affect the distribution of neutrophils without affecting their ability to mobilize at the time of infection. Routine monitoring of complete blood counts is not felt to be useful for preventing bone marrow suppression in patients taking carbamazepine.

Drug-Drug Interactions

Carbamazepine is an enzyme inducer and enhances the metabolism of many drugs that are metabolized by the cytochrome P450 (CYP) system, including itself. Carbamazepine induces and is metabolized extensively by the isoenzyme CYP3A4, and to a lesser extent CYP1A2, CYP2B6, CYP2E1, CYP2C8, CYP2C9 and uridine diphosphate glucuronosyltransferase (UGT) 1A4.[41] Therefore, the metabolism of carbamazepine may be affected by drugs that induce or inhibit these liver microsomal enzymes.[71–73] Carbamazepine also undergoes phase 2 metabolism through UGT2B7 substrate to form an *N*-glucuronide metabolite.[41]

Drugs that are inhibitors of the CYP3A4 isoenzyme will decrease the clearance of carbamazepine due to decreased metabolism. Carbamazepine is reported to be an inhibitor of CYP2C19 as it can increase concentrations of phenytoin, selegiline, and clomipramine.[41] Valproate is an inhibitor of UGT2B7 and may account for the reduction in transformation of the carbamazepine epoxide metabolite to the *trans*-dihydrodiol metabolite.[41] This results in increases of the epoxide concentration when carbamazepine is administered with valproate. Carbamazepine is a substrate and inhibitor of P-glycoprotein, but significant interactions are not likely to occur at concentrations used clinically.[41]

Drugs that are inducers of the CYP P450 system, specifically 3A4, will increase the clearance of carbamazepine due to enhanced metabolism. Tables 11-7 and 11-8 summarize common drug interactions between carbamazepine and other drugs and the expected result.[13,71–113]

Other types of interactions have been described. When chlorpromazine oral solution is administered with carbamazepine suspension a rubbery, orange precipitate results.[3] The effect on bioavailability of either drug is unknown. Therefore, these drugs should not be administered together in this form. When lithium and carbamazepine are used together, there is an increased risk for neurological effects.[2,3] Possible serotonin syndrome may result if carbamazepine is administered concurrently with an MAO inhibitor and combined therapy is contraindicated.[2,3] When used with phenytoin, the concentration of phenytoin may increase or decrease. There is a complex interaction with valproic acid, and the results are unpredictable.[74] Carbamazepine and theophylline induce each other's metabolism resulting in changes in the half-life and plasma concentrations of both drugs.[75] Concurrent use with alcohol may increase the risk of additive CNS effects such as sedation.

Significant amounts of carbamazepine are lost through adsorption if undiluted suspension is administered through polyvinyl chloride nasogastric feeding tubes. Dilution with an equal volume of diluent and flushing after administration minimizes the adsorption.[114] Enteral feedings do not appear to alter the absorption of carbamazepine suspension significantly.[115]

Pharmacodynamic interactions have been reported between carbamazepine and lamotrigine and between carbamazepine and levetiracetam.[116-118] When either lamotrigine or levetiracetam is added to the regimen of patients taking carbamazepine, there is an increase in the incidence of CNS side effects. These effects are not associated with an increase in the concentrations of either the carbamazepine or the 10, 11-epoxide active metabolite. A dosage reduction of carbamazepine may be necessary when these drugs are added. The composite of lacosamide and a traditional sodium channel blocking drug, such as carbamazepine, may increase the incidence of CNS and GI side effects. If this does occur the dose of the sodium channel blocking drug should be decreased.[119]

Table 11-7. Common Carbamazepine Drug Interactions that Impact Concentrations of the Second Drug[13,71–113]

CBZ Increases Concentration	CBZ Decreases Concentration
Clomipramine	Acetaminophen
Primidone	Benzodiazepines (alprazolam, clonazepam, midazolam)
Selegiline	Anticoagulants (warfarin, dicumarol)
Phenytoin	Antifungal agents (fluconazole, itraconazole, ketoconazole)
	Antipsychotics (aripiprazole, clozapine, fluphenazine, haloperidol, olanzapine, risperidone, ziprasidone)
	Dihydropyridine calcium-channel blocking agents (felodipine)
	Corticosteroids (dexamethasone, prednisolone)
	Immunosuppressants (cyclosporine, tacrolimus)
	Doxycycline
	Antiepileptics (ethosuximide, lamotrigine, tiagabine, topiramate, valproate, zonisamide)
	Protease inhibitors (Indinavir)
	Hormonal contraceptives
	Levothyroxine
	Methadone
	Tramadol
	Antidepressants (sertraline, citalopram, escitalopram, duloxetine, bupropion, mirtazapine trazodone, imipramine, amitriptyline, nortriptyline)
	Fentanyl
	Methylphenidate
	Pancuronium bromide, vecuronium
	Statins (atorvastatin, lovastatin, simvastatin)
	β-blockers
	Digoxin

CBZ = carbamazepine, CBZ-E = 10,11-epoxide

Drug–Disease State or Condition Interactions

Children with mixed seizure disorders may have an exacerbation of certain seizure types if carbamazepine therapy is used. It has mild anticholinergic properties and should be used with caution in patients who are sensitive to anticholinergic effects such as the elderly or those who have increased intraocular pressure. Carbamazepine is structurally related to tricyclic compounds. Reports of cardiovascular effects including congestive heart failure, edema, coronary artery disease, arrhythmias, and AV block have been reported.[2] The elderly may also be at an increased risk for SIADH.

Carbamazepine is extensively metabolized in the liver and, therefore, should be used with caution in patients with liver disease. Since carbamazepine (to a very small degree) and its active metabolite are excreted renally, it should be used with some caution in patients with renal disease. Hemodialysis does not affect the clearance of carbamazepine.[120]

Congestive heart failure that causes gut edema may contribute to variable absorption of the drug. Carbamazepine may cause sodium and water retention, aggravating congestive heart failure. Fever (increased metabolism) and pulmonary disease (decreased metabolism) have been associated with alterations of antiepileptic drug clearance. Changes in protein binding and altered metabolism were believed to be responsible for carbamazepine toxicity in patients following cardiothoracic surgery and myocardial infarction.[121]

Table 11-8. Common Drug Interactions that Result in Changes in Carbamazepine Concentrations[13,71–113]

Drug Increases CBZ Concentration	Drug Decreases CBZ Concentration
Acetazolamide	Antineoplastic agents (cisplatin, doxorubicin)
Antifungal agents (fluconazole, itraconazole, ketoconazole)	Rifampin
Antihistamines (loratadine)	Felbamate
Isoniazid	Phenobarbital
Non-dihydropyridine calcium channel blockers (diltiazem, verapamil)	Primidone
Cimetidine	Phenytoin
Danazol	Caffeine
Felbamate (CBZ-E)	
Fluoxetine (CBZ and CBZ-E)	
Fluvoxamine	
Grapefruit juice	
Pomegranate juice	
Protease inhibitors (ritonavir, saquinavir)	
Macrolide antibiotics (clarithromycin and erythromycin but NOT azithromycin)	
Nefazodone	
Niacinamide	
Propoxyphene, dextropropoxyphene	
Valproic acid (CBZ-E)	
Quetiapine	
Omeprazole	
Baclofen	
Gemfibrozil	

CBZ = carbamazepine, CBZ-E = 10,11-epoxide

The clearance of antiepileptic drugs increases during pregnancy, therefore the carbamazepine concentration should be more closely monitored.[122] The need for a dose increase should be anticipated. Following delivery, the clearance returns to normal and the dose may be reduced.[123] Carbamazepine may interfere with some pregnancy tests and is an FDA pregnancy category D medication. However, the benefit of being seizure free may outweigh the risk of fetal abnormalities.

Absorption may be decreased in malnourished patients.[124] Any alterations in the gastrointestinal system could potentially affect the absorption of carbamazepine. Serum thyroid levels may be reduced by carbamazepine although the clinical significance of this is unclear.[2]

Summary

Carbamazepine has been used widely for the treatment of partial and tonic-clonic generalized seizures and is considered a mainstay of therapy. It is often used as a comparator to new products being tested; however, it is not without its limitations. It has shown variable absorption, induces its own metabolism, and is metabolized extensively through the cytochrome P450 system to an active metabolite. Its pharmacokinetics are difficult to predict, and drug interactions are likely to occur.

References

1. Gidal BE, Garnett WR, Graves N. Epilepsy. In: DiPiro JT, Talbert RL, Yee GC, et al., eds. *Pharmacotherapy: A Pathophysiologic Approach*. 7th ed. New York, NY: McGraw Hill; 2008:927-51.

2. Carbamazepine. In: McEvoy GK, ed. *AHFS Drug Information 2010*. Bethesda, MD: American Society of Health-System Pharmacists; 2010:2257-63.
3. Lexi-Comp, Inc. Carbamazepine: drug information. In: Rose, BD, ed. *UpToDate*. Wellesley, MA; 2010.
4. Loiseau P. Carbamazepine: clinical efficacy and use in epilepsy. In: Levy RH, Mattson RH, Meldrum BS. *Antiepileptic Drugs*. 5th ed. New York, NY: Raven Press; 2002:262-2.
5. MacKichan JJ. Carbamazepine. In: Taylor WJ, Caviness MHD, eds. *A Textbook for the Clinical Application of Therapeutic Monitoring*. Irving, TX: Abbott Laboratories; 1986:211-24.
6. Miles MV, Lawless ST, Tennison MB, et al. Rapid loading of critically ill patients with carbamazepine suspension. *Pediatrics*. 1990;86:263-6.
7. Cohen H, Howland MA, Luciano DJ, et al. Feasibility and pharmacokinetics of carbamazepine oral loading doses. *Am J Health-Syst Pharm*. 1998;55:1134-40.
8. Kanner AM, Bourgeois BF, Hasegawa H, et al. Rapid switch over to carbamazepine using pharmacokinetic parameters. *Epilepsia*. 1998;39(2):194-200.
9. Gerardin A, Dobois JP, Moppert J, et al. Absolute bioavailability of carbamazepine after oral administration of a 2% syrup. *Epilepsia*. 1990;31:334-8.
10. Spina E. Carbamazepine: Chemistry, biotransformation, and pharmacokinetics. In: Levy RH, Mattson RH, Meldrum BS, eds. *Antiepileptic Drugs*. 5th ed. New York, NY: Raven Press; 2002:237-46.
11. Wilding IR, Davis SS, Hardy JG, et al. Relationship between systemic drug absorption and gastrointestinal transit after the simultaneous oral administration of carbamazepine as a controlled release system and as a suspension of 15N-labelled drug to healthy volunteers. *Br J Clin Pharmacol*. 1991;32(5):573-9.
12. Hartley R, Forsythe WJ, McLain B, et al. Daily variations in steady-state plasma concentrations of carbamazepine and its metabolites in epileptic children. *Clin Pharmacokinet*. 1991;20:237-44.
13. Thakker KM, Mangat S, Garnett WR, et al. Comparative bioavailability and steady state fluctuations of Tegretol commercial and carbamazepine OROS tablets in adult and pediatric epileptic patients. *Biopharm Drug Disposition*. 1992;13:559-69.
14. Garnett WR, Levy B, McLean AM, et al. Pharmacokinetic evaluation of twice-daily extended release carbamazepine (CBZ) and four times daily immediate release CBZ in patients with epilepsy. *Epilepsia*. 1998;39(3):274-9.
15. Stevens RE, Lim Sakun T, Evans G, et al. Controlled, multidose, pharmacokinetic evaluation of two extended-release carbamazepine formulations (Carbatrol and Tegretol-XR). *J Pharm Sci*. 1998;87:1531-4.
16. Tegretol [package insert]. East Hanover, NJ: Novartis; 2009.
17. McLean A, Browne S, Zhang Y, et al. The influence of food on the bioavailability of a twice-daily controlled release carbamazepine formulation. *J Clin Pharmacol*. 2001;41:183-6.
18. Malhotra, S, Dixit RK, Garg SK. Effect of an acidic beverage (Coca-Cola) on the pharmacokinetics of carbamazepine in healthy volunteers. *Methods Find Exp Clin Pharmacol*. 2002;24:31-3.
19. Riad LE, Chan KKH, Wagner WE, et al. Simultaneous first- and zero-order absorption of carbamazepine tablets in humans. *J Pharm Sci*. 1986;75:897-900.
20. Anon. Carbamazepine and moisture. *Medicom*. 1990;8:442.
21. Anon. Safeguards needed for carbamazepine. *FDA Drug Bull*. 1990;(Apr):5.
22. Pienimaki P, Lampela E, Hakkula J, et al. Pharmacokinetics of oxcarbazepine and carbamazepine in human placenta. *Epilepsia*. 1997;38(3):309-16.
23. Gorodischer R, Burtin P, Verjee Z, et al. Is saliva suitable for therapeutic monitoring of anticonvulsants in children: an evaluation in the routine clinical setting. *Ther Drug Monit*. 1997;19(6):637-42.
24. Baruzzi A, Contin M, Perucca E, et al. Altered serum protein binding of carbamazepine in disease states associated with an increased alpha1 acid glycoprotein concentration. *Eur J Clin Pharmacol*. 1986;31:85-9.
25. Koyama H, Sugioka N, Uno A, et al. Age-related alteration of carbamazepine-serum protein binding in man. *J Pharm Pharmacol*. 1999;51:1009-14.
26. Gianelli M, Gentile S, Verze L, et al. Free drug levels monitoring as a detector of false metabolic refractory epilepsy. *Eur Neurol*. 1988;28:349-53.
27. Koyama H, Sugioka N, Uno A, et al. Effect of glycosylation on carbamazepine-serum protein binding in humans. *J Clin Pharmacol*. 1997;37(11):1048-55.
28. Pearce RE, Vakkalagadda GR, Leeder JS. Pathways of carbamazepine bioactivation in vitro I. Characterization of human cytochromes P450 responsible for the formation of 2- and 3- hydroxylated metabolites. *Drug Metab Dispos*. 2002;30:1170-9.
29. Sumi M, Watari N, Umezawa O, et al. Pharmacokinetic study of carbamazepine and its epoxide metabolite in humans. *J Pharmacobiodyn*. 1987;10:652-61.

30. Tomson T, Almkvist O, Nilsson BY, et al. Carbamazepine-10,11-epoxide in epilepsy: a pilot study. *Arch Neurol.* 1990;47:888-92.

31. Kerr BM, Thummel KE, Wurden CJ, et al. Human liver carbamazepine metabolism. Role of CYP3A4 and CYP2C8 in 10,11 epoxide formation. *Biochem Pharmacol.* 1994;47(11):1969-79.

32. Anderson GD. A mechanistic approach to antiepileptic drug interactions. *Ann Pharmacother*. 1998;32:554-63.

33. Stoner SC, Nelson LA, Lea JW, et al. Historical review of carbamazepine for the treatment of bipolar disorder. *Pharmacotherapy*. 2007;27(1):68-88.

34. Dodson WE. Carbamazepine and oxcarbazepine. In: Pellock JM, Dodson WE, Bourgeois BFD. *Pediatric Epilepsy: Diagnosis and Treatment*. 2nd ed. New York, NY: Demos; 2001:419-32.

35. Robbins DK, Wedlund PJ, Baumann RJ, et al. Inhibition of epoxide hydrolase by valproic acid in epileptic patients receiving carbamazepine. *Br J Clin Pharmacol*. 1990;29:759-62.

36. Mikati MA, Browne TR, Collins JG, et al. Time course of carbamazepine autoinduction. *Neurology*. 1989;39:592-4.

37. Bertilsson L, Tomson T, Tybring G. Pharmacokinetics: time-dependent changes—autoinduction of carbamazepine epoxidation. *J Clin Pharmacol*. 1986;26:459-62.

38. Delgado-Iribarnegaray MF, Santo Bueldga D, Garcia Sanchez MJ, et al. Carbamazepine population pharmacokinetics in children: mixed-effect models. *Ther Drug Monit*. 1997;19(2):132-9.

39. Levy RH, Kerr BM. Clinical pharmacokinetics of carbamazepine. *J Clin Psychiatry*. 1988;49(Suppl): 58-61.

40. Gray AL, Botha JH, Miller R, et al. A model for the determination of carbamazepine clearance in children on mono- and polytherapy. *Eur J Clin Pharmacol*. 1998;54(4):359-62.

41. Hockings N, Pall A, Moody J, et al. The effects of age on carbamazepine pharmacokinetics and adverse effects. *Br J Clin Pharmacol*. 1986;22:725-8.

42. Rowan AJ. Reflections on the treatment of seizures in the elderly population. *Neurology*. 1998;51(5)(*Suppl* 4):S28-33.

43. Thomas RJ. Seizures and epilepsy in the elderly. *Arch Intern Med*. 1997;157(6):605-17.

44. Bernus I, Dickinson RG, Hooper WD, et al. Anticonvulsant therapy in aged patients; clinical pharmacokinetic considerations. *Drugs Aging*. 1997;10(4):278-89.

45. Graves NM, Brundage RG, Wen Y, et al. Population pharmacokinetics of carbamazepine in adults with epilepsy. *Pharmacotherapy*. 1998;18(2):273-81.

46. Reith DM, Hooper WD, Parke J, et al. Population pharmacokinetic modeling of steady state carbamazepine clearance in children, adolescents, and adults. *J Pharmacokinet Biopharm*. 2001;28:79-92.

47. Summers B, Summers RS. Carbamazepine clearance in paediatric epilepsy patients: Influence of body mass, dose, sex and co-medication. *Clin Pharmacokinet*. 1989;17:208-16.

48. Suemaru K, Kawasaki H, Yasuhara K, et al. Steady-state serum concentrations of carbamazepine and valproic acid in obese and lean patients with epilepsy. *Acta Med Okayama*. 1998;52(3):139-42.

49. Kuranari M, Chiba S, Ashikari Y, et al. Clearance of phenytoin and valproic acid is affected by a small body weight reduction in an epileptic obese patient: a case study. *J Clin Pharm Ther*. 1996;21(2):83-7.

50. Reith DM, Appleton DB, Hooper W, et al. The effect of body size on the metabolic clearance of carbamazepine. *Biopharm Drug Dispos*. 2000;21:103-11.

51. Micromedex Healthcare Series, (electronic version). Thomson Micromedex, Greenwood Village, Colorado, USA. Available at: http://0-www.thomsonhc.com.library.uchsc.edu:80 (accessed September 22, 2010).

52. Racine-Poon A, Dubois JP. Predicting the range of plasma carbamazepine concentrations in patients with epilepsy. *Stat Med*. 1989;8:1327-37.

53. Gonzalez ACA, Sanchez MJG, Hurle AD-G. Contribution of serum level monitoring in the individualization of carbamazepine dosage regimens. *Int J Clin Pharmacol Ther Toxicol*. 1988;26:409-12.

54. Garcia MJ, Alonso AC, Maza A, et al. Comparison of methods of carbamazepine dosage, individualization in epileptic patients. *J Clin Pharm Ther*. 1988;13:375-80.

55. Garnett WR, Huffman J, Welsh S. Administration of Carbatrol (carbamazepine extended-release capsules) via feeding tubes. *Epilepsia*. 1999;40(Suppl 7):98.

56. Riss Jr, Kriel RL, Kammer NM, et al. Administration of Carbatrol to children with feeding tubes. *Pediatr Neurol*. 2002;27:193-5.

57. Vasudev A, Tripathi KD, Puri V. Association of drug levels and pharmacokinetics of carbamazepine with seizure control. *Indian J Med Res*. 2000;112:218-23.

58. Holmes GL. Carbamazepine: adverse events. In: Levy RH, Mattson RH, Meldrum BS. *Antiepileptic Drugs*. 5th ed. New York, NY: Raven Press; 2002:285-97.

59. Gilman JT. Carbamazepine dosing for pediatric seizure disorders: the highs and lows. *DICP Ann Pharmacother.* 1991;25:1109-12.

60. Takayanagi K, Hisauchi I, Watanabe J, et al. Carbamazepine induced sinus node dysfunction and atrioventricular block in elderly women. *Japanese Heart J.* 1998;39(4):469-79.

61. Hetzel W. Anticonvulsant treatment in old age—principles and differential indications. *Fortschr Neurol Psychiatr.* 1997;65(6):261-77.

62. Wolkenstein P, Tan C, Le Coeur S, et al. Covalent binding of carbamazepine reactive metabolites to P450 isoforms in the skin. *Chem Biol Interact.* 1998;113(1):39-50.

63. Heyer G, Simon M, Schell H, et al. Dose-dependent pellagroid skin reaction caused by carbamazepine. *Hautarzt.* 1998;49(2):123-5.

64. van Ginneken EE, van der Meer JW, Netten PM, et al. A man with mysterious hypogammaglobulinemia and skin rash. *Neth J Med.* 1999;54(4):158-62.

65. de la Cruz M, Bance M. Carbamazepine induced sensorineural hearing loss. *Arch Otolaryngol Head Neck Surg.* 1999;125(2):225-7.

66. Eijgenraam JW, Buurke EJ, van der Laan JS. Carbamazepine associated acute tubulointerstitial nephritis. *Neth J Med.* 1997;50(1):25-8.

67. McKinney PA, Finkenbine RD, DeVane CL. Alopecia and mood stabilizer therapy. *Ann Clin Psychiatry.* 1996;8(3):183-5.

68. Mabuchi K, Hayashi S, Nitta E, et al. Auditory disturbance induced by carbamazepine administration in a patient with secondary generalized seizure. *Rinsho-Shinkeigaku.* 1995;35(5):553-5.

69. Yoshikawa H, Abe T. Carbamazepine-induced abnormal pitch perception. *Brain Dev.* 2003;25:127-9.

70. Patterson CR, Davies MG. Carbamazepine-induced pemphigus. *Clin Exp Dermatol.* 2003;28:98-9.

71. Ketter TA, Post RM, Worthington K. Principles of clinically important drug interactions with carbamazepine. Part I. *J Clin Psychopharmacol.* 1991;11:198-203.

72. Ketter TA, Post RM, Worthington K. Principles of clinically important drug interactions with carbamazepine. Part II. *J Clin Psychopharmacol.* 1991;11:306-13.

73. Wurden CJ, Levy RH. Carbamazepine: Interactions with other drugs. In: Levy RH, Mattson RH, Meldrum BS. *Antiepileptic Drugs.* 5th ed. New York, NY: Raven Press; 2002:247-61.

74. Valproic acid/carbamazepine. In: Tatro DS, ed. Drug interaction facts. 2011:1897.

75. Theophyllines/carbamazepine. In: Tatro DS, ed. Drug interaction facts. 2011:1743.

76. Spina E, Pisani F, Perucca E. Clinically significant pharmacokinetic drug interactions with carbamazepine: an update. *Clin Pharmacokinet.* 1996;31(3):198-214.

77. Emilien G, Maloteaux JM. Pharmacological management of epilepsy: mechanism of action, pharmacokinetic drug interactions, and new drug discovery possibilities. *Int J Clin Pharmacol Ther.* 1998;36(4):181-94.

78. Riva R, Albani F, Contin M, et al. Pharmacokinetic interactions between antiepileptic drugs: clinical considerations. *Clin Pharmacokinet.* 1996;31(6):470-93.

79. Furukori H, Otani K, Yasuri N, et al. Effect of carbamazepine on the single oral dose pharmacokinetics of alprazolam. *Neuropsychopharmacology.* 1998;18(5):364-9.

80. Otani K, Ishida M, Yasuri W, et al. Interaction between carbamazepine and bromperidol. *Eur J Clin Pharmacol.* 1997;52(3):219-22.

81. Theis JG, Koren G, Daneman R, et al. Interactions of clobazam with conventional antiepileptics in children. *J Child Neurol.* 1997;12(3):208-13.

82. Kelley MT, Walson PD, Cox S, et al. Population pharmacokinetics of felbamate in children. *Ther Drug Monit.* 1997;19(1):29-36.

83. Bartoli A, Guerrini R, Belmonte A, et al. The influence of dosage, age, and co-medication on steady state plasma lamotrigine concentrations in epileptic children: a prospective study with preliminary assessment of correlations with clinical response. *Ther Drug Monit.* 1997;19(3):252-60.

84. Eriksson AS, Hoppu K, Nergardh A, et al. Pharmacokinetic interactions between lamotrigine and other antiepileptic drugs in children with intractable epilepsy. *Epilepsia.* 1996;37(8):769-73.

85. Besag FM, Berry DJ, Newberry JE, et al. Carbamazepine toxicity and lamotrigine: pharmacokinetic or pharmacodynamic interaction? *Epilepsia.* 1998;39(2):183-7.

86. Behar D, Schaller J, Spreat S, et al. Extreme reduction of methylphenidate levels by carbamazepine (letter). *J Am Acad Child Adolesc Psychiatry.* 1998;37(11):1128-9.

87. Backman JT, Olkkola KT, Ojala M, et al. Concentrations and effects of midazolam are greatly reduced in patients treated with carbamazepine or phenytoin. *Epilepsia.* 1996;37(3):253-7.

88. Lucas RA, Gilfiallan DJ, Berrstrom RF. A pharmacokinetic interaction between carbamazepine and olanzapine: observations on possible mechanism. *Eur J Clin Pharmacol*. 1998;54(8):639-43.

89. Sachdeo RC, Sachdeo SK, Walker SA, et al. Steady state pharmacokinetics of topiramate and carbamazepine in patients with epilepsy during monotherapy and concomitant therapy. *Epilepsia*. 1996;37(8):774-80.

90. Alloul K, Whalley DG, Shutway F, et al. Pharmacokinetic origin of carbamazepine-induced resistance to vecuronium neuromuscular blockage in anesthetized patients. *Anesthesiology*. 1996;84(2):330-9.

91. Ono S, Mihara K, Suzuki A, et al. Significant pharmacokinetic interaction between risperidone and carbamazepine: its relationship with CYP2D6 genotypes. *Psychopharmacology (Berlin)*. 2002; 162:50-4.

92. Mula M, Monaaco F. Carbmazepine-risperidone interactions in patients with epilepsy. *Clin Neuropharmacol*. 2002;25:97-100.

93. Steinacher L, Vandel P, Zullino DF, et al. Carbamazepine augmentation in depressive patients nonresponding to citalopram: a pharmacokinetic and clinical pilot study. *Eur Neuropsychopharmacol*. 2002;12:255-60.

94. Pihlsgard M, Elliasson E. Significant reduction of sertraline plasma levels by carbamazepine and phenytoin. *Eur J Clin Pharmacol*. 2002;57:915-6.

95. Khan A, Sha MU, Preskorn SH. Lack of sertraline efficacy probably due to an interaction with carbamazepine. *J Clin Psychiatry*. 2000;61:526-7.

96. Sitsen J, Maris F, Timmer C. Drug-drug interaction studies with mirtazapine and carbamazepine in healthy male subjects. *Eur J Drug Metab Pharmacokinet*. 2001;26:109-21.

97. Schlienger R, Kurmann M, Drewe J, et al. Inhibition of phenprocoumon anticoagulation by carbamazepine. *Eur Neuropsychopharmacol*. 2000;10:219-21.

98. Hugen PW, Burger DM, Brinkman K, et al. Carbamazepine-indinavir interaction causes antiretroviral therapy failure. *Ann Pharmacother*. 2000;34:1348-9.

99. Vaz J, Kulkami C, David J, et al. Influence of caffeine on pharmacokinetic profile of sodium valproate and carbamazepine in normal human volunteers. *Indian J Exp Biol*. 1998;36(1):112-4.

100. Glue P, Banfield CR, Perhach JL, et al. Pharmacokinetic interactions with felbamate: in vitro-in vivo correlation. *Clin Pharmacokinet*. 1997;33(3):214-24.

101. Amsden GW. Erythromycin, clarithromycin, and azithromycin—are the differences real? *Clin Ther*. 1996;18(1):56-72.

102. Cottencin O, Regnaut N, Thevenon-Gignac C, et al. Carbamazepine-fluvoxamine interaction. Consequences for the carbamazepine plasma level. *Encephale*. 1995;21(2):141-5.

103. Garg SK, Kumar N, Bhargava VK, et al. Effect of grapefruit juice on carbamazepine bioavailability in patients with epilepsy. *Clin Pharm Ther*. 1998;64(3):286-8.

104. Bernus I, Dickinson RG, Hooper WD, et al. The mechanism of carbamazepine-valproate interaction in humans. *Br J Clin Pharmacol*. 1997;44(1):21-7.

105. Finch CK, Green CA, Self TH. Fluconazole-carbamazepine interaction. *South Med J*. 2002;95:1099-100.

106. Dixit RK, Chawla AB, Kumar N, et al. Effect of omeprazole on the pharmacokinetics of sustained-release carbamazepine in healthy male volunteers. *Methods Find Exp Clin Pharmacol*. 2001;23:37-9.

107. Desta Z, Soukhova NV, Flockhart DA. Inhibition of cytochrome P450 (CYP450) isoforms by isoniazid: potent inhibition of CYP2C19 and CYP3A4. *Antimicrob Agents Chemother*. 2001;45:382-92.

108. Berbel GA, Latorre IA, Porta EJ, et al. Protease inhibitor-induced carbamazepine toxicity. *Clin Neuropharmacol*. 2000;23:216-8.

109. Kato Y, Fujii T, Mizoguchi N, et al. Potential interaction between ritonavir and carbamazepine. *Pharmacother*. 2000;20:851-5.

110. Patsalos PN, Perucca E. Clinically important drug interactions in epilepsy: interactions between antiepileptic drugs and other drugs. *Lancet Neurology*. 2003;2:473-81.

111. Perucca E. Clinically relevant drug interactions with antiepileptic drugs. *Br J Clin Pharmacol*. 2005;61:246-55.

112. Bazil CW, Pedley TA. Clinical pharmacology of antiepileptic drugs. *Clin Neuropharmacol*. 2003;26:38-52.

113. Hidaka M, Okumura M, Fujita K, et al. Effects of pomegranate juice on human cytochrome P450 3A (CYP 3A) and carbamazepine pharmacokinetics in rats. *Drug Metabolism and Disposition*. 2005;33:644-8.

114. Clark-Schmidt AL, Garnett WR, Lowe DR, et al. Loss of carbamazepine suspension through nasogastric feeding tubes. *Am J Hosp Pharm*. 1990;47:2034-7.

115. Bass J, Miles MV, Tennison MB, et al. Effects of enteral tube feeding on the absorption and pharmacokinetic profile of carbamazepine suspension. *Epilepsia*. 1989;30:364-9.

116. Besang FM, Berry DJ, Pool F, et al. Carbamazepine toxicity with lamotrigine: pharmacokinetic or pharmacodynamic interaction? *Epilepsia*. 1998;39:183-7.

117. Eriksson AS, Boreus LO. No increase in carbamazepine-10,11-epoxide during addition of lamotrigine treatment in children. *Ther Drug Monit.* 1997;19:499-501.

118. Sisodiya SM, Sander JW, Patsalos PN. Carbamazepine toxicity during combination therapy with levetiracetam: a pharmacodynamic interaction. *Epilepsy Res.* 2002;48:217-9.

119. Davies K, Doty P, Eggert-Formella A, et al. Evaluation of lacosamide efficacy and safety as adjunctive therapy in patients receiving traditional sodium channel blocking AEDs. Poster presented at: 63rd Annual Meeting of the American Epilepsy Society (AES); December 4–8, 2009; Boston, MA.

120. Kandrotas RJ, Oles KS, Gal P, et al. Carbamazepine clearance in hemodialysis and hemoperfusion. *DICP Ann Pharmacother.* 1989;23:137-40.

121. Wright PS, Seifert CF, Hampton EM. Toxic carbamazepine concentrations following cardiothoracic surgery and myocardial infarction. *DICP Ann Pharmacother.* 1990;24:822-6.

122. Tomson T, Battino D. Pharmacokinetic and therapeutic drug monitoring of newer antiepileptic drugs during pregnancy and the puerperium. *Clin Pharmacokinet.* 2007;46(3):209-19.

123. Dam M, Christiansen J, Munck O, et al. Antiepileptic drugs: metabolism in pregnancy. *Clin Pharmacokinet.* 1979;4:53-62.

124. Bano G, Raina RK, Sharma DB. Pharmacokinetics of carbamazepine in protein energy malnutrition. *Pharmacology.* 1986;32:232-6.

Chapter 12

*Robert L. Page II**

Digoxin (AHFS 24:04)

In 1785, Sir William Withering published the first accounts of digitalis (dried leaves of the purple foxglove) in cardiovascular medicine.[1] Since that time, digoxin has become well established for use in systolic heart failure (HF) and controlling ventricular response in atrial fibrillation and flutter.[2-4]

Digoxin's mechanism of action is multifaceted. Historically, digoxin's positive inotropic effects were thought to result primarily from inhibition of the sodium-potassium ATPase pump. This inhibition reduces the transmembrane sodium gradient, which indirectly inhibits the sodium-calcium exchanger and thereby allows calcium to accumulate in myocytes. As intracellular calcium increases, so does the heart's contractile force. Over the past decade digoxin has also been noted to alter neurohormonal systems, particularly through the autonomic nervous system. These autonomic effects include a vagomimetic action that is responsible for digoxin's sinoatrial and atrioventricular (AV) nodal effects and an increase in baroreceptor sensitization, which enhances afferent inhibitory activity and diminishes sympathetic nervous system and renin-angiotensin system activities.[5]

Unfortunately, digoxin has a fairly narrow therapeutic range and warrants reasonably cautious dosage determination. It should generally be avoided in patients with sinus node disease, second- or third-degree AV block, accessory AV pathways (Wolff-Parkinson-White syndrome), cardiac amyloidosis, and hypertrophic cardiomyopathy.[6]

Usual Dosage Range in Absence of Clearance-Altering Factors

The loading and maintenance dosage ranges shown in Table 12-1 are based on lean or ideal body weight in patients with normal renal function for their age and on administration of the tablet or elixir form of digoxin, except for neonates.

For adults with normal renal function, the usual approach is administration of a total loading dose of 1–1.5 mg. Approximately 50% of the total load is given as the first dose (e.g., 0.5 mg) followed by 25% (e.g., 0.25 mg) administered at 6- to 8-hour intervals orally or intravenously (IV) after the first dose is given. Once completed, the load is followed by a daily maintenance dose of 0.25 mg/day.[7] Whether given IV or orally, the digoxin load is usually carried out over 24 hours with 3–4 divided doses. This approach is based on the onset of digoxin's effect, which is determined by the rate of distribution to the site of action. For an IV dose, 1–4 hours is required to achieve the full effect from the dose while 2–6 hours is required for an oral dose.[7] Larger loading doses and more aggressive dosing regimens may be required to control the ventricular rate in atrial fibrillation and flutter.[4,8] In patients with heart failure, digoxin loading is not recommended.[2,3]

For patients with impaired renal function (creatinine clearance [CrCl] ≤ 20 ml/min), a smaller loading dose of 0.5 mg given either IV or orally (two 0.25-mg doses 6 hr apart), followed by 0.125 mg/day.[7-9]

Maintenance doses should be based on renal function, patient response, and digoxin concentrations. When used for the management of systolic dysfunction in patients with normal sinus rhythm, digoxin is typically not loaded, but rather initiated at a daily maintenance dose of 0.125 mg or 0.25 mg, depending on renal function. This approach decreases the risk of overshooting digoxin concentrations. Table 12-2 lists proposed maintenance dosages and interval adjustments based on CrCl.[10]

Digoxin is available in a number of different dosage forms, making it convenient to switch forms when necessitated by changing patient condition. Dosage forms are shown in Table 12-3.

It is important to note that the bioavailability of digoxin differs among the dosage forms (Table 12-4) and when patients are changed from one route of administration or dosage form to another, differences in bioavailability should be considered.

*The contributions of Martin L. Job to previous versions of this chapter are acknowledged.

Table 12-1. Loading and Maintenance Doses[7,9]

Dosage Form	Loading Dose[a]	Maintenance Dose[a]
Intravenous		
Premature neonates		
(<4 weeks)	15–30 mcg/kg	5-10 mcg/kg/day[b]
Full-term neonates	10–30 mcg/kg	8-10 mcg/kg/day[b]
Oral (elixir)[c]		
Infants (<2 years)	38–63 mcg/kg	13–15 mcg/kg/day[b]
Children (2–10 years)	25–44 mcg/kg	10–13 mcg/kg/day[b]
Children (>10 years)	10–15 mcg/kg	4–13 mcg/kg/day[d]
Oral (tablets)		
Adults	10–15 mcg/kg[e]	250 mcg/day[d]

[a]Based on ideal body weight (IBW).
[b]Divided into two doses given every 12 hours for children <10 yr.
[c]Doses adjusted according to dosage form bioavailability.
[d]Administered once daily.
[e]Three divided doses.

Table 12-2. CrCl-Based Maintenance Dosages and Interval Adjustments[10]

CrCl	Percent of Normal Recommended Maintenance Dose	Interval
>50 ml/min	100%	24 hr
10–50 ml/min	25%–75%	24–36 hr[a]
<10 ml/min	10%–25%	48 hr

[a]The 36-hr interval is not recommended, due to complicated dosing schedules.

Table 12-3. Dosage Form Availability[7]

Dosage Form	Product
Intravenous	
0.25 mg/ml	Digoxin injection, Lanoxin injection
0.1 mg/ml	Digoxin pediatric injection, Lanoxin injection pediatric
Oral capsules (liquid-filled)	
0.05, 0.1, and 0.2 mg	Lanoxicaps
Oral tablets	
0.125 mg	Digitek
0.125, 0.25 mg	Lanoxin
Oral elixir	
0.05 mg/ml	Digoxin elixir, Lanoxin elixir pediatric

General Pharmacokinetic Information

The various pharmacokinetic parameters for digoxin along with comments relative to the parameter are shown in Tables 12-5 to 12-8.

In adults with CLcr <10 ml/min, the V is 4.8 ± 1.0 L/kg.[15] See the dosing strategies section for estimating V in patients with reduced renal function.

Table 12-4. Bioavailability (*F*) of Dosage Forms[11]

Dosage Form	Bioavailability
Intravenous	100% (1.0)
Intramuscular	IM injection is not recommended
Oral capsules[a,b]	95 ± 13% (0.95)
Oral tablets[a]	75 ± 14% (0.75)
Oral elixir[a]	80 ± 16% (0.80)

[a]Several agents may decrease absorption and erythromycin and tetracycline can increase it. (See section on drug-drug interactions.) Food may reduce the peak concentration achieved without affecting total absorption.
[b]The dose of oral capsules is 80% of that of tablets, allowing for almost equivalent bioavailable dose between the capsules and tablets.

Table 12-5. Pharmacokinetic Parameters[7,11,12]

Parameter	Outcome	Comments
Protein binding	20%–30%	Reduced during hypoalbuminemia but not clinically significant
Distribution	Highly distributed to lean organ tissues (e.g., heart, muscle, kidneys, and liver)	Serum to cardiac tissue approximately 1:100; distribution decreased by co-administration of quinidine and in patients with renal impairment
Excretion (renal unchanged)	50%–70%	Primarily glomerular filtration with some tubular secretion
Elimination (nonrenal)	30%	Primarily through biliary and intestinal tracts with some gut flora elimination; small amount through metabolism; digoxin is a substrate for p-glycoprotein

Table 12-6. Clearance (CL)[13]

Age	Clearance
Neonates[a]	1.8 L/hr/m^2
Infants[a]	11.2 L/hr/m^2
Children[a] (1–12 years)	8 L/hr/m^2
Adults	See dosing strategies

[a]In patients with normal renal function for age.

Table 12-7. Volume of Distribution (*V*)[a,b,13,14]

Age	Volume[a] (Mean ± SD)
Neonates	10.0 ± 1.0 L/kg
Infants	16.3 ± 2.1 L/kg
Children (1–12 years)	16.1 ± 0.8 L/kg
Adults	6.7 ± 1.4 L/kg[b]

[a]When patient weight is used in V calculations, IBW is used for patients whose actual weight > IBW.
[b]The volume of distribution is decreased in patients with renal impairment, so a reduced total loading dose should be used.

Dosing Strategies

Estimating digoxin clearance in adults

For adults (and children >12 years of age), several methods based on population pharmacokinetic parameters have been proposed.

Table 12-8. Half-Life and Time to Steady State[7,13,14,16,17]

Age	Half-Life (Mean ± SD)	Time to Steady State[a]
Premature neonates (<4 weeks)	61 ± 16 hr	225–385 hr
Full-term neonates (<4 weeks)	44 ± 13 hr	157–283 hr
Infants (4 weeks–1 year)	18 ± 9 hr	45–135 hr
Children		
>1–<1.5 years	Not available	Not available
1.5–2.5 years	36 ± 11 hr	124–232 hr
2.5–<7 years	37 ± 16 hr	104–267 hr
7–12 years	Not available[b]	Not available[b]
Adults	36 ± 8 hr	140–220 hr

[a]Five half-lives using ± 1 standard deviation of mean t½.
[b]Although not verified, the half-life (t½) and time to steady state for children 7–12 years old are probably similar to the values found in adults.

Method 1[18,a,b]:

Heart Failure (HF) absent

CL_{dig} = (1.303 × CrCl) + 41 ml/min

(HF present)

CL_{dig} = (1.303 × CrCl) + 20 ml/min

[a]F was assumed to be 0.6 by study authors when calculating clearance.

[b]CL_{dig} and CrCl are expressed in units of ml/min.

Method 2[19,a,b]:

(HF absent)

CL_{dig} = 1.94 L/hr/m^2 + (CrCl × 1.02)

(HF present)

CL_{dig} = 0.78 L/hr/m^2 + (CrCl × 0.88)

[a]F was assumed to be 0.6 by study authors when calculating clearance.

[b]CL_{dig} and CrCl are expressed in units of L/hr/m^2 CrCl is converted from ml/min to L/hr/m^2 by multiplying the CrCl value in ml/min by 0.06 and then dividing by 1.73.

Method 3[20,21,a,b]:

CL_{dig} = 3 L/hr + (0.0546 × CrCl)

(if concomitant quinidine, multiply by 0.56)

[a]F was assumed to be 0.82 by study authors when calculating clearance.

[b]CL_{dig} is expressed in units of L/h while CrCl is in units of ml/min. No conversion of CrCl units is necessary.

Method 1 was developed prior to the identification of the digoxin-quinidine interaction. Since some of the study patients may have been receiving quinidine (and would appear to have lower digoxin clearance), use of these predictors might lead to estimation of lower doses for patients not on quinidine. Method 2 may be a better predictor of digoxin concentrations across all populations.[19,20]

Method 4[22,a,b,c]:

(A predictive performance model based on creatinine clearance values for patients with HF)

D = $Css_{avdesired}$ × [2.22 × (CrCl + 25.7)]

[a]D = dose in mcg/day

[b]Css in mcg/L

[c]CrCl in ml/min

Estimating V in patients with reduced renal function

The following equations adjust volume of distribution estimates based on renal function.

Method 1[23]:

$$V(L/1.73m^2) = V_{min} + V_n(CrCl)/(K_d + CrCl)$$

where

$V_{min} = 226$ L/1.73 m^2

$V_n = 298$ L/1.73 m^2

$K_d = 29.1$ ml/min/1.73 m^2

CrCl in ml/min/1.73 m^2

Method 2[20]:

$$V_{(L)} = [5.05 + (0.0882 \times CrCl)] \times IBW$$

where CrCl is in units of ml/min and IBW is ideal body weight in kg. No unit cancellation is required.

Therapeutic Monitoring

Therapeutic range

The therapeutic range of digoxin (see Table 12-9) varies by what is being treated, though there is question of the value of serum concentrations as a guide to therapeutic benefit in heart failure.[2,3]

Suggested sampling times

Because of digoxin's long half-life and large volume of distribution, concentrations vary only slightly over a few hours, except during the first 4–6 hr after a dose when initial distribution is slow. Concentrations shortly after an intravenous dose can be greater than 10 mcg/L and do not reflect pharmacologic response. Therefore, to ensure that drug distribution is complete and to avoid misinterpretation of the reported concentration, no sampling should occur during the first 8-12 hr after a dose.[28,29] These pre-distribution higher concentrations of digoxin occur with both intravenous and oral administration.

The variation from concentrations just after distribution to the trough concentration before the next dose is usually 30% or less. However, therapeutic monitoring and evaluation of a patient's digoxin clearance will be improved if all concentrations are taken at approximately the same time after doses. A variation in the collection time of only 2–3 hr will generally be inconsequential, making exact timing prior to a dose unnecessary.

For outpatients on a stable dose of digoxin who do not have an obvious change in clearance due to disease state or drug interaction, an annual digoxin concentration measurement is often sufficient.[30] Appointments should be scheduled to ensure that the daily dose has not been taken in the few hours before sampling; if necessary, outpatients can hold the dose for a few hours until sampling is conducted. For hospitalized patients, trough concentrations can usually be scheduled 1–4 hr before the usual morning daily dose.

Assay issues

Digoxin concentrations are predominately measured using commercially available immunoassay methods, which include radioimmunoassay (RIA), fluorescence polarization immunoassay (FPIA), microparticle en-

Table 12-9. Therapeutic Range

Disease or Condition	Therapeutic Range	Comment
Heart failure	0.5–0.8 mcg/L	Most optimal in patients with heart failure (ejection fraction <40%). Concentrations exceeding 1.2 mcg/L are associated with increased mortality.[2,3]
Atrial fibrillation	0.5–2 mcg/L	Patients may require concentrations as high as 3.1 mcg/L to control ventricular response; overlap may occur between therapeutic and toxic ranges; neonates and infants can tolerate higher concentrations than adults, though this may be due in part to endogenous digoxin-like substance assay interference.[24-27]

zyme immunoassay (MEIA), and chemiluminescent immunosorbent assay (ECLIA).[31,32] Due to its ease of use and low expense, the FPIA assay is the more commonly used method for clinical measurement of digoxin concentrations. The digoxin antibodies used in these immunoassays can cross-react with digoxin metabolites, endogenous digoxin-like substances (EDLS), drugs, diagnostic compounds, and certain Chinese medicines or plant products, thereby falsely elevating or decreasing digoxin concentrations. This interference varies among different immunoassay methods and antibody lots.[33] Table 12-10 summarizes agents that may interfere with digoxin immunoassays. EDLS may occur in patients with renal or liver impairment, pregnant women, and neonates.[29,34-36] Various techniques have been developed to eliminate this interference which include extending serum incubation periods, use of ultrafiltration, and combined use of high and low pressure liquid chromatography.[37]

Pharmacodynamic Monitoring

Concentration-related efficacy

Patients with heart failure should be monitored for heart and lung sounds, heart rate, changes in urine output, edema, and neck vein distention. Patients with atrial fibrillation should be monitored for decreased ventricular rate and ECG changes.[2-4] All patients receiving digoxin should have serum creatinine, potassium, magnesium, digoxin concentrations, and general fluid and electrolyte status monitored periodically to avoid toxicity. Changes in status can indicate a need to increase or reduce doses or to monitor digoxin concentrations.[2-4]

Concentration-related toxicity

Toxicity in all patients taking digoxin can be noted as a decrease in heart rate, other ECG changes, and arrhythmias; anorexia, nausea, vomiting, and diarrhea; and visual disturbances.[47] A study of adverse drug events (ADEs) leading to emergency department (ED) visits found that digoxin, along with insulin and warfarin, were

Table 12-10. Potential Digoxin Assay Interactions[29,38-46]

Drug	Effect on Digoxin Concentrations	Comment
Canrenoate	False increase or decrease	May be dose related
Capromab pendetide	False increase	
Ch'an Su	False increase	Interference can be eliminated by measuring unbound digoxin concentrations
Danshen	False increase	Interference can be eliminated by measuring unbound digoxin concentrations
Digoxin immune Fab (ovine)	False increase	Interference can be eliminated by measuring unbound digoxin concentrations
EDLS	False increase	Seen in patients with renal and/or hepatic failure, neonates, and pregnant women in the third trimester
Fluorescein	Invalid results	
Ginseng	False reading	Seen with American, Asian, Indian and Siberian ginseng
Kyushin	False increase	
Lu-Shen-Wan	False increase	Interference can be eliminated by measuring unbound digoxin concentrations
Oleander	False increase	
Steroid hormones: cortisone, dexamethasone, fludrocortisone, hydrocortisone, methylprednisolone, prednisolone, prednisone, progesterone	False increase	
Spironolactone	False increase	May be dose related
Veratrum viride (false hellebore)	False increase	

EDLS = Endogenous digitalis-like substance.

implicated in one in every three estimated ADEs treated in EDs among patients ≥65 years old.[48] These results demonstrate the importance of monitoring for toxicity with digoxin, particularly in elderly patients. Digoxin toxicity can occur within the normal therapeutic range, especially in patients with metabolic derangement (e.g., hypokalemia) or severe underlying disease.[47] Because the volume of distribution is decreased and response to a given concentration is increased in hypothyroidism, patients should be monitored to avoid increased digoxin concentrations and toxicity. Digoxin immune Fab (ovine) is administered to treat life-threatening digoxin toxicity due to iatrogenic or purposeful overdosing. The presence of Fab fragments may interfere with digoxin serum concentration determination. In this situation, ultrafiltration may be used to remove digoxin-bound Fab fragments allowing for a more reliable measurement of the unbound digoxin concentration.[29,47]

Digoxin concentration measurements taken during the distribution phase after digoxin dosing can be quite high and may not be indicative of pharmacologic impact or toxicity.[49] Concentration elevations due to drawing during the distribution phase must not be incorrectly diagnosed and treated with digoxin immune Fab. Signs and symptoms of digoxin toxicity should be present before such treatment.[29,47]

Drug-Drug Interactions

There are a variety of important drug-drug interactions with digoxin. Some are relatively easily avoided, while others are not. Research has shown that ADEs occur with important frequency with digoxin, and interactions that increase the potential for digoxin related toxicity should be carefully monitored or avoided when possible. Potentially important pharmacokinetic and pharmacodynamic digoxin-drug interactions are listed in Table 12-11.

Table 12-11. Digoxin Drug-Drug Interactions[7]

Drug	Effect on Digoxin	Comments
ACE inhibitors	Increased digoxin concentrations	Decreased renal CL.
Amiodarone	Increased digoxin concentrations	Interaction is dose dependent; digoxin concentrations may increase >70%; digoxin dose should be decreased by 25%–50%; reduced renal and nonrenal CL (inhibition of P-gp).
Antacids	Decreased digoxin concentrations	Absorption reduced by 25%. Doses should be separated by ≥2 hours.
AV nodal blocking agents: amiodarone; disopyramide, beta-blockers, flecainide, nondihydropyridine calcium channel blockers, sotalol	Increased risk for heart block	Reduced sinoatrial or AV node conduction.
Carvedilol	Increased digoxin concentrations	Reduced renal and nonrenal CL; increased bioavailability by 9%–20%. May be due to competition for intestinal P-gp; in children, digoxin dose may need to be reduced by 25%.
Cholestyramine	Decreased digoxin concentrations	Absorption reduced (most when given concomitantly). Reduction may be minimized by twice-daily dosing of cholestyramine 8 hours before and after digoxin.
Diltiazem	Increased digoxin concentrations	Reduced renal and nonrenal CL (inhibition of P-gp); interaction is dose dependent.
Dronedarone	Increased digoxin concentrations	Digoxin concentrations may increase 2.5 fold; reduced nonrenal CL (inhibition of P-gp); digoxin dose should be decreased by 50%.
Erythromycin and clarithromycin	Increased digoxin concentrations	Due to inhibition of intestinal and renal P-gp; monitor digoxin concentrations.
Kaolin-pectin	Decreased digoxin concentrations	Time-dependent decrease in absorption (62% when given concomitantly; 20% when given 2 hours apart). Doses should be separated by ≥2 hours.
Itraconazole	Increased digoxin concentrations	Reduced renal and nonrenal CL; reduced *V*. May be due to inhibition of intestinal and renal P-gp; monitor digoxin concentrations.

Table 12-11. (Continued)

Drug	Effect on Digoxin	Comments
Non-potassium sparing diuretics: thiazide and loop	Increased risk for arrhythmias	May be due to reductions in potassium and magnesium.
NSAIDs	Increased digoxin concentrations	Decreased renal CL.
Propafenone	Increased digoxin concentrations of 80% or more	Reduced renal and nonrenal CL; decreased *V*. Interaction is dose dependent; digoxin dose may be reduced by 50%; obtain digoxin concentrations within 48–96 hours of adding or removing propafenone.
Quinidine	Increased digoxin concentrations	Reduced renal CL and tissue binding. Digoxin concentrations should be monitored carefully; digoxin dose may need to be decreased by 50%.
Ranolazine	Increased digoxin concentrations	Reduced nonrenal CL (inhibition of P-gp); digoxin concentrations may increase 1.5 fold.
Rifampin	Decreased digoxin concentrations	Increased nonrenal CL (induction of P-gp and hepatic metabolism
Ritonavir	Increased digoxin concentrations	Reduced renal and nonrenal CL; increased bioavailability. May be due to inhibition of P-gp; monitor digoxin concentrations.
Spironolactone	Increased digoxin concentrations	Reduced renal CL, V, and tissue binding. Monitor digoxin concentrations.
Tetracycline	Increased digoxin concentrations	Increased absorption; reduced intestinal metabolism. Eradication of gut flora (e.g., *Eggerthella lenta*).
Thyroid hormones	Reduced digoxin concentrations	Increased renal and nonrenal CL. May be due to increased expression of P-gp by thyroid hormones.
Verapamil	Increased digoxin concentrations	Reduced renal and extrarenal CL. Interaction is dose dependent; digoxin concentrations may increase 60%–90%; digoxin concentrations may decline over a period of weeks with concomitant therapy; may be due to inhibition of P-gp resulting in decreased digoxin renal tubular elimination.
St. John's Wort	Decreased digoxin concentrations	Reduced absorption. May be mediated by inducing P-gp; monitor clinical response and digoxin concentrations in patients titrated to effective digoxin dose who suddenly discontinue St. John's Wort.

ACE = angiotensin converting enzyme, CL = clearance, NSAID = nonsteroidal anti-inflammatory drug , P-gp = P-glycoprotein, V = volume of distribution.

Drug-Disease/Condition Interactions

Digoxin concentrations may decrease during pregnancy because of increased renal clearance and possible upregulation of p-glycoprotein.[50] Reductions in renal function below the average for age and size lead to lengthening of the half-life and reduction of clearance. Research has shown that there are no significant sex-based differences in digoxin pharmacokinetics when actual or ideal body weight is used to control for dose differences due to weight on concentration outcomes. When adjusted for BMI however, differences were detected.[51]

Patients with hyperthyroidism may have reduced myocardial responsiveness to digoxin therapy. Digoxin response may be improved by treating the hyperthyroidism. The opposite applies when treating hypothyroidism. [2]

Finally, patients carrying polymorphism for the multi-drug-resistance 1 (MDR1) gene that codes for p-glycoprotein may experience a significant increase the bioavailability of digoxin leading to higher digoxin concentrations.[52-54]

References

1. Withering W. An account of the foxglove and some of its medical uses with practical remarks on dropsy and other diseases. In: Willins FA, Keys TE, eds. *Classics of Cardiology*. New York, NY: Henry Schyuman, Dover Publications; 1941:231-51.
2. Lindenfeld J, Albert NM, Boehmer JP, et al. HFSA 2010 Comprehensive Heart Failure Practice Guideline. *J Card Fail.* 2010;16:e1-194.
3. Hunt SA, Abraham WT, Chin MH, et al. 2009 Focused update incorporated into the ACC/AHA 2005 Guidelines for the Diagnosis and Management of Heart Failure in Adults: A Report of the American College of Cardiology Foundation/ American Heart Association Task Force on Practice Guidelines Developed in Collaboration With the International Society for Heart and Lung Transplantation. *J Am Coll Cardiol.* 2009;53:e1-e90.
4. Fuster V, Ryden LE, Cannom DS, et al. ACC/AHA/ESC 2006 Guidelines for the Management of Patients with Atrial Fibrillation: a report of the American College of Cardiology/American Heart Association Task Force on Practice Guidelines and the European Society of Cardiology Committee for Practice Guidelines (Writing Committee to Revise the 2001 Guidelines for the Management of Patients With Atrial Fibrillation): developed in collaboration with the European Heart Rhythm Association and the Heart Rhythm Society. *Circulation.* 2006;114:e257-354.
5. Gheorghiade M, Harinstein ME, Filippatos GS. Digoxin for the treatment of chronic and acute heart failure syndromes. *Acute Card Care.* 2009;11:83-7.
6. Gheorghiade M, van Veldhuisen DJ, Colucci WS. Contemporary use of digoxin in the management of cardiovascular disorders. *Circulation.* 2006;113:2556-64.
7. Digoxin. In: McEvoy, GK ed. *AHFS Drug Information 2010.* Bethesda, MD: American Society of Health System Pharmacists. Available at: http://online.statref.com/Document/Document.aspx?docAddress=7WqlYjrCoMrd4dH7XGSngA%3d%3d&Scroll=57&Index=1&SessionId=12E53DBGVTUKMBWW. Accessed August, 1, 2010.
8. Hornestam B, Jerling M, Karlsson MO, et al. Intravenously administered digoxin in patients with acute atrial fibrillation: a population pharmacokinetic/pharmacodynamic analysis based on the Digitalis in Acute Atrial Fibrillation trial. *Eur J Clin Pharmacol.* 2003;58:747-55.
9. Digoxin. In: Phelps SJ, Hak EB, Crill CM eds. *Pediatric Injectable Drugs.* 9th ed. Bethesda, MD: American Society of Health-System Pharmacists; 2010:140-1.
10. Aronoff GR, Berns JS, Brier ME. Antihypertensive and cardiovascular agents. In: *Drug Prescribing in Renal Failure: Dosing Guidelines for Adults.* 5th ed. Philadelphia, PA: American College of Physicians; 2007:41.
11. Reuning RH, Geraets DR, Rocci ML. Chapter 20: Digoxin. In: Evans WE, Schentag JJ, Jusko WJ, eds. *Applied Pharmacokinetics: Principles of Therapeutic Drug Monitoring.* 3rd ed. Spokane, WA: Applied Therapeutics; 1992:1-48.
12. Igel S, Drescher S, Murdter T, et al. Increased absorption of digoxin from the human jejunum due to inhibition of intestinal transporter-mediated efflux. *Clin Pharmacokinet.* 2007;46:777-85.
13. Morselli PL, Asbael BM, Gomeni R. Digoxin pharmacokinetics during human development. In: Morselli A, Garibatini S, Serini F, eds. *Basic Therapeutic Aspects of Perinatal Pharmacology.* New York, NY: Raven Press; 1975:377-92.
14. Wettrell G. Distribution and elimination of digoxin in infants. *Eur J Clin Pharmacol.* 1977;11:329-35.
15. Cheng JW, Charland SL, Shaw LM, et al. Is the volume of distribution of digoxin reduced in patients with renal dysfunction? Determining digoxin pharmacokinetics by fluorescence polarization immunoassay. *Pharmacotherapy.* 1997;17:584-90.
16. Chow T, Galvin J, McGovern B. Antiarrhythmic drug therapy in pregnancy and lactation. *Am J Cardiol.* 1998;82:58I-62I.
17. Dungan WT, Doherty JE, Harvey C, et al. Tritiated digoxin. 18. Studies in infants and children. *Circulation.* 1972;46:983-8.
18. Koup JR, Greenblatt DJ, Jusko WJ, et al. Pharmacokinetics of digoxin in normal subjects after intravenous bolus and infusion doses. *J Pharmacokinet Biopharm.* 1975;3:181-92.
19. Sheiner LB, Rosenberg B, Marathe VV. Estimation of population characteristics of pharmacokinetic parameters from routine clinical data. *J Pharmacokinet Biopharm.* 1977;5:445-79.
20. Williams PJ, Lane J, Murray W, et al. Pharmacokinetics of the digoxin-quinidine interaction via mixed-effect modeling. *Clin Pharmacokinet.* 1992;22:66-74.
21. Williams PJ, Lane JR, Capparelli EV, et al. Direct comparison of three methods for predicting digoxin concentrations. *Pharmacotherapy.* 1996;16:1085-92.
22. Konishi H, Shimizu S, Chiba M, et al. Predictive performance of serum digoxin concentration in patients with congestive heart failure by a hyperbolic model based on creatinine clearance. *J Clin Pharm Ther.* 2002;27:257-65.
23. Jusko WJ, Szefler SJ, Goldfarb AL. Pharmacokinetic design of digoxin dosage regimens in relation to renal function. *J Clin Pharmacol.* 1974;14:525-35.
24. Chamberlain DA, White RJ, Howard MR, et al. Plasma digoxin concentrations in patients with atrial fibrillation. *Br Med J.* 1970;3:429-32.

25. Halkin H, Radomsky M, Blieden L, et al. Steady state serum digoxin concentration in relation to digitalis toxicity in neonates and infants. *Pediatrics.* 1978;61:184-8.

26. Masuhara JE, Lalonde RL. Serum digoxin concentrations in atrial fibrillation: a review. *Drug Intell Clin Pharm.* 1982;16:543-6.

27. Beasley R, Smith DA, McHaffie DJ. Exercise heart rates at different serum digoxin concentrations in patients with atrial fibrillation. *Br Med J (Clin Res Ed).* 1985;290:9-11.

28. Abad-Santos F, Carcas AJ, Ibanez C, et al. Digoxin level and clinical manifestations as determinants in the diagnosis of digoxin toxicity. *Ther Drug Monit.* 2000;22:163-8.

29. Valdes R, Jr., Jortani SA, Gheorghiade M. Standards of laboratory practice: cardiac drug monitoring. National Academy of Clinical Biochemistry. *Clin Chem.* 1998;44:1096-109.

30. Canas F, Tanasijevic MJ, Ma'luf N, et al. Evaluating the appropriateness of digoxin level monitoring. *Arch Intern Med.* 1999;159:363-8.

31. Spinler SA, Al-Jazairi AS, Cheng JW, et al. Predictive performance study of two digoxin assays in subjects with various degrees of renal function. *Ther Drug Monit.* 2000;22:729-36.

32. Dasgupta A, Kang E, Datta P. A new enzyme-linked chemiluminescent immunosorbent digoxin assay is virtually free from interference of spironolactone, potassium canrenoate, and their common metabolite canrenone. *J Clin Lab Anal.* 2006;20:204-8.

33. Azzazy HM, Duh SH, Maturen A, et al. Multicenter study of Abbott AxSYM Digoxin II assay and comparison with 6 methods for susceptibility to digoxin-like immunoreactive factors. *Clin Chem.* 1997;43:1635-40.

34. Graves SW, Brown B, Valdes R, Jr. An endogenous digoxin-like substance in patients with renal impairment. *Ann Intern Med.* 1983;99:604-8.

35. Graves SW, Valdes R, Jr., Brown BA, et al. Endogenous digoxin-immunoreactive substance in human pregnancies. *J Clin Endocrinol Metab.* 1984;58:748-51.

36. Nikou GC, Vyssoulis GP, Venetikou MS, et al. Digoxin-like substance(s) interfere(s) with serum estimations of the drug in cirrhotic patients. *J Clin Gastroenterol.* 1989;11:430-3.

37. Jones TE, Morris RG. Discordant results from "real-world" patient samples assayed for digoxin. *Ann Pharmacother.* 2008;42:1797-803.

38. Bloom JN, Herman DC, Elin RJ, et al. Intravenous fluorescein interference with clinical laboratory tests. *Am J Ophthalmol.* 1989;108:375-9.

39. Dasgupta A. Herbal supplements and therapeutic drug monitoring: focus on digoxin immunoassays and interactions with St. John's wort. *Ther Drug Monit.* 2008;30:212-7.

40. Datta P, Dasgupta A. Interference of endogenous digoxin-like immunoreactive factors in serum digoxin measurement is minimized in a new turbidimetric digoxin immunoassay on ADVIA 1650 analyzer. *Ther Drug Monit.* 2004;26:85-9.

41. Fushimi R, Yamanishi H, Inoue M, et al. Digoxin immunoassay that avoids cross-reactivity from Chinese medicines. *Clin Chem.* 1995;41:621.

42. McRae S. Elevated serum digoxin levels in a patient taking digoxin and Siberian ginseng. *CMAJ.* 1996;155:293-5.

43. Paterson JR, Weston R, Blackie R, et al. Fluorescein interference in digoxin assay: an isolated case? *Ann Clin Biochem.* 1991;28:314-5.

44. Steimer W, Muller C, Eber B. Digoxin assays: frequent, substantial, and potentially dangerous interference by spironolactone, canrenone, and other steroids. *Clin Chem.* 2002;48:507-16.

45. Bechtel LK, Lawrence DT, Haverstick D, et al. Ingestion of false hellebore plants can cross-react with a digoxin clinical chemistry assay. *Clin Toxicol (Phila).* 2010;48:435-42.

46. Dasgupta A, Kang E, Olsen M, et al. Interference of Asian, American, and Indian (Ashwagandha) ginsengs in serum digoxin measurements by a fluorescence polarization immunoassay can be minimized by using a new enzyme-linked chemiluminescent immunosorbent or turbidimetric assay. *Arch Pathol Lab Med.* 2007;131:619-21.

47. Bauman JL, Didomenico RJ, Galanter WL. Mechanisms, manifestations, and management of digoxin toxicity in the modern era. *Am J Cardiovasc Drugs.* 2006;6:77-86.

48. Budnitz DS, Pollock DA, Weidenbach KN, et al. National surveillance of emergency department visits for outpatient adverse drug events. *JAMA.* 2006;296:1858-66.

49. Longley JM, Murphy JE. Falsely elevated digoxin levels: another look. *Ther Drug Monit.* 1989;11:572-3.

50. Hebert MF, Easterling TR, Kirby B, et al. Effects of pregnancy on CYP3A and P-glycoprotein activities as measured by disposition of midazolam and digoxin: a University of Washington specialized center of research study. *Clin Pharmacol Ther.* 2008;84:248-53.

51. Lee LS, Chan LN. Evaluation of a sex-based difference in the pharmacokinetics of digoxin. *Pharmacotherapy.* 2006;26:44-50.

52. Lowes BD, Buttrick PM. Genetic determinants of drug response in heart failure. *Curr Cardiol Rep.* 2008;10:176-81.
53. Ma JD, Tsunoda SM, Bertino JS, et al. Evaluation of in vivo P-glycoprotein phenotyping probes: a need for validation. *Clin Pharmacokinet.* 2010;49:223-37.
54. Sakurai A, Tamura A, Onishi Y, et al. Genetic polymorphisms of ATP-binding cassette transporters ABCB1 and ABCG2: therapeutic implications. *Expert Opin Pharmacother.* 2005;6:2455-73.

Chapter 13

William R. Garnett, Jacquelyn L. Bainbridge, and Sarah L. Johnson

Ethosuximide (AHFS 28:12.20)

Ethosuximide was approved for marketing by the FDA in 1960 and is only indicated for the treatment of absence seizures alone or in combination with other antiepileptic drugs in patients 3 years of age and older.

Usual Dosage Range in Absence of Clearance-Altering Factors

A loading dose is not needed for the treatment of absence seizures with ethosuximide. The starting dose should be low so that the patient can accommodate to the initial central nervous system (CNS) depression seen with ethosuximide and most antiepileptic drugs (see Table 13-1). The dose should be titrated to the individual patient's response.[1,2]

A once-daily dosage regimen can be used successfully due of the long half-life of ethosuximide. However, gastrointestinal (GI) side effects increase as the dose size increases in some patients. Therefore, ethosuximide may need to be given twice a day.[3,4] Table 13-2 shows the availability of the maintenance dosage forms.

General Pharmacokinetic Information

The pharmacokinetics of ethosuximide are poorly understood, even though it is an old antiepileptic drug and a sensitive and specific assay exists. Ethosuximide has been described as following a one-compartment model with first-order elimination.[2,5]

Absorption

In humans, ethosuximide is well absorbed and peak concentrations are achieved in about 4 hours for adults and in 3–7 hr for children.[2,6] The time to peak concentration is somewhat faster with a single dose than after

Table 13-1. Initial Maintenance Dosages

Dosage Form	Initial Maintenance Dosage[a]
Intravenous	Not available
Oral (capsules and solution)	
Adults and children (> 6 years)	20–40 mg/kg/day
Children (3–6 years)	15–40 mg/kg/day

[a]See dosing strategies section.

Table 13-2. Dosage Form Availability

Dosage Form	Product
Intravenous	Not available
Oral capsules: 250 mg	Zarontin[a]
Oral syrup: 250 mg/5 mL	Zarontin syrup
	Ethosuximide syrup
Oral solution: 250 mg/5 mL	Ethosuximide solution

[a]Available as a generic.

repeated dosing. Absorption from the syrup is faster than from the capsule, but the extent of absorption is the same (see Table 13-3).

Table 13-3. Bioavailability (*F*) of Dosage Forms[5]

Dosage Form	Bioavailability Comments
Intravenous	Not available
Oral capsules and solution	Assumed complete (100%, F = 1)

Distribution

Ethosuximide does not bind to plasma proteins. A cerebrospinal fluid to plasma to saliva ratio of 1 indicates that most of the drug in the plasma is in the unbound form. Ethosuximide is uniformly distributed throughout the body, with the exception of body fat, into which it does not distribute appreciably.

The apparent volume of distribution (*V*) of ethosuximide is approximately 70% of ideal body weight, which is equivalent to total body water. The apparent *V* is 0.69 L/kg in children younger than 10 years of age and 0.62–0.72 L/kg in adults older than 18 years of age (see Table 13-4).[2,7]

Ethosuximide crosses the placenta and passes into breast milk, achieving a concentration similar to that in the mother's plasma.[5] Spinal fluid, saliva, and tears have concentrations similar to that in plasma.

Table 13-4. Volume of Distribution (*V*)

Age	Volume[a]
Children (<10 years)	0.69 L/kg
Adults (>18 years)	0.62–0.72 L/kg

[a]Ideal body weight.

Protein binding

Protein binding of ethosuximide is negligible (0%) in both children and adults.

Elimination and metabolism

Ethosuximide is poorly extracted by the liver and therefore does not undergo first-pass metabolism. The apparent clearance of ethosuximide in normal adults has been estimated at 0.01 ± 0.004 L/hr/kg, which is less than hepatic blood flow and demonstrates that the elimination is not flow dependent (see Table 13-5). Ethosuximide is first hydroxylated and then conjugated to inactive metabolites before being excreted into the urine.[8] CYP3A and CYP2E are primarily involved in ethosuximide metabolism with CYP2B and CYP2C playing a minor role.[8]

Two studies suggested that ethosuximide might display nonlinear clearance at the upper end of the therapeutic range. Smith et al. reported that, in individual patients, successive dose increments of equal size produced disproportionately greater increases in steady state concentrations.[9] Bauer et al. found that 7 of 10 patients demonstrated evidence of nonlinearity.[7] Therefore, the dose and steady state concentration relationship of ethosuximide may vary, especially at the upper end of the therapeutic range.

Table 13-5. Clearance (CL)

Age	Clearance[a]
Children (<10 years)	0.016 L/hr/kg
Adults (>18 years)	0.01 ± 0.004 L/hr/kg

[a]As there is no intravenous form of ethosuximide, clearance calculations are relative to bioavailability of the oral product used (CL/F).

Half-life and time to steady state

The half-life in children has been reported to be ~30 hr versus ~60 hr in adults (see Table 13-6). Although not FDA approved for this patient group, data for neonates derived from case reports indicate that the half-life is between 32 and 41 hr. The half-life of ethosuximide was reported to be unaffected by dose size and to be constant with repeated dosing. However, a 15% decrease in total body clearance has been described between the first dose and steady state and was attributed to a decrease in the non-renal clearance.[2]

Table 13-6. Half-Life and Time to Steady State

Age	Half-Life	Time to Steady State[a]
Children (<10 years)	~30 hr	6 days
Adults (>18 years)	~60 hr	12 days

[a]Based on approximately five half-lives.

Dosing Strategies

Attempts to predict concentrations of ethosuximide associated with doses in epileptic patients have not been very successful. The actual dose of ethosuximide used may depend on the dosage form available. A rough guideline is to initiate therapy with 15 mg/kg/day (maximum of 250 mg/day) in children 3–6 years old and with 500 mg/day in patients older than 6 years. The dose may be increased by 250 mg/day every 4–7 days until seizure control is achieved, the maximum dose of 1.5 g/day has been reached, or side effects become intolerable. The 1.5 g/day dose may be exceeded to achieve concentrations necessary for seizure control if the patient does not have side effects. If side effects occur, the dose of ethosuximide should be reduced. After the patient has been free of absence seizures for 2–4 years, discontinuation of ethosuximide may be attempted; however, dose reduction should occur gradually.

The exact ethosuximide concentration at which a given patient will respond is not predictable, so the dose must be titrated to individual response. While ethosuximide may be assumed to generally follow a first-order pharmacokinetic model, dosage adjustments should be made gradually to allow for patient tolerance. Once steady state has been achieved the patient's response (both efficacy and toxicity) should be assessed.

Therapeutic Range

The therapeutic range of ethosuximide is 40–100 mg/L for the treatment of absence seizures.[1,2] Within this range, 80% of patients will achieve partial control and 60% will become seizure free. However, concentrations up to 150 mg/L or higher may be needed for complete seizure control in some patients. These concentrations have been used without signs of toxicity in some patients, but those with high concentrations should be monitored closely. Factors that predict therapeutic success are: (1) absence seizures as the only seizure type, (2) normal EEG background activity, and (3) normal intelligence.[1,2]

Therapeutic Monitoring

Suggested sampling times and effect on therapeutic range[2]

The indications for monitoring ethosuximide concentrations include:

- A poor response to therapy
- Questionable compliance
- Low doses and good response (to determine if concentrations are also low)
- Initial and chronic maintenance of optimal concentrations

Ethosuximide has a long half-life. This half-life should be considered in determining when to collect blood samples after therapy is initiated or the dosage is changed. The initial sample or the sample after a dosage change should not be drawn for at least 6 days in children or 12 days in adults so that the patient can reach steady state. Samples may be drawn earlier if the patient experiences unexpected side effects.

The long half-life of ethosuximide would generally suggest minimal changes in the peak to trough ratio. However, trough concentrations are recommended for monitoring, particularly if the patient is on a once-a-day regimen, as there is reduced variation in trough concentrations compared to concentrations drawn earlier or at different times in the regimen.

There is no indication that serum ethosuximide concentrations differ from plasma concentrations. Because of the negligible protein binding, there is no indication for determining unbound ethosuximide. The concentration in saliva or tears equals its serum concentration and may be used in some patients if blood sampling is not possible.

The asymmetric center in ethosuximide is quaternary, making racemization unlikely,[10] and metabolism does not appear to be stereo-selective. Therefore, the measurement of total ethosuximide is adequate for therapeutic monitoring.

Once the desired therapeutic response has been achieved, concentrations should be periodically monitored for use as a historical control for that individual patient. A change in response or the onset of unusual side effects indicates a need to monitor concentrations.

Pharmacodynamic Monitoring

Concentration-related efficacy[1,2]

The desired therapeutic end-point for ethosuximide is the abolition of absence seizures and it is a very effective agent as monotherapy for absence seizures. In refractory patients the combination of ethosuximide and valproate may be more effective than either drug alone. Ethosuximide is indicated only for the treatment of absence seizures and may exacerbate other seizure types.

Concentration-related toxicity[11]

Patients should be monitored for ethosuximide side effects. The most frequent side effects, nausea and vomiting, may be related to the dosage size. Other side effects that may be dose or concentration related are abdominal discomfort, anorexia, drowsiness, fatigue, lethargy, dizziness, hiccups, and headache. Headaches may persist after a dosage reduction.

Behavioral and cognitive side effects of ethosuximide are not well documented. Rare side effects include skin rashes, systemic lupus erythematosus, blood dyscrasias, and changes in liver function tests.

Drug-Drug Interactions

Ethanol, haloperidol, loxapine, phenothiazines, and tricyclic antidepressants can decrease the effectiveness of ethosuximide by lowering the seizure threshold and therefore should not be used concurrently.[6] Animal studies indicate that its metabolism may be induced or inhibited, though clinical reports of drug interactions with ethosuximide are rare and often poorly documented. In one report the ratio of ethosuximide concentrations to dose was significantly higher when it was given alone than when it was administered with carbamazepine, primidone, or valproic acid.[12] Barbiturates and phenytoin may also induce metabolism resulting in lower serum concentrations and shorter half-life.[6] Other studies found increased concentrations when ethosuximide was given with valproic acid. Ethosuximide may also result in a lower serum concentration of valproic acid when given concurrently.[8,13] The interaction with valproic acid may be complex and may require the presence of other concurrent antiepileptic drugs or high concentrations of valproic acid.[13–15]

Isoniazid increased ethosuximide concentrations and ethosuximide increased phenytoin concentrations in single-case studies.[16,17]

Drug–Disease State or Condition Interactions

Patients on *hemodialysis* were shown to lose about 50% of their ethosuximide stores during a 6-hr dialysis in one study done in four patients.[18] They were each given a single test dose of 500 mg and the efficacy of removal of ethosuximide was 61% in one patient, 78% in one patient, and close to 100% in two patients. Based on these results, patients on hemodialysis may require increased monitoring post dialysis as well as supplemental dosing.

Pregnancy has been reported to increase the clearance of some antiepileptics, such as lamotrigine, levetiracetam, and oxcarbazepine.[19] Based on two case reports, this effect appears to be true for ethosuximide.[20,21]

Ethosuximide is 80% metabolized by the liver and 20% excreted unchanged. Therefore, although unconfirmed by clinical studies, patients with impaired liver or renal function may require altered dosing.[2]

References

1. Sherwin AL. Succinimides—clinical efficacy and use in epilepsy. In: Levy R, Mattson R, Meldrum B, et al., eds. *Antiepileptic Drugs*. 5th ed. New York: Raven Press; 2002:653-7.
2. Garnett WR. Ethosuximide. In: Taylor WJ, Caviness MHD, eds. *A Textbook for the Clinical Application of Therapeutic Drug Monitoring*. Irving, TX: Abbott Laboratories; 1986:225-35.
3. Dooley JM, Camfield PR, Camfield CS, et al. Once-daily ethosuximide in the treatment of absence epilepsy. *Pediatr Neurol*. 1990;6:38-9.
4. Ethosuximide. In: McEvoy GK, ed. *AHFS Drug Information 2010*. Bethesda, MD: American Society of Health-System Pharmacists. Available at: http://online.statref.com/Document/Document.aspx?docAddress=2gl8oEeUEMvghADOig-evw%3d%3d&Scroll=3&Index=0&SessionId=132CC57KHOJKORWV. Accessed September 22, 2010.
5. Pisani F, Perucca E, Bialer M. Succinimides: Ethosuximide—chemistry, biotransformation, pharmacokinetics, and drug interactions. In: Levy R, Mattson R, Meldrum B, et al., eds. *Antiepileptic Drugs*. 5th ed. New York: Raven Press; 2002:646-51.
6. Gold Standard, Inc. Ethosuximide. *Clinical Pharmacology* [database online]. Available at: http://www.clinicalpharmacology.com. Accessed: September 22, 2010.
7. Bauer LA, Harris C, Wilensky AJ, et al. Ethosuximide kinetics: possible interaction with valproic acid. *Clin Pharmacol Ther*. 1982; 31:741-5.
8. Glauser TA. Ethosuximide. In: Whyllie E, ed. *The Treatment of Epilepsy: Principles and Practice*. 4th ed. Baltimore, MD: Lippincott Williams & Wilkins, 2005:817-28.
9. Smith GA, McKauge L, Dubetz D, et al. Factors influencing plasma concentrations of ethosuximide. *Clin Pharmacokinet*. 1979; 4:38-52.
10. Villen T, Bertilsson L, Sjoqvist F. Nonstereoselective disposition of ethosuximide in humans. *Ther Drug Monit*. 1990; 12:514-6.
11. Galuser TA. Succinimides: adverse effects. In: Levy R, Mattson R, Meldrum B, et al., eds. *Antiepileptic Drugs*. 5th ed. New York: Raven Press; 2002:658-64.
12. Battino D, Cusi C, Franceschetti S, et al. Ethosuximide plasma concentrations: Influence of age and associated concomitant therapy. *Clin Pharmacokinet*. 1982; 7:176-80.
13. Mattson RH, Cramer JA. Valproic acid and ethosuximide interaction. *Ann Neurol*. 1980; 7:583-4.
14. Bourgeois BFD. Combination of valproate and ethosuximide: antiepileptic and neurotoxic interaction. *J Pharmacol Exp Ther*. 1988; 247:1128-32.
15. Pisani F, Narbone MC, Trunfio C, et al. Valproic acid-ethosuximide interaction: a pharmacokinetic study. *Epilepsia*. 1984; 25:229-33.
16. Van Wieringen A, Vriglandt CM. Ethosuximide intoxication caused by interaction with isoniazid. *Neurology*. 1983; 33:1227-8.
17. Dawson GW, Brown HW, Clark BG. Serum phenytoin after ethosuximide. *Ann Neurol*. 1978; 4:583-4.
18. Marbury TC, Lee CC, Perchalski RJ, et al. Hemodialysis clearance of ethosuximide in patients with chronic renal failure. *Am J Hosp Pharm*. 1981; 38:1757-60.
19. Tomson T, Battino D. Pharmacokinetic and therapeutic drug monitoring of newer antiepileptic drugs during pregnancy and the puerperium. *Clin Pharmacokinet*. 2007;46(3):209-19.
20. Koup JR, Rose JQ, Cohen ME. Ethosuximide pharmacokinetics in a pregnant patient and her newborn. *Epilepsia*. 1978; 19:535-9.
21. Rane A, Tulnell R. Ethosuximide in human milk and in plasma of a mother and her nursed infant. *Br J Clin Pharmacol*. 1981; 12:855-8.

Chapter 14

*William E. Dager and A. Joshua Roberts**

Unfractionated Heparin, Low Molecular Weight Heparin (AHFS 20:12.04), and Fondaparinux (AHFS 20:12.04.92)

Heparin (unfractionated and low molecular weight) is used primarily as an anticoagulant to (1) treat active thrombosis, (2) to prevent clot formation in patients at increased risk (e.g., due to surgery, prolonged bed rest, or pregnancy) or during extracorporeal circulation (e.g., hemodialysis, cardiopulmonary bypass and extracorporeal life support [ECLS] in neonates), and (3) in the setting of acute coronary syndromes (ACS). Additionally, unfractionated heparin may help prolong the patency of arterial and venous catheters.

Unfractionated Heparin

Unfractionated heparin (UFH) has been a mainstay of anticoagulant therapy for over 50 years. In many situations, close monitoring and careful dose adjustment is required. It is most commonly administered by intravenous infusions or by intermittent subcutaneous injections. Until recently, the methods used to calibrate heparin units varied between the United States Pharmacopeia (USP) drug monograph and other industrialized nations. In 2009, the USP aligned the heparin unit calibration approach to that of the World Health Organization (WHO) international standardized (IS) unit. This change arose after previous USP standard testing failed to detect tainted lots of heparin that ultimately passed into circulation. This new assay has led the Food and Drug Administration to note the potential for a 10% reduction in heparin USP unit potency when compared to the previous assay and reference standard. The clinical effect of this change is debatable with current consensus suggesting minimal impact.[1]

UFH: Usual Dosage Range in Absence of Clearance-Altering Factors

When UFH therapy is used for active venous thrombosis formation, a loading dose of 70–100 units/kg is typically administered to render an immediate effect in suppressing further expansion of the thrombus. The Eighth American College of Chest Physicians (ACCP) Conference on Antithrombotic and Thrombolytic Therapy: Evidence-Based Guidelines recommend a loading dose of 80 units/kg for treatment of venous embolic disease.[2] Lower loading doses such as 50–70 units/kg have been recommended in the setting of acute coronary syndrome (ACS), especially in situations where Glycoprotein IIb/IIIa inhibitor drug therapy or thrombolytic drug therapy may be co-administered.[3] In selected settings such as high bleeding risk (i.e., stroke) or no emergent need for rapid onset of anticoagulation, a bolus loading dose may not be warranted.

The use of UFH and the dose used should be individualized for each patient since target end-points differ for its various therapeutic uses and assays. The patient's total body weight (TBW) is most commonly used in weight-based dosing approaches though current ACCP guidelines do not address the issue of dosing weight in obese patients (i.e., should ideal body weight [IBW] or TBW be used).[2] Use of an adjusted dosing weight has been suggested to account for obesity (e.g., 30%–40% of the difference between the TBW and IBW is added to the IBW to result in the dosing weight) or modified to their body mass index.[2,4] The use of TBW, and thus a higher dose, is supported by a randomized controlled trial demonstrating that reaching target goals earlier in the treatment course was associated with a reduction in recurrent thromboembolic events.[5] For safety concerns, maximum bolus and maintenance dosing limits should be considered to avoid unintended dosing errors. Depending on the setting of use, loading doses up to 80 units/kg or 5,000 units in the setting of acute

*The authors would like to recognize James B. Groce III and John E. Murphy for their contributions to this chapter in previous editions.

venous thromboembolism (VTE) have been suggested,[6] since doses this high are capable of saturating sites of action in most patients.[7]

Initial continuous infusion UFH maintenance doses can vary depending on the therapeutic indication. Typical starting doses range between 12 and 18 units/kg/hr with titration to the desired aPTT goal.[2,8] Previous studies have shown that using weight adjusted initial maintenance doses have decreased recurrence of thromboembolic events.[5] While not addressed specifically in the guidelines, some authors have suggested an initial maintenance dose cap for patient safety.[9]

UFH: Dosage Form Availability

UFH is available only as a solution for injection. It is usually administered by intravenous (IV) or subcutaneous (SC) routes, but has also been given by inhalation and intrapulmonary instillation.[10] UFH should not be given intramuscularly (IM) as it increases the likelihood of hematoma formation and can cause pain and irritation. Heparin sodium and heparin calcium (the latter not currently available in the United States) for injection are supplied by several manufacturers in concentrations ranging from 1,000 to 20,000 units/ml. Preparations for IV infusion are usually diluted to the desired concentration in either a dextrose or saline solution. Due to the large variation in available concentrations, extreme caution should be exercised in ordering and preparing heparin solutions to avoid errors in dosing.

UFH is also marketed as a heparin sodium flush solution in concentrations of 10–100 units/ml. This flush solution, diluted to 1 unit/ml or less, can be used to maintain the patency of IV catheters. Recent tragic events occurring when incorrect doses were administered for purpose of maintaining patency of IV catheters highlight the importance of creating a system for multiple checks or redundancy for determining that the correct heparin sodium flush concentration has been dispensed or sent from pharmacy.

UFH is heterogeneous with respect to molecular size, anticoagulant activity, and pharmacokinetic properties. The molecular weight of UFH ranges from 3,000 to 30,000 Daltons with a mean of 15,000 Daltons (approximately 45 monosaccharide chains).[6]

UFH: General Pharmacokinetic Information

The pharmacokinetic parameters of UFH have been determined using methods that (1) measure a global coagulation test parameter such as activated partial thromboplastin time (aPTT), (2) directly measure UFH effect by anti-Factor Xa activity, or (3) directly measure neutralization of UFH by protamine titration. Since heparin is an indirect anticoagulant that works thru anti-thrombin (AT), the presence of sufficient AT is necessary for activity.

Absorption

Heparin is not absorbed from the gastrointestinal tract. While bioavailability is 100% after IV administration, it is reduced to roughly 30% after SC administration.[11] SC bioavailability may vary between patient populations, site of injection, and in the presence of vasopressors. Absorption from the SC route is more rapid than would be seen with intramuscular administration. Table 14-1 provides the bioavailability based on the route of administration of UFH.

Distribution

The volume of distribution (V) of UFH closely approximates blood volume at approximately 0.05 to 0.07 L/kg.[12] Estimation of blood volume by the formula V = 0.07 L/kg of body weight provides a reasonable estimate of heparin V when pharmacokinetic calculations are performed. When a large amount of heparin is adminis-

Table 14-1. UFH: Bioavailability (F) of Routes of Administration

Dosage Form	Bioavailability
IV	100% (F = 1)
SC	~20-30% (F = 0.3) (Range 10-90%)

tered during bypass graft surgery, a rebound in anticoagulant effects can occur up to 6 hours after post-surgery protamine neutralization due to redistribution of heparin into the plasma.[13]

Studies employing weight-based nomograms have shown reduced time to therapeutic aPTT when compared to fixed dose nomograms.[5,9] These individualized dosing schemes clearly show that as individual size varies and, by default, V changes, so should the heparin dosing. Some studies suggest additional variables such as age, sex, and height may better approximate the V.[14]

Protein binding

Since heparin products are mixtures of a wide range of molecular weights, pharmacokinetic parameters may vary with the particular preparation used. This variability is caused by UFH's nonspecific binding to proteins and cells. Heparin-binding proteins are quite variable in their concentration during acute illness. These proteins are acute phase reactants and may be elevated in acutely ill patients, accounting for variability in the aPTT results,[15] unpredictable anticoagulant response, and the potential for heparin resistance. These outcomes are demonstrated as a shortening of the aPTT that is seen in some patients. The impact of LMWHs in addressing these problems is discussed later.

Elimination

UFH is cleared by both zero-order and first-order elimination processes. In the saturable, rapid zero-order process, it is metabolized and depolymerized by endothelial cells and macrophages. As for first-order elimination, heparin is cleared renally in a slower, non-saturable process. The half-life of UFH varies from 0.4 to 2.5 hr, increasing as the administered dose increases from 25 to 400 U/kg.[16-18] In addition, patient-specific variables such as age, thromboembolic disease state, hepatic or renal impairment, and obesity, may significantly alter the clearance and volume of distribution (V) of UFH. While hepatic or renal impairment may influence these pharmacokinetic parameters, no significant dosage modification is typically required.

Table 14-2 illustrates the pharmacokinetic parameters for UFH.[10] Differences in parameters may exist depending on whether direct (anti-Factor Xa assay)[10,12,19-21] or indirect (ACT or aPTT)[10,19-26] measurement of the heparin concentration is performed. These differences may account in part for what has been deemed the inter- and intra-patient variability seen in dose responsiveness for patients receiving UFH.

Dosing Strategies

Treating venous thromboembolic disease

For treatment of a venous thromboembolism (VTE), concomitant UFH and warfarin therapy are used, except during early stages of pregnancy or when warfarin is contraindicated. Patients with suspected or confirmed VTE should receive UFH and warfarin as follows.[2]

Suspected VTE[2]

- Obtain baseline aPTT, prothrombin time/international normalized ratio (PT)/(INR), complete blood count (CBC).
- Check for contraindications to heparin therapy.
- Initiate parenteral anticoagulant with UFH (bolus plus infusion or SC), low molecular weight heparin (LMWH), or Fondaparinux at doses typically used for initial management of an acute VTE. Warfarin may not be started until the VTE is confirmed. If the VTE is ruled out, the parenteral agent can be stopped.
- Order imaging study.

Table 14-2. UFH Pharmacokinetic Parameters Assuming a Linear One-Compartment Model

Parameter	Mean Value and/or Range
Clearance (CL)	0.015–0.12 L/h/kg
Volume of distribution (V)	0.07 L/kg (range 0.04–0.14 L/kg)
Half-life (t½)	1.6 hr (range 0.4–2.5 hr)

Confirmed VTE[2]

- Bolus with 80 units/kg IV of UFH and start maintenance infusion at 18 units/kg/hr if a parenteral anticoagulant has not yet been started, and heparin is the chosen agent.
- Check aPTT at 4–8 hr and adjust dose as needed to maintain a range corresponding to a therapeutic heparin concentration. If no bolus is administered an earlier aPTT can be measured. A large bolus can affect the aPTT up to 8 hours after administration, suggesting a greater response of the infusion than is actually occurring. (see Figure 14-1)
- Check platelet count prior to starting therapy, and then on a routine basis (e.g., every 2–3 days for 2 weeks). Carefully monitor patients with a recent exposure to heparin products for potential heparin induced thrombocytopenia (HIT).
- When there is a desire to switch to a LMWH, the LMWH can generally be given at the time the UFH infusion is stopped. An acute thrombus or bleeding are unlikely to occur if there is a slight difference in the time (i.e., 1–2 hours) between stopping the UFH and starting the LMWH. For initiating a UFH infusion for a patient on a LMWH, consider starting the infusion when the next LMWH dose would be administered. A bolus would not typically be required.
- Initiate a vitamin K antagonist (VKA) such as warfarin together with UFH on the first treatment day once a rise in the aPTT has been observed.

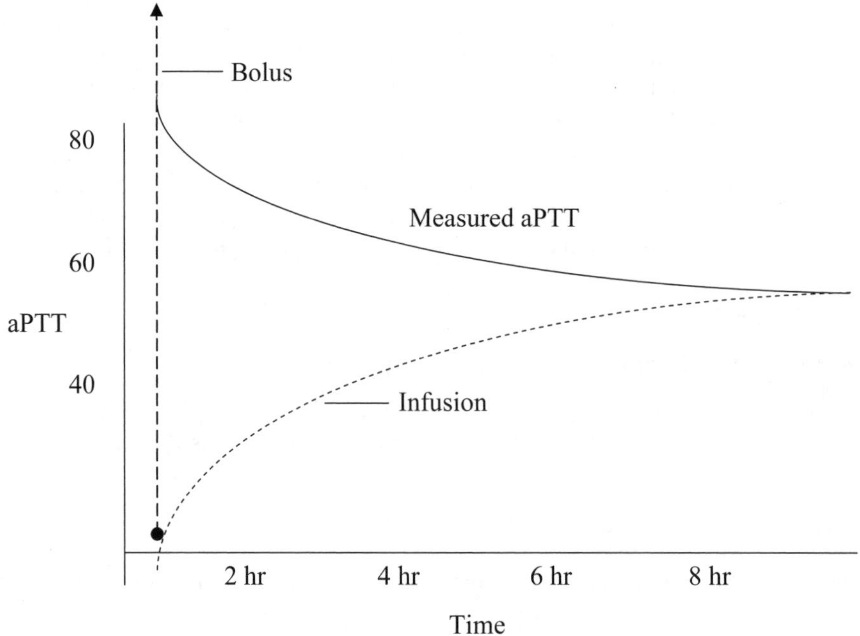

Figure 14-1. Timing of aPTT values when a bolus is given with the initiation or increase in an infusion rate.

Depending on the amount of a bolus (dashed line) administered, the aPTT may rise to a point higher than achieved by the continuous infusion (dotted line). The measured aPTT (solid line) in this situation will then drop over time to a value reflective of the infusion rate. Checking aPTT values earlier than 6 hours after initiating the UFH infusion may be requested in order to determine if an inadequate infusion rate is present (aPTT value close to baseline). When interpreting this "early" aPTT value, it has to be noted that the bolus dose may artificially increase this reading. UFH bolus doses of $>$ 5000 units can also have an effect on aPTT values drawn up to 8 hours later.[27]

Source: Used with permission from: Dager W, Gulseth M, Nutescu E, eds. Anticoagulation Therapy: A Point-Of-Care Guide. Bethesda, MD: American Society of Health-System Pharmacists; 2011.

- Discontinue UFH after a minimum of 4–5 days and when the international normalized ratio (INR) is stable and above 2.0.
- Anticoagulate with warfarin for 3 or more months (patient/disease-state specific). See the warfarin chapter for more extensive discussion of warfarin dosing and monitoring.

Pharmacokinetic dosing approaches

UFH dosing can be adjusted either empirically or by pharmacokinetic calculations using one of several approaches:

1. For practical dosing, the onset of heparin's therapeutic effect can be expedited by a loading dose. This IV bolus dose may be empirically selected (e.g., 2500 to 5000 units) or loading doses may be individualized using the patient's weight, for example 70–100 units/kg. In some instances, the weight-based approach to loading patients is based on the indication for use; in many situations 80 units/kg should suffice in providing a therapeutic aPTT.

   A variety of approaches to continuous dosing have been employed. Empiric dosing of 1000–1300 units/hr may be used.[28] Due to variability in clearance among individuals, use of the lower dose can lead to aPTTs below the therapeutic range, but they may also sometimes be above the targeted range. Other approaches to continuous dosing with UFH include use of weight-based dosing nomograms, for which initiation may vary between 15 and 25 units/kg/hr (ACCP recommends 18 units/kg/hr).[5] In the setting of a PE, doses of 25 units/kg/hr may be necessary due to increased heparin clearance.[24]

   After the patient has been started on UFH, dosing adjustment nomograms can be used to assist in revising the initial weight-based dosing efforts. However, such nomograms should be adapted for a specific aPTT reagent. Examples of dosing adjustment nomograms are depicted in Tables 14-3[29] and 14-4.[5]

Table 14-3. UFH Dosage Adjustment Protocol[a,29]

Patient's aPTT[b]	Repeat Bolus Dose	Hold Infusion (min)	Infusion Rate Change (units/hr)	Timing of Next aPTT
<50	5,000 units[c]	0	+120	6 hr
50–59	0	0	+120	6 hr
60–85	0	0	0	Next morning
86–95	0	0	–80	Next morning
96–120	0	30	–80	6 hr
>120	0	60	–160	6 hr

[a]Starting dose of 5,000 units intravenous bolus followed by 1,300 units/hr (32,000 units/24 hr) as a continuous infusion. An aPTT is performed 6 to 8 hr after the bolus injection; dosage adjustments are made according to protocol, and the aPTT is repeated as indicated in the right-hand column.
[b]Normal range for aPTT with the example reagent where a therapeutic range of 60–85 seconds is equivalent to a heparin concentration of 0.2–0.4 units/ml by whole blood protamine titration or 0.3–0.7 units/ml as a plasma anti-Factor Xa concentration. The therapeutic range varies with the responsiveness (sensitivity) of the particular aPTT reagent to heparin.
[c]When the aPTT is measured at 6–8 hr or longer, steady state can be assumed. An 8-hour aPTT may need to be considered if a larger bolus (e.g., 5,000 units) is given to allow the effects of the bolus to wash out, allowing the aPTT reflect the infusion rate (see Figure 14-1).

Table 14-4. aPTT and Weight-Based Dosing Adjustment Scheme for UFH[a,5,30]

aPTT (seconds)	Infusion Change (units/kg/hr)	Next Action	Repeat aPTT
<35 (<1.2 times normal)	+ 4	Rebolus with 80 units/kg	6 hr
35–45 (1.2–1.5 times normal)	+ 2	Rebolus with 40 units/kg	6 hr
46–70 (1.5–2.3 times normal)	0	0	6 hr[b]
71–90 (2.3–3.0 times normal)	–2	0	6 hr
>90 (>3 times normal)	–3	Hold infusion 1 hr	6 hr

[a]Initial dosing: loading dose is 80 units/kg; maintenance infusion is 18 units/kg/hr (aPTT in 6 hr).
[b]During the first 24 hr, repeat aPTT every 6 hr. Thereafter, monitor aPTT once every morning unless it is outside of the therapeutic range.

Table 14-5 shows outcomes that might be expected if the dosing approaches used in Table 14-4 are employed.

2. For a pharmacokinetic modeling and dosing approach, the infusion rate (R_2) for a target activated clotting time (ACT) [ACT_2] can be estimated from a steady state ACT (ACT_1) on a known UFH dosing rate (R_1) using the formula:[10,16]

$$R_2 = R_1 \times \frac{(\log ACT_2) - (\log ACT_0)}{(\log ACT_1) - (\log ACT_0)}$$

where ACT_0 is the patient's baseline pre-treatment ACT.

3. If aPTT monitoring of heparin's effect is used, doses must be adjusted with the understanding that aPTT rises disproportionately to the heparin dose and concentration in a nonlinear manner. Further, the changes noted in the aPTT with adjustments in UFH doses are relatively unpredictable. Thus, such guidelines are only rough estimates and clinicians may have to frequently deviate from them. Cruickshank et al.[30] described a dosing protocol where 66% and 81% of the patients were above the lower limit of the therapeutic range by 24 and 48 hr, respectively. Of 350 aPTT measurements following the initial dosing adjustments using the protocol however, only 59.4% were within the therapeutic range, while 25.2% were below and 15.4% above the therapeutic range.

4. If anti-Factor Xa heparin activity can be measured concomitantly with coagulation studies, a combined pharmacokinetic-pharmacodynamic model can be used. The target anti-Factor Xa heparin level is determined from the relationship of anti-Factor Xa heparin concentrations and coagulation studies drawn 1 and 4 hr after initiation of UFH.[31] Subsequent UFH infusion rates to achieve the targeted anti-Factor Xa heparin concentrations are then calculated using the pharmacokinetic infusion model developed by Chiou et al.[28]

$$CL = \left(\frac{2R}{(C_1 + C_2)}\right) + \left(\frac{2V(C_1 - C_2)}{(C_1 + C_2)(t_2 + t_1)}\right)$$

where

CL = apparent heparin clearance in units per hour

R = UFH infusion rate in units per hour

V = volume of distribution; equal to patient's estimated blood volume in milliliters (0.07 L/kg)

Table 14-5. Outcomes Noted Using Table 14-4 Dosing Approaches

(N=115; VTE=80)

Time	Standard UFH Bolus: 5,000 units then continuous infusion started at 1,000 units/hr	Weight-Based UFH 80 units/kg load then 18 units/kg/hr (Actual Body Weight)	P value
24 hour aPTT			
Therapeutic	35%	57%	<0.001
Subtherapeutic	58%	15%	<0.001
Supratherapeutic	7%	27%	<0.001
48 hour aPTT			
Therapeutic	44%	65%	<0.001
Subtherapeutic	49%	18%	<0.001
Supratherapeutic	8%	18%	<0.001
Minor/Major Bleeding	2% / 1%	2% / 0%	
Recurrent VTE (3 Mo)	8/32 (25%)	2/41 (5%)	

C_1 = first anti-Factor Xa heparin level, drawn at time 1 (t_1), 1 hr after initiation of UFH (in units/ml)

C_2 = second anti-Factor Xa heparin level, drawn at t_2, 4 hr after initiation of UFH (in units/ml)

The clearance may then be used to determine a dose to produce anti-Factor Xa heparin concentrations in the therapeutic range. This particular model lends itself well to issues regarding disease-state dependent clearance, e.g., in the setting of pulmonary embolism—where clearance has been suggested to be increased.[10] The validity of this dosing approach has been confirmed using plasma heparin concentrations determined by anti-Factor Xa assay, which is more readily adapted to routine clinical applications.[32]

5. UFH dosing also may be estimated using blood volume calculations to estimate V and population half-life estimates (see Table 14-3) to calculate *k*. The correction factors in Table 14-6 can also be used to alter parameters.

   Target anti-Factor Xa heparin concentrations are usually 0.3 to 0.7 units/ml, and UFH doses can be calculated with these formulas[25,33]:

   Loading dose (in units) = (V) × (target heparin concentration × 1000 ml/L) =

   (0.07 L/kg × patient's total body weight) × (0.6 units/ml × 1000 ml/L)

   Maintenance dose (in units/hr) = (target heparin concentration × 1000 ml/L) (V)(k)

   This dosing approach may be particularly useful for morbidly obese patients since obesity has been identified as a factor associated with increased heparin dosage requirements. This has been attributed to the potential for decreased levels of antithrombin (AT) associated with morbid obesity that causes under dosing to be a problem since UFH is dependent on AT as a cofactor to exert its anticoagulant response.[33,34]

6. Determining an SC dose from a currently administered IV infusion:

   Dose SC administered every 12 hours = (Last IV infusion rate/hr x 12) x (1.2)

   "(1.2)" reflects the approximately 20% loss of bioavailability with the SC route.

Table 14-6. Adjustment Factors for Drug–Disease State or Condition Interactions with Comparisons Made to Average DVT Patients[a]

Disease State or Condition	Assay	Clearance	Volume of Distribution[b]	Half-Life
PE	Xa	1.5	1	0.75
	ACT	1	1	1
Liver disease	Xa	1.5	1	0.75
Renal disease	Xa	1	1	1
Hemodialysis	Xa	1	1	1
	ACT	NA[c]	NA[c]	1
Neonates				
>32 weeks	Xa	2.5	1	0.33
≤32 weeks	Xa	2.6	1.3	0.33
	Clotting time	1.6	1.2	0.85
Neonates on ECMO	ACT	5.5	NA[c]	NA[c]
Adults				
Male	ACT	1.1	1	0.85
Female	ACT	0.8	1	1.1
Smoker	ACT	1.2	1	0.67
Nonsmoker	ACT	1	1	1

[a]Standard values for adjustments are CL = 0.03 L/hr/kg, V = 0.07 L/kg, and t½ = 1.6 hr. To correct pharmacokinetic parameters for underlying condition, these values are multiplied by the adjustment factors.

[b]The V of heparin correlates to the patient's blood volume.

[c]NA = Data not available.

The common 250 unit/kg every 12 dose for VTE treatment is based on this concept, 20% over the common 18 units/kg/hr IV infusion rate used in VTE

UFH: Therapeutic Range

Historically, the targeted pharmacologic effect for heparin had been prolongation of the selected clotting test to 1.5–2.5 times the patient's normal baseline value.[2,10,19] It is now observed that use of a standard aPTT therapeutic range of 1.5–2.5 for all reagents and methods of clot detection leads to the systematic administration of subtherapeutic doses of heparin. This is due to limitations of the aPTT test, including wide variation in responsiveness to the anticoagulant in different laboratories that is caused by differences in thromboplastin reagents and coagulometer instruments. Prolongation of the aPTT that is seen with lupus anticoagulant antibodies, certain congenital factor deficiencies, or the presence of oral anticoagulation with warfarin, limits the approach of using a standard aPTT therapeutic range of 1.5–2.5 for dosing decisions. In all circumstances, the therapeutic range should be adapted to the responsiveness of the reagent used (see monitoring section).[35]

The targeted outcome varies with the specific indication for its use (see Table 14-7).[3,22,36-42] Current recommendations of the American College of Chest Physicians and the College of American Pathologists indicate that patients should be treated with continuous IV UFH (CIUFH) to prolong the aPTT to a range that corresponds to a whole-blood heparin concentration of 0.2–0.4 units/ml by protamine titration or 0.3–0.7 units/ml by anti-Factor Xa heparin assay. This approach of targeting a heparin concentration works to overcome the limitations of the global aPTT test previously described. These recommendations are based on well-controlled, randomized trials in patients with both PE and DVT.[3,6]

Several coagulation tests are used for monitoring heparin's effect, and each has different limitations (see Table 14-8).[10,41,44-48] Heparin concentration measurements may be used to reach a target therapeutic range (e.g., 0.3–0.7 units/ml), especially in unusual coagulation situations such as pregnancy where the reliability of clotting

Table 14-7. UFH: Therapeutic End-Points for Specific Treatment Indications

Disease or Condition	Therapeutic Range	Comments
Prevention of catheter clotting	Nonspecific low doses	No studies on survival of catheters related to degree of anticoagulation
ECLS in neonates	ACT 180–240 sec[6,22] Anti-Factor Xa heparin level 0.1–1.0 units/ml[6]	Range apparently based on anecdotal experience and can vary considerably. Fibrinogen, AT levels can decline over time.[43] Any benefits of replacing AT or alterations in the heparin response with AT supplementation are unclear. ACT low-range (ACT-LR) cards may provide more accurate values than high-range (ACT-HR) counterpart; suggest periodic anti-Factor Xa activity
Cardiopulmonary bypass in adults or pediatrics	ACT 400–600 sec[37,38]	Range based on animal studies and anecdotal experience
Hemodialysis	ACT 180–240 sec	
Treatment of DVT and PE	Prolong the aPTT to a range that corresponds to a whole blood heparin concentration of 0.2–0.4 units/ml by protamine titration or plasma anti-Factor Xa activity of 0.3–0.7 units/ml by amidolytic assay	Recommendation based on studies in patients with DVT and PE and on the relationship between the aPTT and effectiveness[2]
Treatment of myocardial infarction (MI)	CIUFH sufficient to prolong the aPTT 1.5–2 times control	With or without thrombolytic therapy having been administered[8]

CIUFH = continuous infusion unfractionated heparin; AT = antithrombin; ACT = activated clotting time; ECLS = extra corporeal life support.

studies is questionable.[42] For DVT or PE, it may be preferable to correlate anti-Factor Xa activity concentrations with a target aPTT.[10,49-51] Pharmacokinetic information derived from anti-Factor Xa activity concentrations may help to achieve therapeutic aPTT values more rapidly.[31]

UFH: Therapeutic Monitoring

Monitoring

The anticoagulant effects of heparin are most frequently monitored by the aPTT, though it is important to be familiar with this global test's shortcomings and their potential impact on reliable interpretation of the results. Dose adjustments are predicated on the results of aPTT values. When UFH is administered in fixed doses, the anticoagulant response varies among patients and within the same patient (inter- and intra-patient variability). This variability is caused by differences in heparin concentrations, neutralizing proteins, and rates of heparin clearance. Traditionally, for many aPTT reagents, therapeutic effect was thought to have been achieved with an aPTT ratio of 1.5–2.5 (measured by dividing the patient's observed aPTT by the mean of the normal laboratory control aPTT). With newer, more sensitive aPTT reagents and differing laboratory instrumentation, the therapeutic range today could be higher, or even change in either direction with a new lot of reagents depending on the sensitivity of the reagent to heparin. For less sensitive reagents the reported aPTT is lower, prompting the necessity of anti-Factor Xa heparin activity determinations.

Since aPTT reagents may vary in their sensitivity, the same aPTT ratio (1.5–2.5) for all reagents should be avoided. The therapeutic range for each aPTT reagent should be calibrated to be equivalent to an anti-Factor

Table 14-8. Coagulation Tests Used To Regulate Heparin Dosing[6,10,44-48]

Test	Range	Advantages	Disadvantages
aPTT	28–42 sec[a] Patient's baseline should be used[b]	DVT and PE studies done using this test; recognized standards available; laboratory control equipment and quality control better; extensive clinical experience	Lacks reproducibility with different instruments, reagents, and laboratories; nonlinear relationship to increasing heparin concentration; loss of accuracy of value above 150 sec
ACT	80–130 sec[a] Patient's baseline should be used[b]	Rapid bedside test; linear increase with heparin concentration in usual therapeutic range; extensive experience in hemodialysis, cardiopulmonary bypass, and ECLS patients	Lacks reproducibility with ACT of >600 sec and with different reagents and instruments; limited clinical trials in DVT or PE patients Affected by ↓ platelets, hemodilution, and hypothermia. The sensitivity and range of heparin intensity can vary between tests. Low-range and high-range kits are available and give different results.[52]
Whole blood heparin anti-Factor Xa concentrations	0.2–0.4 units/ml[c]	Overcomes inadequacies of aPTTs. Useful in heparin resistance and pregnancy.	Relative expense; not available in all institutions.
Plasma heparin anti-Factor Xa concentrations	0.3–0.7 units/ml	Overcomes some inadequacies of aPTTs. Useful in heparin resistance not attributed to low antithrombin, pregnancy, with lupus antibodies, and Antiphospholipid Antibody Syndrome. Less labor intensive than whole blood test.	Relative expense; not available in all institutions. May miss AT deficiency and suggest adequate level of anticoagulation that may not be present. Variability in results can occur between clinical laboratories.

[a]Normal range; varies by manufacturer and instrumentation.
[b]If unavailable or elevated, laboratory control values may be used.
[c]Therapeutic range.
ACT = activated clotting time; ECLS = extra corporeal life support.

Xa heparin activity of 0.2–0.4 units/ml by whole blood (protamine titration) or to an anti-Factor Xa activity (plasma heparin concentration) of about 0.3–0.7 units/ml by amidolytic assay.[53]

Anti-Factor Xa heparin activity concentrations, used by themselves with no reporting of an aPTT value, are another method of monitoring the anticoagulant effects of UFH. This method can be very useful in situations of potential heparin resistance, with the exception of AT deficiency. Elevated levels of fibrinogen or factor VIII, which can suppress aPTT values despite therapeutic heparinization, may not affect the ACT as much. In many cases, existing on-site laboratory instruments may be used to perform these tests and with increased utilization the per-test costs may be reduced, perhaps leading to increased use over time.

While there is evidence relating a higher UFH dose to the likelihood of a bleeding complication, there is also strong evidence supporting the contributions of patient-related factors such as recent surgery, generalized hemostatic abnormalities, peptic ulcers, neoplastic lesions, and use of concomitant antithrombotic medications (e.g., glycoprotein IIb/IIIa inhibitors, thrombolytic agents, and antiplatelet agents) to an increase in the likelihood of bleeding complications.[54] Given these observations, most published guidelines, especially in cardiology settings, advocate a lower dose of UFH when administering antithrombotic agents together. Specific guidelines should be considered when treating the corresponding patient population.[3,8,55]

Suggested sampling times

Specific sampling times for patients receiving UFH therapy vary according to the treatment indication. The times suggested for PE, DVT, extracorporeal circulation, and prophylaxis against venous thrombosis are listed in Table 14-9.[6,56]

Assay issues

The responsiveness of the aPTT to UFH's effect may be impacted by several technical variables that include the type of clot detection system used within the instrumentation and the contact activator and phospholipid composition of the reagent being used. The response of the aPTT to UFH can be reduced in the presence of acute phase reactants such as elevated concentrations of fibrinogen or factor VIII. Antithrombin (AT) deficiency may cause a spurious "shortening" of aPTT that might lead to unnecessary increases in UFH dosing or inappropriately suggest heparin resistance.[6] Clot burden or size, duration of therapy, and concomitant disease states may also affect aPTT responsiveness. In general, the anti-Factor Xa assay may be a better test in the presence of high factor VIII or fibrinogen. However, anti-Factor Xa assays that have antithrombin (AT) added to the test may miss resistance caused by low AT levels in the patient, or provide a higher result than anti-Factor Xa measurements using a test that does not add AT.

UFH: Pharmacodynamic Monitoring—Concentration-Related Efficacy

Thrombus formation, extension, or embolization can be markers of inadequate heparin dosing or the development of heparin-associated thrombocytopenia. Factors that affect heparin concentrations and the anticoagulant

Table 14-9. Suggested Sampling Times for Patients Receiving UFH for Various Indications

Indication	Sampling Time
PE or DVT	Continuous infusion UFH: coagulation test obtained 4-8 hr after start of infusion or after change in infusion rate (4 hours if without bolus and 6–8 hours is bolus given)[a,b]
	Intermittent subcutaneous heparin: coagulation test obtained 6 hr after any dose
Prophylaxis of venous thrombosis	Coagulation test obtained 6 hr after subcutaneous heparin dose
Extracorporeal circulation	Neonatal ECLS or cardiopulmonary bypass: ACT obtained every 30–60 min during dialysis treatment
	Hemodialysis: ACT obtained at least every 60 min during dialysis
	Neonatal ECLS using ACT, aPTT or Anti-Factor Xa heparin activity concentration: per institutional protocol

[a]If heparin is being dosed by a combined pharmacokinetic and pharmacodynamic approach (see pharmacokinetic dosing approaches section), samples for heparin concentrations and clotting studies should be obtained 1, 4, and 12 hr after initiation of a continuous infusion. Doses should be adjusted after 1- and 4-hr samples, and precision should be checked with 12-hr samples.[31,32]
[b]Refer to dosing method 2.

effect relationship include AT, platelet factor 4 (PF4), and the elevated concentrations of factor VIII that can occur in a number of clinical states, including pregnancy, malignancy, acute thrombosis, and major surgery.[50,51] These and other factors are discussed in Table 14-10.[34,57-64]

Table 14-10. Factors to Consider When Interpreting UFH Pharmacodynamics

Factor	Comments
AT (obtained with baseline coagulation studies and on day 3)[34,57-60]	If AT concentrations are notably below normal values for a given age group, heparin may not exert its full anticoagulant effect at usual doses and concentrations (i.e., heparin resistance).[34] Decreased AT predisposes the patient to thrombus formation[34] and PE during heparin therapy for DVT.[57] AT concentrations may fall due to heparin therapy,[57] but AT is easily replaced with administration of blood, plasma, or AT concentrates. Normal AT values are lower in neonates and infants compared to adults.
PF4 (not routinely measured)[61,62]	PF4 neutralizes heparin effect and promotes thrombus formation. When PF4 is increased (e.g., during disseminated intravascular coagulation or immune thrombocytopenia), patients may be relatively heparin resistant.[61,62] Elevated PF4 in plasma also may inactivate heparin in vitro, giving falsely low heparin activity assessments.
Heparin cofactor II (not routinely measured)[63]	This factor plays a minor role when AT concentrations are adequate but can be important if AT deficiency occurs.
Coagulation tests	Correlation of heparin concentrations with coagulation tests shows at least a five-fold variation in clotting tests at the same concentration.[10]
Pregnancy	During the third trimester, pregnant patients display relative heparin resistance and require higher doses.[42]
Circadian effect	Effects of heparin on coagulation tests (both the aPTT and anti-Factor Xa activity) may be greater (up to 50%–60%) at night or during sleeping periods than during the daytime.[64] This suggests the variability is a pharmacokinetic effect instead of an assay issue.

UFH: Pharmacodynamic Monitoring—Concentration-Related Toxicity

Heparin use can lead to a variety of toxic outcomes related or not related to its pharmacological effect. Table 14-11 outlines the various heparin-related toxicities.

Reversing Heparin's Effect

Protamine sulfate is used to neutralize heparin following severe UFH overdosing or severe, unexpected bleeding. Each milligram of protamine sulfate neutralizes approximately 90 units of beef lung heparin sodium, 115 units of heparin sodium derived from porcine intestinal mucosa, or 100 units of heparin calcium. Overdosing with protamine must be avoided as it too can independently promote bleeding. Its administration can also cause severe hypotension and anaphylactoid or anaphylactic reactions. Protamine should be administered slowly over at least 10 minutes to reduce the possibility of anaphylaxis. Outside of reversing heparin after going off cardiopulmonary bypass (CPB), a total single dose of 50 mg should not be exceeded. In CPB, a repeat dose of protamine sulfate may be necessary to neutralize large amounts of heparin given during a procedure or operation and that may re-distribute from the tissues back into the plasma. Prothrombin complex concentrate (PCC) and/or recombinant activated factor VII (rFVIIa) have been used to assist in establishing hemostasis, but these products have no activity to directly neutralize heparin and should not be used as a substitute for protamine sulfate. Table 14-12 provides dosing guidelines for protamine sulfate based on time after UFH dosing.

Because the half-life of IV heparin is relatively short at 60 to 90 min., only heparin given during the preceding several hours needs to be considered when calculating the dose of protamine sulfate. For example, a patient receiving UFH at 1,250 units/hr requires approximately 30 mg of protamine sulfate. Neutralization of UFH given by subcutaneous administration may require a prolonged infusion or repeat doses of protamine sulfate due to continued absorption from the site of administration. The aPTT can be used to assess the effectiveness of protamine sulfate neutralization in reversing the anticoagulant effects of heparin.[6]

Table 14-11. Heparin-Related Toxicities

Toxicity	Monitoring and Detection	Prevention and Management
Major bleeding[65] (leading to blood transfusion, heparin discontinuation, prolonged hospital stay, or death)	Clinical signs depend on site of bleeding. Increased risk correlated with increased dose, but studies of relationship to coagulation tests are limited. Risk factors include female >60 years old, dose of >25 units/kg/hr, concomitant aspirin, heavy alcohol use, increased length of use, and intermittent IV bolus dosing.	Coagulation tests kept below upper limit of targeted therapeutic endpoint. Length of use limited by early initiation of warfarin. Heparin effects reversed with protamine sulfate (see reversing heparin's effect section).
Minor bleeding[65]	Relationship to heparin dose and coagulation studies was noted in some reports. Guaiac-positive stool and bleeding from nose, gums, puncture sites, urine, sputum, etc., occur.	Intramuscular route avoided for medications. Coagulation tests kept below upper limit of targeted therapeutic endpoint.
Thrombocytopenia[66,67]	Direct platelet effect is not dose related, with onset 1–20 (usual 5–9) days after start of heparin. Effect may be transient. Suspect heparin-induced thrombocytopenia (HIT) if there is a 50% decline in baseline platelet count after commencing UFH. Platelet counts should be monitored at least every other day while patient receives heparin.[68]	Use pork intestine heparin instead of beef lung (no longer available in many countries) heparin when possible. Heparin stopped if platelets are <100,000, there is a 50% decline from baseline platelet count, or if bleeding occurs.[67,68]
Thrombosis due to immune thrombocytopenia[66-68]	Triad of decreased platelets, high heparin dose requirements, and formation of arterial thrombi may be present. If platelet count decreases, a functional or activation assay designed to detect HIT related antibodies should be done if possible. Do not await results of confirmatory tests before discontinuing heparin.	Initiate warfarin cautiously and at low dose. Avoid heparin in patients with prior history. If thrombosis is suspected, stop heparin immediately, including flushes and arterial catheters. Initiate FDA-approved direct thrombin inhibitor given as treatment until warfarin effect is adequate[67,68]; warfarin should not initially be used alone[68]
Osteoporosis[6,69]	Problem only occurs with long-term use (>6 months) of doses over 20,000 units/day. Bone films in otherwise at-risk patients may be appropriate.	Risk reduced by assuring adequate calcium intake. May consider use of LMWH.
Hyperkalemia	Monitor K+ at least every 3–4 days during therapy	Fluids and electrolytes adjusted.
Increased aspartate aminotransferase (AST) and alanine aminotransferase (ALT)	Monitoring of laboratory values probably is not routinely necessary	Initiate warfarin and stop heparin as soon as possible. Probably not due to liver disease.
Transient alopecia	No special monitoring necessary	No special treatment performed.
Other side effects Skin lesions Skin necrosis Hypersensitivity Priapism	Observation	Suspect heparin induced thrombocytopenia with thrombotic complication with skin lesions/skin necrosis. Remove all forms of heparin therapy and initiate alternative therapy.

UFH: Drug-Drug Interactions

Heparin does not have definitively identified pharmacokinetic or pharmacodynamic drug interactions, although platelet-inhibiting drugs or drugs irritating to the gastrointestinal tract could in theory lead to complications. Use of the drugs listed in Table 14-13 in patients receiving UFH may warrant adjustments in dosing or sampling procedures.

Table 14-12. Protamine Sulfate Dosing to Reverse UFH Effect

Time after Heparin Dose	Protamine Sulfate Dose[a]
<30 min	1–1.5 mg for each 100 units of heparin in last dose
30–120 min	0.5–0.75 mg for each 100 units of heparin in last dose
>120 min	0.25–0.375 mg for each 100 units of heparin in last dose
Heparin IV infusion	25–50 mg after infusion is stopped

[a]In the event of major bleeding, some clinicians recommend using the lower end of these ranges to avoid potential bleeding caused by excess protamine sulfate. Prescribing directions for protamine sulfate should be carefully followed due to the risks associated with its use. Doses of 50 mg should not be exceeded outside of the operating room. The risk of severe adverse reactions, such as hypotension and bradycardia, can be minimized by administering protamine slowly (i.e., over approximately 10 minutes).

Table 14-13. Heparin-Drug Interactions

Drug	Interaction	Prevention and Management
Nitroglycerin (intravenous)[70,71]	Resistance to anticoagulant effect of heparin	Infuse drugs at different sites. Adjust doses for therapeutic aPTT.
Platelet function inhibitors[72] (e.g., aspirin and nonsteroidal anti-inflammatory agents)	Increased risk of bleeding	Avoid if possible. Salsalate, an alternative anti-inflammatory agent, does not inhibit platelet aggregation.
Decreased in vitro binding of basic and acidic drugs[73] (e.g., propranolol and quinidine; in vivo effect not shown)	Increased lipoprotein lipase activity by heparin increases free fatty acid (FFA) formation, leading to displacement by FFAs.	Heparinized samples should be processed rapidly when analyzing for free (unbound) drug. Interpret results cautiously.
Warfarin[74]	aPTT is prolonged	Heparin dose reduced, if necessary, to prevent excessive aPTT. May consider role of anti-Factor Xa heparin monitoring.
Thrombolytics GPIIb/IIIa antagonists	Risk of bleeding increases	Heparin dose reduced.

UFH: Drug–Disease State or Condition Interactions

UFH's pharmacokinetic parameters may be influenced by a patient's condition or underlying disease state. Table 14-6 provides adjustment factors for several such conditions and disease states.

Summary of UFH Dosing and Monitoring

A combination of UFH (initially) and warfarin is used for the treatment or prevention of VTE disease except during pregnancy or when warfarin is contraindicated. Patients with proven thromboembolic disease should receive therapy with UFH and warfarin and be monitored as follows:

1. Patient specific indication(s) for heparin and warfarin therapy should be addressed and where appropriate, give weight based, nomogram driven, or UFH pharmacokinetic parameter modeled doses to achieve desired outcome of efficacy and safety.
2. Baseline coagulation studies (aPTT, PT/INR, CBC) should be done in all patients prior to initiating therapy. Continue monitoring aPTT at 6-hour intervals and maintain an aPTT range corresponding to a therapeutic anti-Factor Xa heparin concentration. After achieving therapeutic response, daily monitoring of aPTTs is necessary to demonstrate continued efficacy and safety. Alternatively, an anti-Factor Xa heparin activity concentration may be monitored by chromogenic/amidolytic assay methodology in a range of 0.3–0.7 units/ml. Check platelet count at baseline and every other day until day 14, or until UFH is stopped, whichever occurs first.
3. Initiate oral anticoagulation with vitamin K antagonists (VKAs) together with UFH at the time of diagnosis. Adjust subsequent daily dosing based on INR response. Discontinue heparin when the international normalized ratio (INR) is stable and > 2.0; this usually occurs after 5 to 7 days of UFH therapy.[2,75] Note

that if the INR assay does not neutralize the effects of heparin, an elevation in the INR secondary to heparin may occur. See warfarin chapter for details on dosing and monitoring.

4. Monitor for clinical outcomes of efficacy and safety (see Tables 14-10 and 14-11).

Low Molecular Weight Heparins (LMWHs)

LMWHs are now widely used for the prevention and treatment of venous and arterial embolic disease. LMWHs are obtained by fractionating or depolymerizing UFH, which is a heterogeneous mixture of heparin chains with molecular weights of 5,000–30,000 Daltons. The mean molecular weight (Daltons) of LMWHs is approximately 4,000–5,000.

FDA approved indications for the LMWHs vary by manufacturer. Each has been proven to be reasonably safe and effective for the prevention and treatment of venous thromboembolism. LMWHs are used for prevention of DVT after hip replacement, knee replacement, abdominal surgery, and for trauma, oncology, medical, and spinal cord injury patients. In addition, LMWHs are used in the treatment of unstable angina, non-ST elevation myocardial infarction (NSTEMI), DVT, and PE.

The LMWHs are often viewed as a homogeneous group, but their derivation from unfractionated heparin using different methods of enzymatic or hydrolytic cleavage results in different molecular weight profiles for each product. These variations may result in clinically relevant differences in pharmacokinetic and pharmacodynamic effects. Compared with UFH, which has a ratio of anti-Factor Xa to anti-Factor IIa activity of approximately 1:1, the various commercially available LMWHs have anti-Factor Xa to anti-factor IIa ratios varying between approximately 2:1 and 4:1 depending on their molecular size distribution (see Table 14-14).[76] A generic form of enoxaparin was approved for distribution in the United States. Although no comparative phase III clinical trials have been undertaken, the measured activity profile appears to be similar.[77,78]

The pharmacokinetics of UFH and LMWHs differ. LMWHs are less protein bound than UFH. Because of their longer elimination half-lives, some LMWHs may be administered as single daily doses, which can provide certain advantages over UFH.[6] Routine monitoring of coagulation tests (e.g., aPTT) or anti-Factor Xa heparin concentrations during LMWH therapy is generally considered unnecessary and is not routinely recommended.[2,79] Subcutaneous injection of the LMWHs produces only minimal effects on the aPTT. Thus, aPTT values cannot be reliably used to monitor or document efficacy and safety of LMWHs. Anti-Factor Xa assay by either whole blood or plasma determinations can be used, though routine monitoring with this assay is not necessary. The Eighth ACCP Conference on Antithrombotic and Thrombolytic Therapy recommends against routine monitoring with anti-Factor Xa when LMWHs are used for initial treatment of deep venous thrombosis in most settings.[2,6] Anti-Factor Xa heparin activity measurements may be considered in selected populations including pregnancy and pediatrics. Monitoring anti-Factor Xa has been proposed in patients with renal impairment (CrCl < 30 ml/min) because LMWHs are partially eliminated by the kidneys, and in the morbidly obese where response may show increased variation relative to weight-based dosing. However, correlation between measured anti-Factor Xa activity and renal function or weight is poor, limiting the utility of using these measurements for dosing adjustments.[83] Data validating the use of anti-Factor Xa activity for dosing adjustments overall is not currently available, limiting any validity with this approach to management.

If anti-Factor Xa results are used for monitoring, the therapeutic range by chromogenic/amidolytic assay for venous embolic disease treated twice-daily is 0.6–1.0 units/ml.[2,6] This should be measured at the time of peak effect post injection (i.e., 4 hours after subcutaneous administration) for LMWHs. Current data supporting the use of anti-Factor Xa is limited in the setting of acute coronary syndromes. In the setting of elective percutane-

Table 14-14. LMWH Pharmacokinetic and Pharmacodynamic Parameters[79-82]

LMWH	Brand Name	Average Molecular Weight (Daltons)	Percent Bioavailability (F)	Half-Life (hr)	Xa:IIa Binding Affinity Ratio
Dalteparin	Fragmin	5000	87 (0.87)	3	2.7:1
Enoxaparin	Lovenox	4500	92 (0.92)	4.5	3.8:1
Tinzaparin	Innohep	6500	87 (0.87)	3.5	1.9:1

ous coronary intervention (PCI), anti-Factor Xa levels greater than 0.9 units/ml were correlated with increased non-CABG major and minor bleeding, but not major bleeding alone.[84] In the setting of NSTEMI, anti-Factor Xa less than 0.5 units/ml was an independent predictor of increased mortality within 30 days.[85]

LMWH: Usual Dosage Range in the Absence of Clearance-Altering Factors

LMWHs have a longer half-life and more predictable anticoagulant response to weight-adjusted doses than UFH. These characteristics allow some LMWHs to be administered once daily. The actual body weight should be used for dosing, and it is suggested to avoid capping the dose at a certain weight.[86] Dosing of LMWHs is disease state and product specific, with different doses being administered based on the specific indication and product. Table 14-15 shows suggested dosing for product by specific indications.

LMWH: Dosage Form Availability

LMWHs are available only as solutions for injection. Currently FDA approved for SC use, some clinical trials have investigated the IV route of administration for procedural use, emergent situations where immediate effect is needed prior to peak onset of SC route, or instances of questionable SC absorption. LMWHs for injection are supplied in a variety of different concentrations in various delivery devices by their manufacturers. Enoxaparin and dalteparin may be diluted and stored in syringes for use in low weight infants.[91,92]

LMWH: General Pharmacokinetic Information

SC doses of LMWHs are 87% to 92% bioavailable (F = 0.87 to 0.92), which is considerably greater than that of SC doses of UFH (30%; F = 0.3). This may make dose changes unnecessary when converting from SC to IV if IV dosing is approved in the future.[93,94] In selected situations, LMWHs may be administered IV for a more rapid onset of anticoagulation. LMWHs have been shown to achieve heparin activity concentrations (by anti-Factor Xa assay) in the detectable range of 0.5–1.0 units/ml as soon as 30 minutes after SC injection[95] and 3 to 10 min after IV administration of appropriate doses.

This high degree of bioavailability does not appear to hold true in all patient populations. Those medically critically ill[96-98] and critically ill trauma and surgical patients may have altered pharmacokinetics or pharmacodynamics leading to an impaired response to standard dosing as measured by anti-Factor Xa, possibly leading to greater incidence of VTE.[99] Site of administration may also be important. In one analysis, the measured anti-Factor Xa activity of enoxaparin was significantly lower in obese patients when administered in the thigh compared to the abdomen.[100]

The plasma recoveries and pharmacokinetics of LMWHs differ from UFH due to differences in the binding properties of the two sulfated polysaccharides to plasma proteins and endothelial cells. LMWHs bind much less avidly to heparin-binding proteins than UFH, a property that contributes both to the superior bioavailability of

Table 14-15. LMWH Product SC Dosing by Disease-State Indication[79,89]

LMWH	General Surgery Prophylaxis Against DVT	Orthopedic Surgery Prophylaxis Against DVT	DVT Treatment
Dalteparin	5000 units SC daily	2500 units SC daily or 5000 units SC daily	Cancer related DVT; 200 units/kg for the first month followed by 150 units/kg daily for up to 6 months. Therapy beyond 6 months has not been established.[87,88]
Enoxaparin	40 mg SC daily[a]	30 mg SC every 12 hr[a]	1 mg/kg SC every 12 hr[a] or 1.5 mg/kg SC daily[a]
Tinzaparin	Not indicated	Not indicated	175 units/kg SC daily

[a]Dosing guidelines for enoxaparin in patients with severe renal impairment (creatinine clearance <30 ml/min) are as follows: For approved prophylaxis indications (hip and knee replacement, general abdominal surgery and medical prophylaxis) the dose is 30 mg SC daily. For approved treatment indications (acute coronary syndromes and DVT with or without PE) the dose is 1 mg/kg SC daily.[80,86]

For the dosing of enoxaparin in renal failure, analysis was primarily done from patients with Scr values below 2.5. Dosing of enoxaparin when the CrCl is less than 20 ml/min remains unclear beyond regimens explored to maintain the dialysis circuit.[86,90] For tinzaparin of dalteparin, no dosing adjustment is necessary above 20 ml/min.[86]

LMWHs at low doses and their more predictable anticoagulation response in non-critically ill patients. LMWHs also do not bind to endothelial cells (in culture), a property that could account for their longer half-life and dose independent clearance.[76] Active and inactive fragments of LMWHs are partially cleared by the kidney and their half-life is increased in patients with renal failure.[101-103] Pharmacokinetic and pharmacodynamic differences among the LMWHs are shown in Table 14-14.

LMWH: Dosing Strategies

Guidelines for treating and monitoring venous thromboembolism (VTE) with LMWHs

Suspected VTE[2]

- Obtain baseline aPTT, PT/INR, platelet count, and CBC.
- Check for contraindication to heparin therapy.
- For patients with a high clinical suspicion of DVT, ACCP Guidelines (8th edition) recommend initiating treatment with immediate acting parenteral anticoagulant while awaiting the outcome of diagnostic tests. See treatment guidelines for confirmed VTE in UFH and LMWH sections.
- Order imaging study.

Confirmed VTE[2]

- In patients with acute VTE, ACCP recommendations (8th edition) cite initial treatment with LMWH once or twice daily over UFH as an outpatient if possible and as an inpatient if necessary.[2]
- Start VKA (e.g., warfarin) therapy on day 1; adjust subsequent daily dosing according to INR. See warfarin chapter for detailed discussion of warfarin initiation.
- For patients who first received UFH and are now on LMWH, ACCP recommendations (8th edition) suggest platelet count monitoring every 2–3 days from days 4 to day 14, with less frequent monitoring (i.e., once weekly) taking place outside this time period until LMWH is stopped.
- For patients who have only received LMWH and would be considered to have low risk (< 0.1%) for HIT, ACCP (8th edition) recommends that clinicians not use routine platelet count monitoring.[68] However, FDA approved package labeling for the respective LMWHs still suggest continued vigilance against the potential of thrombocytopenia by periodic platelet count determinations.
- Stop LMWH after at least 5–7 days of combined therapy and once the INR is >2 and stable.
- Anticoagulate with VKA for 3 or more months (patient/disease-state specific).

LMWH: Therapeutic Range

LMWHs have been monitored by use of anti-Factor Xa heparin concentrations.[2,104] Desired anti-Factor Xa heparin activity concentrations for twice daily dosing in venous embolic disease are 0.6–1 units/ml[2] and 0.5–1 units/ml for arterial embolic disease and acute coronary syndromes.[85,104,105] For patients receiving once daily dosing, a target range of 1–2 units/ml has been suggested, but no recommendations are currently available due to lack of supporting data.[56] If used, measurements for anti-Factor Xa should be taken 4 hours after an SC dose.[56]

LMWH: Therapeutic Monitoring

LMWHs are not monitored by aPTT determinations. Anti-Factor Xa measurements are not recommended by the manufacturers nor The Eighth ACCP Conference on Antithrombotic and Thrombolytic Therapy for routine monitoring treatment with these agents.

LMWH: Assay Issues

Different assays and instrumentation along with correct measuring of anti-Factor Xa can result in notable differences in reported values. Practitioners should be aware of their institution's methods and how these values compare to other observations or established standards

LMWH: Pharmacodynamic Monitoring—Concentration-Related Efficacy

It is generally accepted that some minimum concentration of LMWH must be maintained to achieve an effective antithrombotic state and that inadequate anticoagulant therapy results in higher rates of thromboembolic disease recurrence. Animal experiments support the concept that a plasma concentration of heparin between 0.2 and 0.4 units/ml (measured by protamine sulfate titration) is necessary to interrupt an ongoing thrombotic process.[106] Studies examining the efficacy of LMWHs for treatment of thromboembolic disease have often used symptomatic recurrent disease as the end-point. No differences in outcomes for recurrence of thromboembolic disease have been noted for LMWHs when compared to titrated UFH.[107,108] For prophylaxis against thromboembolic disease, development of a VTE or bleeding has been end-points for determining lack of efficacy and toxicity.

Much of the literature focused on the utility of anti-Factor Xa measurements for monitoring patients receiving LMWHs gives conflicting information on decisions that should be made with the results. In general, the therapeutic range with this class of agents is wide enough that monitoring is not perceived to be necessary. Post marketing, some special dosing populations have been suggested as potentially benefiting from monitoring anti-Factor Xa activity. Recommendations of the Eighth ACCP Conference on Antithrombotic and Thrombolytic Therapy are to avoid monitoring concentrations for LMWH therapies except in pregnant women, neonates, and children receiving therapeutic doses. The recommendations to avoid monitoring are due in large part to the absence of data correlating anti-Factor Xa values with clinical outcomes.

Caution should be exercised when interpreting measured anti-Factor Xa values. Data suggest a high degree of variability in the measured anti-Factor Xa activity at standard dosing in both obese[83] and normal weight patients. Due to the limited information on dosing in the obese population, common sense would suggest the need for monitoring anti-Factor Xa and adjusting the dose if necessary. Unfortunately, therapeutic outcomes associated with this approach are unknown, and given the variability in assay methods, the potential exists for this approach to lead to either over or under dosing the patient.

LMWH: Pharmacodynamic Monitoring—Concentration-Related Toxicity

The antithrombotic and hemorrhagic effects of LMWHs have been compared with UFH in various experimental animal models. When compared on a gravimetric basis, LMWHs exhibit decreased potential for hemorrhagic episodes in animal models.

Contemporary studies evaluating alternative regimens of continuous infusion unfractionated heparin (CIUFH) versus LMWHs reveal rates of major bleeding ranging from 0 to 7% for CIUFH and rates of fatal bleeding ranging from 0% to 2%. For LMWHs the rates of major bleeding range from 0% to 3% and fatal bleeding from 0% to 0.8%. These data suggest that LMWHs do not result in increased risk of major bleeding compared to UFH.[107] Differences in the relative antithrombotic to hemorrhagic ratios among these polysaccharides might be explained by the observations that LMWHs have less inhibitory effects on platelet function and vascular permeability.[76]

The potential for neuraxial hematoma exists if epidural, spinal anesthesia, or other spinal punctures are performed while patients are anticoagulated for prevention of thromboembolic complications with any of the LMWHs or heparinoids.

LMWHs have been found to have a lessened incidence of thrombocytopenia compared to UFH,[76] but patients with antibodies to UFH may have similar reactions to LMWHs, leading to heparin-induced thrombocytopenia.[68] Because of the high incidence of cross reactivity with heparin antibodies, LMWH should be avoided in patients with HIT.

LMWH: Reversing the Effect of LMWHs

The effect of LMWHs may be partially reversed by protamine sulfate, but care should be taken to avoid overdosing as it may also cause bleeding. Higher sulfated compounds (Tinzaparin > Dalteparin > Enoxaparin) may be neutralized to a greater extent by protamine, but the clinical significance of this is unclear.[109] Administration of protamine can also cause severe hypotension and anaphylactic reactions. Slow intravenous injection of 1 mg of protamine for every 100 anti-Factor Xa International Units of dalteparin or 1 mg of enoxaparin has been recommended by their manufacturers for reversal if less than 8 hours has elapsed since the dose of LMWH. Based on time of dose of the LMWH relative to the hemorrhagic complication, protamine sulfate may not be necessary. Table 14-16 gives guidelines for reversal of LMWHs with respect to time since the last LMWH dose.

Table 14-16. Protamine Doses for Reversal of LMWHs[a]

LMWH	<8 hr	8–12 hr	>12 hr
Dalteparin	1 mg/100 anti-Factor Xa units	0.5 mg/100 anti-Factor Xa units	Not necessary
Enoxaparin	1 mg/1 mg	0.5 mg/1 mg	Not necessary
Tinzaparin	1 mg/100 anti-Factor Xa units	0.5 mg/100 anti-Factor Xa units	Not necessary

[a]Prescribing directions for protamine sulfate should be carefully followed due to the risks associated with its use. Doses of 50 mg of protamine should not be exceeded. The risk of severe adverse reactions, such as hypotension and bradycardia, can be minimized by administering protamine slowly (i.e., over approximately 10 minutes).

LMWH: Drug-Drug Interactions

Similar to UFH, LMWHs do not have definitively identified drug interactions, although platelet-inhibiting drugs or drugs irritating to the gastrointestinal tract could theoretically lead to complications. See Table 14-13 for heparin drug interactions.

LMWH: Drug–Disease State or Condition Interaction

LMWHs bind less avidly than UFH to the acute phase reactant plasma proteins that are often increased during illness. Endogenous plasma proteins, platelet factor 4 (released from activated platelets), and von Willebrand's factor are circulating substances released during illness and clotting respectively. Thromboembolic disease and comorbid conditions account for variability of these plasma proteins that, in turn, causes variable anticoagulant responsiveness with UFH. Such variability is seen less often with LMWHs because of their decreased binding to these acute phase reactant substances and their improved bioavailability.

Smaller doses of LMWHs are used for prophylaxis than for documented thromboembolic disease. As might be expected, low-weight patients treated with fixed prophylaxis doses (non–weight adjusted) of enoxaparin show an increase in exposure (AUC). These patients, and perhaps patients of low weight treated with other LMWHs, should be observed carefully for signs and symptoms of bleeding. The safety and optimal use of prophylactic doses of LMWHs in elderly patients with impaired renal function was evaluated in 125 elderly patients (mean ± SD age 87.5 ± 6.3 years, body weight 56.4 ± 11.9 kg and CrCl 39.8 ± 16.1 ml/min) who received 40 mg daily doses of enoxaparin for up to 10 days.[110] The authors reported that the mean anti-Factor Xa concentration was 0.64 ± 0.23 units/ml (range 0.24–1.5) and concluded that CrCl < 30 ml/min and bodyweight < 50 kg were associated with significantly higher maximal anti-Factor Xa activity. Larger clinical trials assessing the safety of LMWH in elderly patients are needed to determine the clinical relevance of these findings.

Anti-Factor Xa concentrations are not significantly increased when LMWHs are administered to obese patients in doses based on TBW. This observation has been made for enoxaparin in patients with TBW up to 144 kg (body mass index [BMI] = 48); dalteparin in patients with TBW up to 190 kg (BMI = 58); and tinzaparin in patients with TBW up to 165 kg (BMI = 61).[2,86]

Though current product labeling for LMWHs make no specific recommendations for prophylaxis dosing in obese patients (BMI > 30), recommendations of The Seventh ACCP Conference on Antithrombotic and Thrombolytic Therapy state that "in the absence of clear data, it seems prudent to consider a 25% increase in the fixed thromboprophylactic dose of LMWHs in very obese patients."[29] The Eighth ACCP conference suggests that for general surgical patients at higher risk, "higher than standard doses of LMWH" should be used.[111]

There are conflicting data on the use of LMWHs and monitoring anti-Factor Xa activity in renally impaired patients. These include questions on the appropriate cutoff value that defines renal impairment that correlates with an increased risk of bleeding. The Eighth ACCP Conference observed that for this patient population most well-designed studies demonstrated increased anti-Factor Xa activity in patients with diminished renal function and that the pharmacokinetic effect of impaired renal function may differ among LMWHs.[2,6] One analysis showed that once-daily administration of a full dose of enoxaparin did not result in accumulation among non-hemodialysis patients with a CrCl ≤30 ml/min.[83] However, it has been suggested that individuals with CrCl between 30 and 60 ml/min receive a 25% reduction in the dose.[90] The manufacturer's recommendation and Food and Drug Administration approved labeling for enoxaparin suggests a dosage reduction and interval increase (e.g., 30 mg administered SC once daily for any approved prophylaxis indication; 1 mg/kg administered once daily for any approved treatment indication) for patients with CrCl ≤30 ml/min (excluding hemodialysis patients).[80]

Summary of LMWH Dosing and Monitoring

LMWHs represent a breakthrough in the management of venous and arterial thromboembolic disease. Though considerably more expensive, these drugs have better bioavailability, a longer half-life, are easy to administer, require less monitoring, and have a more predictable anticoagulant effect than standard UFH. LMWHs administered subcutaneously and without laboratory monitoring in doses determined by body weight for treatment indications will likely continue to shift management strategies from standard UFH to LMWHs in both inpatient and outpatient settings. The LMWHs along with fondaparinux offer a choice for initiating management in the home setting.

Fondaparinux

Fondaparinux is the 5-sugar moiety analogue of the pentasaccharide binding sequence that allows heparin to exact activity through antithrombin, and it has highly selective anti-Factor Xa activity. It does not appreciably inhibit factor IIa. Unlike UFH or the LMWHs, it is a synthetic compound. Fondaparinux can rapidly bind to AT causing an irreversible conformational change. It is subsequently released, allowing binding to other AT molecules. The absence of the additional chains may diminish its triggering of immune mediated HIT.

Fondaparinux: Dosage Range

Fondaparinux has been studied in several dose response phase II trials. In the management of proximal DVT, no differences were observed between 5 mg, 7.5 mg, and 10 mg dosing regimens for recurrent venous thromboembolism or bleeding events.[112] In the setting of acute coronary syndromes, no differences between 2.5 mg, 4 mg, 8 mg, and 12 mg were seen for the primary end points of death, myocardial infarction, recurrent ischemia, or bleeding. Overall, it appears that there are no differences in response based on doses from 2.5 mg to 10 mg.[112,113] Fondaparinux has been studied in phase III clinical trials using 2.5 mg for VTE prophylaxis in elective knee and hip replacements, hip fracture, acute coronary syndromes, high risk abdominal surgery, and for medical prophylaxis.[114-119] It has also been studied in doses of 5 mg (weight < 50 kg), 7.5 mg (weight 50–99 kg), and 10 mg (> 100 kg) in the treatment of VTE. In general, fondaparinux was found have similar efficacy to CIUFH and enoxaparin with a slight advantage in reducing recurrent thrombotic events, which was balanced by a slight increase in reported bleeding.[120]

Due to its prolonged half-life and renal elimination profile, use in individuals with a CrCl below 30 ml/min is discouraged. In patients with severe renal insufficiency or on hemodialysis, limited information exists on the safe use of fondaparinux. In limited case reports and small case series, a dose of 1.5 mg daily or 2.5 mg every other day has been explored when the CrCl is between 20 to 50 ml/min.[90] In patients on hemodialysis, 0.05 mg/kg prior to hemodialysis has provided adequate anticoagulation, but with a potential for accumulation over time.[121] Additional studies are needed to determine the safest approach to using fondaparinux in severe renal insufficiency. Generally UFH or LMWH may be preferred agents.

Fondaparinux should not be initiated until 6 to 8 hours after joint replacement procedures. In one analysis, no differences in major or minor bleeding or symptomatic VTE were observed between initiating therapy 8 ± 2 hours after surgery compared to the morning after.[122] This provides some option in the initiation of therapy postoperatively. In a meta-analysis of 4 randomized phase III clinical trial for major orthopedic surgery, a 55% reduction (13.7% vs. 6.8%) in thrombus by venography was observed with fondaparinux compared to enoxaparin.[114]

Fondaparinux: Dosage Form Availability

Fondaparinux is supplied only as a solution for injection. While FDA approved for subcutaneous administration, fondaparinux has been administered intravenously for procedural use in clinical trials.

Fondaparinux: General Pharmacokinetic Information

Fondaparinux is rapidly and completely absorbed after SC injection (F = 1) and distributes primarily into the blood (V = 7–11 liters). It is primarily eliminated renally, with 77% excreted unchanged in the urine. It has a relatively long half-life (17–21 hours) and can be administered once daily.[123] Total clearance is approximately 25% lower in patients with a CrCl of 50–80 ml/min, 40% lower when 30 to 50 ml/hr, and 55% lower when less than 30 ml/min. Peak effect is reached approximately 2 hours after SC injection and 10 minutes after IV administration.[124] PT, INR, and aPTT are not typically altered during its use. A linear relationship between the AUC and dose has been observed.[125]

Fondaparinux: Therapeutic Monitoring

Since fondaparinux exerts its anticoagulant effects thru the inhibition of activated factor Xa, it would theoretically be useful to measure anti-Factor Xa activity to assess the degree of effect. A linear correlation with the concentration of fondaparinux and anti-Factor Xa activity has been demonstrated,[126] suggesting that activity could be measured using the anti-Factor Xa activity as a surrogate marker. However, the lack of a dose dependent response or other observed pharmacodynamic measures diminish the potential value of using anti-Factor Xa activity.

Fondaparinux: Reversing the Effect of Fondaparinux

Because of the small molecular size of fondaparinux and the lack of sulfide bonds, protamine is not considered effective in reversing the effects of this drug. The use of rFVIIa has been explored, with some ability to re-establish hemostasis observed for a short period of time.[127-129] In one ex-vivo analysis, low dose prothrombin complex concentrate containing activated clotting factors (FEIBA® 20 units/kg) showed enhanced reversal of anticoagulation over rFVIIa in thrombin production.[130] The suggested explanation is the presence of multiple clotting factors including prothrombin that are already bound to free factor Xa encourages thrombin generation, and that the anti-Factor Xa activity from fondaparinux might inhibit free factor Xa and diminish the impact of rFVIIa.

Fondaparinux: Drug-Condition Interactions

Early observations suggested that fondaparinux might be an option for the treatment or prophylaxis of DVT/PE in patients with heparin-induced thrombocytopenia.[67,68] This may be attributed to the limited ability for the small molecule to trigger platelet factor 4 and the immune mediated response leading to HIT.[131] Single center analysis and case series have also suggested that the lack of a immune response and limited cross reactivity with HIT antibodies make fondaparinux a viable anticoagulation option during management of HIT.[132,133] However, cases of fondaparinux induced HIT have been reported.[134] The ability to administer an agent once daily and avoid more continuous infusion direct thrombin inhibitors has made fondaparinux an attractive option, especially after platelet count recovery and clinical stability has occurred. Given the lack of clinical trials for this use, it is unclear the role fondaparinux has in the management of HIT.

References

1. Smythe MA, Nutescu EA, Wittkowsky AK. Changes in the USP heparin monograph and implications for clinicians. *Pharmacotherapy.* 2010;30(5):428-31.
2. Kearon C, Kahn SR, Agnelli G, et al. Antithrombotic therapy for venous thromboembolic disease: American College of Chest Physicians evidence-based clinical practice guidelines. *Chest.* 2008;133(Suppl 6):454S-545S.
3. Harrington RA, Becker RC, Cannon CP, et al. Antithrombotic therapy for Non–ST-Segment Elevation acute coronary syndromes: American College of Chest Physicians evidence-based clinical practice guidelines. *Chest.* 2008;133(Suppl 6);670S-707S.
4. Riney JN, Hollands JM, Smith JR, et al. Identifying optimal initial infusion rates for unfractionated heparin in morbidly obese patients. *Ann Pharmacotherapy.* 2010;44(7-8):1141-51.
5. Raschke RA, Reilly BM, Guidry JR, et al. The weight-based heparin nomogram compared with a "standard care" nomogram: a randomized controlled trial. *Ann Intern Med.* 1993;119(9):874-81.
6. Hirsh J, Bauer KA, Donati MB, et al. Parenteral anticoagulants: American College of Chest Physicians evidence-based clinical practice guidelines. *Chest.* 2008;133(Suppl 6):141S-159S.
7. Laslett L, White R. Predictors of the effect of heparin during cardiac catheterization. *Cardiology.* 1995;86(5):380-3.
8. Goodman SG, Menon V, Cannon CP, et al. Acute ST-segment elevation myocardial infarction: American College of Chest Physicians evidence-based clinical practice guidelines. *Chest.* 2008;133(Suppl 6):708S-775S.
9. Yee WP, Norton LL. Optimal weight base for a weight-based heparin dosing protocol. *Am J Health Syst Pharm.* 1998;55(2):159-62.
10. Cipolle RJ, Rodvold KA. Heparin. In: Evans WE, Schentag JJ, Jusko WJ, eds. *Applied Pharmacokinetics: Principles of Therapeutic Drug Monitoring.* 2nd ed. Spokane, WA: Applied Therapeutics; 1986:908-43.

11. Bara L, Billaud E, Gramond G, et al. Comparative pharmacokinetics of a low molecular weight heparin (PK 10 169) and unfractionated heparin after intravenous and subcutaneous administration. *Thromb Res.* 1985;39:631-36.
12. Kandrotas RJ, Gal P, Douglas JB, et al. Heparin pharmacokinetics during hemodialysis. *Ther Drug Monit.* 1989;11(6):674-9.
13. Teoh KH, Young E, Blackall MH, et al. Can extra protamine eliminate heparin rebound following cardiopulmonary bypass surgery? *J Thorac Cardiovasc Surg.* 2004;128(2):211-9.
14. Rosborough TK. Monitoring unfractionated heparin therapy with antifactor Xa activity results in fewer monitoring tests and dosage changes than monitoring with the activated partial thromboplastin time. *Pharmacotherapy.* 1999;19:760–6.
15. Young E, Prins MH, Levine MN, et al. Heparin binding to plasma proteins, an important mechanism for heparin resistance. *Thromb Haemost.* 1992;67(6):639-43.
16. de Swart CA, Nijmeyer B, Roelofs JM, et al. Kinetics of intravenously administered heparin in normal humans. *Blood.* 1982;60(6):1251-8.
17. Olsson P, Lagergren H, Ek S. The elimination from plasma of intravenous heparin: an experimental study on dogs and humans. *Acta Med Scand.* 1963;173:619-30.
18. Bjornsson TO, Wolfram BS, Kitchell BB. Heparin kinetics determined by three assay methods. *Clin Pharmacol Ther.* 1982;31:104-13.
19. McDonald MM, Jacobson LJ, Hay WW, et al. Heparin clearance in the newborn. *Pediatr Res.* 1981;15(7):1015-8.
20. Simon TL, Hyers TM, Gaston JP, et al. Heparin pharmacokinetics: increased requirements in pulmonary embolism. *Br J Haematol.* 1978;39:111-20.
21. Hirsh J, van Aken WG, Gallus AS, et al. Heparin kinetics in venous thrombosis and pulmonary embolism. *Circulation.* 1976;53:681–95.
22. Green TP, Isham-Schopf B, Irmiter R, et al. Inactivation of heparin during extracorporeal circulation in infants. *Clin Pharmacol Ther.* 1990;48:148-54.
23. Estes JW. Kinetics of the anticoagulant effect of heparin. *JAMA.* 1970;212(9):1492-5.
24. Cipolle RJ, Seifert RD, Nellan BA, et al. Heparin kinetics: variables related to disposition and dosage. *Clin Pharmacol Ther.* 1981;29(3):387-93.
25. Perry PJ, Herron GR, King JC. Heparin half-life in normal and impaired renal function. *Clin Pharmacol Ther.* 1974;16(3):514-9.
26. Bull BS, Korpman RA, Huse WM, et al. Heparin therapy during extracorporeal circulation. *J Thorac Cardiovasc Surg.* 1975;69(5):674-84.
27. Dager W. Unfractionated heparin. In: Dager W, Gulseth M, Nutescu E, eds. *Anticoagulation Therapy: A Point-Of-Care Guide.* Bethesda, MD: American Society of Health-System Pharmacists; 2011.
28. Chiou WL, Gadella MA, Peng GW. Method for the rapid estimation of the total body clearance and adjustment of dosage regiments in patients during a constant-rate intravenous infusion. *J Pharmacokinet Biopharm.* 1978;6(2):135-51.
29. Hirsh J, Raschke R. Heparin and low-molecular-weight-heparin: the seventh ACCP conference on antithrombotic and thrombolytic therapy. *Chest.* 2004;126(3 Suppl):188S-203S.
30. Cruickshank MK, Levine MN, Hirsh J, et al. A standard heparin nomogram for the management of heparin therapy. *Arch Intern Med.* 1991;151(2):333-7.
31. Groce JB, Gal P, Douglas JB, et al. Heparin dosage adjustment in patients with deep-vein thrombosis using heparin concentrations rather than activated partial thromboplastin time. *Clin Pharm.* 1987;6(3):216-22.
32. Kandrotas RJ, Gal P, Douglas JB, et al. Rapid determination of maintenance heparin infusion rates with the use of non-steady-state heparin concentrations. *Ann Pharmacother.* 1993;27(12):1429-33.
33. Ellison MJ, Sawyer WT, Mills TC. Calculation of heparin dosage in a morbidly obese woman. *Clin Pharm.* 1989;8(1):65-8.
34. Thaler E, Lechner K. Antithrombin III deficiency and thromboembolism. *Clin Haematol.* 1981;10(2):369-90.
35. Raschke R, Hirsh J, Guidry JR. Suboptimal monitoring and dosing of unfractionated heparin in comparative studies with low-molecular-weight heparin. *Ann Intern Med.* 2003;138(9):720-3.
36. Young JA, Kisker CT, Doty DB. Adequate anticoagulation during cardiopulmonary bypass determined by activated clotting time and the appearance of fibrin monomer. *Ann Thorac Surg.* 1978;26(3):231-40.
37. Cohen JA. Activated coagulation time method for control of heparin is reliable during cardiopulmonary bypass. *Anesthesiology.* 1984;60:121-4.
38. Basu D, Gallus A, Hirsh J, et al. A prospective study of the value of monitoring heparin treatment with the activated partial thromboplastin time. *N Engl J Med.* 1972;287(7):324-7.
39. Hull RD, Raskob GE, Hirsh J, et al. Continuous intravenous heparin compared with intermittent subcutaneous heparin in the initial treatment of proximal-vein thrombosis. *N Engl J Med.* 1986;315:1109–14.

40. Taberner DA, Poller L, Thomson JM, et al. Randomized study of adjusted versus fixed low dose heparin prophylaxis of deep vein thrombosis in hip surgery. *Br J Surg.* 1989 Sep;76(9):933-5.

41. Leyvraz PF, Richard J, Bachmann F, et al. Adjusted versus fixed-dose subcutaneous heparin in the prevention of deep-vein thrombosis after total hip replacement. *N Engl J Med.* 1983;309(16):954-8.

42. Hahn CL. Pulsatile heparin administration in pregnancy: a new approach. *Am J Obstet Gynecol.* 1986;155(2):283-7.

43. Urlesberger B, Zobel G, Zenz W, et al. Activation of the clotting system during extracorporeal membrane oxygenation in term newborn infants. *J Pediatr.* 1996;129(2):264-8.

44. Brandt JT, Triplett DA. Laboratory monitoring of heparin. Effect of reagents and instruments on the activated partial thromboplastin time. *Am J Clin Pathol.* 1981;76(4 Suppl):530-7.

45. Banez EI, Triplett DA, Koepke J. Laboratory monitoring of heparin therapy—the effect of different salts of heparin on the activated partial thromboplastin time. *Am J Clin Pathol.* 1980;74(4 Suppl):569-74.

46. Bain B, Forster T, Sleigh B. Heparin and the activated partial thromboplastin time--a difference between the in-vitro and in-vivo effects and implications for the therapeutic range. *Am J Clin Pathol.* 1980;74(5):668-73.

47. Hattersley PG. Progress report: the activated coagulation time of whole blood (ACT). *Am J Clin Pathol.* 1976;66(5):899-904.

48. Uden DL, Payne NR, Kriesmer P, et al. Procedural variables which affect activated clotting time test results during extracorporeal membrane oxygenation therapy. *Crit Care Med.* 1989;17(10):1048-51.

49. Hasegawa H, Oguma Y, Takei H, et al. Assay of heparin in plasma using a chromogenic substrate and its clinical applications. *Jpn Heart J.* 1980;21(3):367-80.

50. Holm HA, Abildgaard U, Larsen ML, et al. Monitoring of heparin therapy: should heparin assays also reflect the patient's antithrombin concentration? *Thromb Res.* 1987;46(5):669-75.

51. Kandrotas RJ. Heparin pharmacokinetics and pharmacodynamics. *Clin Pharmacokinet.* 1992;22(5):359-74.

52. Gosselin RC, Smythe MA. Coagulation laboratory considerations. In: Dager W, Gulseth M, Nutescu E, eds. *Anticoagulation Therapy: A Point-of-Care Guide.* Bethesda, MD: American Society of Health-System Pharmacists; 2011.

53. Brill-Edwards P, Ginsberg JS, Johnston M, et al. Establishing a therapeutic range for heparin therapy. *Ann Intern Med.* 1993;119(2):104-9.

54. Schulman S, Beyth RJ, Kearon C, et al. Hemorrhagic complications of anticoagulant and thrombolytic treatment: American College of Chest Physicians evidence-based clinical practice guidelines. *Chest.* 2008;133(Suppl 6):257S-298S.

55. Braunwald E, Antman EM, Beasley JW, et al. ACC/AHA guideline update for the management of patients with unstable angina and non-ST-segment elevation myocardial infarction—2002: summary article. *Circulation.* 2002;106(14):1893-900.

56. Laposata M, Green D, Van Cott EM, et al. College of American Pathologists Conference XXXI on laboratory monitoring of anticoagulant therapy: the clinical use and laboratory monitoring of low-molecular-weight heparin, danaparoid, hirudin and related compounds, and argatroban. *Arch Pathol Lab Med.* 1998;122(9):799-807.

57. Holm HA, Kalvenes S, Abildgaard U. Changes in plasma antithrombin (heparin cofactor activity) during intravenous heparin therapy: observations in 198 patients with deep venous thrombosis. *Scand J Haematol.* 1985;35(5):564-9.

58. Rosenberg RD. Heparin, antithrombin, and abnormal clotting. *Annu Rev Med.* 1978;29:367-78.

59. Rosenberg RD. Biochemistry of heparin antithrombin interactions, and the physiologic role of this natural anticoagulant mechanism. *Am J Med.* 1989;87(3B):2S-9S.

60. Batist G, Bothe A, Bern M, et al. Low antithrombin III in morbid obesity: return to normal with weight reduction. *J Parenter Enteral Nutr.* 1983;7(5):447-9.

61. Triplett DA. Heparin: biochemistry, therapy, and laboratory monitoring. *Ther Drug Monit.* 1979;1(2):173-97.

62. Levine SP, Sorenson RR, Harris MA, et al. The effect of platelet factor 4 (PF4) on assays of plasma heparin. *Br J Haematol.* 1984;57(4):585-96.

63. Andersson TR, Bangstad H, Larsen ML. Heparin cofactor II, antithrombin and protein C in plasma from term and preterm infants. *Acta Paediatr Scand.* 1988;77(4):485-8.

64. Decousus HA, Croze M, Levi FA, et al. Circadian changes in anticoagulant effect of heparin infused at a constant rate. *Br Med J (Clin Res Ed).* 1985;290(6465):341-4.

65. Levine MN, Hirsh J. Hemorrhagic complications of anticoagulant therapy. *Semin Thromb Hemost.* 1986;12(1):39-57.

66. Nelson JC, Lerner RG, Goldstein R, et al. Heparin-induced thrombocytopenia. *Arch Intern Med.* 1978;138(4):548-52.

67. Dager WE, Dougherty JA, Nguyen PH, et al. Heparin-induced thrombocytopenia: treatment options and special considerations. *Pharmacotherapy.* 2007;27(4):564-87.

68. Warkentin TE, Greinacher A, Koster A, et al. Treatment and prevention of heparin-induced thrombocytopenia: American College of Chest Physicians evidence-based clinical practice guidelines. *Chest.* 2008;133(6 Suppl):340S-380S.

69. Griffith GC, Nichols G, Asher JD, et al. Heparin osteoporosis. *JAMA.* 1965;193:91-4.
70. Habbab MA, Haft JI. Heparin resistance induced by intravenous nitroglycerin. A word of caution when both drugs are used concomitantly. *Arch Intern Med.* 1987;147(5):857-60.
71. Becker RC, Corrao JM, Bovill EG, et al. Intravenous nitroglycerin-induced heparin resistance: a qualitative antithrombin III abnormality. *Am Heart J.* 1990;119(6):1254-61.
72. Clifton GD, Smith MD. Thrombolytic therapy in heparin-associated thrombocytopenia with thrombosis. *Clin Pharm.* 1986;5(7):597-601.
73. Colburn WA. Pharmacologic implications of heparin interactions with other drugs. *Drug Metab Rev.* 1976;5(2):281-93.
74. Mungall D, Floyd R. Bayesian forecasting of APTT response to continuously infused heparin with and without warfarin administration. *J Clin Pharmacol.* 1989;29(11):1043-7.
75. Hull RD, Raskob GE, Rosenbloom D, et al. Heparin for 5 days as compared with 10 days in the initial treatment of proximal venous thrombosis. *N Engl J Med.* 1990;322(18):1260-4.
76. Weitz JI. Low-molecular-weight heparins. *N Engl J Med.* 1997;337(10):688-98.
77. Ofosu FA. The United States Food and Drug Administration approves a generic. *Clin Appl Thromb Hemost.* 2011;17(1):5-8.
78. Fareed J, Adiguzel C, Thethi I. Differentiation of parenteral anticoagulants in the prevention and treatment of venous thromboembolism. *Thromb J.* 2011;9(1):5.
79. Heparins. In: McEvoy GK, ed. *AHFS Drug Information 2011.* Bethesda, MD: American Society of Health-System Pharmacists; 2011.
80. Lovenox [package insert]. Bridgewater, NJ : Sanofi-Aventis Pharmaceuticals, Inc.; 2009.
81. Fragmin [package insert]. New York, NY: Pfizer Inc.; 2007.
82. Innohep [package insert]. Boulder, CO: Pharmion Corporation; 2007.
83. Bazinet A, Almanric K, Brunet C, et al. Dosage of enoxaparin among obese and renal impairment patients. *Thromb Res.* 2005;116(1):41-50.
84. Montalescot G, Cohen M, Salette G, et al. Impact of anticoagulation levels on outcomes in patients undergoing elective percutaneous coronary intervention: insights from the STEEPLE trial. *Eur Heart J.* 2008;29(4):462-71.
85. Montalescot G, Collet JP, Tanguy ML, et al. Anti-Xa activity relates to survival and efficacy in unselected acute coronary syndrome patients treated with enoxaparin. *Circulation.* 2004;110(4):392-8.
86. Nutescu EA, Spinler SA, Wittkowsky A, et al. Low-molecular-weight heparins in renal impairment and obesity: available evidence and clinical practice recommendations across medical and surgical settings. *Ann Pharmacother.* 2009;43(6):1064-83.
87. Lee AY, Levine MN, Baker RI, et al. Low-molecular-weight heparin versus a coumarin for the prevention of recurrent venous thromboembolism in patients with cancer. *N Engl J Med.* 2003;349(2):146-53.
88. Lee AY, Rickles FE, Julian JA, et al. Randomized comparison of low molecular weight heparin and coumarin derivatives on the survival of patients with cancer and venous thromboembolism. *J Clin Oncol.* 2005;23(10):2123-9.
89. Hirsh J. *Low Molecular Weight Heparins.* St. Louis, MO: B.C. Decker; 1999.
90. Dager WE, Kiser TH. Systemic anticoagulation considerations in chronic kidney disease. *Adv Chronic Kidney Dis.* 2010;17(5):420-7.
91. Dager WE, Gosselin RC, King JH, et al. Anti-Xa stability of diluted enoxaparin for use in pediatrics. *Ann Pharmacother.* 2004;38(4):569-73.
92. Goldenberg NA, Jacobson L, Hathaway H, et al. Anti-Xa stability of diluted dalteparin for pediatric use. *Ann Pharmacother.* 2008;42(4):511-5.
93. Cziraky MJ, Spinler SA. Low-molecular-weight heparins for the treatment of deep-vein thrombosis. *Clin Pharm.* 1993;12(12):892-9.
94. Hoppensteadt D, Walenga JM, Fareed J. Low molecular weight heparins. An objective overview. *Drugs Aging.* 1992;2(5):406-22.
95. Cohen M, Demers C, Gurfinkel EP, et al. A comparison of low-molecular-weight heparin with unfractionated heparin for unstable coronary artery disease. Efficacy and Safety of Subcutaneous Enoxaparin in Non-Q-Wave Coronary Events Study Group. *N Engl J Med.* 1997;337(7):447-52.
96. Mayr AJ, Dünser M, Jochberger S, et al. Antifactor Xa activity in intensive care patients receiving thromboembolic prophylaxis with standard doses of enoxaparin. *Thromb Res.* 2002;105(3):201-4.
97. Dörffler-Melly J, de Jonge E, Pont AC, et al. Bioavailability of subcutaneous low-molecular-weight heparin to patients on vasopressors. *Lancet.* 2002;359(9309):849-50.
98. Priglinger U, Delle Karth G, Geppert A, et al. Prophylactic anticoagulation with enoxaparin: Is the subcutaneous route appropriate in the critically ill? *Crit Care Med.* 2003;31(5):1405-9.

99. Malinoski D, Jafari F, Ewing T, et al. Standard prophylactic enoxaparin dosing leads to inadequate anti-Xa levels and increased deep venous thrombosis rates in critically ill trauma and surgical patients. *J Trauma.* 2010;68(4):874-80.

100. Hacquard M, Mainard D, de Maistre E, et al. Influence of injection site on prophylactic dose enoxaparin bioavailability in obese patients. *J Thromb Haemost.* 2007;5(Suppl 2):P-M-669.

101. Boneu B, Caranobe C, Cadroy Y, et al. Pharmacokinetic studies of standard unfractionated heparin, and low molecular weight heparins in the rabbit. *Semin Thromb Hemost.* 1988;14(1):18-27.

102. Caranobe C, Barret A, Gabaig AM, et al. Disappearance of circulating anti-Xa activity after intravenous injection of standard heparin and of a low molecular weight heparin (CY 216) in normal and nephrectomized rabbits. *Thromb Res.* 1985;40(1):129-33.

103. Palm M, Mattsson C. Pharmacokinetics of heparin and low molecular weight heparin fragment (Fragmin) in rabbits with impaired renal or metabolic clearance. *Thromb Haemost.* 1987;58(3):932-5.

104. Abbate R, Gori AM, Farsi A, et al. Monitoring of low-molecular-weight heparins in cardiovascular disease. *Am J Cardiol.* 1998;82(5B):33L-36L.

105. Pollack CV, Roe MT, Peterson ED. 2002 update to the ACC/AHA guidelines for the management of patients with unstable angina and non-ST-segment elevation myocardial infarction: implications for emergency department practice. *Ann Emerg Med.* 2003;41(3):355-69.

106. Chiu HM, Hirsh J, Yung WL, et al. Relationship between the anticoagulant and antithrombotic effects of heparin in experimental venous thrombosis. *Blood.* 1977;49(2):171-84.

107. Levine M, Gent M, Hirsh J, et al. A comparison of low-molecular-weight heparin administered primarily at home with unfractionated heparin administered in the hospital for proximal deep-vein thrombosis. *N Engl J Med.* 1996;334(11):677-81.

108. Koopman MM, Prandoni P, Piovella F, et al. Treatment of venous thrombosis with intravenous unfractionated heparin administered in the hospital as compared with subcutaneous low-molecular-weight heparin administered at home. The Tasman Study Group. *N Engl J Med.* 1996;334(11):682-7.

109. Crowther MA, Berry LR, Monagle PT, et al. Mechanisms responsible for the failure of protamine to inactivate low-molecular-weight heparin. *Br J Haematol.* 2002;116(1):178-86.

110. Mahe I, Gouin-Thibault I, Drouet L, et al. Elderly medical patients treated with prophylactic dosages of enoxaparin: influence of renal function on anti-Xa activity level. *Drugs Aging.* 2007;24(1):63-71.

111. Geerts WH, Bergqvist D, Pineo GF, et al. Prevention of venous thromboembolism: American College of Chest Physicians Evidence-Based Clinical Practice Guidelines (8th Edition). *Chest.* 2008;133(6 Suppl):381S-453S.

112. Treatment of proximal deep vein thrombosis with a novel synthetic compound (SR90107A/ORG31540) with pure anti-factor Xa activity: A phase II evaluation. The Rembrandt Investigators. *Circulation.* 2000;102(22):2726-31.

113. Simoons ML, Bobbink IW, Boland J, et al. A dose-finding study of fondaparinux in patients with non-ST-segment elevation acute coronary syndromes: the Pentasaccharide in Unstable Angina (PENTUA) Study. *J Am Coll Cardiol.* 2004;43(12):2183-90.

114. Turpie AG, Bauer KA, Eriksson BI, et al. Fondaparinux vs. enoxaparin for the prevention of venous thromboembolism in major orthopedic surgery: a meta-analysis of 4 randomized double-blind studies. *Arch Intern Med.* 2002;162(16):1833-40.

115. Fifth Organization to Assess Strategies in Acute Ischemic Syndromes Investigators, Yusuf S, Mehta SR, et al. Comparison of fondaparinux and enoxaparin in acute coronary syndromes. *N Engl J Med.* 2006;354(14):1464-76.

116. Yusuf S, Mehta SR, Chrolavicius S, et al. Effects of fondaparinux on mortality and reinfarction in patients with acute ST-segment elevation myocardial infarction: the OASIS-6 randomized trial. *JAMA.* 2006;295(13):1519-30.

117. Eriksson BI, Lassen MR, PENTasaccharide in HIp-FRActure Surgery Plus Investigators. Duration of prophylaxis against venous thromboembolism with fondaparinux after hip fracture surgery: a multicenter, randomized, placebo-controlled, double-blind study. *Arch Intern Med.* 2003;163(11):1337-42.

118. Agnelli G, Bergqvist D, Cohen AT, PEGASUS investigators. Randomized clinical trial of postoperative fondaparinux versus perioperative dalteparin for prevention of venous thromboembolism in high-risk abdominal surgery. *Br J Surg.* 2005;92:1212-20.

119. Cohen AT, Davidson BL, Gallus AS, et al. Efficacy and safety of fondaparinux for the prevention of venous thromboembolism in older acute medical patients: randomised placebo controlled trial. *BMJ.* 2006;332(7537):325-9.

120. Davidson BL, Büller HR, Decousus H, et al. Effect of obesity on outcomes after fondaparinux, enoxaparin, or heparin treatment for acute venous thromboembolism in the Matisse trials. *J Thromb Haemost.* 2007;5(6):1191-4.

121. Douketis J, Cook D, Meade M, et al. Prophylaxis against deep vein thrombosis in critically ill patients with severe renal insufficiency with the low-molecular-weight heparin dalteparin: an assessment of safety and pharmacodynamics: the DIRECT study. *Arch Intern Med.* 2008;168(16):1805-12.

122. Colwell CW, Kwong LM, Turpie AG, et al. Flexibility in administration of fondaparinux for prevention of symptomatic venous thromboembolism in orthopaedic surgery. *J Arthroplasty.* 2006;21(1):36-45.

123. Hawkins D. Clinical trials with factor Xa inhibition in the prevention of postoperative venous thromboembolism. *Am J Health-Syst Pharm.* 2003;60(22 Suppl 7):S6-10.

124. Vuillemenot A, Schiele F, Meneveau N, et al. Efficacy of a synthetic pentasaccharide, a pure factor Xa inhibitor, as an antithrombotic agent--a pilot study in the setting of coronary angioplasty. *Thromb Haemost.* 1999;81(2):214-20.

125. Donat F, Duret JP, Santoni A, et al. The pharmacokinetics of fondaparinux sodium in healthy volunteers. *Clin Pharmacokinet.* 2002;41(Suppl 2):1-9.

126. Klaeffling C, Piechottka G, Daemgen-von Brevern G, et al. Development and clinical evaluation of two chromogenic substrate methods for monitoring fondaparinux sodium. *Ther Drug Monit.* 2006;28(3):375-81.

127. Bijsterveld NR, Moons AH, Boekholdt SM, et al. Ability of recombinant factor VIIa to reverse the anticoagulant effect of the pentasaccharide fondaparinux in healthy volunteers. *Circulation.* 2002;106(20):2550-4.

128. Lisman T, Bijsterveld NR, Adelmeijer J, et al. Recombinant factor VIIa reverses the in vitro and ex vivo anticoagulant and profibrinolytic effects of fondaparinux. *J Thromb Haemost.*2003;1(11):2368-73.

129. Young G, Yonekawa KE, Nakagawa PA, et al. Recombinant activated factor VII effectively reverses the anticoagulant effects of heparin, enoxaparin, fondaparinux, argatroban, and bivalirudin ex vivo as measured using thromboelastography. *Blood Coagul Fibrinolysis.*2007;18(6):547-53.

130. Desmurs-Clavel H, Huchon C, Chatard B, et al. Reversal of the inhibitory effect of fondaparinux on thrombin generation by rFVIIa, aPCC and PCC. *Thromb Res.* 2009;123(5):796-8.

131. Greinacher A, Alban S, Omer-Adam MA, et al. Heparin-induced thrombocytopenia: a stoichiometry-based model to explain the differing immunogenicities of unfractionated heparin, low-molecular-weight heparin, and fondaparinux in different clinical settings. *Thromb Res.* 2008;122(2):211-20.

132. Grouzi E, Kyriakou E, Panagou I, et al. Fondaparinux for the treatment of acute heparin-induced thrombocytopenia: a single-center experience. *Clin Appl Thromb Hemost.* 2010;16(6):663-7.

133. Lobo B, Finch C, Howard A, et al. Fondaparinux for the treatment of patients with acute heparin-induced thrombocytopenia. *Thromb Haemost.* 2008;99(1):208-14.

134. Warkentin TE, Maurer BT, Aster RH. Heparin-induced thrombocytopenia associated with fondaparinux. *N Engl J Med.* 2007;356(25):2653-5.

Chapter 15

Paul E. Nolan, Jr., and Toby C. Trujillo

Lidocaine (AHFS 24:04.04.08)

Lidocaine is a class IB antiarrhythmic that is also used as a local anesthetic, analgesic, and anticonvulsant.[1] In usual serum concentrations lidocaine's cardiac electrophysiologic effects are largely limited to the His-Purkinje system and ventricular myocardium. It has minimal effects on the autonomic nervous system. Lidocaine is most often used as an alternative to other antiarrhythmic drugs in the treatment of symptomatic or life-threatening ventricular arrhythmias. Lidocaine is generally not indicated for the treatment of supraventricular arrhythmias.

Lidocaine is no longer recommended as initial treatment of isolated ventricular premature beats, couplets, or nonsustained ventricular tachycardia or as prophylaxis against ventricular arrhythmias in the setting of acute coronary syndrome/acute myocardial infarction (ACS/MI).[2] The rationale for this change in practice is that overall mortality may not be altered and may, actually, be increased.[2-6] Furthermore, the frequency of adverse effects attributed to prophylactic lidocaine are significantly greater than placebo.[2,7]

With respect to other arrhythmias, recently updated guidelines for advanced cardiac life support (ACLS) neither support nor refute the use of lidocaine in the management of defibrillation-resistant ventricular tachycardia/fibrillation (VT/VF) that fails to respond to amiodarone.[8] In the setting of ACS/MI lidocaine may be useful in terminating unstable sustained monomorphic VT with normal or low left ventricular ejection fractions as well as polymorphic VT with or without prolonged baseline QT interval.[9] However, it appears relatively ineffective in terminating hemodynamically stable, sustained monomorphic ventricular tachycardia that is unrelated to ACS/MI.[10-12] Additional antiarrhythmic uses for lidocaine include acute termination of Wolff-Parkinson-White syndrome with atrial fibrillation;[13] lidocaine-sensitive atrial tachycardia;[14] verapamil-sensitive idiopathic left ventricular tachycardia;[15] and prevention of reperfusion ventricular fibrillation following release of aortic cross-clamping in patients undergoing coronary artery bypass graft surgery.[16]

Usual Dosage Range in Absence of Clearance-Altering Factors

The dosage ranges in Table 15-1 are suggested for the treatment of ventricular arrhythmias; dosages should be adjusted according to individual requirements.[1]

Lidocaine also can be administered via an endotracheal tube or intraosseously during cardiac arrest.[1,8,17]

Dosage Form Availability

All listed preparations are intended for cardiac use (Table 15-2). Lidocaine preparations containing epinephrine (intended for anesthesia) should never be used for cardiac or anticonvulsant purposes. All lidocaine parenteral preparations are available as the hydrochloride salt and provide 86% lidocaine base (**S = 0.86**).

Table 15-3 gives the absorption of various dosage forms and administration methods. Since the intramuscular method of drug administration avoids the first-pass metabolism of the liver, bioavailability should be similar to that for intravenous lidocaine. The deltoid muscle is preferred for intramuscular administration, resulting in a superior rate and extent of absorption compared to the gluteus and vastus lateralis muscles.[18,19]

Although the oral bioavailability of lidocaine averages 39% in patients without hepatic impairment, a large intersubject variability exists due to first-pass hepatic metabolism.[20] Therapeutic lidocaine concentrations may not be rapidly and predictably attained in many patients, thus preventing its use as an oral agent.

Table 15-1. Suggested Dosage Ranges for the Treatment of Ventricular Arrhythmias[1]

Dosage Form	Initial Dosage (Lidocaine Hydrochloride)
Intravenous (bolus)	
Children (<18 years)[a]	For ACLS: 1 mg/kg, up to a maximum of 100 mg; a second dose of 0.5–1 mg/kg should be given if there is greater than a 15-minute delay from the time of the initial bolus to the start of the continuous infusion (see below). Alternatively 0.5–1 mg/kg dose via slow intravenous push at 25–50 mg/min; dose may be repeated every 3–5 min if needed; total loading dose should not exceed 3–5 mg/kg.
Adults (≥18 years)	For cardiac arrest secondary to either ventricular fibrillation or pulseless ventricular tachycardia: 1 to 1.5 mg/kg; then 0.5 to 0.75 mg/kg repeated every 5–10 minutes up to a total of 3 doses or up to 3 mg/kg. For initial treatment of (other) ventricular arrhythmias: 50–100 mg (0.7 to 1.4 mg/kg) or alternatively 1–1.5 mg/kg either at a rate of 25–50 mg/min; supplemental doses of 25–50 mg or 0.5–0.75 mg/kg every 5–10 minutes up to a maximum total loading dose of 3 mg/kg may be administered if the desired clinical response is not achieved; total dose should not exceed 300 mg in a 1-hour period.
Intraosseous dosing	Refer to intravenous bolus dosing guidelines.
Intravenous (maintenance)	
Children (<18 years)	Infusion of 10–50 μg/kg/min; with an additional 0.5–1 mg/kg bolus if clinically indicated.
Adults (≥18 years)	Infusion of 20–50 μg/kg/min (approximately 1–4 mg/min in 70 kg adult) depending on patient's clinical condition; if the arrhythmia recurs, a small bolus of 0.5 mg/kg followed by an increase in the infusion rate may be warranted.
Intramuscular	
Children (<18 years)	Not FDA-approved.
Adults (≥18 years)	300 mg (4.3 mg/kg in a 70 kg adult) injected into deltoid muscle (or lateral thigh if autoinjector device is used), with dose repeated in 60–90 min if clinically indicated.
Endotracheal[b]	
Children (< 18 years)	2-3 mg/kg flushed with 5 ml of 0.9% sodium chloride followed by 5 assisted manual ventilations.
Adults (≥ 18 years)	2 to 2.5 times the recommended IV dose and diluted in 5–10 ml of 0.9% sodium chloride or sterile water.
Oral	Not applicable.

[a]Controlled clinical studies to establish dosing schedules for lidocaine in pediatric patients have not been conducted.
[b]Optimal endotracheal doses of lidocaine for either adult or pediatric patients have not been established.

Table 15-2. Dosage Form Availability by Product[1]

Dosage Form	Product
Intravenous (bolus): 10 and 20 mg/ml	Various manufacturers
Intravenous (for infusion preparation) 100 mg/ml (1 g) and 200 mg/ml (1 or 2 g)	Various manufacturers
Intravenous (premixed infusion solution)	
4 mg/ml (1 or 2 g) in dextrose 5%	Various manufacturers
8 mg/ml (2 or 4 g) in dextrose 5%	Various manufacturers
Oral	Not available

Table 15-3. Bioavailability (*F*) of Dosage Forms

Dosage Form	Bioavailability Comments
Intravenous[20]	100% ($F = 1$)
Intramuscular	Absolute bioavailability not determined
Oral[20]	91% ± 6% for hepatically impaired patients ($F = 0.91$)
	39% ± 5% for normal patients ($F = 0.39$)

General Pharmacokinetic Information

Distribution

Following intravenous administration, the disposition of lidocaine is usually described by an open, two-compartment model.[21] However, some studies best describe lidocaine disposition by a three-compartment model.[21,22] For this chapter, a two-compartment model is assumed.

Volume of Distribution (*V*)[17,23,30]

Lidocaine is widely distributed into body tissue following distribution from the central compartment (i.e., heart, lungs, and kidneys). Table 15-4 presents the volume of distribution after administration of a single lidocaine dose to different patient populations.

Table 15-4. Volume of Distribution of Lidocaine

Population	Volume (Mean ± SD)
Adults[23]	$V_c = 0.50 \pm 0.21$ L/kg
	$V_\beta = 1.66$ L/kg[a]
	$V_{ss} = 1.32 \pm 0.27$ L/kg
Adults (endotracheal tube)[17]	$V_\beta = 1.06 \pm 0.54$ L/kg
Children[24,25]	$V_c = 0.31 \pm 0.07$ L/kg
	$V_\beta = 1.10 \pm 0.11$ L/kg
	$V_{ss} = 1.18 \pm 0.36$ L/kg
Neonates[26]	$V_\beta = 2.75 \pm 1.61$ L/kg
Elderly males[27]	$V_\beta = 2.91 \pm 0.88$ L/kg
Elderly females[27]	$V_\beta = 3.45 \pm 0.79$ L/kg
Morbidly obese adult males[28]	$V_\beta = 2.67 \pm 0.82$ L/kg[b]
Morbidly obese adult females[28]	$V_\beta = 2.88 \pm 1.03$ L/kg[b]
Chronic CHF[29]	$V_c = 0.30$ L/kg[c]
	$V_{ss} = 0.88$ L/kg[c]
Chronic hepatic dysfunction[29]	$V_c = 0.61$ L/kg[c]
	$V_{ss} = 2.31$ L/kg[c]
Chronic renal failure[29]	$V_c = 0.55$ L/kg[c]
(receiving hemodialysis)	$V_{ss} = 1.20$ L/kg[c]
Severe trauma[30]	$V_c = 0.26 \pm 0.15$ L/kg[d]
	$V_{ss} = 0.72 \pm 0.28$ L/kg[d]

[a]Calculated using $V_\beta = (CL_{total})/k$.
[b]Based on actual body weight.
[c]Only mean data reported.
[d]Patients had no prior history of significant cardiac, pulmonary, hepatic, or renal disease.
Vc = volume of central compartment; Vss = volume steady-state.

Elimination

Determination of the total body or systemic clearance (CL_{total} or $CL_{systemic}$) of lidocaine depends on the method of administration. Compared to a single intravenous bolus dose, the CL_{total} decreases during a prolonged (longer than 24 hr) constant-rate infusion (i.e., time-dependent pharmacokinetics).[22,31,32] The magnitude of the reduction in CL_{total} of lidocaine with a continuous infusion may depend on its absolute duration as well as on the patient's underlying clinical condition.

The mechanism for the time-dependent decline in CL_{total} of lidocaine is a reduction in the intrinsic clearance of lidocaine mediated either by lidocaine itself[33] or by monoethylglycinexylidide (MEGX), its principal metabolite.[34]

Lidocaine is extensively hepatically metabolized via sequential deethylation steps by several cytochrome P450 isozymes: CYP3A4, CYP3A5, and CYP1A2.[21,35-39] CYP1A2 may be principally responsible for lidocaine biotransformation at clinically relevant lidocaine concentrations in individuals with normal hepatic function.[38,39] The hepatic extraction ratio is high, ranging from 62% to 81% of the dose administered.[20] As with other highly extracted drugs, hepatic blood flow appears to be the primary determinant of clearance.[40,41] However, changes in lidocaine clearance also can result from hepatic enzyme induction or inhibition.[21,41] Therefore, alterations in either hepatic blood flow or intrinsic hepatic metabolic capacity can influence the elimination of lidocaine.

The hepatic metabolism of lidocaine results in the formation of two active metabolites, MEGX and glycinexylidide (GX) (Table 15-5).[34,42,47] MEGX may contribute to both the therapeutic and toxic effects, whereas GX may contribute to the toxicity.

Conditions that decrease lidocaine clearance also may potentially decrease MEGX clearance, resulting in increased adverse effects secondary to accumulation of MEGX.[34,43] On the other hand, patients with renal impairment may be at greater risk of adverse effects secondary to accumulation of GX.[43,44]

Protein binding

Protein binding of lidocaine depends on many variables, including drug concentration, type and concentration of plasma proteins, sample collection method, pH, and quantification method.[21] Lidocaine exhibits concentration-dependent binding; that is, the degree of binding decreases as the total (bound plus unbound) drug concentration increases.[48] Although lidocaine binds to albumin (approximately 25%), alpha-1-acid glycoprotein (AAG), an acute phase reactant, serves as the primary binding protein (approximately 50%).

The concentration of AAG may be significantly altered by disease, stress, or other clinical situations.[49-57] Decreased concentrations of AAG result in a higher unbound fraction of lidocaine (increased free drug concentration) and possibly increased pharmacologic and/or toxic effects at any given total lidocaine concentration. Conversely, increased AAG levels decrease the proportion of unbound (active) drug and may decrease the pharmacologic effect at any given total lidocaine concentration.

Displacement of lidocaine bound to AAG by another basic drug (e.g., disopyramide, quinidine, propranolol, and tricyclic antidepressants) may result in a higher free fraction of lidocaine, but without significant enhancement of the pharmacologic or toxic effect.[50-52,58]

Table 15-5. Formation and Activity of Lidocaine Metabolites[34,42-47]

Compound	Amount Excreted in Urine[a]	Antiarrhythmic Activity	Pro-Convulsant Activity
Lidocaine	2%	Yes	Yes
MEGX	4%	Yes	Yes
GX	2.5%	No[b]	Yes
4-OH 2,6-xylidine	73%	No	No
Others	10%–20%	No	No

[a]Percentage of administered lidocaine dose.
[b]GX has only 10% of the antiarrhythmic activity of lidocaine. GX's antiarrhythmic activity is not clinically significant.

Clearance (CL)

The clearance of lidocaine in different patient populations determined during different administration techniques are presented in Table 15-6. Aging as well as a variety of diseases and body conditions alter lidocaine clearance.

Half-Life and Time to Steady State

Unless otherwise specified, the half-lives and anticipated times to steady state in Table 15-7 are based on intravenous bolus dosing. As previously described, clearance decreases with prolonged infusions of lidocaine, thus increasing the half-life and time to steady state.[31,32] When time to steady state is assessed, the method of drug administration must be considered along with patient population characteristics.[19,31,32]

Dosing Strategies

The optimal dosing strategy for lidocaine should rapidly achieve and consistently maintain therapeutic concentrations. However, the multicompartmental disposition characteristics of lidocaine, the interpatient variability in its pharmacokinetics, and its relatively narrow therapeutic index make designing a dosing strategy somewhat difficult.

Loading doses of lidocaine are required to quickly attain adequate concentrations within the central compartment. Following distribution in the central compartment, lidocaine rapidly moves into the peripheral

Table 15-6. Clearance of Lidocaine[17,23,24,26,28-30,59-62]

Population[a]	Clearance (Mean ± SD)	Mode of Administration
Adults[23]	0.72 ± 0.15 L/hr/kg	Single dose
Adults[31]	0.51 ± 0.13 L/hr/kg	Continuous infusion
Adults (endotracheal tube)[17]	0.55 ± 0.18 L/hr/kg	Single dose
Children[24]	0.71 ± 0.2 L/hr/kg	Single dose
Neonates[26]	0.61 ± 0.38 L/hr/kg	Single dose
Morbidly obese adult males[28]	0.69 ± 0.22 L/hr/kg[b]	Single dose
Morbidly obese adult females[28]	0.68 ± 0.17 L/hr/kg[b]	Single dose
Chronic CHF[29]	0.38 L/hr/kg[c]	Single dose
Chronic CHF[59]	0.23 ± 0.08 L/hr/kg	Continuous infusion
Mild to moderate chronic CHF[59]	0.35 L/hr/kg[c]	Continuous infusion
Severe chronic CHF[59]	0.12 L/hr/kg[c]	Continuous infusion
Chronic hepatic dysfunction[29] (hepatic dysfunction level unspecified)	0.42 ± 0.19 L/hr/kg	Single dose
Child-Pugh Class A hepatic dysfunction[60]	0.41 L/hr/kg[c]	Single dose
Child-Pugh Class B hepatic dysfunction[60]	0.31 L/hr/kg[c]	Single dose
Child-Pugh Class C hepatic dysfunction[60]	0.25 L/hr/kg[c]	Single dose
Chronic renal failure (with dialysis)[29]	0.82 L/hr/kg[c]	Single dose
Chronic renal failure without dialysis[61] (CrCl<30 mL/min/1.73m^2)	0.36 ± 0.15 L/hr/kg	Single dose
Acute myocardial infarction without heart failure[62]	0.54 ± 0.12 L/hr/kg[d]	Continuous infusion
Acute myocardial infarction with heart failure[62]	0.33 ± 0.09 L/hr/kg[d]	Continuous infusion
Severe trauma[30]	0.40 ± 0.10 L/hr/kg	Single dose

[a]Most studies had small numbers of patients.
[b]Based on actual body weight.
[c]Only mean data reported.
[d]Blood to plasma conversion applied.

Table 15-7. Half-Life and Time to Steady State for Lidocaine

Population	Terminal Half-Life (Mean ± SD)	Time to Steady State[a]
Adults[23]	1.6 ± 0.4 hr	6–10 hr
Adults (endotracheal tube)[17]	1.2 ± 0.5 hr	3.5–8.5 hr
Children[24]	1.0 ± 0.3 hr	3.5–6.5 hr
Neonates[26]	3.2 ± 0.1 hr	15.5–16.5 hr
Elderly males[27]	2.7 ± 0.5 hr	11–16 hr
Elderly females[27]	2.3 ± 0.6 hr	8.5–14.5 hr
Morbidly obese adult males[28]	2.7 ± 0.8 hr	9.5–17.5 hr
Morbidly obese adult females[28]	3.0 ± 1.0 hr	10–20 hr
Chronic CHF[29]	1.9 hr[b]	9.5 hr
Chronic hepatic dysfunction[29] (degree of hepatic dysfunction unspecified)	4.9 hr[b]	24.5 hr
Child-Pugh Class A hepatic dysfunction[60]	2.2 hr[c]	11.0 hr
Child-Pugh Class B hepatic dysfunction[60]	5.6 hr[c]	28.0 hr
Child-Pugh Class C hepatic dysfunction[60]	7.8 hr[c]	39.0 hr
Chronic renal failure (with hemodialysis)[29]	1.3 hr[b]	6.5 hr
Chronic renal failure (CrCl<30 mL/min/1.73m^2) (without hemodialysis)[61]	4.6 ± 1.7 hr	14.2–31.3 hr
Severe trauma[30]	1.5 ± 0.6 hr	4.5–10.5 hr
Acute myocardial infarction without heart failure[63]	3.2 ± 0.5 hr[d]	13.5–18.5 hr
Acute myocardial infarction with heart failure[64]	10.2 ± 5.3 hr[d]	24.5–77.5 hr

[a]Time to steady state estimated using + and –1 SD of the mean t ½ and assuming steady state is achieved in five half-lives.
[b]Only mean data reported.
[c]Only mean data listed because of large SD.
[d]Continuous infusion of longer than 24 hr.

compartment, so subtherapeutic concentrations may be observed until the maintenance infusion reaches steady state. This "therapeutic gap" may require additional bolus doses or other dosing interventions to maintain efficacious concentrations. The therapeutic gap may occur during a critical timeframe when adequate drug concentrations.[65,66] While numerous dosing schemes have been tested for lidocaine,[1,8,65,69] Table 15-8 focuses on seven representative methods for clinical application.

The efficacy of lidocaine as an antiarrhythmic agent is directly linked to the rapid achievement and maintenance of therapeutic lidocaine concentrations.[21] For example avoiding the therapeutic gap may be critical during the first few hours following myocardial infarction when the incidence of lethal or potentially lethal arrhythmias is greatest.[70] Salzer et al. reported comparative data for the percentage of time that total lidocaine concentrations were within the therapeutic range (2–4 mg/L) in a small number of patients dosed using Methods 1–4a.[66] They concluded that Method 4a resulted in total lidocaine concentrations within the stated therapeutic range nearly 80% of the time. Riddell et al. reported that all eight of their subjects dosed using Method 5 maintained total concentrations between 1.5 and 5 mg/L 100% of the time.[67]

These dosing regimens serve only as guidelines for lidocaine administration. To achieve optimal efficacy, maintenance infusion rates always must be adjusted according to the patient's underlying clinical condition and other clearance-altering factors.

Each of these methods has both advantages and disadvantages. Although Method 5 requires no human intervention once the drug delivery system is set up, preparation of the delivery system is somewhat complicated and time consuming. The complexity of this method limits its utility in many hospital settings. Methods 3 and 4 require interventions to adjust infusion rates but do not require specialized delivery systems. Method 4a provides acceptable concentration-time results that are better than those achieved with Methods 1–3. Both Methods 4a and 4b are relatively simple to administer and require minimal nursing intervention. Ultimately,

Table 15-8. Lidocaine Hydrochloride Dosing Methods[1,8,65,69]

Method	Bolus Dose and Timing	Loading Infusion	Maintenance Infusion
1. Single bolus plus infusion technique[65-67]	100 mg initially	NA	120 mg/hr
2. Multiple bolus plus infusion technique[65-67]	100 mg initially 50 mg at 20 min	NA	120 mg/hr
3. Two-step infusion technique[65,66]	NA	200 mg over 25 min	120 mg/hr
4a. Two-step bolus plus infusion technique[66,67]	1.5 mg/kg (100 mg) plus simultaneous loading infusion	0.12 mg/kg/min for 25 min (or 200 mg over 25 min)	1.8 mg/kg/hr (120 mg/hr)
4b. Two-step bolus plus infusion technique[68]	75 mg plus simultaneous loading infusion	150 mg over 20 min	120 mg/hr
5. Exponentially declining infusion technique[67-69]	92 mg	8.3 mg/min exponentially declining to maintenance infusion rate	120 mg/hr
6. ACLS bolus technique for cardiac arrest due to VF or pulseless VT[8]	1.5 mg/kg followed by additional bolus of 0.5 to 0.75 mg/kg if necessary for refractory VT/VF; total dose should not exceed 3 mg/kg (or >200–300 mg) during a 1-hour period	NA	120–240 mg/hr (Note: Guidelines recommend only bolus therapy in cardiac arrest; however, it is reasonable to continue with an infusion of lidocaine if the drug was associated with restoration of a stable rhythm.)
7. Endotracheal administration[1,8,a]	3.0 to 3.75 mg/kg (i.e., 2 to 2.5 times recommended IV dose)	NA	NA

[a]Endotrachial administration has sometimes been used during cardiac arrest in situations where peripheral venous access was not possible.

the choice of method should be determined by available personnel, equipment, and facilities in addition to the patient's clinical condition.[66,67,69]

Therapeutic Range

When a therapeutic range for lidocaine is determined, it is important to note that plasma, serum, and whole blood concentrations are not interchangeable. For conversion from blood (C_b) to serum (C_s) concentrations, a factor of 1.3 should be applied[48]:

$$C_s = (C_b)\,(1.3)$$

The usual therapeutic range in serum is 1.5–6 mg/L (of total drug)[70] or 0.5–2 mg/L (of free or unbound drug).

Suggested Sampling Times and Effect on Therapeutic Range

Assessment or confirmation of suspected lidocaine toxicity is the most likely clinical situation for which lidocaine concentrations may be measured. Other circumstances may include:[21,71]

- Patient at increased risk for developing lidocaine toxicity (e.g., patient with cardiogenic shock, moderate to severe CHF, severe hepatic disease or severe renal insufficiency and not receiving hemodialysis).
- Patient concomitantly receiving medications with potential for clinically major or moderate drug interactions. (See Drug-Drug Interactions section.)
- Prolonged infusion (longer than 24 hr), especially in patients with underlying disease states or conditions that may decrease lidocaine clearance.

- Patient requiring doses that exceed the usual maximum recommended amount.
- Research investigation.

Table 15-9 provides suggestions for sample collection times.[71]

Table 15-9. Sample Collection Times

Monitoring Goal	Suggested Sampling Time
Assessment of efficacy	1–2 hr following initiation of therapy in patients who fail to respond[a]
Dosage adjustment	12–24 hr following initiation of therapy to assess steady state concentration
	24–48 hr following initiation of ongoing continuous infusion to avoid drug accumulation resulting from time-dependent reduction in clearance
Confirmation of toxicity	When clinical signs and symptoms of suspected lidocaine toxicity appear

[a]Failure to respond may result from the "therapeutic gap," high systemic lidocaine clearance, or intrinsic resistance to lidocaine therapy.

Pharmacodynamic Monitoring: Concentration-Related Efficacy and Toxicity

Lidocaine serum concentrations associated with the control of ventricular arrhythmias have generally fallen in the range of 1.5 to 6 mg/L.[70,72] Adverse effects with lidocaine principally involve the central nervous system (CNS) or cardiovascular (CV) system. CNS effects include confusion, dizziness, slurred speech, numbness of the lips and tongue, diplopia, tremor, severe nausea and vomiting, and seizures. Cardiovascular adverse effects include sinus bradycardia, sinus arrest, and atrioventricular conduction disturbances. Adverse effects have been weakly correlated to bound and unbound lidocaine concentrations.[7,21] In Table 15-10, possible signs of toxicity are correlated to total serum lidocaine concentrations.

Drug-Drug Interactions

Pharmacokinetic drug-drug interactions affecting lidocaine largely result from drug-induced alterations in hepatic clearance. Hepatic clearance depends on three factors[41]:

- free fraction of the drug
- hepatic blood flow
- intrinsic metabolic clearance

For lidocaine, drug-induced decreases in hepatic blood flow would be expected to produce more clinically important interactions (moderate to major), whereas drug-induced changes in lidocaine intrinsic clearance or in lidocaine free fraction appear less significant (mild to moderate). An exception would be the effects of fluvoxamine, a potent inhibitor of CYP1A2, which decreases the total body clearance of lidocaine by 40% to 60%.[39] Drug-drug interactions with lidocaine are listed in Table 15-11 along with the postulated mechanism

Table 15-10. Lidocaine Concentration-Toxicity Correlation

Total Serum Lidocaine Concentration	Underlying Toxicity
<1.5 mg/L	Idiosyncratic
1.5–4 mg/L	Mild CNS and cardiovascular (CV) effects
>4 mg/L	Mild CNS toxicity[a]; cardiovascular toxicity[b] more common with pre-existing CV disease present
>6 mg/L	Major CNS[c] and cardiovascular depressant effects
>8 mg/L	Seizures, obtundation, hypotension, respiratory depression, and decreased cardiac output

[a]Mild CNS toxicity includes somnolence, dizziness, numbness, slurred speech, and confusion.
[b]Cardiovascular toxicity includes sinus bradycardia, sinus arrest, atrioventricular conduction disturbances, hypotension, and decreased cardiac output.
[c]Major CNS toxicity includes severe confusion, severe slurred speech, tremor, diplopia, respiratory arrest, and seizure.

and clinical significance of the interactions. Although there appear to be no clinical reports regarding the effects of lidocaine on the pharmacokinetics of other agents, lidocaine may be anticipated to diminish the clearance of drugs metabolized by CYP1A2 given the *in vitro* inhibitory effects of lidocaine on the function of this isozyme.[73]

Maintenance infusion rates may have to be adjusted for lidocaine when it is administered concomitantly with drugs that result in interactions of moderate or major clinical significance. Table 15-11 also provides suggestions for initial dosage reductions associated with drug-drug interactions for patients with normal hepatic function. Careful monitoring for clinical signs and symptoms of lidocaine toxicity is also recommended. Furthermore, the extent of any drug interaction may increase in the presence of other clearance-altering factors, which may necessitate additional dose adjustments. However, in patients with advanced hepatic dysfunction (i.e., Child-Pugh Class C), the coadministration of fluvoxamine did not result in additional decreases in the total body clearance of lidocaine relative to the non-fluvoxamine condition.[39] Similar findings also have been reported for erythromycin, an inhibitor of CYP3A4.[74]

Drug–Disease State or Condition Interactions

Congestive heart failure (CHF)

A significant inverse relationship exists between cardiac index and lidocaine concentrations.[78] For example, in adult patients the increasing severity of CHF results in an increased potential for drug accumulation and decreased dosing requirements.[59]

For adults with mild to moderate CHF (i.e., presence of S_3 gallop and basilar pulmonary rales), an initial maintenance infusion of 1.4 mg/kg/hr is suggested to achieve steady state lidocaine serum concentrations of approximately 4 mg/L.[59] For patients with severe CHF (i.e., pulmonary edema or cardiogenic shock), the initial maintenance infusion should be 0.6 mg/kg/hr to achieve steady state concentrations of about 4 mg/L. As always, careful individual assessment of efficacy and toxicity is prudent. Loading doses may need to be reduced due to smaller central volume in patients with CHF.[59]

Table 15-11. Drug-Drug Interactions with Lidocaine[31,38,39,73-90]

Interacting Agent	Interaction	Significance and Initial Dosage Change Recommendations
Amiodarone[75-77]	Likely due to inhibition of CYP3A4-mediated metabolism	Mild to moderate: decrease lidocaine infusion rate by 20%
Beta-adrenergic blockers[31,78-80]	Decreases in hepatic blood flow and intrinsic metabolism of lidocaine; more likely to occur with lipophilic β-adrenergic blockers and those without intrinsic sympathomimetic activity	Moderate to major: decrease lidocaine infusion rates by 30% when coadministered with metoprolol and 40% to 50% with propranolol
Cimetidine[81-83]	Likely due to decreases in hepatic blood flow; V_{ss} of lidocaine also decreased; interaction only occurs with orally administered cimetidine	Mild to moderate: decrease lidocaine infusion rate by 15% to 25%
Erythromycin[74,84,85]	Concentrations of lidocaine and MEGX metabolite increased, likely due to inhibition of CYP3A4-mediated metabolism	Mild to moderate: decrease lidocaine infusion rate by 10% to 20%
Fluvoxamine[38,39,85]	Likely due to inhibition of CYP1A2-mediated metabolism	Moderate to major: decrease lidocaine infusion rate by 40% to 60%
Mexiletine[73,86]	CL_{total} of lidocaine decreased; V of lidocaine decreased; possible inhibition of CYP1A2-mediated metabolism and possible displacement from tissue binding sites	Mild to moderate: decrease lidocaine infusion rate by 20% to 25%
Propafenone[87]	CL_{total} decreased and may be accompanied by increased CNS adverse effects	Mild: decrease lidocaine infusion rate by 10%
Ciprofloxacin[88]	Probably via inhibition of CYP1A2-mediated metabolism	Mild to moderate: decrease lidocaine infusion rate by 20%
Rifampin[89,90]	CL_{total} of lidocaine increased due to induction by rifampin of CYP3A4- or CYP1A2-mediated metabolism of lidocaine	Mild to moderate: increase lidocaine infusion rate by 15% in patients with normal hepatic function

Acute myocardial infarction (AMI)

For adult patients with AMI without CHF, a constant rate infusion of 2.6 mg/kg/hr should achieve steady state concentrations of about 4 mg/L.[62] Patients with AMI and CHF require lower continuous infusion rates.[62] Therefore, an initial continuous infusion rate of 1.5 mg/kg/hr is suggested for this population. Furthermore, loading doses may need to be reduced approximately 40% because of a decreased central volume of distribution.[29]

AAG concentrations increase following AMI.[51] The implications of altered binding were previously addressed (see General Pharmacokinetic Information section). Since binding alterations are unpredictable and may not be of great clinical significance, especially in patients receiving short-term or prophylactic lidocaine, empiric dosage adjustment recommendations are not needed. However, clinical parameters should be carefully monitored, with appropriate reductions in lidocaine dosages made based on clinical response and lidocaine concentrations when available.

Hepatic disease

Chronic hepatic disease generally diminishes lidocaine clearance.[29,39,60,74] Due to the anticipated reduction in protein binding for this patient population, a continuous infusion should be initiated at 1.3 mg/kg/hr for steady state serum concentrations of around 3 mg/L.[29] The degree of hepatic dysfunction as determined by Child-Puch classification will influence the choice of the initial infusion rate.[39,60,74]

An additional consideration for patients with hepatic dysfunction receiving lidocaine is the potential accumulation of the active metabolite MEGX. This accumulation may increase the risk for developing toxicity despite "therapeutic" concentrations.[34]

Renal disease

Since lidocaine is almost exclusively hepatically eliminated in healthy humans, renal dysfunction is generally thought to have little effect on its disposition and elimination.[21] Two studies have reported no significant effects of chronic renal dysfunction on systemic clearance.[29,43] These studies suggest that loading and maintenance doses of lidocaine do not require adjustment in patients with chronic renal failure. However, they only examined patients with chronic renal failure undergoing long-term hemodialysis. Another study showed that clearance of lidocaine is significantly decreased in patients with severe chronic renal insufficiency (i.e., creatinine clearance <30 mL/min/1.73 m^2) not undergoing hemodialysis.[61] Therefore, reductions in lidocaine infusion rates should be anticipated in this patient population.

Morbid obesity

IBW should be used for the calculation of bolus dosing, and ABW should be used for the calculation of continuous intravenous infusion rate.[28]

Advanced age (elderly)

Compared to young adult control subjects, the elderly have an increased volume of distribution and a decreased clearance of lidocaine.[27] There may be gender-specific effects on the distribution and clearance of lidocaine with volume of distribution and clearance higher in elderly females compared to elderly males, although not to a statistically significant degree.[27]

Severe trauma

Adult patients with severe trauma (but without a history of clinically significant pre-trauma heart, lung, liver, or kidney disease) given single IV doses of lidocaine to suppress the stress response associated with endotracheal intubation or bronchoscopy show about 33% decreases in lidocaine total body clearance and approximately 50% decreases in volume of distribution of lidocaine.[30]

Pregnancy and lactation

Lidocaine is currently listed as Risk Category BM.[91] Although lidocaine rapidly crosses the placenta to the fetus, observational clinical studies where lidocaine was administered to the mother any time during the pregnancy, found no evidence of an association between the use of lidocaine with large categories of major or minor fetal malformations or to individual birth defects.[91] Though small amounts of lidocaine are excreted into breast milk with concentrations approximately 40% of maternal serum concentrations, it is considered to be compatible with breast feeding by The American Academy of Pediatrics.[91]

References

1. Class Ib Antiarrhythmics. Lidocaine. In: McEvoy GK, ed. *AHFS Drug Information 2010*. Bethesda, MD: American Society of Health-System Pharmacists; 2010:1646-50.
2. O'Connor RE, Bossaert L, Arntz H-R, et al. 2010 International Consensus on Cardiopulmonary Resuscitation and Emergency Cardiovascular Care Science with Treatment Recommendations. Part 9: Acute Coronary Syndromes. *Circulation*. 2010;122[suppl 2]:S422-S465.
3. MacMahon S, Collins R, Peto R, et al. Effects of prophylactic lidocaine in suspected acute myocardial infarction. *JAMA*. 1988;260(13):1910-6.
4. Hine LK, Laird N, Hewitt P, et al. Meta-analytic evidence against prophylactic use of lidocaine in acute myocardial infarction. *Arch Intern Med.* 1989;149(12):2694-8.
5. Alexander JH, Granger CB, Sadowski Z, et al. Prophylactic lidocaine use in acute myocardial infarction: incidence and outcomes from two international trials. *Am Heart J.* 1999;137(5):799-805.
6. Sadowski ZP, Alexander JH, Skrabucha B, et al. Multicenter randomized trial and a systematic overview of lidocaine in acute myocardial infarction. *Am Heart J.* 1999;137(5):792-8.
7. Rademaker AW, Kellen J, Tam YK, et al. Character of adverse effects of prophylactic lidocaine in the coronary care unit. *Clin Pharmacol Ther*. 1986;40(1):71-80.
8. Morrison LJ, Deakin CD, Morley PT, et al. 2010 International Consensus on Cardiopulmonary Resuscitation and Emergency Cardiovascular Care Science with Treatment Recommendations. Part 8: Advanced Life Support. *Circulation*. 2010;122[suppl 2]:S345-S421.
9. Zipes DP, Camm AJ, Borgrefe M, et al. ACC/AHA/ESC 2006 guidelines for management of patients with ventricular arrhythmias and the prevention of sudden cardiac death. *J Am Coll Cardiol*. 2006;48(5):e247-e346.
10. Nasir N, Taylor A, Doyle TK, et al. Evaluation of intravenous lidocaine for the termination of sustained monomorphic ventricular tachycardia in patients with coronary artery disease with and without healed myocardial infarction. *Am J Cardiol.* 1994;74(12):1183-6.
11. Gorgels APM, van den Dool A, Hofs A, et al. Comparison of procainamide and lidocaine in terminating sustained monomorphic ventricular tachycardia. *Am J Cardiol.* 1996;78(1):43-6.
12. Komura S, Chinushi M, Furushima H, et al. Efficacy of procainamide and lidocaine in terminating sustained monomorphic ventricular tachycardia. *Circ J.* 2010;74:864-9.
13. Josephson ME, Kastor JA, Kitchen JG. Lidocaine in Wolff-Parkinson-White Syndrome with atrial fibrillation. *Ann Intern Med.* 1976;84(1):44-5.
14. Chiale PA, Franco DA, Selva HO, et al. Lidocaine-sensitive atrial tachycardia: Lidocaine-sensitive, rate-related, repetitive atrial tachycardia: a new arrhythmogenic syndrome. *J Am Coll Cardiol.* 2000;36(5):1637-45.
15. Tsuchiya T, Okumura K, Honda T, et al. Effects of verapamil and lidocaine on two components of the re-entry circuit of verapamil-sensitive idiopathic left ventricular tachycardia. *J Am Coll Cardiol.* 2001;37(5):1415-21.
16. Ayoub CM, Sfeir PM, Bou-Khalil P, et al. Prophylactic amiodarone versus lidocaine for prevention of reperfusion ventricular fibrillation after release of aortic cross-clamp. *Eur J Anaesthesiol.* 2009;26(12):1056-60.
17. Raehl CL. Endotracheal drug therapy in cardiopulmonary resuscitation. *Clin Pharm.* 1986;5(7):572-9.
18. Cohen LS, Rosenthal JE, Horner DW, et al. Plasma levels of lidocaine after intramuscular injection. *Am J Cardiol.* 1972;29(4):520-3.
19. Schwartz ML, Meyer MB, Covino BG, et al. Antiarrhythmic effectiveness of intramuscular lidocaine: influence of different injection sites. *J Clin Pharmacol.* 1974;14(2):77-83.
20. Huet PM, Lelorier J, Pomier G, et al. Bioavailability of lidocaine in normal volunteers and cirrhotic patients. *Clin Pharmacol Ther.* 1979;25(2):229-30.
21. Benowitz NL, Meister W. Clinical pharmacokinetics of lidocaine. *Clin Pharmacokinet.* 1978;3(3):177-201.
22. Morgan DJ, Horowitz JD, Louis WJ. Prediction of acute myocardial disposition of antiarrhythmic drugs. *J Pharm Sci.* 1989;78(5):384-8.
23. Burm AG, De Boer AG, Van Kleef JW, et al. Pharmacokinetics of lidocaine and bupivacaine and stable isotope labeled analogues: a study in healthy volunteers. *Biopharm Drug Dispos.* 1988;9(1): 85-95.
24. Burrows FA, Lerman J, LeDez KM, et al. Pharmacokinetics of lidocaine in children with congenital heart disease. *Can*

J Anaesth. 1991;38(2):196-200.

25. Finholt DA, Stirt JA, DiFazio CA, et al. Lidocaine pharmacokinetics in children during general anesthesia. *Anesth Analg.* 1986;65(3):279-82.
26. Mihaly GW, Moore RG, Triggs EJ, et al. The pharmacokinetics and metabolism of the anilide local anaesthetic in neonates. I. Lignocaine. *Eur J Clin Pharmacol.* 1978;13(2):143-52.
27. Abernethy DR, Greenblatt DJ. Impairment of lidocaine clearance in elderly male subjects. *J Cardiovasc Pharmacol.* 1983;5(6):1093-6.
28. Abernethy DR, Greenblatt DJ. Lidocaine disposition in obesity. *Am J Cardiol.* 1984;53(8):1183-6.
29. Thomson PD, Melmon KL, Richardson KA, et al. Lidocaine pharmacokinetics in advanced heart failure, liver disease and renal failure in humans. *Ann Intern Med.* 1973;78(4):499-508.
30. Berkenstadt H, Mayan H, Segal E, et al. The pharmacokinetics of morphine and lidocaine in nine severe trauma patients. *J Clin Anesth.* 1999;11(8):630-4.
31. Ochs HR, Carstens G, Greenblatt DJ. Reduction in lidocaine clearance during continuous infusion and by coadministration of propranolol. *N Engl J Med.* 1980;303(7):373-7.
32. Bauer LA, Brown T, Gibaldi M, et al. Influence of long-term infusions on lidocaine kinetics. *Clin Pharmacol Ther.* 1982;31(4):433-7.
33. Saville BA, Gray MR, Tam YK. Evidence for lidocaine-induced enzyme inactivation. *J Pharm Sci.* 1989;78(12):1003-8.
34. Thomson AH, Elliott HL, Kelman AW, et al. The pharmacokinetics and pharmacodynamics for lignocaine and MEGX in healthy subjects. *J Pharmacokinet Biopharm.* 1987;15(2):101-15.
35. Bargetzi MJ, Aoyama T, Gonzalez FJ, et al. Lidocaine metabolism in human liver microsomes by cytochrome P450IIIA4. *Clin Pharmacol Ther.* 1989;46(5):521-7.
36. Huang W, Lin YS, McConn DJ, et al. Evidence of significant contribution from CYP3A5 to hepatic drug metabolism. *Drug Metab Dispos.* 2004;32(12):1434-45.
37. Wang JS, Backman MT, Taavitsainen P, et al. Involvement of CYP1A2 and CYP3A4 in lidocaine n-demethylation and 3 hydroxylation in humans. *Drug Metab Dispos.* 2000;28(8):959-65.
38. Wang JS, Backman JT, Wen X, et al. Fluvoxamine is a more potent inhibitor of lidocaine metabolism than ketoconazole and erythromycin in vitro. *Pharmacol and Toxicol.* 1999;85(5):201-5.
39. Orlando R, Piccoli P, De Martin S, et al. Cytochrome P450 1A2 is a major determinant of lidocaine metabolism in vivo: effects of liver function. *Clin Pharmacol Ther.* 2004;75(1):80-8.
40. Bennett PN, Aarons LJ, Bending MR, et al. Pharmacokinetics of lidocaine and its deethylated metabolite: dose and time dependency studies in man. *J Pharmacokinet Biopharm.* 1982;10(3):265-81.
41. Wilkinson GR, Shand DG. A physiological approach to hepatic drug clearance. *Clin Pharmacol Ther.* 1975;18(4):377-90.
42. Narang PK, Crouthamel WG, Carliner NH, et al. Lidocaine and its active metabolites. *Clin Pharmacol Ther.* 1978;24(6):654-62.
43. Collinsworth KA, Strong JM, Atkinson AJ, et al. Pharmacokinetics and metabolism of lidocaine in patients with renal failure. *Clin Pharmacol Ther.* 1975;18(1):59-64.
44. Strong JM, Mayfield DE, Atkinson AJ, et al. Pharmacological activity, metabolism, and pharmacokinetics of glycinexylidide. *Clin Pharmacol Ther.* 1975;17(2):184-94.
45. Burney RG, DiFazia CA, Peach MJ, et al. Anti-arrhythmic effects of lidocaine metabolites. *Am Heart J.* 1974;88(6):765-9.
46. Blumer J, Strong JM, Atkinson AJ Jr. The convulsant potency of lidocaine and its N-dealkylated metabolites. *J Pharmacol Exp Ther.* 1973;186(1):31-6.
47. Boyes RN, Scott DB, Jebson PJ, et al. Metabolism of lidocaine in man. *Clin Pharmacol Ther.* 1971;12(1):105-16.
48. Tucker GT, Boyes RN, Bridenbaugh PO, et al. Binding of anilide-type local anesthetics in human plasma. I. Relationships between binding, physicochemical properties, and anesthetic activity. *Anesthesiology.* 1970;33(3):287-303.
49. Drayer DE, Lorenzo B, Werns S, et al. Plasma levels, protein binding, and elimination data of lidocaine and active metabolites in cardiac patients of various ages. *Clin Pharmacol Ther.* 1983;34(1):14-22.
50. Routledge PA. The plasma protein binding of basic drugs. *Br J Clin Pharmacol.* 1986;22(5):499-506.
51. Routledge PA, Stargel WW, Wagner GS, et al. Increased alpha-1-acid glycoprotein and lidocaine disposition in myocardial infarction. *Ann Intern Med.* 1980;93(5):701-4.
52. Routledge PA, Barchowsky A, Bjornsson TD, et al. Lidocaine plasma protein binding. *Clin Pharmacol Ther.* 1980;27(3):347-51.
53. Gillis AM, Yee YG, Kates RG. Binding of antiarrhythmic drugs to purified human a1-acid glycoprotein. *Biochem Pharmacol.* 1985;34(24):4279-82.
54. Giardina EGV, Khether R, Freilich D, et al. Time course of alpha-1-acid glycoprotein and its relation to myocardial

enzymes after acute myocardial infarction. *Am J Cardiol*. 1985;56(4):262-5.

55. Barry M, Keeling PW, Weir D, et al. Severity of cirrhosis and the relationship of a1-acid glycoprotein concentration to plasma protein binding of lidocaine. *Clin Pharmacol Ther*. 1990;47(3):366-70.
56. Lerman J, Strong AH, LeDez KM, et al. Effects of age on the serum concentration of a1-acid glycoprotein and the binding of lidocaine in pediatric patients. *Clin Pharmacol Ther*. 1989;46(2):219-25.
57. McNamara PJ, Slaughter RL, Visco JP, et al. Effect of smoking on binding of lidocaine to human serum proteins. *J Pharm Sci*. 1980;69(6):749-51.
58. Goolkasian DL, Slaughter RL, Edwards DJ, et al. Displacement of lidocaine from serum a1-acid glycoprotein binding sites by basic drugs. *Eur J Clin Pharmacol*. 1983;25(3):413-7.
59. Zito RA, Reid PR. Lidocaine kinetics predicted by indocyanine green clearance. *N Engl J Med*. 1978;298(21):1160-3.
60. Wójcicki J, Kozłowski K, Droździk M, et al. Lidocaine elimination in patients with liver cirrhosis. *Acta Poloniae Pharmaceutica*. 2002;59(4):321-4.
61. De Martin S, Orlando R, Bertoli M, et al. Differential effect of chronic renal failure on the pharmacokinetics of lidocaine in patients receiving and not receiving hemodialysis. *Clin Pharmacol Ther*. 2006;80(6):597-606.
62. Bax ND, Tucker GT, Woods HF. Lignocaine and indocyanine green kinetics in patients following myocardial infarction. *Br J Clin Pharmacol*. 1980;10(4):353-61.
63. Lelorier J, Grenon D, Latour Y, et al. Pharmacokinetics of lidocaine after prolonged intravenous infusions in uncomplicated myocardial infarction. *Ann Intern Med*. 1977;87(6):700-6.
64. Prescott LF, Adjepon-Yamoah KK, Talbot RG. Impaired lignocaine metabolism in patients with myocardial infarction. *Br Med J*. 1976;1(6015):939-41.
65. Greenblatt DJ, Bolognini V, Koch-Weser J, et al. Pharmacokinetic approach to the clinical use of lidocaine intravenously. *JAMA*. 1976;236(3):273-7.
66. Salzer LB, Weinreb AB, Marina RJ, et al. A comparison of methods of lidocaine administration in patients. *Clin Pharmacol Ther*. 1981;29(5):617-24.
67. Riddell JG, McAllister CB, Wilkinson GR, et al. A new method for constant plasma drug concentration: application to lidocaine. *Ann Intern Med*. 1984;100(1):25-8.
68. Stargel WW, Shand DG, Routledge PA, et al. Clinical comparison of rapid infusion and multiple injection methods for lidocaine loading. *Am Heart J*. 1981;102(5):872-6.
69. Sebaldt RJ, Nattell S, Kreeft JH, et al. Lidocaine therapy with an exponentially declining infusion. Clinical evaluation of an optimized dosing technique. *Ann Intern Med*. 1984;101(5):632-4.
70. Lie KI, Wellens HJ, Van Capelle FJ, et al. Lidocaine in the prevention of primary ventricular fibrillation. A double-blind, randomized study of 212 consecutive patients. *N Engl J Med*. 1974;291(25):1324-6.
71. Pieper JA, Johnson KE. Lidocaine. In: Evans WE, Schentag JJ, Jusko WJ, eds. *Applied Pharmacokinetics: Principles of Therapeutic Drug Monitoring*. Vancouver, WA: Applied Therapeutics;1992:21:1-37.
72. Gianelly R, von der Groeben JO. Spivack AP, et al. Effect of lidocaine on ventricular arrhythmias in patients with coronary heart disease. *N Engl J Med*. 1967;277(23):1215-9.
73. Wei X, Dai R, Zhai S, et al. Inhibition of human liver cytochrome P-450 1A2 by the class IB antiarrhythmics mexiletine, lidocaine, and tocainide. *J Pharmacol Exp Ther*. 1999;289(2):853-8.
74. Orlando R, Piccoli P, De Martin S, et al. Effect of the CYP3A4 inhibitor erythromycin on the pharmacokinetics of lignocaine and its pharmacologically active metabolites in subjects with normal and impaired liver function. *Br J Clin Pharmacol*. 2003;55(1):86-93.
75. Fruncillo RJ, Kozin SH, Digregorio GJ. Effect of amiodarone on the pharmacokinetics of phenytoin, quinidine, and lidocaine in the rat. *Res Commun Chem Pathol Pharmacol*. 1985;50(3):451-4.
76. Siegmund JB, Wilson JH, Imhoff TE. Amiodarone interaction with lidocaine. *J Cardiovasc Pharmacol*. 1993;21(4):513-5.
77. Ha HR, Candinas R, Stieger B, et al. Interaction between amiodarone and lidocaine. *J Cardiovasc Pharmacol*. 1996;28(4):533-9.
78. Stenson RE, Constantino RT, Harrison DC. Interrelationships of hepatic blood flow, cardiac output and blood levels of lidocaine in man. *Circulation*. 1971;43(2):205-11.
79. Conrad KA, Byers JM 3rd, Finley PR, et al. Lidocaine elimination: effects of metoprolol and of propranolol. *Clin Pharmacol Ther*. 1983;33(2):133-8.
80. Bax ND, Tucker GT, Lennard MS, et al. The impairment of lignocaine clearance by propranolol—major contribution from enzyme inhibition. *Br J Clin Pharmacol*. 1985;19(5):597-603.
81. Feely J, Wilkinson GR, McAllister CB, et al. Increased toxicity and reduced clearance of lidocaine by cimetidine. *Ann Intern Med*. 1982;96(5):592-4.

82. Berk SI, Gal P, Bauman JL, et al. The effect of oral cimetidine on total and unbound serum lidocaine concentration in patients with suspected myocardial infarction. *Int J Cardiol*. 1987;14(1):91-4.

83. Powell JR, Foster JR, Patterson JH, et al. Effect of duration of lidocaine infusion and route of cimetidine administration on lidocaine pharmacokinetics. *Clin Pharm*. 1986;5(12):993-8.

84. Isohanni MH, Neuvonen PJ, Palkama VJ, et al. Effect of erythromycin and itraconazole on the pharmacokinetics of intravenous lignocaine. *Eur J Clin Pharmacol*. 1998;54(7):561-5.

85. Olkkola KT, Isohanni MH, Hamunen K, et al. The effect of erythromycin and fluvoxamine on the pharmacokinetics of intravenous lidocaine. *Anesth Analg*. 2005;100(5):1352-6.

86. Maeda Y, Funakoshi S, Nakamura M, et al. Possible mechanism for pharmacokinetic interaction between lidocaine and mexiletine. *Clin Pharmacol Ther*. 2002;71(5):389-97.

87. Ujhelyi MR, O'Rangers EA, Fan C, et al. The pharmacokinetic and pharmacodynamic interaction between propafenone and lidocaine. *Clin Pharmacol Ther.* 1993;53(1):38-48.

88. Isohanni MH, Ahonen J, Neuvonen PJ, et al. Effect of ciprofloxacin on the pharmacokinetics of intravenous lidocaine. *Eur J Anaesth*. 2005;22(10):795-9.

89. Li AP, Rasmussen A, Xu L, et al. Rifampicin induction of lidocaine metabolism in cultured human hepatocytes. *J Pharmacol Exp Ther*. 1995;274(2):673-7.

90. Reichel C, Skodra T, Nacke A, et al. The lignocaine metabolite (MEGX) liver function test and P-450 induction in humans. *Br J Clin Pharmacol*. 1998;46(6):535-9.

91. Briggs GG, Freeman RK, Yaffe SJ. *Drugs in Pregnancy and Lactation: A Reference Guide to Fetal and Neonatal Risk*. 8th ed. Philadelphia, PA: Lippincott Williams & Wilkins, a Wolters Kluwer business; 2008:1049-51.

Chapter 16

Giulia Ghibellini and Stanley W. Carson

Lithium (AHFS 28:28)

Lithium is a monovalent cation (1 mmol/L = 1 mEq/L) that is indicated in the treatment of manic episodes of manic-depressive illness and for maintenance therapy to prevent or diminish the intensity of subsequent episodes in those manic-depressive patients with a history of mania.[1]

Lithium is also used as monotherapy and combination therapy for acute bipolar depression.[2,3] Off-label uses include borderline personality disorder, traumatic brain injury, improvement of neutrophil count, prophylaxis of cluster headache, premenstrual tension, bulimia, alcoholism, syndrome of inappropriate secretion of antidiuretic hormone, tardive dyskinesia, hyperthyroidism, postpartum affective psychosis, and corticosteroid-induced psychosis.[4,5] Its neuroprotective properties lead to study lithium for applications in acute head injuries and chronic neurodegenerative disorders.[6-10]

Lithium shares properties of physiologic cations, particularly sodium (Na^+) and potassium (K^+), and all are regulated in the kidney in a similar fashion. Previous theories regarding the mechanism of action of lithium held that Li^+ was likely substituted for these cations in the body, thereby improving ion dysregulation, modifying monamine neurotransmitter signaling, or interacting with second messengers such as adenyl cyclase, inositol phosphate, or protein kinase C systems.[11,12] Recent advances suggest lithium may inhibit glycogen synthase kinase-3, which phosphorylates and inhibits nuclear factors that regulate cell growth and protection programs, thereby preventing apoptosis and enhancing neuroplasticity and cellular resilience.[10] Taken altogether these mechanisms may augment cellular homeostasis and may be neuroprotective.[10,13]

Lithium concentrations are closely related to therapeutic response and side effects. Changes in fluid and sodium balance due to changes in the glomerular filtration rate (GFR) or renal tubular reabsorption of lithium and/or sodium are of particular importance and can affect lithium pharmacokinetics. Consideration of drug-drug interactions or drug-drug disease state or condition interactions is also important when monitoring patients receiving lithium. Because of lithium's relatively narrow therapeutic index, periodic lithium concentration determinations are essential to achieve optimal therapeutic response with minimal side effects.

Usual Dosage Range in Absence of Clearance-Altering Factors

The following dosage recommendations are guidelines for the initiation of lithium therapy. Acute and maintenance dosage regimens should be individualized for all patients and guided by lithium concentration determinations. Patients with reduced renal function, and therefore diminished renal clearance of lithium, need lower doses.

Acute therapy

Recommendations for initiation of lithium for acute therapy are given in Table 16-1. In adults, acute lithium therapy is initiated with 300–600 mg of lithium carbonate tablets or capsules three times daily. Sustained-

Table 16-1. Lithium Dosing Recommendations for Initiation of Acute Therapy[14]

Population	Dosage[a] Oral Tablets, Capsules, or Syrup
Children (<18 years)	15–60 mg/kg daily[b]
Adults (19–59 years)	900–1800 mg/day (~15 mg/kg)
Elderly (>59 years)	600–900 mg/day[c]

[a]Dosage should be given in divided doses and titrated to achieve therapeutic serum lithium concentrations based on clinical response and patient tolerance.
[b]Not FDA approved for use in children below 12 years of age.
[c]The elderly may have altered lithium clearance due to reduced renal function and concomitant medications.

release products may be initiated with 600–900 mg daily, with an increase to 1200–1800 mg daily on day 2 of therapy.[14] Loading doses are not commonly used.[15-17] Dosage regimens should be individually titrated to desired concentrations and clinical response of the patient. For most individuals an increase of 300 mg (or 8 mEq) equates to an increase of approximately 0.3 ± 0.1 mEq/L in steady state lithium concentration.[16,17] Titrating initial dosage regimens over several days may minimize initial side effects.

Maintenance therapy

Currently, there are no standardized guidelines for the use of long-term lithium therapy for prophylaxis or prevention of relapse (i.e., maintenance) after an acute bipolar episode. Traditionally, the criteria for the initiation of maintenance lithium therapy have been the requirement of two or three episodes of mania or depression in a 5-year period, however the American Psychiatric Association recommends maintenance therapy after a single manic episode.[16] The decision to initiate maintenance or prophylaxis therapy should be made with the following considerations: frequency and severity of episodes, seasonality of prior episodes, prior response to other bipolar medication, and possible consequences of relapse. Lithium dosage regimens for maintenance or prophylactic therapy are usually lower than those used for acute therapy (900 to 1200 mg daily) with target trough lithium concentrations of approximately 0.6–0.8 mEq/L (see Table 16-2).[14,16,18,19] Several studies suggest that concentrations > 0.7–0.8 mEq/L may be more likely to result in a positive response; however, individual patients may respond well to lower concentrations, particularly those who do not tolerate concentrations in the upper part of the therapeutic range (see Therapeutic Range for additional details).[19] Once- or twice-daily dosing schedules that simplify the maintenance regimen may enhance long-term adherence to treatment. It has been suggested to decrease maintenance doses slowly to minimize the risk of relapse in previously stable patients who require dose reduction.[16,19,20]

Table 16-2. Lithium Dosing Recommendations for Initiation of Maintenance Therapy[14]

Population	Dosage[a] Oral Tablets, Capsules, or Syrup
Children (<18 years)	150–300 mg/day[b]
Adults (19–59 years)	900–1200 mg/day
Elderly (>59 years)	600–900 mg/day[c]

[a]Dosage should be given in divided doses and titrated to achieve therapeutic serum lithium concentrations based on clinical response and patient tolerance.
[b]Not approved for use in children below 12 years of age by FDA.
[c]The elderly may have altered lithium clearance due to reduced renal function and concomitant medications.

Dosage Form Availability

Lithium salts are available in a number of dosage forms.[21] Lithium carbonate is the most commonly formulated salt and has the longest stability and shelf life. The use of different salts does not generally affect the pharmacokinetics of lithium. Injectable lithium preparations are not available for clinical use in the United States.[22] Lithium is most commonly administered by the oral route as the carbonate or citrate salt. Because lithium is a monovalent ion, lithium concentrations are reported as milliequivalents per liter (mEq/L) or millimoles per liter (mmol/L) rather than in the more familiar concentration term of milligrams per liter (mg/L). Dosages are listed as millimole (mmol) equivalents of lithium carbonate (300 mg lithium carbonate = 8.12 mmol Li^{++} = 8.12 mEq Li^{++}; 5 ml lithium citrate = 8.0 mmol Li^{++} = 8.0 mEq Li^{++}).[14] Lithium is available in capsules, immediate and prolonged release tablets, and oral syrup formulations; a summary of available lithium products is given in Table 16-3.

General Pharmacokinetic Information

Absorption

Lithium is readily absorbed in the gastrointestinal tract, primarily in the jejunum and ileum with some inherent intra- and interindividual variability.[23,24] Oral solutions of lithium are the most rapidly absorbed, with peak concentrations occurring within 15–45 minutes. Nearly complete absorption of immediate-release lithium carbonate tablets and capsules occurs within 1–6 hr after dosing, with peak lithium concentrations occurring

Table 16-3. Lithium Dosage Form Availability

Formulation/Brand	Salt Form S = 1.0	Dosage Unit (1 mEq = 1 mmol)	F
Oral tablets			
Generic lithium carbonate	Carbonate	300 mg/8.12 mEq	~1.0
Oral capsules			
Generic lithium carbonate	Carbonate	150 mg/4.06 mEq	~1.0
Generic lithium carbonate		300 mg/8.12 mEq	~1.0
Generic lithium carbonate		600 mg/16.24 mEq	~1.0
Extended-release tablets			
Generic lithium carbonate	Carbonate	300 mg/8.12 mEq	~1.0
Lithobid (slow release)		300 mg/8.12 mEq	0.8
Generic lithium carbonate		450 mg/12.18 mEq	0.97
Oral syrup			
Generic lithium citrate		5 ml/8 mEq	1.0

within 0.5–3 hr. Absorption from extended-release products is typically prolonged with peak concentrations occurring within 4–12 hr after dosing.[14]

The presence of food may significantly delay the rate of lithium absorption due to slower gastric emptying into the intestinal tract, but it does not affect the extent of absorption. Administering immediate-release preparations with food may be used as a strategy to minimize potential side effects associated with rapidly increasing lithium concentrations sometimes seen with these products.[25,26] Controlled-release products also are associated with lower and sustained plasma concentrations, and this may reduce the occurrence of these concentration-related side effects.[24,27]

Bioavailability (F) of dosage forms

Since an intravenous preparation is not available in the United States, the oral syrup dosage form is usually used as the reference product to calculate bioavailability of other oral dosage forms and is assumed to be 100% bioavailable. The bioavailability from the immediate-release, sustained-release, and syrup lithium formulations is very high and ranges from 80%–104%.[28] Lithium carbonate capsules and tablets are 95%–100% absorbed. Extended-release lithium carbonate tablets are 60%–90% absorbed.[14] Food does not appear to affect the bioavailability of lithium.[23,24] A comparison of lithium citrate syrup and lithium capsules found no significant differences in lithium concentrations at steady state.[29]

Distribution

Lithium is widely distributed in the body, with initial distribution into the extracellular fluid followed by gradual accumulation in tissues. Lithium more rapidly distributes into the central compartment (e.g., heart, lung, kidney) and less rapidly into peripheral compartments (e.g., brain, bone, muscle, and thyroid).[14] Lithium also distributes into saliva and erythrocytes, and concentration measurements at these sites have been suggested for surrogate measures of toxicity and/or noncompliance. However, considerable variability in these concentrations limit their usefulness in routine clinical practice.[30,31] Lithium crosses into the placenta with similar concentrations in maternal and fetal serum. Lithium concentrations in breast milk are approximately 33%–50% of that in maternal serum, and high lithium concentrations have been reported in infant serum following breast feeding. Therefore, babies of mothers receiving lithium and breast-feeding should be closely monitored.[1,32-36] Lithium does not bind to plasma proteins.

A two-compartment, open pharmacokinetic model classically describes the disposition of lithium. In clinical practice, the early distributional phase may be obscured by prolonged absorption of lithium from tablets and capsules and sparse blood sampling and, therefore, appear as a one-compartment model (monoexponential elimination).[28]

The volume of the central compartment approximates 25%–40% of body weight, with the combined central and peripheral compartments comprising 123% of body weight.[37-39] The apparent steady state volume of distribution (V_β or V_{area}) was approximately 0.8 L/kg with micro-rate constants of 0.24 hr−1 (k_{12}) and 0.19 hr−1 (k_{21}) in normal volunteers.[37] Additional studies indicate that the volume of distribution for lithium typically ranges from 0.5–1.2 L/kg.[17,37,38,40,41] There is an age-dependent reduction in volume of distribution, probably due in part to decreased total body water and lean body mass seen with advancing age.[42,43] In one study, the volume of distribution in elderly subjects was reportedly 20%–40% lower compared with healthy, young volunteers.[42] Table 16-4 provides typical estimates for volume of distribution by age. A recent population PK analysis on single dose lithium pharmacokinetics in children 7–17 years of age[41] confirmed the volume of distribution range previously reported by Vitiello.[44] When fat free mass was included in the model as a covariate this explained most of the variability in the estimates of V and CL in children, in good accordance with previous results in elderly and obese patients.[41]

Table 16-4. Lithium Volume of Distribution Estimates by Age

Population	Volume of Distribution (Mean ± SD)
Children and adolescents[44]	0.93 ± 0.25 L/kg[a]
Adults (19–59 years)[37,53]	0.85 ± 0.25 L/kg[a]
Elderly (>59 years)[42]	0.53 ± 0.12 L/kg[a]

[a]Based on ideal body weight.

Elimination

Lithium is primarily eliminated in urine as the free ion and is not metabolized. Lithium clearance is largely renal, with saliva, sweat, and feces accounting for minor amounts (<5%).[45] The lithium ion is completely filtered across the glomerular membrane, similar to sodium and potassium, and is 80% reabsorbed via the proximal renal tubules. Lithium clearance is directly proportional to GFR and blood flow to the kidney and is ~20% of creatinine clearance (CrCl).[46] Estimates for lithium clearance by age are given in Table 16-5. Lithium clearance decreases in parallel with age-related decreases in GFR, which is approximately 10 ml/min per decade after 30 years of age.[47] Based on a population pharmacokinetic study, lean body weight and CrCl are important predictors of lithium clearance.[48] Circadian rhythm changes in GFR, CrCl, and lithium clearance all result in higher daytime clearances and variations in elimination half-life, which may affect therapeutic concentration monitoring.[28] The clearance of lithium also appears similar in children compared with adults.[44,41] Modest decreases in glomerular filtration rate occasionally occur in patients receiving long-term lithium therapy, but a causal relationship has not been established. Lithium may also inhibit its own clearance via its effects on antidiuretic hormone and aldosterone.[49,50]

Increases in lithium concentrations occur with sodium depletion or with a low-salt diet secondary to enhanced proximal tubular reabsorption of the lithium ion.[51,52] Renal excretion of lithium does not appear to be enhanced by increasing water intake or acidification of urine. Drug-drug interactions or drug–disease state/conditions that result in changes in GFR or in the reabsorption of lithium and/or sodium are likely to affect lithium clearance and should be considered when designing or modifying lithium regimens.[28,53]

Table 16-5. Lithium Clearance Estimates by Age[a]

Population	Clearance (Mean)[b]
Children and adolescents[41,44]	0.021 L/hr/kg
Adults (19–59 years)[37,53]	0.024 L/hr/kg
Elderly (>59 years)[42]	0.015 L/hr/kg

[a]In patients with normal renal function for age.
[b]Based on 70 kg weight.

Half-life and time to steady state

Lithium exhibits biphasic elimination (two-compartment model). The elimination half-life of lithium is dependent on volume of distribution and clearance rates, and possibly on duration of therapy. Table 16-6 provides estimates for half-life and time to steady state concentrations by age. In patients with normal renal function, the initial ($t_{1/2\alpha}$) and terminal half-lives ($t^{1/2}_{\beta}$) have been reported as 0.8–1.2 hr and 20–27 hr, respectively, after single dose administration; however, the initial (distributional) phase is typically not adequately characterized in clinical practice. For clinical purposes, the disposition of lithium can be estimated by a single terminal half-life (one-compartment model).[54]

In patients with normal renal function the mean terminal $t_{1/2}$ ranged from 16 to 30 hr after multiple dosing.[37,38,40,55] Treatment duration has been associated with increases in elimination half-life. Significantly longer half-lives have been reported in patients receiving continuous lithium therapy for more than 1 year compared with those receiving therapy for less than 1 year (2.4 vs. 1.7 days).[56] Lithium-associated nephrotoxicity or changes in lithium transport across red cell membranes over time may account for these effects.[57,58] Longer elimination half-lives of 36 hr and 40–50 hr have been reported in elderly patients and in those with impaired renal function, respectively. The elimination half-life of lithium in children (9 to 12 years) was 17.9 hr after a single 300-mg oral lithium dose.[44] However a recent population PK analysis of lithium kinetics in children after a single dose determined this shorter half-life to be an artifact of the noncompartmental analysis and a higher lower limit of quantification (LLOQ).[41] In this new study it was concluded that when taking into account the concentration time profiles of all subjects simultaneously and considering concentrations below the quantification limit by population PK analysis, the allometrically scaled clearance in children was within the range of values reported for adults. The authors concluded that the differences in lithium PK parameters between children and adults might be explained by including the effect of body weight.

Table 16-6. Lithium Half-Life and Time to Steady State Estimates by Age[a]

Population	Half-life (Mean ± SD)	Time to Steady State[b] (Range)
Children and adolescents[41, 44]	27± 11 hr	80-190 hr
Adults (19–59 years)[37,53]	22 ± 7 hr	75–145 hr
Elderly (>59 years)[42]	27 ± 8 hr	95–175 hr

[a]In patients with normal renal function for age.
[b]Five half-lives were assumed for steady state, using ± 1 standard deviation of the mean half-life.

Dosing strategies

Dose prediction methods

Numerous equations and dosage prediction methods have been proposed to help clinicians identify an appropriate lithium dose for desired therapeutic concentrations. While many methods use lithium concentrations and a specific pharmacokinetic model, some use principles of population pharmacokinetics to relate patient characteristics to changes in lithium clearance.

Comparative evaluations of some dose prediction methods are available.[59-68] For example, in a comparative study, three dose prediction methods (i.e., the Zetin, Pepin, and Jermain methods) described below yielded more precise estimates than an empiric method for dosing lithium. The Jermain method was more precise at predicting steady state concentrations within 20% of actual lithium concentrations measurements from doses.[68] However, no one method was significantly better than another.

When lithium clearance is estimated or determined from measured concentrations, the clinician can select the dose (D) and dosage interval (τ) necessary to achieve the target trough (12 hr) steady state concentration (approximated by Css_{av}; see Equation 7 in the Introduction). When patients are at steady state and lithium pharmacokinetic parameters are stable, lithium dosages can be adjusted proportionately to reach the desired concentration.

Dosage prediction using the traditional pharmacokinetic method

Lithium exhibits linear pharmacokinetics that can be adequately described with a one-compartment model following oral dosing. The following equation may be used to estimate the dose required to produce a 12-hr trough concentration at steady state when an individual's lithium clearance is known or can be estimated.

$$D = \frac{CL \times \tau \times Css_{av}}{S \times F}$$

where D = dose (mEq), CL = clearance of lithium (L/h), τ = dosing interval (h), Cssav = average steady state concentration (mEq/L), F = fraction absorbed (~90% for most patients), and S = salt form (1).[57] The dose is then converted from mEq to mg.

Though rarely done, a patient's individual elimination half-life can be determined directly from two or more lithium concentrations obtained in the post-absorptive, post-distributive phase following an oral dose.[69] The multiple-point prediction method of Perry and colleagues employs a 1200-mg test dose, 12-, 24-, and 36-hr post dose concentration determinations, and direct estimation of the patient's individual elimination half-life.[70]

Dosage prediction by a priori demographics

The most common characteristics used for prediction methods include estimations of renal function, age, and body weight as represented by the method of Zetin et al.[71]

$$\begin{aligned} \text{Dose (mg/day)} &= 486.9 + (746.83 \times \text{desired concentration}) \\ &\quad - (10.08 \times \text{age}) + (5.95 \times \text{weight}) + (92.01 \times \text{status}) \\ &\quad + (147.8 \times \text{sex}) - (74.73 \times \text{TCA}) \end{aligned}$$

where desired concentration is in mEq/L, age in years, actual body weight in kg; status is 1 for inpatient, 0 for outpatient; sex is 1 for male and 0 for female; and TCA is 1 for concomitant tricyclic anti-depressant (TCA) administration or otherwise 0 for none.

Terao et al.[72] proposed an a priori demographic method based on stepwise multiple linear regression and blood urea nitrogen (BUN) as a measurement of renal function:

$$\begin{aligned} \text{Dose (mg/day)} &= 100.5 + (752.7 \times \text{desired concentration}) - (3.6 \times \text{age}) \\ &\quad + (7.2 \times \text{actual body weight}) - (13.7 \times \text{BUN}) \end{aligned}$$

where desired concentration is in mEq/L, age in years, weight in kg, and blood urea nitrogen (BUN) in mg/dl.

Dosage prediction by lithium renal clearance estimation

Pepin et al.[73] devised a prediction method based on their population pharmacokinetic findings that lithium clearance CL_{Li} is related to estimated creatinine clearance (CrCl); however, this method is not consistently precise or accurate.[59,74]

$$CL_{Li} = 0.235 \times \text{CrCl}$$

Units for CL_{Li} are the same as those used for CrCl.

The method of Jermain et al.[48] predicts lithium clearance based on population pharmacokinetics. It was developed using nonlinear fixed-effects models (NONMEM):

$$CL_{Li} = [0.0093\ (\text{L/hr/kg}) \times \text{LBW}] + (0.0885 \times \text{CrCl})$$

where LBW is the lean body weight in kg (see Chapter 3, Table 3-1, for lean body weight equation) and CrCl is the estimated creatinine clearance *in liters per hour.* This method suggests that LBW and CrCl are the most important predictors of lithium clearance. Age is not directly represented in this method, but decreases in CrCl and changes in total body water and muscle mass, as reflected in the lean body weight, likely account for the changes in lithium clearance usually attributed to age. This method yielded a coefficient of variation for predicted lithium clearance of about 24% and gave fairly accurate predictions of steady state lithium concentrations (coefficient of variation, 16%).

Dosage prediction by population pharmacokinetics and measured concentration(s)

The classic dosing chart of Cooper et al.[75] is based on population clearance values for lithium and uses a 600-mg standard release lithium carbonate test dose and a single 24-hr lithium concentration. This method does not predict a specific lithium concentration but provides a dose that is likely to result in a lithium concentration within the appropriate therapeutic range as indicated by a nomogram. The clinical utility and limitations of this method have been reviewed elsewhere.[76,77] The following equation may be used as an alternative to the nomogram.

$$Li^{+}\ (\text{mmol/day}) = e^{4.80 - (7.5 \times C_{test})}$$

where Ctest is equal to the 24-hr lithium concentration following the 600-mg test dose. Note that subtle differences in reported Ctest values lead to large differences in dose prediction using this method.

Perry and colleagues reported on both single-point and multiple-point prediction methods based on their findings of a significant correlation between observed lithium concentrations and predicted steady state concentrations.[70,78] Their single point method uses a 1200-mg test dose and a 24-hr post dose concentration determination, with use of a nomogram to predict steady state lithium concentrations.

Therapeutic Range

Some controversy exists regarding a standard therapeutic range for lithium; this is due, in part, to the search for the lowest possible range effective in maintenance and prophylaxis therapies.[16] The therapeutic ranges shown in Table 16-7 are generally accepted. In patients with acute mania, more than 90% of patients respond at lithium concentrations <1.2 mEq/L. Higher concentrations (1.2–1.5 mEq/L) may be required in selected patients. No definitive study is available to show a relationship between lithium concentrations and clinical response in children. However, several studies that evaluated lithium in children/adolescents showed that though mean lithium concentrations in the adult range were achieved, concentrations were not different between responders and nonresponders. Until more information is available, lithium concentration recommendations for children/adolescents are similar to that of adults.[79-81] Similarly, despite a limited amount of clinical data, lower target concentrations (0.5–0.8 mEq/L) are often recommended in elderly patients, primarily in an effort to minimize side effects.[82,83]

According to the most recent guidelines for the treatment of bipolar disorder, the therapeutic range traditionally targeted for lithium is 0.6–0.8 mEq/L for maintenance and prophylaxis therapies for patients with bipolar illness.[16] Several studies evaluating lower target concentrations (<0.7 mEq/L) indicate that the risk of relapse was substantially higher, and patients maintained in the lower portion of the therapeutic range had fewer satisfactory responses.[84-88] Maintaining higher lithium concentrations (0.8–1.0 mEq/L) may increase the likelihood of successful prophylactic treatment, but some patients do respond at lower concentrations.[89,90] Similarly, small changes in concentrations (0.2–0.3 mEq/L) may be clinically significant and substantially affect relapse rates.[16,19,85,89] Appropriate therapeutic drug monitoring and use of sound pharmacokinetic principles to more precisely target desired lithium concentrations may be beneficial.

Table 16-7. Proposed Therapeutic Range for Lithium[16]

Disease or Condition	Therapeutic Range
Acute mania	0.5–1.2 mEq/L
Prophylaxis of mania and/or depression	0.6–0.8 mEq/L

Therapeutic Monitoring

Suggested sampling times and effect on therapeutic range

Considerable efforts have been made to standardize the sampling time for steady state lithium concentration determinations.[17] Several factors including daily lithium schedule, timing of sampling, patient compliance, diurnal variation, lithium preparation, and changes in salt intake, renal function, hydration status, and concomitant medication all may affect measured lithium concentrations.[19] Based on divided daily dosing schedules (two, three, or four times daily) the conventional lithium concentration determination is a 12-hr (±30 min) post dose trough concentration, collected after the evening dose but before the morning dose (hold the morning dose if necessary). This 12-hr time point is arbitrary but usually occurs in the post absorption and post distribution phase, thus minimizing the intra- and interindividual variability in lithium measurements over time. If an 8-hour post dose trough concentration time point is used, then lithium concentrations would be higher than the standard 12-hour concentration and therefore would affect interpretation.

In the case of once-daily dosing, there are much greater peak-to-trough fluctuations around the average steady state lithium concentration compared with the same daily dosage given in divided doses. Therefore, the 12-hr lithium concentration measurement may be higher and a 24-hr trough lithium concentration may be lower than the standard 12-hr concentration measurements obtained after a divided daily dosing schedule. A 10% to 26% increase in the standard 12-hr lithium concentrations may be expected with a change to a once-daily dosing schedule using the same total daily dose.[91] As shown in Figure 16-1, simulated steady state lithium concentration-time profiles using the same lithium dosage divided into different daily schedules illustrate the variability of the 12-hr lithium concentration determination due to differences in dosing interval. The 12-hr lithium concentration measurements were 1.37 versus 1.07, 1.00, and 0.96 mEq/L when the same daily dose was given once-daily versus divided into two, three, or four doses, respectively.[28] Current therapeutic ranges assume multiple daily dosage regimens, and no therapeutic range has been established for once-daily regimens.

Concentration measurement frequency

Because lithium concentrations are closely related to therapeutic response and side effects, the use of lithium concentration monitoring is an important clinical tool to manage patients receiving lithium. Therapeutic drug monitoring can be used to monitor efficacy, toxicity, compliance, and accuracy of prediction models. In acute mania, initial 12-hr lithium trough concentrations should be performed once or twice weekly until the desired therapeutic concentration is achieved, with continued follow-up monitoring at least every 3 to 6 months, or as necessary during periods of therapeutic nonresponse or appearance of side effects in acutely manic patients.[16] A conventional monitoring method for the once-daily dosage patient is to identify the 12-hr lithium concentration that is therapeutic for that individual and to carefully screen for side effects, toxicity, or relapse of manic symptoms.

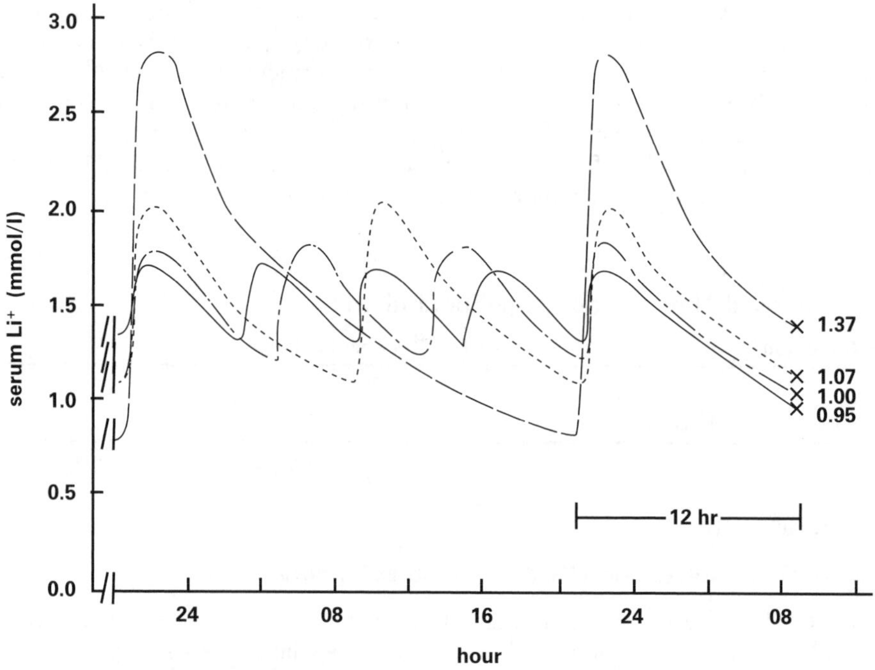

Figure 16-1. Simulated steady state serum lithium (S_{Li}) concentration-time profiles of identical lithium doses divided into one, two, three, or four doses illustrate the variability of 12-hr S_{Li} concentrations due solely to differences in dosage interval.

Source: *Reprinted with permission from reference 28.*

Current practice guidelines for the treatment of patients with bipolar disorder also recommend that lithium concentrations be obtained at least every 3 to 6 months during maintenance therapy in stable patients.[16,92] More frequent monitoring may be required with changes in fluid and electrolyte balance, unstable renal function, or if toxicity is a concern. Other laboratory monitoring parameters and information for patient and family counseling can be found elsewhere.[15,93]

A treatment initiation and monitoring scheme for patients receiving lithium is shown in Figure 16-2.

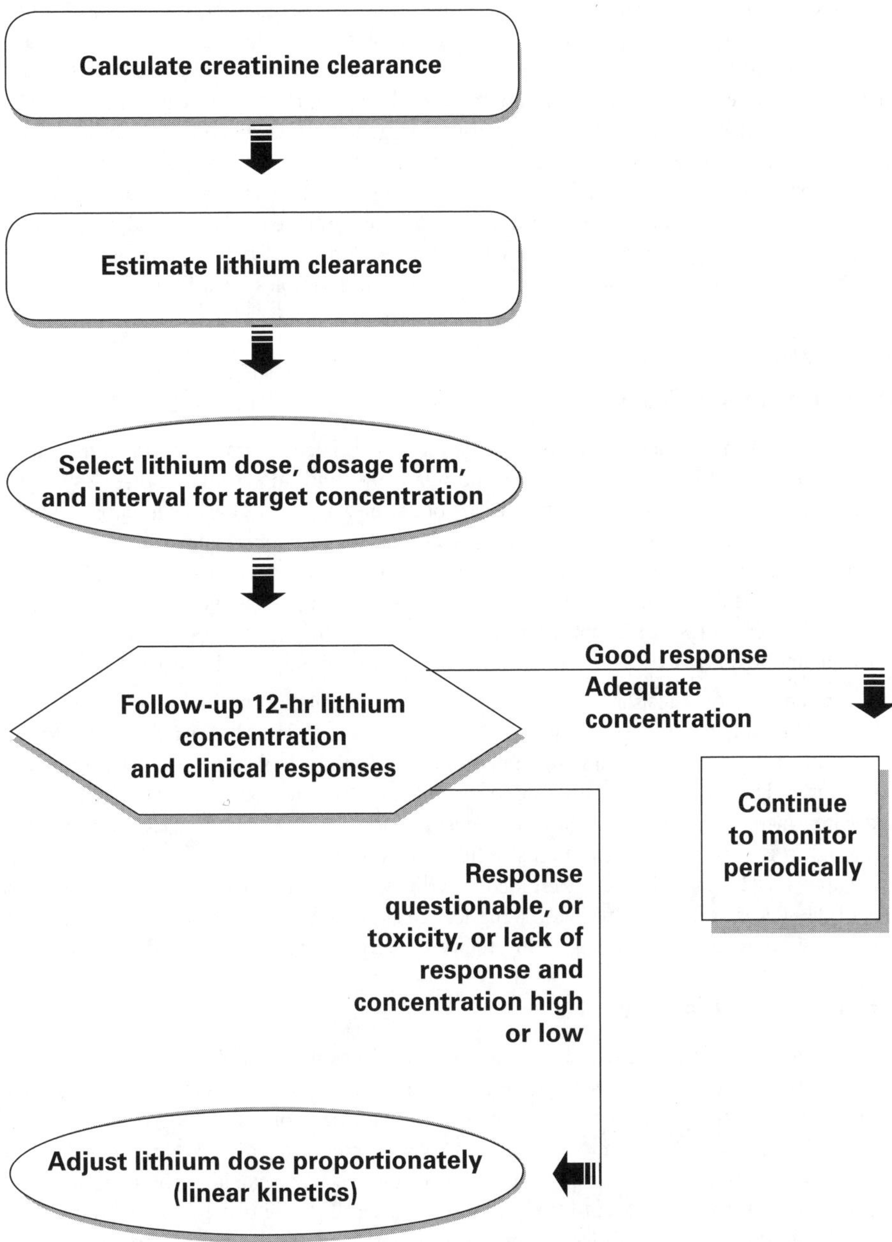

Figure 16-2. General scheme for therapeutic drug monitoring of lithium therapy in patients with bipolar disorder.

Assay issues

Plasma or serum may be used to determine lithium concentrations; both provide similar results. Bioassay methods for lithium include flame photometry and atomic absorption. Both are commonly used in the determination of lithium concentrations in biofluids and provide comparable results.[62,94]

A third methodology used to determine lithium concentrations is the ion-specific or ion-selective electrode (ISE) analyzer.[95-97] Recently, several spectrophotometric and colorimetric methods have also been evaluated to monitor lithium serum concentrations; the advantage of these methodologies is that they are fast and easy to perform and often require only small volumes of sample, however, hemoglobin can interfere with the determinations and these methods are applied only to serum samples.[98-101] A methodology based on capillary zone electrophoresis with indirect detection has been described in the literature.[102] This method is more time consuming than ion-selective electrodes or flame photometry; however, the sophisticated separation mechanism prior to detection excludes potential interferences from endogenous and exogenous compounds present in the sample. Therefore it is proposed to be used as a confirmatory tool in controversial analysis or non-standard samples such as forensic specimens. Finally a new methodology based on a microchip capillary electrophoresis method has been developed to analyze minute amounts of blood with the final goal to allow for self-monitoring at home from simple capillary blood obtained by finger stick.[103] In order to avoid interferences, sample tubes containing lithium-heparin should not be used to collect biofluid samples for lithium determinations.[104]

Pharmacodynamic Monitoring

Concentration-related efficacy

The application of pharmacokinetic principles to monitor pharmacodynamic responses in clinical practice assumes that the response is objective, reversible, and relatively rapid. In psychiatric diseases, some evaluated responses may fail to meet all of these assumptions. Response measurements evaluated in patients with psychiatric illness typically are affected by subjective rating scales, delayed responses (days or weeks), and significant placebo effects. Thus, percent of response or relative risk of relapse at a particular drug concentration may be used to account for these discrepancies. In patients receiving lithium, target symptom response is most often used to gauge the effectiveness of lithium therapy. Improvements in manic or depressive symptoms, such as sleep patterns, agitation, and anxiety, are good indicators of lithium efficacy (Table 16-8).

Due to the heterogeneity of response in the bipolar patient population, the optimal lithium concentration for individual patients may vary depending on the indicated use. Different target concentrations have been suggested to manage acute mania, maintain remission, or provide prophylaxis against future episodes (see Therapeutic Range). The paradigm of using the lowest effective dose to limit the appearance of side effects is widely held when managing patients on lithium. Several studies have shown that as lithium concentrations increase from 0.3 to 1.4 mEq/L, the risk of relapse decreases and the incidence of side effects increases.[84,85,105] The risk of relapse was 2.6 times higher when median lithium concentrations (12-hr post dose) were targeted in the range of 0.4–0.6 mEq/L compared with a higher target range of 0.8–1.0 mEq/L.[86] This finding suggests considerable variation in clinical response within the typical concentration range of 0.5–1.2 mEq/L.

Concentration-related toxicity

Lithium toxicities appear to increase with increasing lithium concentrations (Table 16-9). Toxicity most often occurs with 12-hr trough concentrations greater than 1.5 mEq/L, but side effects may occur in some patients at therapeutic concentrations. Mild and transient effects such as fine tremor, nausea, diarrhea, muscle weakness, polyuria, and polydipsia can be seen at concentrations of less than or equal to 1.5 mEq/L. Moderate toxicity usually occurs at concentrations of 1.5 to 2.5 mEq/L, with more severe toxicities observed at trough concentrations greater than 2.5 mEq/L. Concentrations above 3.0–3.5 mEq/L are usually considered life threatening; hemodialysis, the most effective extrarenal clearance mechanism, should be considered.[57,107]

Drug-Drug Interactions

A number of lithium drug-drug interactions are associated with effects on fluid and/or sodium balance, thus GFR and sodium excretion are of particular importance. An extensive review of lithium drug interactions is reported elsewhere.[108] Drugs causing a decrease in GFR or a compensatory increase in sodium reabsorption

Table 16-8. Therapeutic Response Sequence Following Initiation of Lithium Therapy[106]

Manic Symptoms

1–3 weeks
Decrease in pressured speech
Decreases in hostile or assaultive behaviors

2–3 weeks
Improved thought pattern disturbances

2–4 weeks
Increased attention to appearance or hygiene

1–2 months
Less grandiosity
Less irritability

Depressive Symptoms

2–4 weeks
Improved motor and mental activities
Improved sleep pattern
Decrease in any psychotic features

1–2 months
Improved mood

result in reduced lithium clearance and elevated lithium concentrations. Examples of this type of lithium-drug interaction include the non-thiazide, thiazide, and loop diuretics; nonsteroidal anti-inflammatory agents; angiotensin-converting enzyme inhibitors; platinum-containing chemotherapeutics; and iodides (Table 16-10). When assessing the impact of these drug-drug interactions, adjustment factors can be used to estimate changes in pharmacokinetic parameters. For example, angiotensin converting enzyme inhibitors may decrease lithium clearance by 30% in patients ≥50 years of age, while caffeine or theophylline may increase lithium clearance by 20%–25%. Because there is considerable interindividual variation in drug-drug interactions with lithium, these adjustment factors should be used with caution.

Other drugs that have been reported to interact with lithium include antipsychotics, anticonvulsants, selective-serotonin receptor antagonists, calcium-channel blockers, antibiotics, and neuromuscular-blocking agents.[116-119] Several case reports or series also have suggested potential lithium interactions with tetracycline, metronidazole, diazepam, opiates, beta-adrenergic antagonists, topiramate, levofloxacin, doxycycline, methyldopa, digoxin, mefenamic acid, angiotensin receptor blockers, and possibly minocycline.[14,117,120-129]

Drug–Disease State Interactions and Special Populations

Disease state or condition interactions with lithium are often related to an individual's renal function and usually to GFR and/or sodium excretion. Disease states or conditions that increase GFR, such as pregnancy or excess fluid administration, are likely to increase lithium clearance, resulting in shorter half-lives and lower lithium concentrations.

Children typically have increased renal function and higher excretion rates compared with adults and may require higher lithium doses per kilogram of body weight to achieve therapeutic concentrations. Compared to other treatments there are more data available for lithium than for any other medication in children for bipolar disorder. Even though only limited data are available in children receiving lithium, the clinical response has ranged from 50% to 100% in various studies.[16,44,80,152-156] Lithium is not approved for use in children below 12 years of age and, therefore, should be used with special caution.

Conversely, conditions such as advancing age or renal impairment are associated with a decrease in GFR. Alterations in total body water and lean muscle mass that accompany aging are associated with a reduced volume of distribution and higher lithium concentrations. Conditions that result in a compensatory increase in sodium reabsorption, such as dehydration, increase lithium reabsorption and decrease lithium clearance,

Table 16-9. Concentration-Related Toxicity Associated with Lithium Therapy[109-115]

Concentration-Related Toxicity[a]	Comment
Potential side effects observed with therapeutic concentrations Agitation Cog-wheel rigidity Confusion Delirium Dysarthria Increased deep tendon reflexes Memory impairment Seizures	Measure lithium concentration; consider reduction in dose.
Mild toxicity (>1.5 mEq/L) Fatigue Fine tremors of the limbs Gastrointestinal disturbances Muscle weakness	Measure lithium concentration; interview patient regarding changes in diet, health, or concomitant medications; consider reduction in dose.
Moderate toxicity (1.5–2.5 mEq/L) Ataxia Coarse tremors Dysarthria Headaches Hyperthermia Impaired sensorium Increased deep tendon reflexes Lethargy Nystagmus Sedation	Measure lithium concentration; interview patient regarding changes in diet, health, or concomitant medications; consider reduction in dose; consider supportive care to correct any fluid imbalance.
Severe toxicity (>2.5 mEq/L) Basal ganglia dysfunction Coarse tremors Delirium Respiratory complication Seizures Death	Occurs in overdose, in patients receiving high lithium doses, and with concomitant illnesses; hold doses and consider use of hemodialysis or peritoneal dialysis; reduce dose unless efficacy shown to be compromised at lower concentration.

[a]Toxicities that occur at lower concentrations may also occur at higher concentrations.

leading to increased lithium concentrations. Lithium should be used cautiously in patients with restricted sodium intake. Patients with underlying cardiovascular or thyroid disease should be monitored for signs and symptoms of dysrhythmia while receiving lithium since sinus nodal arrhythmias may occur. When assessing the impact of these disease state or condition interactions, adjustment factors can be used to estimate changes in pharmacokinetic parameters (Table 16-11). For example, dehydration may decrease lithium clearance to 81% of normal while pregnancy may increase it 2-fold.

Dialysis

Lithium may be removed by either hemodialysis or peritoneal dialysis; rebound increases in lithium concentrations may occur for up to 8 hr after dialysis.[14,163,164]

Pregnancy

The Food and Drug Administration classify lithium as a Category D drug as there is evidence of human fetal risk, but benefits to the pregnant woman may outweigh the risk. Untreated pregnant women are at increased risk of relapse, and the high incidence of post-partum affective disorders poses some question regarding the discontinuation of prophylactic therapy. Current recommendations suggest avoiding first-trimester exposure if possible.[165]

Table 16-10. Selected Lithium-Drug Interactions and Adjustment Factors

Drug	Affected Pharmacokinetic Parameter	Adjustment Factor[a]
Thiazide diuretics[130-135]	Renal clearance	0.32–0.74
Angiotensin converting enzyme	Renal clearance	<50 years, 0.87
(ACE) inhibitors[116,136]		≥50 years, 0.69
Nonsteroidal anti-inflammatory		
Agents[137,138]	Renal clearance	0.33–1
Celecoxib[138-141]	Renal clearance	0.43–0.95[b]
Diclofenac[138,141]	Renal clearance	0.53–0.80
Flurbiprofen[138-142]	Renal clearance	0.84–0.92
Ibuprofen[138,143]	Renal clearance	0.60–1.1
Indomethacin[138,144]	Renal clearance	0.62–0.83
Ketorolac[138,145]	Renal clearance	0.64–0.79
Mefenamic acid[138]	Renal clearance	0.25[b]
Meloxicam[138]	Renal clearance	0.71
Naproxen[138,146,147]	Renal clearance	0.67–1
Phenylbutazone[138]	Renal clearance	0.87
Piroxicam[138]	Renal clearance	0.26–0.79
Sulindac[c,138]	Renal clearance	0.50–0.71[b]
Cisplatin/fluids[148,149]	Renal clearance	1.6
	Half-life	0.25–0.50
Theophylline[150]	Renal clearance	1.21
Caffeine[53]	Renal clearance	1.2–1.25
Sodium-containing intravenous fluids[117,151]	Renal clearance	1.2

[a]Adjustment factor is the fraction of usual dose (or clearance or half-life) that would be suggested in cases where both drugs are used concomitantly.
[b]Adjustment factor based on one or more individual case reports.
[c]Transient changes in lithium plasma concentrations after sulindac administration returned to baseline with continued sulindac treatment.

Fetal exposure to lithium in the first trimester is associated with a 1/1000 to 1/2000 risk of developing Ebstein's anomaly of the tricuspid valve. The risk in the general population is 1/20,000. The risk for this very rare malformation remains very low, and other recent studies concluded that the use of lithium during pregnancy did not increase the number of congenital malformations.[36,165] Because GFR increases and creatinine clearance may double during pregnancy, lithium dosage requirements will likely increase in the third trimester. Careful monitoring of lithium concentrations during pregnancy and after delivery is essential. Lithium concentrations should be monitored at least monthly, along with thyroid and electrolyte measurements, during pregnancy.[165,166] Subsequent downward titration by 25%–30% or discontinuation of lithium immediately prior to delivery will decrease the risks of neonatal toxicity and toxicity due to rapid postpartum shifts in plasma volume.[167,168]

Lithium concentrations in breast milk are approximately 50% of the maternal concentrations, and because an infant's renal status is immature, any lithium ingested from breast milk may be cleared slowly.[168] In a study of 10 maternal-infant pairs of carefully selected patients with bipolar disorder, breast milk concentrations averaged approximately 50% of maternal trough concentrations (10–14 hours post-dose) and infant concentrations averaged approximately 50% of breast milk concentrations. There were no reports of treatment emergent adverse events or behavioral effects in the infants.[169,170] Nevertheless, infants should be carefully monitored for hypotonia, lethargy, cyanosis, hydration status, renal function, thyroid function, and perhaps lithium concentration if breast fed.[165]

Table 16-11. Selected Lithium-Disease State or Condition Interactions and Adjustment Factors

Population	Affected Pharmacokinetic Parameter	Adjustment Factor
Acute mania[157]	Renal clearance	0.6
Pregnancy[33,34]	Clearance	2
Elderly[37,42,158]	Renal clearance	0.6–0.7
	Distribution volume	0.6–0.8
Dehydration[158]	Renal clearance	0.8[a]
Low-salt diet[159,160]	Renal clearance	<1.0
Obesity[161]	Renal clearance	1.5
	Distribution volume	0.6
Lithium therapy for >1 year[158]	Half-life	1.3–1.4[b]
Strenuous exercise[162]	Renal clearance	1.2[a]

[a]Lithium clearance based on single concentration in case reports.
[b]Not consistent in all studies.

Summary

The therapeutic goal of lithium pharmacotherapy is to return the patient to an appropriate level of psychosocial functioning and remission of the disorder. Clinically, lithium disposition is consistent with a one-compartment model following oral dosing, with a linear pharmacokinetic profile. Lithium is primarily cleared through the kidney, and changes in renal clearance significantly affect lithium pharmacokinetics. Target 12-hr trough concentrations are 0.5–1.2 mEq/L for acute mania and 0.6–0.8 mEq/L for prophylaxis of bipolar disorder. Potential drug interactions caused by concomitant drug therapy, disease states, or conditions that alter GFR or sodium reabsorption should be reviewed when initiating and assessing lithium pharmacotherapy. Overall, optimal lithium therapy should be guided by targeted lithium concentration monitoring and clinical response of the patient.

References

1. Eskalith [package insert]. Research Triangle Park, NC: GlaxoSmithkline. 2003.
2. Bauer M, Adli M, Bschor T, et al. Lithium's emerging role in the treatment of refractory major depressive episodes: augmentation of antidepressants. *Neuropsychobiology*. 2010; 62:36-42.
3. Grunze H, Vieta E, Goodwin G, et al. The World Federation of Societies of Biological Psychiatry (WFSBP) Guidelines for the biological treatment of bipolar disorders: update 2010 on the treatment of acute bipolar depression. *World J Biol Psychiatry.* 2010;11:81-109.
4. Lithium Monograph. In: *Drugs Facts and Comparisons E Answers*. Wolters Kluwer Health, Inc. 2010. Accessed July 29, 2010.
5. Thase ME, Sachs GS. Bipolar depression: pharmacotherapy and related therapeutic strategies. *Biol Psychiatry*. 2000;48:558-72.
6. Cipriani A, Pretty H, Hawton K, et al. Lithium in the prevention of suicidal behavior and all-cause mortality in patients with mood disorders: a systematic review of randomized trials. *Am J Psychiatry*. 2005;162:1805-19.
7. Davis KL, Charney D, Coyle JT, et al., eds. *Neuropsychopharmacology: The Fifth Generation Of Progress*. Philadelphia, PA: Lippincott, Williams & Wilkins; 2002.
8. Ipser J, Stein DJ. Systematic review of pharmacotherapy of disruptive behavior disorders in children and adolescents. *Psychopharmacology*. 2007;191:127-40.
9. Wada A, Yokoo H, Yanagita T, et al. Lithium: Potential therapeutics against acute brain injuries and chronic neurodegenerative diseases. *J Pharmacol Sci*. 2005;99:307-21.
10. Young W. Review of lithium effects on brain and blood. *Cell Transplantation*. 2009; 18:951-75.
11. Risby ED, Hsiao JK, Manji HK, et al. The mechanisms of action of lithium. II. Effects on adenylate cyclase activity and beta-adrenergic receptor binding in normal subjects. *Arch Gen Psychiatry*. 1991;48:513-24.

12. Marmol F. Lithium: Bipolar disorder and neurodegenerative diseases possible cellular mechanisms of the therapeutic effects of lithium. *Prog Neuro-Psychophamacol Biol Psychiatry.* 2008;32:1761-71.
13. Gould TD, Quiroz JA, Singh J, et al. Emerging experimental therapeutics for bipolar disorder: insights from the molecular and cellular actions of current mood stabilizers. *Molecular Psychiatry*. 2004;9:734-55.
14. Lithium salts. In: McEvoy GK, ed. *AHFS Drug Information 2011*. Bethesda, MD: American Society of Health-System Pharmacists; 2011:2566-75.
15. Keck PE, Jr., McElroy SL, Bennett JA. Pharmacologic loading in the treatment of acute mania. *Bipolar Disord.* 2000;2:42-6.
16. Hirschfeld RMA. *Guideline Watch: Practice Guideline for the Treatment of Patients with Bipolar Disorder.* Arlington, VA: American Psychiatric Association; 2005.
17. Amdisen A. Serum level monitoring and clinical pharmacokinetics of lithium. *Clin Pharmacokinet.* 1977;2:73-92.
18. Geddes JR, Burgess S, Hawton K, et al. Long-term lithium therapy for bipolar disorder: systematic review and meta-analysis of randomized controlled trials. *Am J Psychiatry.* 2004;161:217-22.
19. Sproule B. Lithium in bipolar disorder: can drug concentrations predict therapeutic effect? *Clin Pharmacokinet.* 2002;41:639-60.
20. Baldessarini RJ, Tondo L, Viguera AC. Discontinuing lithium maintenance treatment in bipolar disorders: risks and implications. *Bipolar Disord.* 1999;1:17-24.
21. Lithium. In: Anon. 2010 Physicians Desk Reference. Williston, VT: PDR Network LLC; 2010.
22. Amdisen A. Sustained release preparations of lithium. In: Johnson FN, ed. *Lithium Research and Therapy*. London: Academic Press; 1975.
23. Amdisen A, Sjorgren J. Lithium absorption from sustained-release tablets (Duretter). *Acta Pharm Suec.* 1968;5:465-72.
24. Diamond JM, Ehrlich BE, Morawski SG, et al. Lithium absorption in tight and leaky segments of intestine. *J Membr Biol.* 1983;72:153-9.
25. Ereshefsky L, Gilderman AM, Jewett CM. Lithium therapy of manic depressive illness. Part II: Monitoring. *Drug Intell Clin Pharm.* 1979;13:492-7.
26. Shopsin B, Sathananthan G, Gershon S. Plasma renin response to lithium in psychiatric patients. *Clin Pharmacol Ther.* 1973;14:561-4.
27. Ehrlich BE, Diamond JM. Lithium absorption: implications for sustained-release lithium preparations. *Lancet.* 1983;1:306.
28. Carson S. Lithium. In: Evans WE, Schentag JJ, Jusko WJ, eds. *Applied Pharmacokinetics: Principles of Therapeutic Drug Monitoring.* 3rd ed. Spokane, WA: Applied Therapeutics; 1992:34-1-34-26.
29. Heiman MF, Schwabach G, Tupin J. Liquid lithium vs. solid lithium: an open, cross-over, pilot study comparing oral preparations. *Dis Nerv Syst.* 1976;37:9-11.
30. Mendels J, Frazer A. Intracellular lithium concentration and clinical response: towards a membrane theory of depression. *J Psychiatr Res.* 1973;10:9-18.
31. Gengo F, Frazer A, Ramsey TA, et al. The lithium ratio as a guide to patient compliance. *Compr Psychiatry.* 1980;21:276-80.
32. Ayd FJ. Excretion of psychotropic drugs in human breast milk. *Int Drug Ther Newsletter.* 1973;8:33.
33. Schou M, Amdisen A. Lithium and pregnancy. 3. Lithium ingestion by children breast-fed by women on lithium treatment. *Br Med J.* 1973(a);2:138.
34. Schou M, Amdisen A, Steenstrup OR. Lithium and pregnancy. II. Hazards to women given lithium during pregnancy and delivery. *Br Med J.* 1973(b);2:137-8.
35. Yoshida K, Smith B, Kumar R. Psychotropic drugs in mothers' milk: a comprehensive review of assay methods, pharmacokinetics and of safety of breast-feeding. *J Psychopharmacol.* 1999;13:64-80.
36. Gentile S. Prophylactic treatment of bipolar disorder in pregnancy and breastfeeding: focus on emerging mood stabilizers. *Bipolar Disorders*. 2006;8:207-20.
37. Nielsen-Kudsk F, Amdisen A. Analysis of the pharmacokinetics of lithium in man. *Eur J Clin Pharmacol.* 1979;16:271-7.
38. Lehmann K, Merten K. Elimination of lithium in dependence on age in healthy subjects and patients with renal insufficiency. *Int J Clin Pharmacol.* 1974;10:292-8.
39. Thornhill DP. Comparison of ordinary and sustained release lithium carbonate in manic patients. *Br J Pharmacol.* 1978;5:352.
40. Perry PJ, Dunner FJ, Hahn RL, et al. Lithium kinetics in single daily dosing. *Acta Psychiatr Scand.* 1981;64:281-94.
41. Findling RL, Landersdorfer CB, Kafantaris V, et al. First-dose pharmacokinetics of lithium carbonate in children and adolescents. *J Clin Psychopharmacol.* 2010;30:404-10.
42. Karki SD, Carson SW, Gagnon A. Evaluation of total body water and disposition of lithium in elderly patients. *Lithium.* 1992;3:29-33.

43. Sproule BA, Hardy BG, Shulman KI. Differential pharmacokinetics of lithium in elderly patients. *Drugs Aging.* 2000;16:165-77.

44. Vitiello B, Behar D, Malone R, et al. Pharmacokinetics of lithium carbonate in children. *J Clin Psychopharmacol.* 1988;8:355-9.

45. Jefferson JW, Greist JH. General pharmacology. In: Jefferson JW, Griest JH, eds. *Primer of Lithium Therapy.* Baltimore, MD: Williams and Wilkins: 1977;95-6.

46. Thomsen K, Schou M. Renal lithium excretion in man. *Am J Physiol.* 1968;215:823-7.

47. Lindeman RD. Trace minerals and the kidney: an overview. *J Am Coll Nutr.* 1989;8:285-91.

48. Jermain DM, Crismon ML, Martin ES. Population pharmacokinetics of lithium. *Clin Pharm.* 1991;10:376-81.

49. Boton R, Gaviria M, Batlle DC. Prevalence, pathogenesis, and treatment of renal dysfunction associated with chronic lithium therapy. *Am J Kidney Dis.* 1987;10:329.

50. Jorkasky DK. Lithium-induced renal disease: a prospective study. *Clin Nephrol.* 1988;30:293.

51. Davis JM, Fann WE. Lithium. *Ann Rev Pharmacol.* 1971;11:285-302.

52. Platman SR, Fieve RR. Lithium retention and excretion. The effect of sodium and fluid intake. *Arch Gen Psychiatry.* 1969;20:285-9.

53. Carson SW, Gagnon A, Bahkai Y. Pharmacokinetic and pharmacodynamic effects of caffeine on lithium disposition. *Pharmacotherapy.* 1989;9:196-7.

54. Nelson RW, Cohen JL. Plasma and erythrocyte kinetic considerations in lithium therapy. *Am J Hosp Pharm.* 1976;33:658-64.

55. Taright N, Mentre F, Mallet A, et al. Nonparametric estimation of population characteristics of the kinetics of lithium from observational and experimental data: individualization of chronic dosing regimen using a new Bayesian approach. *Ther Drug Monit.* 1994;16:258-69.

56. Goodnick PJ, Fieve RR. Plasma lithium level and inter-episode functioning in bipolar disorder. *Am J Psychiatry.* 1985;142:761-2.

57. Ereshefsky L, Jann MW. Lithium. In: Mungall D, ed. *Applied Clinical Pharmacokinetics.* New York, NY: Raven Press; 1983:245-70.

58. Grunfeld J-P, Rossier BC. Lithium nephrotoxicity revisited. *Nat Rev Nephrol.* 2009;5:270-6.

59. Browne JL, Patel RA, Huffman CS, et al. Comparison of pharmacokinetic procedures for dosing lithium based on analysis of prediction error. *Drug Intell Clin Pharm.* 1988;22:227-31.

60. Browne JL, Huffman CS, Golden RN. A comparison of pharmacokinetic versus empirical lithium dosing techniques. *Ther Drug Monit.* 1989;11:149-54.

61. Cummings MA, Haviland MG, Cummings KL, et al. Lithium dose prediction: a prospective case series. *J Clin Psychiatry.* 1988;49:373.

62. Karki SD, Carson SW, Holden JMC. Effect of assay methodology on the prediction of lithium maintenance dosage. *Drug Intell Clin Pharm.* 1989;23:372-5.

63. Lobeck F, Nelson MV, Evans RL, et al. Evaluation of four methods for predicting lithium dosage. *Clin Pharm.* 1987;6:230-3.

64. Lobeck F. A review of lithium dosing methods. *Pharmacotherapy.* 1988;8:248-55.

65. Markoff RA, King M Jr. Does lithium dose prediction improve treatment efficiency? Prospective evaluation of a mathematical method. *J Clin Psychopharmacol.* 1992;12:305-8.

66. Nelson MV. Comparison of three lithium dosing methods in 950 "subjects" by computer simulation. *Ther Drug Monit.* 1988;10:269-74.

67. Williams PJ, Browne JL, Patel RA. Bayesian forecasting of serum lithium concentrations. Comparison with traditional methods. *Clin Pharmacokinet.* 1989;17:45-52.

68. Wright R, Crismon ML. Comparison of three a priori methods and one empirical method in predicting lithium dosage requirements. *Am J Health-Syst Pharm.* 2000;57:1698-702.

69. Carson SW, DeVane CL. Estimation of half-life and exponential decay using a nomogram. *Am J Hosp Pharm.* 1983;40:1696-8.

70. Perry PJ, Alexander B, Dunner FJ, et al. Pharmacokinetic protocol for predicting serum lithium levels. *J Clin Psychopharmacol.* 1982;2:114-8.

71. Zetin M, Garber D, De Antonio M, et al. Prediction of lithium dose: a mathematical alternative to the test-dose method. *J Clin Psychiatry.* 1986;47:175-8.

72. Terao T, Okuno K, Okuno T, et al. A simpler and more accurate equation to predict daily lithium dose. *J Clin Psychopharmacol.* 1999;19:336-40.

73. Pepin SM, Bake DE, Nance KS, et al. Lithium dosage calculation from age, sex, height, weight and serum creatinine.

Paper presented at 15th Annual ASHP Midyear Clinical Meeting. San Francisco, CA; 1980 Dec 9.

74. Stip E, Dufresne J, Boulerice B, et al. Accuracy of the Pepin method to determine appropriate lithium dosages in healthy volunteers. *J Psychiatry Neurosci.* 2001;26:330-5.
75. Cooper TB, Bergner PE, Simpson GM. The 24-hour serum lithium level as a prognosticator of dosage requirements. *Am J Psychiatry.* 1973;130:601-3.
76. Gengo F, Timko J, D'Antonio J, et al. Prediction of dosage of lithium carbonate: use of a standard predictive method. *J Clin Psychiatry.* 1980;41:319-20.
77. Peterse JW, Havenaar JM, van Rijn HJ. Possible hazard in use of priming dose to determine lithium dosage. *Am J Psychiatry.* 1999;156:157-8.
78. Perry PJ, Prince RA, Alexander B, et al. Prediction of lithium maintenance doses using a single point prediction protocol. *J Clin Psychopharmacol.* 1983;3:13-7.
79. Davanzo PA, McCracken JT. Mood stabilizers in the treatment of juvenile bipolar disorder: advances and controversies. *Child Adolesc Psychiatr Clin N Am.* 2000;9:159-82.
80. Geller B, Cooper TB, Sun K, et al. Double-blind and placebo-controlled study of lithium for adolescent bipolar disorders with secondary substance dependency. *J Am Acad Child Adolesc Psychiatry.* 1998;37:171-8.
81. McClellan J, Werry J. Practice parameters for the assessment and treatment of children and adolescents with bipolar disorder. American Academy of Child and Adolescent Psychiatry. *J Am Acad Child Adolesc Psychiatry.* 1997;36(suppl 10):157S-76S.
82. Shulman KI, Herrmann N. The nature and management of mania in old age. *Psychiatric Clin North Am.* 1999;22:649-65.
83. Young RC. Treatment of geriatric mania. In: Shulman KI, Tohen M, Kitcher SP, eds. *Mood Disorders Across the Life Span.* New York, NY: John Wiley & Sons, Inc.; 1996:411-25.
84. Prien RF, Caffey EM, Jr., Klett CJ. Relationship between serum lithium level and clinical response in acute mania treated with lithium. *Br J Psychiatry.* 1972;120:409-14.
85. Gelenberg AJ, Carroll JA, Baudhuin MG, et al. The meaning of serum lithium levels in maintenance therapy of mood disorders: a review of the literature. *J Clin Psychiatry.* 1989;(suppl 50):17-22; discussion 45-7.
86. Gelenberg AJ, Kane JM, Keller MB, et al. Comparison of standard and low serum levels of lithium for maintenance treatment of bipolar disorder. *N Engl J Med.* 1989;321:1489-93.
87. Solomon DA, Ristow WR, Keller MB, et al. Serum lithium levels and psychosocial function in patients with bipolar I disorder. *Am J Psychiatry.* 1996;153:1301-7.
88. Waters B, Lapierre Y, Gagnon A, et al. Determination of the optimal concentration of lithium for the prophylaxis of manic-depressive disorder. *Biol Psychiatry.* 1982;17:1323-9.
89. Hopkins HS, Gelenberg AJ. Serum lithium levels and the outcome of maintenance therapy of bipolar disorder. *Bipolar Disord.* 2000;2:174-9.
90. Vestergaard P, Licht RW, Brodersen A, et al. Outcome of lithium prophylaxis: a prospective followup of affective disorder patients assigned to high and low serum lithium levels. *Acta Psychiatr Scand.* 1998;98:310-5.
91. Mitchell PB. Therapeutic drug monitoring of psychotropic medications. *Br J Pharmacol.* 2001;52:45S-54S.
92. Ng F, Mammen OK, Wilting I, et al. The International Society for Bipolar Disorders (ISBD) consensus guidelines for the safety monitoring of bipolar disorder treatments. *Bipolar Disorders.* 2009;11:559-95.
93. Carson SW, Foslien-Nash C. Lithium pharmacotherapy. *US Pharm.* 1990;15:H1-H10.
94. Lippmann S, Regan W, Manshadi M. Plasma lithium stability and a comparison of flame photometry and atomic absorption spectrophotometry analysis. *Am J Psychiatry.* 1981;138:1375-7.
95. Bertholf RL, Savory MG, Winborne KH, et al. Lithium determined in serum with an ion-selective electrode. *Clin Chem.* 1988;34(7):1500-2.
96. Sampson M, Ruddel M, Elin RJ. Lithium determinations evaluated in eight analyzers. *Clin Chem.* 1994;40(6):869-72.
97. Greffe J, Gouget B. Red cell effects on lithium measurements by ion-selective electrode. *Scand J Clin Lab Invest Suppl.* 1996;224:187-91.
98. Lyon AW, Whitley C, Eintracht SL. Analytic evaluation and application of a novel spectrophotometric serum lithium method to a rapid response laboratory. *Ther Drug Monit.* 2004;26(1):98-101.
99. Christenson RH, Mandichak JJ, Duh SH, et al. Clinical performance characteristics of a new photometric lithium assay: a multicenter study. *Clin Chim Acta.* 2003;327(1-2):157-64.
100. Gorham JD, Walton KG, McClellan AC, et al. Evaluation of a new colorimetric assay for serum lithium. *Ther Drug Monit.* 1994;16(3):277-80.
101. Gruson D, Lallali A, Furlan V, et al. Evaluation of a new lithium colorimetric assay performed on the Dade Behring Dimension® X-pand™ system. *Clin Chem Lab Med.* 2004;42(9):1066-8.

102. Pascali JP, Sorio D, Bortolotti F, et al. Rapid determination of lithium in serum samples by capillary electrophoresis. *Anal Bioanal Chem.* 2010;396:2543-6.

103. Floris A, Staal S, Lenk S, et al. A prefilled, ready-to-use electrophoresis based lab-on-a-chip device for monitoring lithium in blood. *Lab Chip.* 2010;10:1799-806.

104. Quattrocchi FP, May B, Ackerman L. Green-top test tubes and lithium concentration. *Drug Intell Clin Pharm.* 1988;22:79.

105. Stokes PE, Shamoian CA, Stoll PM, et al. Efficacy of lithium as acute treatment of manic-depressive illness. *Lancet.* 1971;1:1319-25.

106. Carlson GA. The stages of mania. *Arch Gen Psychiatry.* 1973;28:221-8.

107. Hansen HE, Amdisen A. Lithium intoxication. (Report of 23 cases and review of 100 cases from the literature.) *Q J Med.* 1978;47:123-44.

108. Finley PR, Warner MD, Peabody CA. Clinical relevance of drug interactions with lithium. *Clin Pharmacokinet.* 1995;29:172-91.

109. Amdisen A. Clinical and serum level monitoring in lithium therapy and lithium intoxication. *J Anal Toxicol.* 1978;2:193-202.

110. Amdisen A. Clinical features and management of lithium poisoning. *Med Toxicol Adverse Drug Exp.* 1988;3:18-32.

111. Gadallah MF, Feinstein EI, Massry SG. Lithium intoxication: clinical course and therapeutic considerations. *Mineral Electrolyte Metab.* 1988;14:146-9.

112. Rifkin A, Klein DF, Quitkin F. Organic brain syndrome during lithium carbonate treatment. *Compr Psychiatry.* 1973;14:251.

113. Reisberg B, Gershon S. Side effects associated with lithium therapy. *Arch Gen Psychiatry.* 1979;36:879-87.

114. Simard M, Gumbiner B, Lee A, et al. Lithium carbonate: a case report and review of the literature. *Arch Intern Med.* 1989;149:36-46.

115. Speirs G, Hirsch SR. Severe lithium toxicity with "normal" serum concentrations. *Br Med J.* 1978;1:815-6.

116. Finley PR, O'Brien JG, Coleman RW. Lithium and angiotensin-converting enzyme inhibitors: evaluation of a potential interaction. *J Clin Psychopharmacol.* 1996;16:68-71.

117. Pinninti NR, Zelinski G. Does topiramate elevate serum lithium levels? *J Clin Psychopharmacol.* 2002;22:340.

118. Katona CL. Psychotropics and drug interactions in the elderly patient. *Int J Geriatr Psychiatry.* 2001;16 Suppl 1:S86-90.

119. Wilting I, Movig KL, Moolenaar M, et al. Drug-drug interactions as a determinant of elevated lithium serum levels in daily clinical practice. *Bipolar Disord.* 2005;7(3):274-80.

120. Takahashi H, Higuchi H, Shimizu T. Severe lithium toxicity induced by combined levofloxacin administration. *J Clin Psychiatry.* 2000;61(12):949-50.

121. Miller SC. Doxycycline-induced lithium toxicity. *J Clin Psychopharmacol.* 1997;17(1):54-5.

122. Byrd GJ. Lithium carbonate and methyldopa: apparent interaction in man. *Clin Toxicol.* 1977;11(1):1-4.

123. Yassa R. Lithium-methyldopa interaction. *CMAJ.* 1986;134(2):141-2.

124. Jonnalagadda J, Saito E, Kafantaris V. Lithium, minocycline, and pseudotumor cerebri. *J Am Acad Child Adolesc Psychiatry.* 2005;44(3):209.

125. Cooper SJ, Kelly JG, Johnston GD, et al. Pharmacodynamics and pharmacokinetics of digoxin in the presence of lithium. *Br J Clin Pharmacol.* 1984;18:21-5.

126. Shelley RK. Lithium toxicity and mefenamic acid. A possible interaction and the role of prostaglandin inhibition. *Br J Psychiatry.* 1987;151:847-8.

127. Blanche P, Raynaud E, Kerob D, et al. Lithium intoxication in an elderly patient after combined treatment with losartan (letter). *Eur J Clin Pharmacol.* 1997;52:501.

128. Aruna AS. Lithium toxicity secondary to lithium-losartan interaction. *J Pharmacy Techol.* 2009;25(2):89-93

129. Su Y-P, Chang C-J, Hwang T-J [letter to editor]. Lithium intoxication after valsartan treatment. *Psych Clin Neurosci.* 2007;61:204.

130. Atherton JC, Green R, Higgins A, et al. Lithium clearance in healthy humans: effects of sodium intake and diuretics. *Kidney Int Suppl.* 1990;28:S36-8.

131. Boer WH, Koomans HA, Beutler JJ, et al. Small intra- and large inter-individual variability in lithium clearance in humans. *Kidney Int.* 1989;35:1183-8.

132. Himmelhoch JM, Poust RI, Mallinger AG, et al. Adjustment of lithium dose during lithium-chlorothiazide therapy. *Clin Pharmacol Ther.* 1977;22:225-7.

133. Solomon K. Combined use of lithium and diuretics. *South Med J.* 1978;71:1098-9, 1104.

134. Dorevitch A, Baruch E. Lithium toxicity induced by combined amiloride HCl-hydrochlorothiazide administration. *Am*

J Psychiatry. 1986;143:257-8.

135. Chambers G, Kerry RJ, Owen G. Lithium used with a diuretic. *Br Med J.* 1977;2:805-6.
136. Juurlink DN, Mamdani MM, Kopp A, et al. Drug-induced lithium toxicity in the elderly: a population-based study. *J Am Geriatr Soc.* 2004;52(5):794-8.
137. Ragheb M. The clinical significance of lithium-nonsteroidal anti-inflammatory drug interactions. *J Clin Psychopharmacol.* 1990;10:350-4.
138. Phelan KM, Mosholder AD, Lu S. Lithium interaction with the cyclooxygenase 2 inhibitors rofecoxib and celecoxib and other nonsteroidal anti-inflammatory drugs. *J Clin Psychiatry.* 2003;64(11):1328-34.
139. Rossat J, Maillard M, Nussberger J, et al. Renal effects of selective cyclooxygenase-2 inhibition in normotensive salt-depleted subjects. *Clin Pharmacol Ther.* 1999;66:76-84.
140. Celebrex Prescriber Information, Pfizer Inc., February 2007.
141. Monji A, Maekawa T, Miura T, et al. Interactions between lithium and non-steroidal antiinflammatory drugs. *Clin Neuropharmacol.* 2002;25:241-2.
142. Hughes BM, Small RE, Brink D, et al. The effect of flurbiprofen on steady state plasma lithium levels. *Pharmacotherapy.* 1997;17:113-20.
143. Baldessarini RJ, Tondo L, Hennen J, et al. Is lithium still worth using? An update of selected recent research. *Harv Rev Psychiatry.* 2002;10:59-75
144. Frolich JC, Leftwich R, Ragheb M, et al. Indomethacin increases plasma lithium. *Br Med J.* 1979;1:1115-6.
145. Cold JA, ZumBrunnen TL, Simpson MA, et al. Increased lithium serum and red blood cell concentrations during ketorolac coadministration. *J Clin Psychopharmacol.* 1998;18:33-7.
146. Ragheb M, Powell AL. Lithium interaction with sulindac and naproxen. *J Clin Psychopharmacol.* 1986;6:150-4.
147. Levin GM, Grum C, Eisele G. Effect of over-the-counter dosages of naproxen sodium and acetaminophen on plasma lithium concentrations in normal volunteers. *J Clin Psychopharmacol.* 1998;18:237-40.
148. Pietruszka LJ, Biermann WA, Vlasses PH. Evaluation of cisplatin-lithium interaction. *Drug Intell Clin Pharm.* 1985;19:31-2.
149. Parfrey PS, Ikeman R, Anglin D, et al. Severe lithium intoxication treated by forced diuresis. *Can Med Assoc J.* 1983;129:979-80.
150. Cook BL, Smith RE, Perry PJ, et al. Theophylline-lithium interaction. *J Clin Psychiatry.* 1985;46:278-9.
151. Holstad SG, Perry PJ, Kathol RG, et al. The effects of intravenous theophylline infusion versus intravenous sodium bicarbonate infusion on lithium clearance in normal subjects. *Psychiatry Res.* 1988;25:203-11.
152. Spina E, Perucca E. Clinical significance of pharmacokinetic interactions between antiepileptic and psychotropic drugs. *Epilepsia.* 2002;43(suppl 2):37-44.
153. Jefferson JW. The use of lithium in childhood and adolescence: an overview. *J Clin Psychiatry.* 1982;43:174-7.
154. Birch NJ. Bone side-effects of lithium. In: Johnson FN, ed. *Handbook of Lithium Therapy.* Baltimore, MD: University Park Press: 1980;365-71.
155. Khandelwal SW, Varma VK, Srinivisa Murthy R. Renal function in children receiving long-term lithium prophylaxis. *Am J Psychiatry.* 1984;141:278-9.
156. Lena B. Lithium therapy in hyperaggressive behavior in adolescence. In: Sandler M, ed. *Pharmacology of Aggression.* New York, NY: Raven Press; 1979:197-203.
157. Almy GL, Taylor MA. Lithium retention in mania. *Arch Gen Psychiatry.* 1973;29:232-4.
158. Wallin L, Alling C, Aurell M. Impairment of renal function in patients on long-term lithium treatment. *Clin Nephrol.* 1982;18:23-8.
159. Tonks CM. Lithium intoxications induced by dieting and saunas. *Br Med J.* 1977;2:1396-7.
160. Demers RG, Heninger GR. Sodium intake and lithium treatment in mania. *Am J Psychiatry.* 1971;128:100-4.
161. Reiss RA, Haas CE, Karki SD, et al. Lithium pharmacokinetics in the obese. *Clin Pharmacol Ther.* 1994;55:392-8.
162. Jefferson JW, Greist JH, Clagnaz PJ, et al. Effect of strenuous exercise on serum lithium level in man. *Am J Psychiatry.* 1982;139:1593-5.
163. Scharman EJ. Methods used to decrease lithium absorption or enhance elimination. *Clin Toxicol.* 1997;35:601-8.
164. Eyer F, Pfab R, Felgenhauer N, et al. Lithium poisoning: pharmacokinetics and clearance during different therapeutic measures. *J Clin Psychopharmacol.* 2006;26:325-30.
165. Viguera AC, Cohen LS. The course and management of bipolar disorder during pregnancy. *Psychopharmacol Bull.* 1998;34:339-46.
166. Llewellyn A, Stowe ZN. Psychotropic medications in lactation. *J Clin Psychiatry.* 1998;59(Suppl 2):41-52.
167. Llewellyn A, Stowe ZN, Strader JR, Jr. The use of lithium and management of women with bipolar disorder during

pregnancy and lactation. *J Clin Psychiatry.* 1998;59(Suppl 6):57-64; discussion 65.

168. Cohen LS, Rosenbaum JF. Psychotropic drug use during pregnancy: weighing the risks. *J Clin Psychiatry.* 1998;59(Suppl 2):18-28.

169. Viguera AC, Newport DJ, Ritchie J, et al. Lithium in breast milk and nursing infants: clinical implications. *Am J Psychiatry.* 2007;164:342-5.

170. Grandjean EM, Aubry JM. Lithium: updated human knowledge using an evidence-based approach: part III: clinical safety. *CNS Drugs.* 2009;23(5):397-418.

Chapter 17

Kimberly B. Tallian and Douglas M. Anderson

Phenobarbital (AHFS 28:12.04 and 28:24.04)

Although the use of phenobarbital has declined in favor of newer, nonbarbiturate medications, it remains an agent of choice in a variety of central nervous system disorders. Properly administered, phenobarbital continues to afford safe and effective therapy to many patients in a reliable and convenient fashion. Approved uses include febrile seizures in children and all forms of epilepsy except absence seizures.[1] Some frequent uses, which are not FDA approved, include prevention of seizures associated with intracranial hemorrhage in preterm neonates, treatment of essential tremor in adults, and cerebral salvage related to traumatic and/or hypoxic brain injury.[2]

Usual Dosage Range in Absence of Clearance-Altering Factors[3,4]

Phenobarbital exhibits a predictable pharmacokinetic profile with a relatively wide therapeutic window. As a result, dosing protocols are often used with satisfactory results. The dosing recommendations in Table 17-1, based on average pharmacokinetic parameters, should produce concentrations in the therapeutic range for most patients. However, significant interpatient variation necessitates therapeutic monitoring.

Once-daily dosing at bedtime is preferred to minimize daytime sedation and increase compliance in ambulatory patients.[5,6] If the clinical situation allows, initial sedation may be minimized by starting therapy with 25% of the desired maintenance dose and increasing it weekly by another 25% until the full maintenance dose is achieved.[7] Since phenobarbital exhibits first-order elimination, linear relationships exist between dose adjustments and resultant drug concentrations during steady state conditions.

For intravenous and intramuscular routes, the sodium salt of phenobarbital is used, which has a *salt fraction* (*S*) of approximately 0.9 (91% phenobarbital). Intravenous phenobarbital loading doses have been reported to cause hypotension, particularly in neonates (possibly an effect of the propylene glycol in the product). However, recommended loading doses should be safe if administered at less than 50 mg/min in adults.[3] In neonates and children, phenobarbital should not be administered intravenously at a rate greater than 1 mg/kg/min with a maximum of 30 mg/min.[6] Phenobarbital's slow elimination precludes the need for continuous intravenous infusions or sustained-release products (see Table 17-2 for product availability).

Table 17-1. Loading and Maintenance Doses by Age Group

Age Group	Loading Dose[a,b]	Maintenance Doses[a]
Neonates (<2 weeks)	15–25 mg/kg	2–4 mg/kg/day
Infants (2 weeks–<1 year)	15–25 mg/kg	5 mg/kg/day
Children		
1–<5 years	10–20 mg/kg	4.5 mg/kg/day
5–<10 years	10–20 mg/kg	3.6 mg/kg/day
10–<15 years	10–20 mg/kg	2.9 mg/kg/day
15–<19 years	10–20 mg/kg	2.5 mg/kg/day
Adults (19–65 years)	10–20 mg/kg	2 mg/kg/day
Geriatrics (>65 years)	10–20 mg/kg	1.1–2 mg/kg/day

[a]Oral (capsules, tablets, and elixir), intravenous, and intramuscular.
[b]IV loading doses should be administered at <50 mg/min in adults and <1 mg/kg/min or ≤30 mg/min in children.[3]

Table 17-2. Dosage Form Availability[8]

Dosage Form	Product
Intravenous and intramuscular	
30, 60, 65, and 130 mg/ml	Phenobarbital sodium injection (Elkins-Sinn, Wyeth-Ayerst)
130 mg/ml	Luminal Sodium (Sanofi Winthrop)
Oral capsules	
16 mg	Solfoton (ECR Pharm.)
Oral elixir	
15 mg/5 ml	Various manufacturers
20 mg/5 ml	Various manufacturers
Oral tablets	
15, 16, 30, 60, 100 mg	Various manufacturers

General Pharmacokinetic Information

Absorption

Phenobarbital is slowly but completely absorbed. Oral products are most often >90% bioavailable (F = 1) (Table 17-3). With oral dosage forms, large single doses over 750 mg may exhibit delayed or reduced absorption in adults due to the insolubility of phenobarbital crystals that form and remain for some time in the GI (gastrointestinal) tract. Drugs or diseases that affect GI motility may influence the rate of absorption. The effect on the extent of absorption is unclear. The presence of food apparently does not affect the extent of absorption.

Distribution

Phenobarbital's volume of distribution ranges from 0.5 to 1 L/kg (Table 17-4). Volumes relative to body weight are largest at birth through infancy, decline slightly in childhood, and reach the lowest L/kg population values in adults. Significant variation may exist within each age group, due in part to fluctuation of plasma proteins and a correlation with pH.[4] A weak acid, phenobarbital has a pKa of 7.3, approximating plasma pH. Increases in plasma or urine pH may increase clearance and vice versa.

Distribution occurs in a biphasic manner, normally reaching the beta phase about 2 hours after administration.[6] At this time point after an intravenous dose, CNS concentrations approximate the serum unbound concentrations and range from 43% to 60% of serum values.[4] As a result of slow distribution into the CNS, phenobarbital has not historically been used for status epilepticus. However, one study found phenobarbital's efficacy comparable to that of benzodiazepines.[9]

Phenobarbital has been associated with reduced cognitive outcomes for children if given during pregnancy and should be avoided.[10] It also readily crosses placental tissue and achieves fetal concentrations approximately equal to that of the mother[3,11] but may exceed the mother's concentration based on reduced fetal elimination.[11] Data regarding excretion into breast milk varies with 1.5%–41% of maternal phenobarbital *serum* concentrations detected in *breast milk*.[4,12] Only large doses are reported to produce clinically significant concentrations and resultant sedation in nursing infants and neonates.[13]

Table 17-3. Bioavailability (F) of Dosage Forms[4,8]

Dosage Form	Bioavailability	Comments
Intramuscular	100% (F = 1)	Onset of action within 30 min; time to peak concentrations ≤3 hr
Intravenous	100% (F = 1)	Immediate onset of action
Rectal	90% (F = 0.9)	Faster rate of absorption than oral or intramuscular routes
Oral (capsules, tablets, elixir)	90%–100% (F = 0.90–1)	Time to peak variable (~2 hr)

Protein binding

Phenobarbital binds primarily to albumin in the plasma with the free (unbound) fraction affected by albumin concentration. This effect appears to be clinically significant only when combined with renal failure and acidosis.[5,14] The degree of protein binding is affected by age (Table 17-4). The unbound fraction increases with hypoalbuminemia and hyperbilirubinemia[3,4] and may be as high as 90% of the total plasma concentration at birth, followed by a gradual decline to 70% after 1 week.[3]

Table 17-4. Volume of Distribution and Protein Binding by Age Group

Age	Volume (Mean ± SD)[4,12]	Protein Binding (Mean ± SD)
Neonates (<2 weeks)[a]	0.96 ± 0.02 L/kg	37 ± 17%
Infants and children (2 weeks–19 years)	0.63 ± 0.09 L/kg	51%
Adults and geriatrics (>19 years)	0.61 ± 0.05 L/kg	51%

[a]Volume may be increased by ECMO. One case reported a volume of 1.2 L/kg.[15]

Clearance

Following slow but essentially complete absorption, phenobarbital undergoes extensive non-first-pass, non-dose-dependent biotransformation by hepatic microenzymes into inactive metabolites. Phenobarbital is a potent inducer of CYP3A4, CYP1A2, CYP2B6, CYP2C, and CYP2D6 hepatic enzymes, requiring approximately 1 week for the effects of induction to be observed.[16] Although some enterohepatic cycling occurs, fecal excretion does not significantly affect clearance.[4]

Renal excretion of unchanged drug is urine flow and pH dependent (increasing with alkaline urine) and varies from 20% to 40% of a dose in patients with normal renal function. Combined diuresis and alkalinization can increase renal clearance up to fourfold.[4]

Although hepatic disease may decrease phenobarbital clearance, renal excretion apparently increases with impaired hepatic function, thereby averting severe reductions in clearance.[8] Likewise, renal insufficiency, even in end-stage disease, appears to have little effect on phenobarbital concentrations because of increased hepatic metabolism.[3]

Phenobarbital clearance can be affected by certain drugs, disease states, and age (see sections on drug–drug interactions and drug–disease state or condition interactions). A CYP2C19 hepatic enzyme genetic polymorphism is reported to slightly reduce clearance of phenobarbital in some Japanese adults. One study demonstrated an average of 18.8% reduction in clearance in the 8% of patients expressing the phenotype.[17]

The clearance values presented in Table 17-5 can be assumed in the absence of disease or drug interactions.[3,18,19]

Half-Life and Time to Steady State[1,18,20]

Phenobarbital's half-life and time to steady state are age group dependent (Table 17-6) and can be affected by certain drug interactions and disease states (see sections on drug–drug interactions and drug–disease state or condition interactions).

Table 17-5. Clearance and Fraction Excreted Unchanged by Age Group

Age	Clearance (Mean ± SD)	Fraction of Parent Drug Excreted in Urine
Neonates and infants (<1 year)	0.0047 ± 0.0002 L/hr/kg	~0.2[a]
Children (1–<19 years)	0.0082 ± 0.0031 L/hr/kg	0.2–0.4
Adults (19–65 years)	0.0056 ± 0.0026 L/hr/kg	0.24–0.5
Geriatrics (>65 years)	0.0024 L/hr/kg	Not available

[a]This value was reported to be greater than or equal to 0.6 during the first week of life.

Table 17-6. Half-Life and Time to Steady State by Age Group

Age	Half-Life (Mean ± SD)	Time to Steady State[a,b]
Neonates (<2 weeks)	111 ± 34 hr	16–30 days
Infants (2 weeks–<1 year)	63 ± 5 hr	12–14 days
Children (1–<19 years)	69 ± 3 hr	14–15 days
Adults and geriatrics (>19 years)	96 ± 13 hr[b]	17–23 days

[a]Time to steady state estimated using + and – 1 SD of the mean t½ and assuming steady state is achieved in five half-lives.
[b]May be higher for patients over 65 years.

Therapeutic Range

Of the patients whose seizure activity responds to phenobarbital, 84% respond at concentrations of 10–40 mg/L.[4] These concentrations are generally considered the therapeutic range. However, patient response should be the definitive guide for dosage adjustment. Behavioral effects may occur in the absence of overt signs of clinical toxicity, especially in children.[19] One study showed that 42% of children treated with phenobarbital developed behavioral disturbances, namely hyperactivity and somnolence.[21] Once phenobarbital was discontinued, improvement and resolution of symptoms were observed in 73% of these patients. Although the study found no correlation between these disturbances and phenobarbital concentrations, maintaining this population at the lowest effective concentration remains desirable pending further research. Table 17-7 provides additional condition-specific therapeutic ranges that have been reported.

Drug Monitoring Assay Considerations

While determinations of phenobarbital serum concentrations remain the standard for therapeutic drug monitoring, studies have shown saliva sample assay to be an acceptable alternative to venipuncture under certain

Table 17-7. Condition-Specific Therapeutic Ranges

Clinical Condition	Recommended Therapeutic Range	Comments
Febrile convulsions	16–30 mg/L[4]	A 6-month recurrence rate of <4% was demonstrated at these concentrations versus 21% at ≤15 mg/L or with no drug.[7] Prophylaxis following febrile convulsion may only be necessary when complicated by underlying neurologic disorders, prolonged febrile seizures, or family history of nonfebrile seizures.[4]
Hypoxic ischemic seizures in neonates (perinatal asphyxia)	>30 mg/L initially	20–30 mg/L may be acceptable 24–48 hr after birth; may require lower maintenance doses due to longer than usual half-life.[20]
Antenatal therapy to prevent intracranial hemorrhage in preterm infants	10–15 mg/L	Conflicting studies exist with regard to efficacy. A dose of 780 mg IV given to the mother up to 1 hr prior to delivery was shown to achieve recommended neonatal concentrations in 24 of 26 neonates.[22]
Generalized tonic-clonic seizures	10–25 mg/L	10 mg/L has improved EEGs (but not necessarily controlled seizures) in 90% of patients.[7] Due to increased incidence of adverse effects, concentrations should generally not exceed 30 mg/L unless required for seizure control in refractory patients.[24]
Refractory status epilepticus	≥70 mg/L	May be employed without consideration of maximum dose or concentration (ICU required).[25] This treatment has initiation advantages over high-dose benzodiazepines and phenytoin, as well as a more predictable pharmacokinetic profile.
Cerebral salvage from hypoxic or traumatic brain damage	>75 mg/L[3]	These concentrations may induce barbiturate coma, particularly in nonhabituated patients.[7]

conditions. This method is noninvasive, less expensive than serum determinations, and has a high correlation between saliva and plasma across a wide range of concentrations in patients ≥8 years of age (patients studied were also receiving concurrent carbamazepine and phenytoin).[26] Saliva samples can be also useful for monitoring medication compliance and in situations where repeat sampling is necessary. Several factors, however, can influence the medication concentrations in saliva such as salivary flow rate and pH, sampling conditions, and contamination. Regardless of sample type, most phenobarbital assays are performed using fluorescence polarization immunoassay.

Suggested Sampling Times and Effect on Therapeutic Range[3,7]

Since the peak to trough fluctuation is minimal during normal dosing intervals, sampling time after a dose at steady state is not usually critical. However, sampling times relative to dose administration should be fairly consistent when comparing to previous values. A post loading dose measurement at approximately 2–3 hr following administration is helpful in confirming therapeutic concentrations and can allow for determination of a patient's volume of distribution. If the clinical situation warrants, a concentration may be repeated in 3–4 days to determine if the maintenance dose is sufficient. If the loading dose concentration was satisfactory, a decrease from the post load value may indicate the need for a larger maintenance dose and vice versa. This second concentration may not reflect steady state conditions due to the long t½ of phenobarbital.

To document acceptable steady state values, another concentration may be obtained 2–4 weeks after initiation of therapy or dose adjustments. Sampling should be repeated when known enzyme inhibitors or inducers are added, adjusted, or discontinued. Concentrations should be determined if seizure control is lost or toxicity is suspected. More frequent monitoring may be required during pregnancy and for 8 weeks following delivery.

Pharmacodynamic Monitoring—Concentration-Related Efficacy

The efficacy of therapy for seizure disorders is usually determined by seizure frequency, though the absence of seizures may not be the therapeutic endpoint for some conditions. Noncompliance must always be considered with patients receiving anticonvulsants since noncompliance rates range from 25%–75%.[27] For intracranial hemorrhage or ischemic cerebral lesions in neonates, therapy should be directed primarily by serial EEGs instead of seizure patterns or phenobarbital concentrations.[28]

Pharmacodynamic Monitoring—Concentration-Related Toxicity[3,7,31-33]

Toxicity with phenobarbital therapy can present as either neurologic or non-neurologic adverse effects. *Neurologic effects* may or may not be concentration related. Table 17-8 lists several concentration-related neurologic adverse effects. Neurologic adverse effects that may occur without regard to concentration are sedation (in naïve patients), neonatal feeding disorders, sexual dysfunction, and behavioral abnormalities (including lethargy, sleep disorders, hyperactivity in children, irritability, depression, and suicide-risk). See Table 17-9 for *non-neurologic* adverse effects.

Table 17-8. Phenobarbital Concentration-Related Neurologic Adverse Effects[28]

Adverse Effect	Phenobarbital Concentration
Sedation[a]	≥5 mg/L
Impaired cognition (with or without sedation)[b]	>19 mg/L
Decreased neonatal feeding, respirations, and muscle tone[b]	>30 mg/L
Sedation, slowness, and ataxia[b]	35–80 mg/L
Potential coma[b]	≥65 mg/L
Coma without reflexes (potentially lethal)[b]	≥80 mg/L

[a]In nonhabituated patients.
[b]In habituated or nonhabituated patients.

Table 17-9. Non-Neurological Adverse Effects of Chronic Phenobarbital Therapy[a,26,29]

Adverse Effect	Relative Frequency	Monitoring Parameter
Folate deficiency	52%	Folate concentrations
Fetal vitamin K deficit from maternal phenobarbital therapy	<50%	Neonatal coagulation studies
Gingival hyperplasia	16%	Increased frequency of dental exams to monitor for developing caries and gingivitis
Vitamin D deficiency	10%	Calcium and alkaline phosphatase concentrations
Shoulder-hand syndrome	<6%	If bone joint or bone pain are present, therapy should be reevaluated
Hepatotoxicity	<1%	No monitoring is necessary unless overt signs of hepatotoxicity exist

[a]In general, non-neurologic adverse effects lack a clear relationship to phenobarbital concentration and most often present during chronic therapy.

Drug-Drug Interactions

Certain drugs may either increase or decrease phenobarbital concentrations (see Table 17-10). Although conflicting studies exist, phenytoin seldom affects phenobarbital concentrations in a significant manner.[31,33] Newer anticonvulsants such as gabapentin and levetiracetam do not appear to affect, or be affected by, phenobarbital concentrations.[37,38]

Phenobarbital has been shown to induce the metabolism of many medications through its induction effect on various cytochromes (CYP). Table 17-11 provides a list of medications known to be metabolized by various CYPs and therefore potentially impacted by co-administration with phenobarbital.

Drug–Disease State or Condition Interactions

A limited number of disease states and conditions have been reported to alter phenobarbital clearance. The known effects of certain disease states and clinical conditions on phenobarbital pharmacokinetics are listed in Table 17-12.

Table 17-10. Drugs Affecting Phenobarbital Concentrations

Drug	Clearance Factor[a]	Mechanism of Interaction
Chloramphenicol[34,b]	0.6	Competitive inhibition of hepatic metabolism
Methsuximide[34,b]	<1	Competitive inhibition of hepatic metabolism
Propoxyphene[34,b]	0.8	Competitive inhibition of hepatic metabolism
Valproic acid[14]	0.7	Competitive inhibition of hepatic metabolism
Bicarbonate[3,7,34,39]	>1	Decreased tubular reabsorption
Charcoal with sorbitol[39,40]	>1	Adsorption of oral phenobarbital or during enterohepatic cycling
Charcoal without sorbitol[39,40]	≥1.5	Adsorption of oral phenobarbital or during enterohepatic cycling
Pyridoxine[20,b]	1.4	Unknown
Rifampin[20]	>1	Hepatic induction
Thioridazine/mesoridazine[20,c]	1.3	Hepatic induction

[a]When multiplied by normal phenobarbital clearance, this factor adjusts clearance for the particular drug interaction. Clearance factors <1 lead to increases in phenobarbital concentrations while factors >1 lead to decreases.
[b]Anecdotal data, or from small study populations. Reliability of clearance factor or clinical significance of interaction is not well substantiated.
[c]A similar interaction may exist with other phenothiazines.

Table 17-11. CYP Enzymes Induced by Phenobarbital and Drugs That May Have Reduced Concentrations in the Presence of Phenobarbital[a,16,31,35,37]

CYP3A4	CYP2D6	CYP2B6	CYP2C	CYP1A2
Alprazolam	Amitriptyline	Bupropion	S-Warfarin	Clozapine
Beta-blockers (except sotalol)	Amphetamine	Cyclophosphamide	Topiramate	Fluvoxamine
Calcium channel blockers	Aripiprazole	Efavirenz	Voriconazole	Griseofulvin
Carbamazepine	Atomoxetine	Ifosfamide		Olanzapine
Cimetidine	Carvedilol	Methadone		Ondansetron
Chlorpheniramine	Chlorpheniramine			Propranolol
Clonazepam	Chlorpromazine			Tacrine
Corticosteroids	Clomipramine			Theophylline
Cyclosporine	Codeine			Tizanidine
Diazepam	Desipramine			Verapamil
Digoxin	Dextromethorphan			Zolmitriptan
Disopyramide	Donepezil			
Donepezil	Duloxetine			
Etoposide	Flecainide			
Haloperidol	Fluoxetine			
HMG CoA reductase Inhibitors	Fluvoxamine			
Indinavir	Haloperidol			
Itraconazole	Imipramine			
Ketoconazole	Lidocaine			
Lamotrigine	Methadone			
Lidocaine	Metoclopramide			
Losartan	Mexilletine			
Macrolide antibiotics	Montelukaste			
Methadone	Nortriptyline			
Midazolam	Ondansetron			
Nelfinavir	Oxycodone			
Ondansetron	Paroxetine			
Oral contraceptives	Phenothiazines			
Phenytoin	Propafenone			
Quetiapine	Propranolol			
Quinidine	Risperidone			
Quinine	Tamoxifen			
Risperidone	Tramadol			
Ritonavir	Venlafaxine			
Saquinavir				
Sildenafil				
Sirolimus				
Tacrolimus				
Tamoxifen				
Taxol				
Tetracyclines				
Tiagabine				

Table 17-11. (Continued)

CYP3A4	CYP2D6	CYP2B6	CYP2C	CYP1A2
Trazodone				
Triazolam				
Valproic				
Vincristine				
Voriconazole				
Zaleplon				
Ziprasidone				
Zolpidem				
Zonisamide				

[a]Any drug metabolized by these enzymes may be subject to enhanced clearance due to induction of the enzymes by phenobarbital.

Table 17-12. Conditions That Alter Phenobarbital Pharmacokinetics[a]

Clinical Condition	Effect on Clearance	Effect on Half-Life
Hepatic dysfunction[4]		
Cirrhosis[b]	Decreased	Extended
Acute viral hepatitis[b]	No change	No change
Renal failure[3]		
Mild or moderate[b,c]	No change	No change
Severe[b,c]	Decreased	Increased
Hepato-renal[b]	Decreased	Increased
Hemodialysis (4 hr)[d]	~30% of drug removed	Not available
Peritoneal dialysis[e]	~7.5%–15% of drug removed[d]	Not available
Pregnancy[3,4,f]	Increased	Decreased
Perinatal asphyxia (Apgar <5 at 5 min)[17,b]	Reported to be 0.0048 ± 0.0018 L/hr/kg	Reported to be 148 ± 55 hr
Prolonged starvation[4,b]	Increased	Decreased

[a]Little data exist regarding changes in V in these conditions. However, with perinatal asphyxia, V has been reported to increase by 13%.
[b]A decrease in albumin may cause an increase in free (unbound) fraction of drug.
[c]Studies to date do not suggest that dosage adjustments are necessary for moderate to severe renal failure.[3] Little data exist regarding hepatorenal disease.
[d]One third of daily phenobarbital dose should be replaced after hemodialysis.[3] Clearance may be higher with more recent, high-efficiency hemodialyzers (up to 50% in one case report[41]).
[e]The effect of peritoneal dialysis on phenobarbital clearance is unpredictable. Patients may require more frequent serum concentration monitoring to guide dosing.[3] In phenobarbital toxicity, removal may be increased with 5% albumin dialysate.[42]
[f]Clearance may gradually increase through gestation before returning to baseline within 4–8 weeks following delivery.[3]

References

1. Baulac M. Phenobarbital and other barbiturates: Clinical efficacy and use in epilepsy. In: Levy RH, Mattson RH, Meldrum BS, et al., eds. *Antiepileptic Drugs*. 5th ed. New York, NY: Raven Press; 2002:514-21.
2. Crowther CA, Crosby DD, Henderson-Smart DJ. Phenobarbital prior to preterm birth for preventing neonatal periventricular hemorrhage. *Cochrane Database Syst Rev.* 2010;20(1):CD000164. http://www.ncbi.nlm.nih.gov/pubmed/20091502. Accessed December 5, 2010.
3. Gal P. Phenobarbital and primidone. In: Taylor WJ, Diers Caviness MH, eds. *A Textbook for the Clinical Application of Therapeutic Drug Monitoring*. Irving, TX: Abbott Laboratories Diagnostics Division; 1986:237-52.
4. Anderson GD. Phenobarbital and other barbiturates: Chemistry, biotransformation, and pharmacokinetics. In: Levy

RH, Mattson RH, Meldrum BS, et al., eds. *Antiepileptic Drugs*. 5th ed. New York, NY: Raven Press; 2002:496-503.

5. Wroblewski BA, Garvin WH Jr. Once-daily administration of phenobarbital in adults: clinical efficacy and benefit. *Arch Neurol.* 1985;42:699-700.
6. Taketomo CK, Hodding JH, Kraus DM. Phenobarbital. In: *Pediatric Dosage Handbook*. 13th ed. Hudson, NY: LexiComp; 2006.
7. Davis AG, Mutchie KD, Thompson JA, et al. Once daily dosing with phenobarbital in children with seizure disorders. *Pediatrics.* 1981;68:824-7.
8. Phenobarbital. In: McEvoy GK, ed. *AHFS Drug Information 2011*. Bethesda, MD: American Society of Health-System Pharmacists; 2011.
9. Shaner MD, McCurdy SR, Hering M, et al. Treatment of status epileptics: a prospective comparison of diazepam and phenytoin versus phenobarbital and optional phenytoin. *Neurology.* 1988;38:202-7.
10. Harden CL, Meado KJ, Pennell PB, et al. Management issues for women with epilepsy—focus on pregnancy (an evidence-based review): II. Teratogenesis and perinatal outcomes. *Epilepsia.* 2009;50(5):1237-46.
11. Nau H, Kuhnz W, Egger HJ, et al. Anticonvulsants during pregnancy and lactation: transplacental, maternal, and neonatal pharmacokinetics. *Clin Pharmacokinet.* 1982;7:508-43.
12. Landrum-Michalets E. Update: Clinically significant cytochrome P-450 drug interactions. *Pharmacotherapy.* 1998;18(1):84-112.
13. Pugh CP. Phenytoin and phenobarbital protein binding alterations in a uremic burn patient. *Drug Intell Clin Pharm.* 1987;21:264-7.
14. Patel IH, Levy RH, Cutler R. Phenobarbital–valproic acid interaction. *Clin Pharmacol Ther.* 1980;27:515-21.
15. Elliot ES, Buck ML. Phenobarbital dosing and pharmacokinetics in a neonate receiving extracorporeal membrane oxygenation. *Ann Pharmacother.* 1999;33:419-29.
16. Thummel KE, Shen DD. Design and optimization of dosage regimens: Pharmacokinetic data. In: Hardman JG, Linbird LE, et al., eds. *Goodman & Gilman's Pharmacological Basis of Therapeutics*. 10th ed. Columbus, OH: McGraw-Hill; 2001: Appendix II: 1917-2023.
17. Mamiya K, Hadama A, Yukawa E, et. al. CYP2C19 polymorphism effect on phenobarbitone pharmacokinetics in Japanese patients with epilepsy: analysis by population pharmacokinetics. *Eur J Pharmacol.* 2000;55:821-5.
18. Beghi E. Phenobarbital and other barbiturates: Clinical efficacy and use in nonepileptic disorders. In: Levy RH, Mattson RH, Meldrum BS, et al., eds. *Antiepileptic Drugs*. 5th ed. New York, NY: Raven Press; 2002:522-7.
19. Fahim MF, King TM. Effect of phenobarbital on lactation in the nursing neonate. *Am J Obstet Gynecol.* 1968;101:1103.
20. Phenobarbital. In: Drugdex Information System, Micromedex, Inc.; 2010.
21. Wolf S, Forsythe A. Behavior disturbance, phenobarbital, and febrile seizures. *Pediatrics.* 1978;61:729-31.
22. McNamara JO. Drugs effective in the therapy of the epilepsies. In: Hardman JG, Linbird LE, et al., eds. *Goodman & Gilman's Pharmacological Basis of Therapeutics*. 11th ed. Columbus, OH: McGraw-Hill; 2006.
23. Hole JW. Adequacy of antenatal phenobarbital dosing for neonatal intraventricular hemorrhage prophylaxis. *J Perinatol.* 1996;16(2):160.
24. Donn SM, Grasela TH, Goldstein GW. Safety of a higher loading dose of phenobarbital in the term newborn. *Pediatrics.* 1985;75:1061-4.
25. Crawford TO, Mitchell WG, Fishman LS, et al. Very-high-dose phenobarbital for refractory status epilepticus in children. *Neurology.* 1998;38:1035-40.
26. Gorodischer R, Burtin P, Verjee Z, et al. Is saliva suitable for therapeutic monitoring of anticonvulsants in children: An evaluation in the routine clinical setting. *Ther Drug Mon.* 1997;19(6):637-42.
27. Specht U, Elsner H, May TW, et al. Postictal serum levels of antiepileptic drugs for detection of noncompliance. *Epilepsy Behav.* 2003(4):487-95.
28. Pugh C, Garnett W. Current issues in the treatment of epilepsy. *Clin Pharm.* 1991;10:335-58.
29. Gurbuz T, Tan H. Oral health status in epileptic children. *Pediatrc Int.* 2010;52(2):279-83.
30. Connell J, Dozeer R, DeVries L, et al. Clinical and EEG response to anticonvulsants in neonatal seizures. *Arch Dis Child.* 1989;64:459-64.
31. Rizack MA, ed. *Adverse Drug Interactions Program for Windows*. New Rochelle, NY: The Medical Letter; 2007.
32. Hamoda HM, Guild DJ, Gumlak S, et al. Association between attention-deficit/hyperactivity disorder and epilepsy in pediatric populations. *Expert Rev Neurother.* 2009;9(12):1747-54.
33. Olesen JB, Hansen PR, Erdal J, et al. Antiepilpetic drugs and risk of suicide: a nationwide study. *Pharmacoepidemiol Drug Saf.* 2010;19(5):516-24.
34. Leeder SJ. Phenobarbital: Interactions with other drugs. In: Levy RH, Mattson RH, Meldrum BS, et al., eds. *Antiepileptic*

Drugs. 5th ed. New York, NY: Raven Press; 2002:504-13.

35. Omiecinski CJ, Remmel RP, Hosagrahara VP. Forum: Concise review of the cytochrome P450s and their roles in toxicology. *Toxicol Sci*. 1999;48:151-6.
36. Reddy DS. Clinical pharmacokinetic interactions between antiepileptic drugs and hormonal contraceptives. *Expert Rev Clin Pharmacol*. 2010;3(2):183-92.
37. Neurontin (Gabapentin) Data on File. Pfizer Pharmaceuticals 2007.
38. Keppra (Levetiracetam) Data on File. UCB Pharma, Inc. 2006.
39. Frenia ML, Schauben JL, Wears RL, et al. Multiple-dose activated charcoal compared to urinary alkalinization for the enhancement of phenobarbital elimination. *J Toxicol Clin Toxicol*. 1996;34(2):169-75.
40. Berg MS, Rose JQ, Vivister DE, et al. Effect of charcoal and sorbitol-charcoal suspension on the elimination of intravenous phenobarbital. *Ther Drug Monit*. 1987;9:41-7.
41. Palmer BF. Effectiveness of hemodialysis in the extracorporeal therapy of phenobarbital overdose. *Am J Kid Dis*. 2000;36:640-3.
42. Berman LB, Vogelsang P. Removal rates for barbiturates using two types of peritoneal dialysis. *New Engl J Med*. 1964;270:77-80.

Chapter 18

Michael E. Winter

Phenytoin and Fosphenytoin (AHFS 28:12.12)

Phenytoin, a hydantoin-derivative anticonvulsant, is indicated for the treatment of tonic-clonic and complex partial seizures and for seizure prophylaxis following neurosurgery. Phenytoin also exhibits antiarrhythmic properties similar to those of lidocaine but is seldom if ever used as an antiarrhythmic.

Usual Dosage Range in Absence of Clearance-Altering Factors

Loading dose[1-7]

When a rapid therapeutic concentration is desired, a loading dose is recommended. Because of the slow absorption characteristics of phenytoin, the loading dose is often administered by the intravenous route.

The maximum intravenous infusion rate of phenytoin sodium injection in neonates is 0.5 mg/kg/min, children, and adolescents is 1 mg/kg/min. In adults, the maximum infusion rate is 50 mg/min. Fosphenytoin, administered as phenytoin equivalents (PE), has a maximum administration rate of 1.5 mg PE/kg/min for neonates, 3 mg PE/kg/min for children and adolescents, and for adults the maximum infusion rate is 150 mg PE/min.

For children, adolescents, and adults, oral loading doses are usually given in 5 mg/kg increments every 2 hr until the total dose has been administered (Table 18-1). The usual adult dose is 1000 mg (approximately 15 mg/kg multiplied by 70 kg), given in 400-, 300-, and 300 mg doses, each separated by 2 hr.

Maintenance dose[1-3,8,9]

In infants, children, and adolescents, the total daily dose (Table 18-2) is usually divided into equal doses and given at evenly spaced intervals of 6, 8, or 12 hr. In adults, the usual initial daily dose is 300 mg given once a day at bedtime (for the once-daily schedule, phenytoin sodium extended must be used).

Table 18-1. Loading Doses

Age	Loading Dose
Neonates and infants (<1 year)	15–20 mg/kg
Children (1–<12 years)	15–18 mg/kg
Adolescents (≥12 years), adults, and geriatrics	15–18 mg/kg

Table 18-2. Maintenance Doses

Age	Maintenance Dosage
Neonates (<4 weeks)	3–5 mg/kg/day[a]
Infants (4 weeks–<1 year)	4–8 mg/kg/day[a]
Children (1–<12 years)	4–10 mg/kg/day[a]
Adolescents (12–<18 years)	4–8 mg/kg/day[a]
Adults and geriatrics (≥18 years)	4–7 mg/kg/day

[a]Usually given in divided doses.

Dosage Form Availability[1-3,10-16]

Phenytoin is available in the acid or sodium salt form and as the phosphate ester prodrug (fosphenytoin) of phenytoin. The sodium salt has a salt fraction (S) of approximately 92% phenytoin (**S = 0.92**) and 8% sodium. Phenytoin sodium is available both intravenously and as a capsule. Phenytoin as the acid form is available as a suspension or chewable tablet (**S = 1**). Fosphenytoin is available only as an injectable dosage form that can be administered either intravenously or intramuscularly. Fosphenytoin is labeled as milligrams of phenytoin equivalents (PE) of phenytoin sodium injection and therefore the S factor for fosphenytoin PE to calculate the milligrams of acid phenytoin is 0.92.

Phenytoin sodium injection contains propylene glycol, a cardiac depressant. The maximum recommended infusion rate is 50 mg/min for adults and 0.5 mg/kg/min for neonates and 1 mg/kg/min for older children is primarily due to this cardiac depressant. Patients receiving phenytoin sodium injection should be monitored for bradycardia, hypotension, and, if ECG is available, widened PR, QRS, or QT intervals as indications of myocardial depression. In most instances the actual infusion rate is about ½ to ¼ of the usually recommended maximum. If phenytoin sodium injection is diluted prior to infusion, normal saline should be used as other IV diluents result in rapid precipitation. Fosphenytoin does not contain propylene glycol and therefore can be administered more rapidly (maximum recommended infusion rate for adults is 150 mg/min). However, bradycardia and hypotension can still occur and transient pruritus is relatively common. Therefore, cardiovascular monitoring is required and infusion rates of less than 150 mg/min should be considered. Fosphenytoin, while requiring refrigeration for storage, is more soluble than phenytoin for injection and when reconstituted can be prepared in either dextrose or saline solution. While fosphenytoin is probably a better parenteral product, with fewer side effects, many institutions limit its use because it is significantly more expensive,

Daily doses of phenytoin injectable (fosphenytoin and intravenous sodium phenytoin) and oral acid phenytoin (chew tabs and suspension) should be divided. Phenytoin sodium extended may be dosed once daily but in children even if the extended product is used the daily doses are often divided. In addition, to minimize phenytoin concentration fluctuations and potential gastrointestinal disturbances, single daily doses of phenytoin sodium extended greater than 6 mg/kg/day also may need to be divided.

The suspension form requires complete dispersion and accurate volume delivery to ensure accurate dose administration. The suspension should be shaken vigorously prior to administration (1–2 min if the container has not been used for some time).

Intramuscular (IM) administration of phenytoin sodium injection is not recommended. Although absorption following intramuscular administration is probably complete, it is erratic due to precipitation at the injection site. Absorption of IM fosphenytoin appears to be complete with peak phenytoin concentrations occurring approximately 30 minutes after injection. However, the intravenous route is still preferred for fosphenytoin and phenytoin sodium injection when rapid achievement of phenytoin concentration is the goal (e.g., acute seizures or status epilepticus). Table 18-3 gives the available dosage forms.

General Pharmacokinetic Information

Absorption[1,2,5,8,17-26]

Although all dosage forms of phenytoin are assumed to have a bioavailability of 100%, phenytoin has capacity-limited metabolism; as a result, bioavailability studies are difficult to interpret. Unless the capacity-limited metabolism is carefully considered in the bioavailability analysis, drug products with the same fraction absorbed but having different rates of absorption can appear to have different bioavailabilities. In addition since phenytoin is a weak acid with limited water solubility, its absorption is slow and peak concentrations are delayed for several hours following oral administration.

The time to achieve peak concentration is both product and dose dependent. The suspension and chewable tablets appear to be absorbed more rapidly than capsules. Furthermore, the rate of absorption and time to peak concentration are dose dependent. Single Dilantin doses of 400, 800, and 1600 mg achieve peak concentrations at approximately 8, 13, and 30 hr after administration, respectively. Peak concentrations following these oral doses are on average only about half of what would be expected after administration of single intravenous doses. The reduced peak concentration following large oral doses is most likely the result of slow absorption rather than a reduced extent of absorption.

Table 18-3. Available Dosage Forms

Dosage Form	Product
Phenytoin sodium injection	
50 mg/mL	Phenytoin sodium injection
Fosphenytoin injection	
50 mg PE/mL	Cerebyx
Oral capsules	
Phenytoin sodium extended:	
30 mg	Dilantin and generic
100 mg	Dilantin and generic
200 mg and 300 mg	Phenytek and generic
Oral phenytoin chewable tablets	
50 mg	Dilantin Infatab
Oral phenytoin suspension	
125 mg/5 mL	Dilantin-125
	Phenytoin suspension

While data indicate that the phenytoin suspension is completely absorbed in most patients, two notable exceptions are neonates and patients receiving liquid nutritional support (e.g., nasogastric feedings). The reason for the low phenytoin concentrations in these two patient populations following oral administration of the suspension is unclear, and, although debated, the most likely explanation is a decreased bioavailability.

While there are a number of generic brands of phenytoin, some care should be taken when, for cost or supply reasons, there is a change in manufacturer. Some evidence suggests there may be differences between brands of phenytoin in the therapeutic response i.e. increased seizure frequency. It is not clear whether the differences observed are due to inconsistent intake with a high fat meal or a more intrinsic issue with the extent of absorption. In any case, if the brand of phenytoin is changed, careful monitoring of both clinical response and concentrations is probably warranted.

Distribution

Volume of distribution (*V*).[1,3,8,27-29] The volume of distribution for phenytoin (see Table 18-4) is calculated in part by using plasma concentrations. Any factor that alters plasma protein binding can alter the concentration and, therefore, the apparent volume of distribution. The phenytoin that is displaced from the albumin binding sites, while a large percent of the plasma concentration, is only a small percent of the total amount of phenytoin in the body. The "extra" phenytoin that is not bound to the albumin is rapidly distributed into the tissues and as a result the bound concentration decreases but the unbound concentration, tissue concentrations and pharmacologic effect are relatively unchanged. The decrease in plasma bound phenytoin with no change in the unbound phenytoin concentration results in an equally offsetting increase in the apparent volume of distribution. Therefore, no change in loading dose is required in patients with altered plasma binding.

Loading Dose = (Total Concentration) (volume of distribution)

Since phenytoin is a relatively lipid-soluble drug, obese patients have a larger volume of distribution (in liters) equal to:

$$V_{(\text{obese in L})} = 0.65\,{}^{\text{L}}\!/\!_{\text{kg}}[(IBW) + 1.33(ABW - IBW)] \qquad \text{(Eq. 1)}$$

where *ABW* is actual body weight in kg and *IBW* is ideal body weight in kg. Ideal body weight can be calculated by the following:

$$IBW_{\text{males}}(\text{kg}) = 50 + [(2.3)(H - 60)] \qquad \text{(Eq. 2)}$$

and

$$IBW_{\text{females}}(\text{kg}) = 45.5 + [(2.3)(H - 60)] \qquad \text{(Eq. 3)}$$

where H is the patient's height in inches.

Table 18-4. Volume of Distribution

Age	Volume (Mean ± SD)
Neonates and infants (<1 year)	1 ± 0.3 L/kg
Children (≥1 year), adults, and geriatrics[a]	0.65 ± 0.2 L/kg

[a]The geriatric population is more likely to have decreased serum albumin and therefore a larger apparent volume of distribution. The altered binding that results in a larger volume of distribution will be offset by a lower observed total phenytoin concentration and therefore no change in the usual loading dose is required.

Protein binding.[1-3,8,30-36] Phenytoin is bound primarily to albumin in the plasma (fraction bound in plasma equals 0.9), though less than 5% of the total body phenytoin is bound to albumin. As a result, changes in plasma binding have little impact on the unbound plasma concentration, tissue stores, and pharmacologic response.

Most clinical assays measure the total (total = bound + unbound) phenytoin concentrations. Therefore, alterations in plasma binding require adjustment for the change in the bound concentration. The two factors most commonly associated with altered phenytoin plasma protein binding are hypoalbuminemia and end-stage renal failure (i.e., patients receiving dialysis). While there are several methods available, phenytoin concentrations reported (C_{reported}) in these patients can be adjusted to represent the phenytoin concentration anticipated under normal plasma protein binding ($C_{\text{normal binding}}$) conditions by using Equations 4 and 5 below.

For low albumin and creatinine clearance greater than 25 ml/min:

$$C_{\text{normal binding}} = \frac{C_{\text{reported}}}{\left[(0.9)\left(\frac{\text{albumin}}{4.4}\right)\right] + 0.1} \qquad \text{(Eq. 4)}$$

For normal or low albumin and patient receiving dialysis:

$$C_{\text{normal binding}} = \frac{C_{\text{reported}}}{\left[(0.9)(0.48)\left(\frac{\text{albumin}}{4.4}\right)\right] + 0.1} \qquad \text{(Eq. 5)}$$

where

$C_{\text{normal binding}}$ = total phenytoin concentration that would be observed if patient had normal protein binding (90% bound)

C_{reported} = patient's total phenytoin concentration reported by laboratory (represents decreased plasma protein binding)

albumin = patient's albumin concentration in grams per deciliter

These equations should only be used as a guide or approximation because considerable variability has been reported.

Valproic acid in concentrations exceeding 30–40 mg/L displaces phenytoin from plasma albumin. Equation 6 (revised slightly from the original for consistency with similar equations throughout the text) can provide an estimate of the phenytoin concentration in normal plasma binding (90% bound):

$$C_{\text{normal binding}} = \frac{[0.1 + (0.001 \times C_{\text{valproic acid}})] \times C_{\text{reported}}}{0.1} \qquad \text{(Eq. 6)}$$

where C_{valproic} acid and C_{reported} are the measured concentrations of valproic acid and total phenytoin, respectively, obtained at the same time and C_{normal} binding is the total phenytoin concentration that would have been measured if valproic acid was not present.

It is the C_{normal} binding concentration that should be used when comparing the phenytoin concentration to the usual therapeutic range of 10 to 20 mg/L. In addition when performing pharmacokinetic calculations it is the C_{normal} binding that should usually be used as most of the equations have other pharmacokinetic parameters that assume normal plasma binding (volume of distribution, Km, etc.).

Equation 6 does have some limits. One of the most common is that the valproic acid and phenytoin concentrations have to be obtained at the same time. In addition equation 6 is not valid when there are factors other than valproic acid that also alter the phenytoin binding, e.g. hypoalbuminemia or end stage renal failure.

Elimination

Clearance (CL).[1,3,27,37-41] Renal elimination accounts for less than 5% of phenytoin clearance and is generally considered to be negligible. Phenytoin is cleared primarily (over 95%) by hepatic metabolism, which is capacity limited. Clinically important implications of this clearance include

- Css_{av} is not proportional to the maintenance dose (see Equations 8 and 9).
- Time to steady state (accumulation) is not three to five half-lives. (For a more detailed discussion, refer to the half-life and time to steady state section.)

This capacity-limited clearance is illustrated by

$$CL_{\text{phenytoin}} = \frac{V_{\max}}{K_m + Css_{av}} \qquad \text{(Eq. 7)}$$

where Vmax is the maximum rate (or velocity) of metabolism, and K_m is the concentration at which metabolism is occurring at half the maximum rate. Note that the clearance of phenytoin is dependent on the concentration and decreases with rising concentration. This non-linear relationship can then be used to calculate maintenance doses and steady state concentrations:

$$\left(\frac{(S)(F)(D)}{\tau}\right) = \frac{(V_{\max})(Css_{av})}{K_m + Css_{av}} \qquad \text{(Eq. 8)}$$

$$Css_{av} = \frac{(K_m)\left(\frac{(S)(F)(D)}{\tau}\right)}{V_{\max} - \left(\frac{(S)(F)(D)}{\tau}\right)} \qquad \text{(Eq. 9)}$$

Depending on the specific values of $V_{\max}$ and K_m used in these equations, a wide range of maintenance doses and steady state concentrations can be calculated. Since reported values of $V_{\max}$ and K_m (Table 18-5) vary widely, care should be taken that any calculated dose is reasonable for the patient in question. Phenytoin concentration monitoring is also appropriate to refine or adjust initial dose recommendations.

Pharmacogenomics.[42-46] Phenytoin is eliminated primarily by hepatic metabolism. Approximately 90% is by CYP 2C9 and 10% by CYP 2C19. Patients who are deficient in CYP 2C9 have a limited ability to metabolize phenytoin and are at risk for toxicity when receiving usual phenytoin maintenance doses. Unfortunately prior knowledge of a patient's genotype is uncommon. Patients with a limited ability to metabolize phenytoin are often identified only after they have developed high phenytoin concentrations and demonstrated clinical side effects or toxicity. Monitoring of clinical symptoms and phenytoin concentrations coupled with knowledge of

Table 18-5. Reported Values of V_{max} and K_m

Age	K_m (Mean ± SD)	V_{max} (Mean ± SD)[a]
Neonates and infants (<1 year)[b]	b	b
Children		
6 months–<4 years	6.6 ± 4.2 mg/L	14 ± 4.2 mg/kg/day
4–<7 years	6.8 ± 3.5 mg/L	10.9 ± 3.0 mg/kg/day
7–<10 years	6.5 ± 3.0 mg/L	10.1 ± 2.6 mg/kg/day
Adolescents (10–16 years)[c]	5.7 ± 2.7 mg/L	8.3 ± 2.8 mg/kg/day
Adults (18–≤59 years)	4.3 ± 3.5 mg/L	7.0 ± 3.0 mg/kg/day
Geriatrics (>59 years)[d]	5.8 ± 2.3 mg/L	7.0 ± 3.0 mg/kg/day

[a]For obese patients, the maximum velocity of drug elimination (Vmax) for phenytoin probably should be based on ideal body weight (IBW).
[b]Estimates for Vmax and Km in neonates and infants up to 1 year are uncertain. Some data suggest an initial slow rate of metabolism followed by a rapid increase in the ability to eliminate phenytoin over the first 3 months following birth. The limited data available suggest a Km of 4–6 mg/L and a Vmax of 10–13 mg/kg/day.
[c]Data unavailable for the 17-year-old.
[d]The limited data available suggest that Km and Vmax are similar to adults.

the nonlinear accumulation pattern for phenytoin should help to identify patients who are 2C9 deficient before they accumulate excessive concentrations.

Half-Life and time to steady state[1,3,47]

The relationship of half-life to a drug's accumulation or decline is applicable only to first-order drugs, i.e., those with a constant clearance and volume of distribution. Since the elimination of phenytoin is capacity limited and clearance decreases with increasing concentrations (see Elimination section), estimating time to achieve steady state is a complex process. Under certain conditions, accumulation can be slow and may continue for a prolonged period.

Equation 10 can be used to estimate the time necessary to achieve 90% of the steady state concentration:

$$t_{90\%} = \left(\frac{(K_m)(V)}{\left[V_{max} - \left(\frac{(S)(F)(D)}{\tau} \right) \right]^2} \right) \left[(2.3 \times V_{max}) - (0.9)\left(\frac{(S)(F)(D)}{\tau} \right) \right] \quad \text{(Eq. 10)}$$

where the following units apply:

V *in* L, K_m *in mg/L*, V_{max} *in mg/day, and dose/τ in mg/day*

The accuracy of Equation 10 and the calculated time to steady state depends on the values used for V_{max}, K_m, and V. When literature estimates or uncertain patient-specific values are used, the actual steady state concentration and time to achieve 90% of steady state may be considerably different than the calculated values. The errors are especially large when the anticipated steady state concentrations are high or the time to 90% of steady state is long. In addition, compliance to the prescribed dosage regimen is an important variable.

The time required for a phenytoin concentration to decline from an initial concentration ($C_{initial}$) to a lower concentration (C) is described by Equation 11, which assumes that no absorption occurs in the time between $C_{initial}$ and C:

$$t = \frac{\left[(K_m)\left(\ln\left(\frac{C_{initial}}{C}\right)\right)\right] + (C_{initial} - C)}{\left(\frac{V_{max}}{V}\right)} \quad \text{(Eq. 11)}$$

where the following units apply:

K_m, C and $C_{initial}$ in mg/L; V_{max} in mg/day; V in L; and t in days.

As long as the phenytoin concentrations are much greater than K_m (4 to 5 times higher than K_m), the rate of phenytoin elimination approaches and is only slightly less than *V*max, the maximum rate of metabolism. Under these conditions, the time required to decline from *C*initial to *C* is determined primarily by *V*max and *V*. Therefore, at high concentrations the daily decline in the phenytoin concentration can be estimated by using *V*max/*V*. Using this approach, the expected maximum decline in phenytoin concentration for the average patient with phenytoin concentrations greater than 15 mg/L would be approximately 10 mg/L/day, i.e., (*V*max/*V* = 7 mg/kg/day divided by 0.65 L/kg).

Therapeutic Range[1,48,49]

For seizure disorders, the therapeutic range is 10–20 mg/L of total (bound + unbound) phenytoin in patients with normal binding. Approximately 50% of patients show decreased seizure frequency with phenytoin concentrations equal to or greater than 10 mg/L, and almost 90% respond with concentrations equal to or greater than 15 mg/L. It should be remembered that the target concentrations of 10 to 20 mg/L represent unbound or free phenytoin concentrations of 1 to 2 mg/L. It is the unbound drug that is in equilibrium with the tissue and pharmacologic receptors.

Phenytoin also is reported to be effective in some neurological (non-seizure) disorders. However, most cases are anecdotal, with little or no reference to phenytoin concentrations.

Therapeutic Monitoring[1,3,8,31,50-55]

Suggested sampling times

The time of sampling depends on the clinical situation as well as the route and/or dosage form. As a general rule, intravenous loading doses are reasonably reliable in achieving the desired phenytoin concentrations, but oral loading and oral or intravenous maintenance regimens are less predictable.

When fosphenytoin or phenytoin sodium injection is administered parenterally, sampling should not be performed during the hydrolysis or distribution phase (i.e., within 2 hr after the end of infusion or within 4 hr of an intramuscular fosphenytoin injection) (Table 18-6).

After a *maintenance regimen is started*, the first sample should be obtained within 3 to 4 days (not steady state) to ensure that concentrations are not too low or high for a prolonged period. Then, sampling should be performed with decreasing frequency if concentrations are acceptable and stable or every 3 to 4 days if the maintenance dose must be changed or if phenytoin concentrations are declining or increasing.

At *steady state*, the sampling interval is debatable during stable chronic therapy. Sampling probably should be done every 7 to 14 days in the acute care setting and every 1 to 6 months in ambulatory patients.

Following a *change in status* (e.g., change in route, maintenance dose, dosage form, or addition of drugs known to alter metabolism or absorption), phenytoin concentrations should be monitored in a manner similar to when a regimen is started. In addition, the appearance of side effects or breakthrough seizures would warrant obtaining a phenytoin concentration.

Analytical methods.[31,50-62] While there are many assay techniques available, immunologic methods are by far the most common in clinical practice. Most are either fluorescence polarization (FPIA) or enzyme multiplied (EMIT) assay techniques. These methods are usually specific but on occasion have cross-reactivity with phenytoin metabolites or other drugs. In uremia, phenytoin metabolites can accumulate and cross-react, but for the most part these problems have been resolved by the development of more specific antibodies that rec-

Table 18-6. Suggested Sample Times

Administered Dose	Suggested Sampling Time
Loading dose:	
Intravenous (phenytoin sodium injection	
or fosphenytoin)	>2 hr after end of infusion[a]
Intramuscular (fosphenytoin)	>4 hr after injection
Oral	About 24 hr after loading dose
Maintenance dose:	
Oral single daily dose	Trough recommended[b]
Intravenous (divided dose)	Trough
Oral divided dose	Trough recommended

[a]Concentration measurements not necessarily recommended but may be useful for assessing V. If V appears to be unusually large, consider potential of decreased protein binding.
[b]Morning sampling time is probably acceptable with bedtime dosing if time of sampling after dose is consistent.

ognize only the parent compound. Sampling soon after administration of fosphenytoin results in inaccurate estimates of the actual phenytoin concentration. Samples that are obtained early will contain both fosphenytoin and phenytoin. With time, the fosphenytoin in the sample will be hydrolyzed to phenytoin. As a result the phenytoin concentration will increase and the fosphenytoin concentration will decrease so that the sample no longer reflects the phenytoin concentration at the original time of sampling.

The usual assay error for clinical samples in the normal therapeutic range is approximately 5% to as much as 10%. While this error is acceptable for clinical monitoring it should be kept in mind that significant errors can occur with this non-linear drug, especially when extrapolating to higher or lower concentrations. In addition, improper collection or storage of samples can lead to invalid assay results. Caution should be used when the reported assay results are inconsistent with the clinical picture.

Monitoring unbound or free concentrations would seem to be a logical approach considering the known problems with altered plasma binding of phenytoin. However, use of unbound phenytoin concentrations is relatively uncommon in clinical practice. This may be attributed to the fact that most patients do not experience significant alterations in their plasma binding. In addition assay procedures that measure unbound concentrations are more expensive, and there is limited data supporting the use of unbound phenytoin concentrations. When unbound concentrations are measured, it is important to adjust the assay procedure to increase assay sensitivity. Most assays have a percent error and a fixed error. In the case of phenytoin the fixed error is usually in the range of 1 mg/L. An error of 1 mg/L is acceptable when measuring concentrations of 10 to 20 mg/L but would not be acceptable when measuring the unbound concentrations of 1 to 2 mg/L that would be associated with the usual total concentrations of 10 to 20 mg/L. The fixed error of approximately 1 mg/L is also a problem when considering dose adjustment based on concentrations of less than 5 mg/L. Nonetheless, the clinician should always consider the possibility of altered binding and how, if present, altered binding would affect the relationship between the measured total phenytoin concentration (bound + unbound) and the patient's clinical response.

Pharmacodynamic Monitoring[1-3]

Concentration-related efficacy

In the treatment of seizures, efficacy directly relates to seizure frequency and improvement of EEG findings. In patients who are being treated prophylactically or whose seizures are infrequent, assessing the adequacy of therapy based on the number or frequency of seizures is difficult.

Concentration-related toxicity

The concentrations associated with the various side effects listed below are only approximate guidelines; many patients experience significant side effects at much lower concentrations or no side effects at considerably higher concentrations. These differences may be due to individual susceptibility or sensitivity to phenytoin or, possibly, to alterations in plasma protein binding and as a result an underestimate of the unbound phenytoin concentration.

How often a patient should be monitored for concentration-related side effects depends on the course of treatment and the stability of the patient's clinical status and phenytoin concentrations. For example, the patient should be observed continuously and blood pressure and heart rate should be monitored very frequently when intravenous loading doses are administered.

Nystagmus and a simple assessment of mental status (e.g., "How do you feel?" "Are you tired or sleepy?") are easily checked every time an outpatient is examined or daily in the acute care setting.

Nystagmus. Nystagmus is a tremor or slight twitching of the eye. This is one of the clinical signs that practitioners are looking for when they ask patients to hold their head still and follow their finger with their eyes as they move their finger from side to side. Nystagmus can be progressive and be present only on a far lateral gaze at phenytoin concentrations of 15 to over 20 mg/L to present when the patient is looking straight ahead at concentrations greater than 50 mg/L. Some patients have baseline nystagmus that is unrelated to phenytoin while others do not develop nystagmus until phenytoin concentrations are well above the usual therapeutic range. Although nystagmus is frequently used to document the presence of phenytoin, it is not generally considered to be a toxic symptom and by itself is not a reason to adjust the phenytoin dose.

CNS depression. This side effect can vary from mild sedation to an inability to concentrate to confusion to coma. Most patients experience relatively mild effects at concentrations of 5–15 mg/L; others tolerate phenytoin concentrations greater than 20 mg/L. Ataxia and impaired motor function are usually observed with phenytoin concentrations greater than 20 mg/L and become more frequent and obvious at concentrations greater than 30 mg/L. It is unclear whether patients, with time, develop true tolerance to CNS effects or simply learn to accept them.

Non-concentration-related side effects

Some side effects may be more associated with the duration of phenytoin therapy. They include hypertrichosis, coarsening of facial features, folate deficiency, glucose intolerance, gingival hyperplasia, vitamin D deficiency, osteomalacia, peripheral neuropathy, and very rarely systemic lupus erythematosus.

The presence of propylene glycol in intravenous phenytoin sodium injection has been reported to cause myocardial depression, hypotension, bradycardia, and widened PR, QRS, and QT intervals. Without propylene glycol, phenytoin has less effect on the myocardium, hence, the more rapid infusion rate for fosphenytoin. However, bradycardia and hypotension still occur with fosphenytoin but are usually less profound than with phenytoin sodium injection. When cardiovascular side effects occur during IV administration, the usual approach is to decrease or stop the infusion.

Drug-Drug Interactions

Numerous drugs are reported to interact with phenytoin, but capacity-limited metabolism makes assessment of these interactions difficult. For example, a 10% change in *Vmax* may have relatively little impact on a steady state phenytoin concentration of 5 mg/L but a significant effect on a steady state concentration of 15 mg/L. Likewise, small changes in absorption have similar effects on low and high steady state phenytoin concentrations. As Css_{av} becomes much greater than K_m, the maintenance dose approaches *Vmax*. Under these conditions, a small change in either the maintenance dose or the *Vmax* can result in disproportionate changes in the new steady state concentration.

Because of the potential for very small changes in metabolism or absorption to alter phenytoin concentrations significantly, patients should be closely monitored following any change in their regimen.

Table 18-7 is a partial list of drugs that influence phenytoin. Emphasis is given to those drugs most likely to alter phenytoin pharmacokinetics and/or to be encountered in the clinical setting. Since it is eliminated primarily by hepatic metabolism with approximately 90% by CYP 2C9 and 10% by CYP 2C19, drugs that inhibit or induce these enzymes might be expected to cause drug-drug interactions with phenytoin.

Drug–Disease State or Condition Interactions

As with drug-drug interactions, the effects of disease states on phenytoin therapy are difficult to quantify. In addition it should be recognized that phenytoin might alter the effects of other drugs. As examples, cyclosporine, hormonal contraceptives and voriconazole all may have reduced effectiveness when phenytoin is added, presumably due to enzyme induction. The following are disease states and drugs that are known to alter the pharmacokinetics of phenytoin.

Hepatic disease—cirrhosis[96,97]

Phenytoin is eliminated from the body primarily by hepatic metabolism. Therefore, patients with significant hepatic disease may require reduced maintenance doses. These patients frequently also have hypoalbuminemia, which alters the reported total phenytoin concentration. The reported phenytoin concentration can be "adjusted" by using Equation 4. The altered albumin has little effect on the loading dose required to achieve therapeutic unbound plasma and tissue concentrations (see volume of distribution section).

Renal failure[32,86,97]

Patients with end-stage renal failure (i.e., receiving dialysis) have a decreased plasma phenytoin binding affinity for albumin. They also usually have low serum albumin. These factors, which greatly affect the reported

Table 18-7. Drugs Influencing Phenytoin Pharmacokinetics

Drug	Effect on Phenytoin Concentration	Mechanism
Amiodarone[63,64]	Increase	Inhibition of metabolism
Antacids[a,65-67]	Decrease	Decreased absorption
Carbamazepine[68,69]	Increase or decrease	Induction of metabolism
Chloramphenicol[70]	Increase	Inhibition of metabolism
Cimetidine[71]	Increase	Inhibition of metabolism
Ciprofloxacin[72,73]	Increase	Inhibition of metabolism
Disulfiram[74,75]	Increase	Inhibition of metabolism
Fluconazole[76]	Increase	Inhibition of metabolism
Fluoxetine[77]	Increase	Inhibition of metabolism
Folic acid[78-80]	Decrease	Induction of metabolism
Isoniazid[81-82]	Increase	Inhibition of metabolism (most significant in phenotypically slow acetylators)
Phenobarbital[b,83,84]	Increase or decrease	Inhibition or induction of metabolism
Rifampin[85]	Decrease	Induction of metabolism
Salicylates[c,86]	Decrease	Plasma protein displacement
Sertraline[87]	Increase	Inhibition of metabolism
Sulfonamides[88,89]	Increase	Inhibition of metabolism; plasma protein displacement
Ticlopidine[90,91]	Increase	Inhibition of metabolism
Trimethoprim[92]	Increase	Inhibition of metabolism
Valproic acid[d,33,93,94]	Decrease	Plasma protein displacement
Voriconazole[95]	Increase	Inhibition of metabolism

[a]A decrease in absorption is not consistently observed. Both drugs should not be administered at the same time; antacid and phenytoin doses should be taken at least 2 hr apart whenever possible.
[b]The direction of change (if any) for the phenytoin concentration depends on which phenobarbital effect is predominant (i.e., induction or inhibition of metabolism).
[c]Plasma protein displacement results in a decrease in the reported total phenytoin concentration but has little effect on the unbound phenytoin concentration or therapeutic effect.
[d]Valproic acid displaces phenytoin from its plasma protein binding. It is not clear, however, as to whether valproic acid also inhibits phenytoin metabolism.

total concentration, have little influence on the unbound phenytoin concentration and the therapeutic effect. Therefore, patients with renal failure should initially receive normal loading and maintenance doses.

Equation 5 can be used to approximate the total phenytoin concentration that would be observed in end-stage renal failure patients on dialysis if they had normal plasma protein binding ($C_{\text{normal binding}}$). The $C_{\text{normal binding}}$ concentration should be compared to the usual therapeutic range and the potential for phenytoin to produce either therapeutic or toxic effects.

Obesity[29,98]

In obese patients, the ideal or non-obese weight probably correlates best with metabolism and, therefore, V_{max} and maintenance doses. Although using the non-obese weight to estimate the initial maintenance dose for the obese patient is recommended, plasma concentration monitoring is important, as significant variations have been observed. Loading doses require some adjustment because phenytoin has significant lipid solubility and an increased volume of distribution in obese patients. As stated earlier (see volume of distribution section), the volume of distribution (in liters) in obese patients can be calculated using Equation 1.

Malabsorption[18-21,25,99]

There is little direct evidence that phenytoin is incompletely absorbed (see bioavailability of dosage forms section). However, patients with diarrhea or rapid GI transit may have incomplete phenytoin absorption, especially if they take large single doses resulting in prolonged absorption.

AIDS[100,101]

Seizure disorders are common in patients with HIV/AIDS, and phenytoin is commonly used for control of seizures in this patient population. Many clinicians believe that AIDS patients achieve low concentrations while receiving normal phenytoin doses. These observations may be because many patients with AIDS have a low serum albumin, GI disorders, and rapid GI transit due to other drug therapy or infectious disease processes resulting in decreased plasma binding, decreased bioavailability, or both.

Pregnancy and lactation[79,80,102-112]

Most women (>90%) who have epilepsy and continue phenytoin throughout their pregnancy deliver normal babies. However, infants born to women with epilepsy and receiving phenytoin are about two to three times more likely to have some type of congenital defect. The benefits of continuing phenytoin usually outweigh the risks to the fetus if the mother develops uncontrolled seizures.

Decreases in phenytoin concentrations during pregnancy have been reported. The reason for the decrease is unclear but proposed mechanisms include decreased bioavailability, decreased plasma binding, and increased maternal and/or fetal metabolism. In addition, folate depletion or supplementation may also influence phenytoin metabolism. During pregnancy, phenytoin therapy should be monitored closely to ensure optimal therapeutic control of the seizure disorder.

Critically ill[113-115]

Critically ill patients are complex and dynamic with regard to their clinical status and physiology. There is conflicting evidence as to whether or not this patient population has decreased, relatively normal, or increased metabolic capacity. In addition these patients are likely to have altered renal function, hypoalbuminemia, and the presence of displacing drugs and as a result an alteration in phenytoin plasma binding. For these reasons critically ill patients require frequent plasma monitoring of phenytoin and may be candidates for measuring unbound phenytoin concentrations if exhibiting an unusual clinical response.

References

1. Winter ME, Tozer TN. Phenytoin. In: Burton ME, Shaw LM, Schentag JJ, et al., eds. *Applied Pharmacokinetics & Pharmacodynamics: Principles of Therapeutic Drug Monitoring.* 4th ed. Baltimore, MD: Lippincott Williams & Wilkins; 2006:463-90.
2. Woodbury DM, Penry JK, Pippenger CE, eds. *Antiepileptic Drugs.* New York, NY: Raven Press; 1982:191-281.

3. Winter ME. Phenytoin. In: Winter ME. *Basic Clinical Pharmacokinetics*. 5th ed. Philadelphia, PA: Lippincott, Williams & Wilkins; 2010:355-402.
4. Wilder BJ, Serrano EE, Ramsay RE. Plasma phenytoin levels after loading and maintenance doses. *Clin Pharmacol Ther.* 1973;14:797-801.
5. Jung D, Powel JR, Walson P, et al. Effect of dose on phenytoin absorption. *Clin Pharmacol Ther.* 1980;28:479-85.
6. Swadron SP, Rudis MI, Azimian K, et al. A comparison of phenytoin-loading techniques in the emergency department. *Acad Emerg Med.* 2004;11:244-52.
7. Rudis MI, Touchette DR, Swadron SP, et al. Cost-effectiveness of oral phenytoin, intravenous phenytoin and intravenous fosphenytoin in the emergency department. *Ann Emerg Med.* 2004;43:386-400
8. Thummel KE, Shen DD, Isoherranen N, et al. Appendix II: Design and optimization of dosage regimens: pharmacokinetic data. In Bruton LL, Lazo JS, Purke KL, eds. *Goodman and Gilman's The Pharmacologic Basis of Therapeutics.* 11th ed. New York, NY: McGraw-Hill; 2005.
9. Privitera MD. Clinical rules for phenytoin dosing. *Ann Pharmacother.* 1993;27:1169-73.
10. Fischer JH, Cwik MJ, Luer MS, et al. Stability of fosphenytoin sodium with intravenous solutions in glass bottles, polyvinyl chloride bags, and polypropylene syringes. *Ann Pharmacother.* 1997;31:553-9.
11. Knapp LE, Kugler AR. Clinical experience with fosphenytoin in adults: pharmacokinetics, safety, and efficacy. *J Child Neurol.* 1988;13(Suppl 1):S15-8.
12. Fosphenytoin. In: McEvoy GK. *AHFS Drug Information 2010.* Bethesda, MD: American Society of Health-System Pharmacists; 2010:2252-4.
13. Phenytoin and Phenytoin Sodium. In: McEvoy GK. *AHFS Drug Information 2010.* Bethesda, MD: American Society of Health-System Pharmacists; 2010:2254-7.
14. Facts and Comparisons 4.0 [database online], Wolters Kluwer Health, Inc.; 2010.
15. Pryor FM, Gidal B, Ramsay RE, et al. Fosphenytoin: Pharmacokinetics and tolerance of intramuscular loading doses. *Epilepsia.* 2001;42:245-50.
16. Browne TR. Fosphenytoin (Cerebyx) *Clin Neuropharmacol.* 1997;20:1-12.
17. McCauley DL, Tozer TN, Winter ME. Time for phenytoin concentration to peak: consequences of first-order or zero-order absorption. *Ther Drug Monitor.* 1989;11:540-2.
18. Faraji B, Yu PP. Serum phenytoin levels of patients on gastrostomy tube feeding. *J Neuroscience Nurs.* 1998;30:55-9.
19. Dec KU, Hast CE, Dunnigan KJ, et al. Bioavailability of phenytoin acid and phenytoin sodium with enteral feedings. *Pharmacother.* 1998;18:637-45.
20. Kitchen D, Smith D. Problems with phenytoin administration in neurology/neurosurgery ITU patients receiving enteral feeding. *Seizure* 2001;10:265-8.
21. Yeung SCSA, Ensom, MHH. Phenytoin and enteral feedings: Does evidence support an interaction? *Ann Pharmacother.* 2000;34:896-905.
22. Wilder BJ, Leppik I, Hietpas TJ, et al. Effect of food on absorption of Dilantin Kapseals and Mylan extended phenytoin sodium capsules. *Neurology.* 2001;57:582-9.
23. O'Hagan M, Wallace SJ. Enteral formula feeds interfere with phenytoin absorption. *Brain and Development.* 1994;16:165-7.
24. Koak KK, Haas CE, Dunningan KJ, et al. Bioavailability of phenytoin acid and phenytoin sodium with enteral feedings. *Pharmacother*. 1998;18:637-45.
25. Rodman DP, Stevenson TL, Ray TR. Phenytoin malabsorption after jejunostomy tube delivery. *Pharmacother*. 1995;15:801-5.
26. Berg MJ, Gross RA, Tomaszewski KJ, et al. Generic substitution in the treatment of epilepsy: case evidence of breakthrough seizures. *Neurology.* 2008;71:525-30.
27. Bauer LA, Blouin RA. Phenytoin Michaelis-Menten pharmacokinetics in Caucasian pediatric patients. *Clin Pharmacokinet.* 1983;8:454-9.
28. Bauer LA, Blouin RA. Age and phenytoin kinetics in adult epileptics. *Clin Pharmacol Ther.* 1982;31:301-4.
29. Abernethy DR, Greenblatt DJ. Phenytoin disposition in obesity. Determination of loading dose. *Arch Neurol.* 1985;42:568-71.
30. Benet LZ, Hoener BA. Changes in plasma protein binding have little clinical relevance. *Clin Pharmacol Ther.* 2002; 71:115-211.
31. Barre J, Didey F, Delion F, et al. Problems in therapeutic drug monitoring: free drug level monitoring. *Ther Drug Monit.* 1988;10:133-43.
32. Liponi DF, Winter ME, Tozer TN. Renal function and therapeutic concentrations of phenytoin. *Neurology.* 1984 Mar;34(3):395-7.

33. Kerrick JM, Wolff DL, Graves NM. Predicting unbound phenytoin concentrations in patients receiving valproic acid: a comparison of two prediction methods. *Ann Pharmacother.* 1995;29:470-4.

34. Iwamoto T, Kagawa Y, Naito Y, et al. Clinical evaluation of plasma free phenytoin measurement and factors influencing its protein binding. *Biopharm Drug Dispos.* 2006;27:77-84.

35. Mlynarek ME, Peterson EL, Zarowitz BJ. Predicting unbound phenytoin concentrations in the critically ill neurosurgical patient. *Ann Pharmacother.* 1996;30:219-23.

36. Anderson GD, Pak C, Doane KW, et al. Revised Winter-Tozer equation for normalized phenytoin concentrations in trauma and elderly patients with hypoalbuminemia. *Ann Pharmacother.* 1997;31:279-84.

37. Chiba K, Ishizaki T, Miura H, et al. Michaelis-Menten pharmacokinetics of diphenylhydantoin and applications in the pediatric age patient. *J Pediatr.* 1980;96:479-84.

38. Grasela TH, Sheiner LB, Rambeck B, et al. Steady-state pharmacokinetics of phenytoin from routinely collected patient data. *Clin Pharmacokinet.* 1983;8:355-64.

39. Deleu D, Aarons L, Ahmed IA. Estimation of population pharmacokinetic parameters of free phenytoin in adult epileptic patients. *Arch Med Res.* 2005;36:49-53. Erratum in: *Arch Med Res.* 2005;36:186.

40. Kidd RS, Curry TB, Gallagher S, et al. Identification of a null allele of CYP2C9 in an African-American exhibiting toxicity to phenytoin. *Pharmacogenetics.* 2001;11:803-8.

41. Wang B, Wang J, Huang SQ, et al. Genetic polymorphism of human cytochrome P 450 2C9 gene and its clinical significance. *Curr Drug Metab.* 2009;10:781-834.

42. Brandolese R, Scordo MG, Spina E, et al. Severe phenytoin intoxication in a subject homozygous for CYP2C9*3. *Clin Pharmacol Ther.* 2001;70:391-4.

43. Giancarlo GM, Venkatakrishnan K, Granda BW, et al. Relative contributions of CYP2C9 and 2C19 to phenytoin 4-hydroxylation in vitro: inhibition by sulfaphenazole, omeprazole, and ticlopidine. *Eur J Clin Pharmacol.* 2001;57:31-6.

44. Lee CR, Goldstein JA, Pieper JA. Cytochrome P450 2C9 polymorphisms: a comprehensive review of the in-vitro and human data. *Pharmacogenetics.* 2002;12:251-63.

45. Yukawa E, Mamiya K. Effect of CYP2C19 genetic polymorphism on pharmacokinetics of phenytoin and phenobarbital in Japanese epileptic patients using non-linear mixed effects model approach. *J Clin Pharm Ther.* 2006;31:275-82.

46. Desta Z, Zhao X, Shin JG, et al. Clinical significance of the cytochrome P450 2C19 genetic polymorphism. *Clin Pharmacokinet.* 2002;41:913-58.

47. Vozeh S, Follath F. Nomographic estimation of time to reach steady-state serum concentrations during phenytoin therapy. *Eur J Clin Pharmacol.* 1980;17:33-5.

48. Buchtal F, Svensmark O, Schiller JP. Clinical and electroencephalographic correlation with serum levels of diphenylhydantoin. *Arch Neurol.* 1960;2:624-30.

49. Reynolds EH, Shorvon SD, Galbraith AW, et al. Phenytoin monotherapy for epilepsy: a long-term prospective study, assisted by serum level monitoring in previously untreated patients. *Epilepsia.* 1981;22:485-8.

50. Warner A, Privitera M, Bates D. Standards of laboratory practice: antiepileptic drug monitoring. *Clin Chem.* 1998; 44:1085-95.

51. Yukawa E. Optimization of antiepileptic drug therapy. The importance of serum drug concentration monitoring. *Clin Pharmacokinet.* 1996;31:120-30.

52. Kugler AR, Annesley TM, Nordblom GD, et al. Cross-reactivity of fosphenytoin in two human plasma phenytoin immunoassays. *Clin Chem.* 1998;44:1474-80.

53. Levine M, Chang T. Therapeutic drug monitoring of phenytoin. Rationale and current status. *Clin Pharmacokinet.* 1990;19:341-58.

54. Eadie MJ. Therapeutic drug monitoring-antiepileptic drugs. *Br J Clin Pharmacol.* 2001;52 Suppl:11S-20S.

55. Dasgupta A. Usefulness of monitoring free (unbound) concentrations of therapeutic drugs in patient management. *Clinica Chimica Acta* [serial online]. 2006;377:1-13. Available from: Science Direct, Amsterdam, The Netherlands. Accessed August 3, 2010.

56. Datta P, Scurlock D, Dasgupta A. Analytic performance evaluation of a new turbidimetric immunoassay for phenytoin on the ADVIA 1650 analyzer: effect of phenytoin metabolite and analogue. *Ther Drug Monit.* 2005;27:305-8.

57. Rainey PM, Rogers KE, Roberts WL. Metabolite and matrix interference in phenytoin immunoassays. *Clin Chem.* 1996;42:1645-53.

58. Steijns LSW, Bouw J, van der Weide J. Evaluation of fluorescence polarization assays for measuring valproic acid, phenytoin, carbamazepine and phenobarbital in serum. *Ther Drug Monit.* 2002;24:432-5.

59. Green PJ, Vlasses PH, Frauenhoffer SM, et al. Phenytoin can be measured reliably in uremic patients by immunoassay. *Clin Chem.* 1983;29:737.

60. Roberts WL, Annesley TM, De BK, et al. Performance characteristics of four free phenytoin immunoassays. *Ther Drug*

Monit. 2001;23:148-54.

61. Roberts, WL, De, BK, Coleman, JP, et al. Falsely increased immunoassay measurements of total and unbound phenytoin in critically ill uremic patients receiving fosphenytoin. *Clin Chem.* 1999;45:829-37.
62. Soldin, SJ, Wang E, Verjee Z, et al. Phenytoin overview-metabolite interference in some immunoassays could be clinically important: results of a College of American Pathologist Study. *Archives of Pathology & Laboratory Medicine.* December 2003. Available from: Archives of Pathology and Laboratory Medicine, on line. Accessed November 17, 2010.
63. Nolan PE Jr., Marcus FI, Hoyer GL, et al. Pharmacokinetic interaction between intravenous phenytoin and amiodarone in healthy volunteers. *Clin Pharmacol Ther.* 1989;46:43-50.
64. Shackleford EJ, Watson FT. Amiodarone-phenytoin interaction. *Drug Intell Clin Pharm.* 1987;21:921.
65. Garnett WR, Carter BL, Pellock JM. Bioavailability of phenytoin administered with antacids. *Ther Drug Monit.* 1979;1:435-7.
66. O'Brien WM, Orme ML, Breckenridge AM. Failure of antacids to alter the pharmacokinetics of phenytoin. *Br J Clin Pharmacol.* 1978;6:276-7.
67. Smart HL, Somerville KW, Williams J, et al. The effects of sucralfate upon phenytoin absorption in man. *Br J Clin Pharmacol.* 1985;20:238-40.
68. Molholm-Hansen J, Siersbaek-Nielsen K, Skovsted L. Carbamazepine-induced acceleration of diphenylhydantoin and warfarin metabolism in man. *Clin Pharmacol Ther.* 1971;12:539-43.
69. Brown TR, Szabo GK, Evans JE, et al. Carbamazepine increases phenytoin serum concentrations and reduces phenytoin clearance. *Neurology.* 1988;38:1146-50.
70. Harper JM, Yost RL, Stewart RB, et al. Phenytoin-chloramphenicol interaction: a retrospective study. *Drug Intell Clin Pharm.* 1979;13:425-9.
71. Phillips P, Hansky J. Phenytoin toxicity secondary to cimetidine administration. *Med J Aust.* 1984;141:602.
72. Pollak PT, Slayter KL. Hazards of doubling phenytoin dose in the face of an unrecognized interaction with ciprofloxacin. *Ann Pharmacother.* 1997;31:61-4.
73. Dillard ML. Ciprofloxacin-phenytoin interaction. *Ann Pharmacother.* 1992;26:263.
74. Olesen OV. Disulfiram (Antabuse) as inhibitor of phenytoin metabolism. *Acta Pharmacol Toxicol.* 1966;24:317-22.
75. Brown CG, Kaminsky MJ, Feroli ER, et al. Delirium with phenytoin and disulfiram administration. *Ann Emerg Med.* 1983;12:310-3.
76. Blum RA, Wilton JH, Hilloigoss DM, et al. Effect of fluconazole on the disposition of phenytoin. *Clin Pharmacol Ther.* 1991;49:420-5.
77. Jalil P. Toxic reaction following the combined administration of fluoxetine and phenytoin: two case reports. *J Neurol Neurosurg Psychiatry.* 1992;55:412.
78. Lewis DP, Van Dyke DC, Willhite LA, et al. Phenytoin-folic acid interaction. *Ann Pharmacother.* 1995;29:726-35.
79. Seligmann H, Potasman I, Weller B, et al. Phenytoin-folic acid interactions: a lesson to be learned. *Clin Neuropharmacol.* 1999;22:268-72.
80. Berg MJ, Stumbo PJ, Chenard CA, et al. Folic acid improves phenytoin pharmacokinetics. *J Am Dietetic Assn.* 1995;95:352-6.
81. Miller RR, Porter J, Greenblatt DJ. Clinical importance of the interaction of phenytoin and isoniazid. *Chest.* 1979;75:356-8.
82. Brennan RW, Dehejia H, Kutt H, et al. Diphenylhydantoin intoxication attendant to slow inactivation of isoniazid. *Neurology.* 1970;20:687-9.
83. Kutt H, Haynes J, Verebely K, et al. The effect of phenobarbital on plasma diphenylhydantoin level and metabolism in man and in rat liver microsomes. *Neurology.* 1969;19:611-6.
84. Morselli PL, Rizzo M, Garaltini S, et al. Interaction between phenobarbital and diphenylhydantoin in animals and in epileptic patients. *Ann NY Acad Sci.* 1971;179:88-107.
85. Kay L, Kampmann JP, Svendsen TL, et al. Influence of rifampicin and isoniazid on the kinetics of phenytoin. *Br J Clin Pharmacol.* 1985;20:323-6.
86. Odar-Cederlof I, Borga O. Impaired plasma protein binding of phenytoin in uremia and displacement effect of salicylic acid. *Clin Pharmacol Ther.* 1976;20:36-47.
87. Haselberger MB, Freedman LS, Tolbert S. Elevated serum phenytoin concentrations associated with coadministration of sertraline. *J Clin Psychopharmacol.* 1997;17:107-9.
88. Lumholtz B, Siersbaek-Nielsen K, Skovsted L, et al. Sulfamethizole-induced inhibition of diphenylhydantoin, tolbutamide and warfarin metabolism. *Clin Pharmacol Ther.* 1975;17: 731-4.
89. Lunde PKM, Rane A, Yaffe SJ. Plasma protein binding of diphenylhydantoin in man. Interaction with other drugs and the effect of temperature and plasma dilution. *Clin Pharmacol Ther.* 1970;11:846-55.

90. Privitera M, Welty TE. Acute phenytoin toxicity followed by seizure breakthrough from a ticlopidine-phenytoin interaction. *Arch Neurol.* 1996;53:1191.

91. Donahue S, Flockhart, DA, Abernethy, DR. Ticlopidine inhibits phenytoin clearance. *Clin Pharmacol Therap.* 1999;66:563-8.

92. Hansen JM, Kampmann JP, Siersbaek-Nielsen K, et al. The effect of different sulfonamides on phenytoin metabolism in man. *Acta Med Scand Suppl.* 1979;624:106-10.

93. Mattson RH, Cramer JA, Williamson PD, et al. Valproic acid in epilepsy: clinical and pharmacological effects. *Ann Neurol.* 1978;3:20-5.

94. Monks A, Richens A. Effect of single doses of sodium valproate on serum phenytoin levels and protein binding in epileptic patients. *Clin Pharmacol Ther.* 1980;27:89-95.

95. Purkins L, Wood N, Ghahramani P, et al. Coadministration of voriconazole and phenytoin: pharmacokinetic interaction, safety, and toleration. *Br J Clin Pharmacol.* 2003;56:37-44.

96. Wallace S, Brodle MJ. Decreased drug binding in serum from patients with chronic hepatic disease. *Eur J Clin Pharmacol.* 1976;9:429-32.

97. Aweeka FT, Gottwald MD, Gambertoglio JG, et al. Pharmacokinetics of fosphenytoin in patients with hepatic or renal disease. *Epilepsia.* 1999;40:777-82.

98. de Oca GM, Gums JG, Robinson JD. Phenytoin dosing in obese patients: two case reports. *Drug Intell Clin Pharm.* 1988;22:708-10.

99. Bauer LA. Interference of oral phenytoin absorption by continuous nasogastric feedings. *Neurology.* 1982;32:570-72.

100. Toler SM, Wilkerson MA, Porter WH, et al. Severe phenytoin intoxication as a result of altered protein binding in AIDS. *Drug Intell Clin Pharm.* 1990;24:698-700.

101. Wong MC, Suite ND, Labar DR. Seizures in human immunodeficiency virus infection. *Arch Neurol.* 1990;47:640-2.

102. Briggs GG, Freeman RK, Yaffe SJ. *Drugs in Pregnancy and Lactation.* 5th ed. Baltimore, MD: Williams & Wilkins; 1998:859-63.

103. Chen SS, Perucca E, Lee JN, et al. Serum protein binding and free concentrations of phenytoin and phenobarbitone in pregnancy. *Br J Clin Pharmacol.* 1982;13:547-52.

104. van der Klign E, Schobben F, Bree TB. Clinical pharmacokinetics of antiepileptic drugs. *Drug Intell Clin Pharm.* 1980;14:647-85.

105. Nau H, Kuhnz W, Egger HJ, et al. Anticonvulsants during pregnancy and lactation: transplacental, maternal and neonatal pharmacokinetics. *Clin Pharmacokinet.* 1982;7:508-43.

106. Horning MG, Stillwell WG, Nowling J, et al. Identification and quantification of drugs and drug metabolites in human breast milk using GC-MS-COM methods. *Mod Probl Pediatr.* 1975;15:73-9.

107. Committee on Drugs, American Academy of Pediatrics. The transfer of drugs and other chemicals into human milk. *Pediatrics.* 1994;93:137-50.

108. Bruno MK, Harden CL. Epilepsy in pregnant women. *Curr Treat Options Neurol.* 2002;4:31-40.

109. McAuley JW, Anderson GD. Treatment of epilepsy in women of reproductive age: pharmacokinetic considerations. *Clin Pharmacokinet.* 2002;41:559-79.

110. Kjær D, Horvath-Puhó E, Christensen J, et al. Use of phenytoin, phenobarbital, or diazepam during pregnancy and risk of congenital abnormalities: a case-time-control study. *Pharmacoepidemiology Drug Safety* [serial online]. 2006;16:181-8. Available from: Wiley InterScience, Hoboken, NJ. Accessed July 7, 2010.

111. Tomson T. Gender aspects of pharmacokinetics of new and old AEDs: pregnancy and breastfeeding. *Ther Drug Monit.* 2005;27:718-21.

112. Pennell PB. Antiepileptic drug pharmacokinetics during pregnancy and lactation. *Neurology.* 2003;61:S35-42.

113. Boucher BA, Rodman JH, Fabian TC, et al. Disposition of phenytoin in critically ill trauma patients. *Clin Pharm.* 1987;6:881-7.

114. Boucher BA, Rodman JH, Jaresko GS, et al. Phenytoin pharmacokinetics in critically ill trauma patients. *Clin Pharmacol Ther.* 1988;44:675-783.

115. McKindley DS, Boucher BA, Hess MM, et al. Effect of acute phase response on phenytoin metabolism in neurotrauma patients. *J Clin Pharmacol.* 1997;37:129-239.

Chapter 19

Robert L. Page II and John E. Murphy

Procainamide (AHFS 24:04)

Procainamide is a class IA antiarrhythmic agent initially approved in 1950 for the treatment of life-threatening ventricular arrhythmias and less severe but symptomatic ventricular arrhythmias in carefully selected patients. With the advent of newer antiarrhythmic agents, procainamide has fallen to second or even third line therapy.[1,2] However, it is used intravenously to acutely convert patients to normal sinus rhythm with atrial fibrillation and/or flutter; for termination of ventricular arrhythmias in pregnant women; and as provocative pharmacological challenge during electrophysiological risk assessment.[3-6] Based on its mechanism of action, procainamide decreases myocardial excitability, contractility, and conduction velocity.

Procainamide clearance is dependent on both hepatic metabolism (50%) and renal elimination of unchanged drug (40%–60%).[7,8] Hepatic metabolism is mainly via phase II acetylation by polymorphic N-acetyltransferase (NAT2) leading to the primary active metabolite, N-acetyl procainamide (NAPA). In the population, NAT2 exhibits a bimodal genetic polymorphism distribution in which patients may be considered either "slow acetylators" or "rapid acetylators."[7,8] Additionally, cytochrome P450 (CYP 450) 2D6 may also play a role in the formation of other metabolites. Due to the complexities of procainamide pharmacokinetics, the suggested dosages should be considered as initial guides. Doses should be individualized based on patient response and appropriate monitoring.[8]

In this chapter the following age groups will be used:

Neonates (<30 days)

Infants (30 days–<1 year)

Children (1–12 years)

Adolescents (13–18 years)

Adults (>18–75 years)

Older geriatrics (>75 years)

Usual Dosage Range in Absence of Clearance-Altering Factors

As of November 2007, all oral formations of procainamide, the immediate release capsules and extended release tablets, have been discontinued. Only the intravenous solution is available on the market.

Procainamide can be administered intramuscularly or intravenously in the acute setting. When procainamide is administered intravenously, it is common to administer a loading dose prior to a continuous intravenous infusion. Table 19-1 provides usual doses and intervals for procainamide therapy.

As seen in Table 19-2, only the intravenous solution is presently available.

General Pharmacokinetic Information

Absorption

Intravenous procainamide has a bioavailability of ~100% (F = 1.0) with peak concentrations observed within ~2 minutes (Table 19-3).[7]

Distribution[9-11]

Procainamide distributes extensively into lean body tissue and poorly into adipose tissue. In obese patients, the volume of distribution at steady state appears to correlate best with ideal body weight (IBW). The volume of distribution in medically treated heart failure patients and controls are similar. Volumes of distribution for

Table 19-1. Usual Dosage Range in the Absence of Clearance-Altering Factors[7,12,23,35]

Dosage Form	Dose[a]	Interval (hr)
Intramuscular		
Neonates and infants	Not available	
Children	20–30 mg/kg/day (ABW); not to exceed 4 g/day	4–6 hr
Adolescents	Not available	
Adults	50 mg/kg/day (ABW)	3–6 hr
Older geriatrics[b]	Not available	
Intravenous		
Neonates and infants	Not available	
Children	Load: 2–6 mg/kg (IBW); (max 100 mg) over 5 min; may repeat every 5–10 min to a total of 15 mg/kg or max dose of 500 mg over 30 min	
	Maintenance dose: 50–100 mg/kg/day (IBW); not to exceed 2 g/day	4 hr
	OR	
	Load: 10–15 mg/kg (IBW); over 30–60 min followed by continuous infusion	
	Continuous infusion: 0.20–0.12 mg/kg/min (ABW); not to exceed 2 g/day	
Adolescents	Not available	
Adults	Load: 12–17 mg/kg (IBW); or 100 mg every 5 min (until control of arrhythmia or toxicity) at maximum rate of 50 mg/min	
	Continuous infusion: 1–6 mg/min	
	Intermittent infusion: 50 mg/kg/day	3–6 hr
	(ABW); at maximum rate of 50 mg/min	
Older geriatrics[b]	Not available	

[a]Divide daily dose by number of doses to be given per day. When dose guidelines are not available for a specific group, the term *not available* is used. Clinicians may wish to use the nearest guidelines or be initially more conservative.
[b]Maintenance doses appear to be lower than adult doses; therefore, the dose should be based on clinical response and procainamide concentrations.
ABW = actual body weight; IBW = ideal body weight.

Table 19-2. Dosage Form Availability[7,12,23,35]

Dosage Form	Dosage Strengths	Products
Parenteral[a]	100 mg/ml, 500 mg/ml	Various manufacturers

[a]This product should be diluted with dextrose 5% or normal saline prior to intravenous administration to facilitate control of administration rate.

Table 19-3. Bioavailability (F) of Dosage Form[7,12,23,35]

Dosage Form	Bioavailability Comments
Intravenous	100% (F = 1) with peak concentrations achieved at end of intermittent infusion
Intramuscular	100% (F = 1) with peak concentrations achieved within 45–60 min; absorption rate half-life of 10–17 min

various age groups are listed in Table 19-4. The protein binding of procainamide is approximately 15%–20% and for NAPA is 10%.

Metabolism[10,12-14]

The percentage of procainamide metabolized by the liver in normal subjects is approximately 50%. The majority of procainamide's metabolism results from hepatic acetylation by polymorphic NAT2, leading to the formation of NAPA. CYP450 2D6 appears to play a significant role in the N-oxidation of procainamide as well as in the

N-deethylation of procainamide. Para-aminobenzoic acid (PABA) is an inactive metabolite of procainamide.

The following clearance values are guidelines in patients with normal renal function for age when suggested dosing strategies cannot be used (Table 19-5).

In patients with New York Heart Association Class II–III heart failure on digoxin, diuretics, and ACE inhibitors, CL_{total} appears to be similar to controls (0.61 L/hr/kg versus 0.53 L/hr/kg), although earlier studies suggested a 25%–50% decrease in the metabolic clearance of procainamide in non-optimally treated heart failure patients.[11] In obese patients, clearance appears to correlate best with actual body weight (ABW).[15,16] Preterm infants appear to have a lower mean clearance rate (0.31 ± 0.02 L/hr/kg) compared to those born at term (0.49 L/hr/kg + 0.02 L/hr/kg).[17]

Half-life and time to steady state

Table 19-6 lists the distribution and terminal elimination half-lives and the time to steady state in various populations.

Table 19-4. Volume of Distribution[7,10,12,41]

Age	Volume (Mean ± SD)
Neonates and infants	Data are lacking
All other age groups	2 ± 0.4 L/kg (IBW)

IBW = ideal body weight.

Table 19-5. Population Clearance Values[15,17,20]

Age	Total Clearance[a] (Mean + SD)
Neonates	Pharmacokinetic data are limited but available data suggest clearance is slightly lower than in children and adults. One retrospective study (n = 20) reported a clearance of 0.37 ± 0.20 L/hr/kg.
Infants	Data are lacking.
Children	1.16 ± 0.12 L/hr/kg[b]
	Pharmacokinetic data are limited, but available data suggest increased clearance in comparison to adults. One small study (n = 6) reported a clearance of 0.56 ± 0.12 L/ /kg/hr.[b]
Adolescents	Not available.
Adults	
Fast acetylators	0.56 L/hr/kg[b]
Slow acetylators	0.44 L/hr/kg[b]

[a]Values will be significantly lower in patients with renal dysfunction.
[b]Based on actual body weight (ABW).

Table 19-6. Mean Half-Life and Time to Steady State[7,12,13,16,23,41]

Age	Distribution Half-Life (min)	Terminal Half-Life (hr)	Time to Steady State (hr)
Neonates	Not available		
Children[a]	5	1.7	<12
Adolescents (13–<18 years)	Not available		
Adults[b]	5	3	12–24
Older geriatrics	>5	>3	>12–24

[a]The small amount of data available suggests that the procainamide half-life in children is significantly shorter than adult estimates.
[b]Average half-life in adults is 3 hr. Fast acetylators have a half-life near 2.5 hr while slow acetylators have a half-life of approximately 5 hr.

N-Acetylprocainamide (NAPA)[18-20]

The contribution of NAPA to the overall antiarrhythmic activity of procainamide is usually of limited clinical importance, although in some patients (e.g., those with renal impairment) it may be appropriate to monitor NAPA concentrations. Limited data exist on concentration-toxicity relationships for NAPA even though cardiac toxicity may result when NAPA concentrations exceed 30 mg/L. NAPA concentrations above 30 mg/L have also been reported to have little additional antiarrhythmic effect.

Both the procainamide concentration and acetylation clearance determine the NAPA production. The acetylation clearance of procainamide is based on the acetylation phenotype (see dosing strategies section). NAPA concentrations may accumulate dramatically in patients with poor renal function. NAPA clearance is 77%–87% renal and 13%–23% nonrenal. A 6-hr half-life for NAPA is about average in normal renal function. Patients with poor renal function may have a half-life of 30 hr or more. The NAPA volume of distribution (V) is ~1.5 L/kg.

Elimination[21,22]

The organic anion transport and organic cation transport (OCT) systems are two of the major families of renal drug transport systems in humans. Procainamide and NAPA are organic cations that are transported by OCT in the kidney. Specifically, procainamide is a substrate for human OCT1, OCT2, and OCT3 transporters. The percentage of procainamide excreted unchanged in patients with normal renal function ranges from 40% to 60%. As renal clearance is approximately three times creatinine clearance (CrCl), proximal tubular secretion appears to be involved in the renal elimination process in addition to glomerular filtration. Distal tubular reabsorption is clinically insignificant. However, as procainamide is a weak base, marked increases in urine pH can decrease renal elimination of procainamide.

Dosing strategies[7,10-12,16,23,24]

Procainamide therapy can be initiated using standard doses for the population with consideration of possible factors that might alter normal clearance (e.g., reduced renal function). It is also possible to estimate a dosage regimen based on predicted procainamide and NAPA clearance or to predict procainamide and NAPA concentrations that might result from a given dosage regimen using these predicted clearances.

Population-based predictors of procainamide clearance (CL)

Procainamide is cleared by renal and metabolic mechanisms as illustrated by the equation

$$CL_{total} = CL_{renal} + CL_{metabolism}$$

In adult patients with normal renal function, approximately half of the clearance is renal while half is due to nonrenal metabolism. A normal CL_{renal} can be assumed to be approximately 0.27 L/hr/kg or three times the CrCl. The $CL_{metabolism}$ value consists of both acetylation clearance ($CL_{acetylation}$) and a nonrenal, nonacetylated metabolic clearance. The $CL_{acetylation}$ value is based on the acetylation phenotype. For *fast acetylators*, $CL_{acetylation}$ is approximately 0.19 L/hr/kg. For *slow acetylators*, it is approximately 0.07 L/hr/kg. Therefore, an average $CL_{acetylation}$ can be assumed to be approximately 0.13 L/hr/kg. Approximately 50% of the African American and Caucasian populations in the United States are *fast acetylators*, while the other 50% are *slow acetylators*. Asian patients tend to be *fast acetylators* (80%–90%). The nonrenal, nonacetylated metabolic clearance appears to be 0.1 L/hr/kg. The average $CL_{metabolism}$ in fast and slow acetylators is, therefore, 0.29 L/hr/kg (0.19 + 0.1) and 0.17 L/hr/kg (0.07 + 0.1), respectively. An average $CL_{acetylation}$ would be 0.23 L/hr/kg (0.13 + 0.1). The total procainamide clearance (CL_{renal} + $CL_{metabolism}$) in normal renal function is then 0.56 L/hr/kg in fast acetylators and 0.44 L/hr/kg in slow acetylators.

The above information then can be translated as

$$CL_{total} = 3(CrCl) + [(CL_{acetylation} + 0.1\ L/hr/kg)(ABW)]$$

where CrCl is expressed in L/hr and $CL_{acetylation}$ in L/hr/kg.

The predicted clearance may be used to determine a dose to produce desired steady state procainamide concentrations using the following equation:

$$D = \frac{\tau \times CL_{procainaide} \times Css_{avDesired}}{S \times F}$$

The following predictions are useful for estimating NAPA production and NAPA concentrations based on the procainamide doses administered in an *adult* population. There is limited information on NAPA production in children.

NAPA production (the "dose" of NAPA)

Rate of conversion = $(Css_{av\ procainamide})(CL_{acetylation})$

where $CL_{acetylation}$ = 0.07 L/hr/kg (slow), 0.13 L/hr/kg (average), or 0.19 L/hr/kg (fast).

In Asian patients use fast acetylation value. In African American and Caucasian patients use average unless acetylator status is known.

NAPA clearance (CL) prediction

The clearance of NAPA is based primarily on renal function but also in part on nonrenal mechanisms. This can be represented by the equation:

$$CL_{total} = CL_{renal} + CL_{nonrenal}$$

Average renal and nonrenal clearance values in patients with normal renal function are:

$$CL_{total} = 0.17 \text{ L/h/kg (ABW)} + 0.033 \text{ L/h/kg (ABW)}$$

$$= 0.2 \text{ L/h/kg (ABW)}$$

For patients with reduced renal function, the following method may be used to predict NAPA clearance:

$$CL_{total} = 1.6(CrCl) + [(0.025 \text{ L/hr/kg})(ABW)]$$

where CrCl and CL_{total} are expressed in L/h.

To estimate the NAPA concentration, the following formula may be used:

$$Css_{NAPA} = \frac{\text{Rate of conversion}_{NAPA}}{CL_{total\ NAPA}}$$

Therapeutic Monitoring

Therapeutic range[25-27]

The therapeutic range for procainamide is 4–10 mg/L. In the reported studies, therapy was effective in 85% of cardiac patients with premature ventricular beats with concentrations of 4–8 mg/L. Ten percent of patients may receive added benefit with concentrations up to 12 mg/L but at the cost of possible serious toxicities. However, there have been reports of patients warranting concentrations between 15–20 mg/L without adverse effects. These higher concentrations may be needed in patients with sustained ventricular tachycardia. Concentrations of NAPA correlated with efficacy have been reported between 5–30 mg/L. Most laboratories will routinely measure both procainamide and NAPA concentrations from the same sample. Some laboratories may sum the two concentrations of procainamide and NAPA and compare this value to a therapeutic range (often reported a 10–30 mg/L). However, this particular practice should be discouraged, as the molar units of the two chemicals need to be used for this method to be valid. Furthermore, both procainamide and NAPA have completely different electrophysiological behaviors, thus it is counterintuitive to use the sum of both chemicals.

Suggested sampling times[22,25,27]

With continuous infusion, sampling at any time during the infusion is appropriate once steady state is achieved. Careful clinical monitoring for efficacy and toxicity is always required. Because NAPA competes with renal tubular secretion of procainamide and is pharmacologically active, both the parent drug and its metabolite should be monitored in cases of decreased kidney function. In addition, procainamide concentrations can provide useful information for dosage adjustments when needed, especially when obtained at steady state. Steady state concentrations for both procainamide and NAPA is not observed until at least 18 hr in patients with good renal function and as long as a week in renal impairment due to the long NAPA half-life. Procainamide concentrations probably should be obtained following changes in a patient's clinical status, changes in the dosage regimen, when significantly interacting drugs are added or deleted, or when signs of toxicity or inadequate response occur.

Assays[19,27-31]

Blood, anticoagulated with heparin, ethylenediaminetetraacetic acid (EDTA), or oxalate, may be used to recover NAPA and procainamide samples. Samples are considered stable for 24 hr at 2°C to 8°C and for 1–2 weeks at –20°C. Measurement of procainamide and NAPA concentrations from saliva has been proposed as an alternative to obtaining blood samples. However, the saliva to plasma concentration ratio shows considerable inter- and intra-individual variability, thus making this method of measurement of little clinical use.

Fluorescence polarization immunoassay (TDX®) and enzyme multiplied immunoassay technique (EMIT®) are the two most commonly used commercial, immunochemical, automated assays for measuring NAPA and procainamide concentrations. Both methods require separate determinations of procainamide and NAPA on the same serum or plasma sample. Elevations of hemoglobin, lipids, and bilirubin can interfere with the reading of immunoassay results. In cases where the sample may be hemolyzed, lipemic, and/or icteric, chromatographic methods (high performance liquid chromatography or gas liquid chromatography), which are not affected by these factors, can be employed to allow simultaneous measurement of procainamide and NAPA. Table 19-7 summarizes agents that may interfere with procainamide immunoassays.

Pharmacodynamic Monitoring

Concentration-related efficacy

The following are useful indicators of procainamide efficacy:

- Conversion of atrial arrhythmia to normal sinus rhythm.
- Heart rate normalization.
- Electrocardiograph (ECG) normalization.
- Suppression of sustained ventricular arrhythmias.

Concentration-related toxicity

Elevated concentrations of procainamide have been associated with toxicities. The exact relationship between NAPA concentrations and toxicity is not clearly established. Although some of the cardiac side effects of procainamide can be seen at concentrations considered to be in the therapeutic range, a variety of more serious and potentially lethal effects are more common at concentrations above 30 mg/L for procainamide plus NAPA. (See Table 19-8.)

In addition to concentration-related toxicities, procainamide has been associated with a serious, non concentration-related systemic lupus erythematosus (SLE)-like syndrome. Procainamide-induced SLE appears to occur during maintenance therapy, primarily in slow acetylators. About 60%–70% of patients on procainamide develop antinuclear antibody (ANA) titers after 1–12 months of therapy, and 15%–20% of these patients develop signs and symptoms of SLE.[32] As procainamide is only available intravenously and not orally, it is expected that the overall incidence of SLE associated with the drug will drop. Common symptoms include polyarthralgia, arthritis, and pleuritic pain. Fever, myalgia, skin lesions, and pericarditis as well as cardiac tamponade also occur. ANA titers should be monitored regularly in patients on long-term therapy or when lupus-like reactions occur. The clinical signs and symptoms of drug-induced SLE usually diminish several days to weeks after

Table 19-7. Potential Procainamide Assay Interactions[19,27-31]

Agent	Effect on Procainamide and/or NAPA Concentration(s)	Comment
Antibodies to E. coli beta-galactosidase	False elevation in procainamide concentrations	
Hyperbilirubinemia (>30 mg/dL)[a]	False elevation in procainamide concentrations	Chromatographic methods should be considered
HAMA	False elevation in procainamide concentrations	
Elevated hemoglobin (>1000 mg/dL)[a]	False decrease or increase in procainamide concentrations	Due to photometric interference; chromatographic methods should be considered
Intravenous lipid preparations (>5 g/L)[a]	False elevation in procainamide concentrations	Due to photometric interference; chromatographic methods should be considered
Lidocaine	False decrease in procainamide and NAPA concentrations	Occurs only with supra-therapeutic doses of lidocaine; inhibits fluorescence of procainamide and NAPA
Meprobamate	False decrease in procainamide and NAPA concentrations	Occurs only with supra-therapeutic doses of meprobamate; inhibits fluorescence of procainamide and NAPA
Metronidazole	False elevation in procainamide concentrations	Only documented with HPLC
Propranolol	False elevation in procainamide and NAPA concentrations	Enhances fluorescence of procainamide and NAPA
Hypertriglyceridemia (>2000 mg/dL)[a]	False elevation in procainamide concentrations	Due to photometric interference; chromatographic methods should be considered

HAMA = human anti-mouse antibodies; HPLC = high performance liquid chromatography; NAPA=N-acetylprocainamide.
[a]Specific value varies between various immunoassays

Table 19-8. Concentration-Related Toxicities[7,12,23,35]

Minor Toxicities (8–12 mg/L)	Major Toxicities (>12 mg/L)
GI disturbances	≥20% decrease in arterial pressure[a]
Malaise, weakness	>30% prolongation of PR, QRS, and QT intervals[b]
Dizziness, giddiness	Development of new arrhythmias
<20% decrease in arterial pressure[a]	Cardiac arrest
10%–30% prolongation of PR, QRS, and QT intervals[b]	

GI = gastrointestinal.
[a]Frequent blood pressure monitoring is needed when therapy is initiated; monitoring can be less frequent when maintenance therapy is established.
[b]Continuous ECG monitoring is needed with intravenous dosing and frequent monitoring is required during initiation of maintenance therapy; occasional monitoring is required during maintenance therapy.

procainamide therapy is discontinued.[33] One study suggested that the presence of antiguanosine antibodies may indicate patients at risk for developing procainamide-induced SLE.[34]

Toxicities related to the intravenous infusion rate of procainamide are hypotension and bradycardia. However, these toxicities generally can be avoided if procainamide is infused at a rate of 50 mg/min or less.[7,12,23,35]

Serious idiosyncratic reactions are rare but include:

- Angioneurotic edema
- Maculopapular rash

- Granulomatous hepatitis
- Agranulocytosis
- Leukopenia
- Thrombocytopenia

Patients should know the signs and symptoms of neutropenia, including sore throat, fever, malaise, and other symptoms of infection. Routine blood counts should be performed frequently during the first 3 months of therapy due to the increased incidence of neutropenia during this time. Periodic blood counts also should be performed throughout maintenance therapy. A drop in the neutrophil count to less than 2000 cells/mm^3 requires immediate attention.

Drug-Drug Interactions[7,12,23,35-40]

Significant drug-drug interactions and their mechanisms are listed in Table 19-9.

Table 19-9. Significant Pharmacokinetic and Pharmacodynamic Drug-Drug Interactions[7,12,23,35-40,42,43]

Drug	Effect	Mechanism
Amiodarone[a]	Increase in procainamide concentration by 40%–60%	Inhibition of both hepatic and renal clearance of procainamide
Belladonna	Increase in anticholinergic side effects (severe dry mouth, constipation, decreased urination, excessive sedation, blurred vision)	Additive anticholinergic effect
Cimetidine[b,c]	Increase in procainamide concentration and NAPA concentration by 20%–40% each	Reduced tubular secretion of procainamide and NAPA
Class IA, IC, III antiarrhythmics; antipsychotics; phenothiazines; macrolides; tricyclic antidepressants; other QT prolonging medications	QT prolongation, torsades de pointes, cardiac arrest	Additive cardiac effects
Dronedarone	Increased dronedarone concentrations leading to QT prolongation; increased procainamide concentrations	Decreased renal and hepatic clearance by procainamide; decreased renal and hepatic clearance by dronedarone
Ethanol	Increase in NAPA concentration and decrease in procainamide concentration (chronic use)	Enhanced acetylation of procainamide
Levofloxacin[c]	Increase in procainamide and NAPA concentrations	Decrease in procainamide and NAPA renal clearance by 21%–26%
Metformin	Increased metformin concentrations	Decreased renal clearance by procainamide
Neuromuscular blocking agents	Excessive, prolonged neuromuscular blockade	Decreased acetylcholine release by procainamide
Ofloxacin[a]	Increase in procainamide AUC and peak concentration by 20%–25%	Decreased renal clearance of procainamide
Para-aminobenzoic acid	Increase in NAPA concentration and $t_{1/2}$	Decreased NAPA renal clearance
Quinidine[b]	Increase procainamide concentrations	Reduced renal and metabolic clearance
Ranitidine[c]	Increase in procainamide and NAPA concentrations by 10%–20%	Decreased renal clearance
Trimethoprim[a]	Increase in procainamide concentration by 50%–60% and NAPA concentration by 50%	Interference with renal secretion of procainamide and NAPA; inhibition of metabolism of procainamide

[a]Procainamide concentrations should be monitored when this drug is added to therapy.
[b]The procainamide dose may need to be reduced if the response to procainamide and NAPA is enhanced.
[c]Procainamide and NAPA concentrations should be monitored when this drug is added to therapy.

Table 19-10. Disease State and Condition Interactions[7,9,10,12,23,24,35,41]

Disease State or Condition	Clearance	Volume of Distribution	Half-Life
Renal disease	Decreased[a]	Same	Increased[a]
Obesity[b]	Use ABW	Use IBW	Not available
Advanced age (>70 years)[c]	Decreased	Not available	Increased

[a]Magnitude depends on degree of renal dysfunction.
[b]Obese patients apparently have increased renal clearance of procainamide. Therefore, the patient's ABW should be used to predict clearance. The volume of distribution in obese patients appears to correlate best with IBW.
[c]Data suggest that renal clearance declines to a greater extent than expected based on the age-related decrease in glomerular filtration rate (refer to clearance section).

Drug–Disease State or Condition Interactions[7,9,10,12,23,24,35,41]

Several disease states can alter the pharmacokinetics and pharmacodynamics of procainamide and NAPA. These disease state interactions are listed in Table 19-10. Renal disease decreases procainamide clearance with no notable change in the volume of distribution; therefore, an increase in the procainamide half-life is expected. One study suggested a one-third dose reduction for patients with moderate cardiac or renal impairment.[4] An additional one third dose reduction is suggested for patients with severe renal impairment. Since 85% of NAPA's total body clearance is due to renal clearance, NAPA accumulates to a greater extent than procainamide in patients with renal failure.

References

1. Zipes DP, Camm AJ, Borggrefe M, et al. ACC/AHA/ESC 2006 guidelines for management of patients with ventricular arrhythmias and the prevention of sudden cardiac death: a report of the American College of Cardiology/American Heart Association Task Force and the European Society of Cardiology Committee for Practice Guidelines (Writing Committee to Develop Guidelines for Management of Patients With Ventricular Arrhythmias and the Prevention of Sudden Cardiac Death). *J Am Coll Cardiol.* 2006;48:e247-346.
2. Fuster V, Ryden LE, Cannom DS, et al. ACC/AHA/ESC 2006 guidelines for the management of patients with atrial fibrillation: full text: a report of the American College of Cardiology/American Heart Association Task Force on practice guidelines and the European Society of Cardiology Committee for Practice Guidelines (Writing Committee to Revise the 2001 guidelines for the management of patients with atrial fibrillation) developed in collaboration with the European Heart Rhythm Association and the Heart Rhythm Society. *Europace.* 2006;8:651-745.
3. Adamson DL, Nelson-Piercy C. Managing palpitations and arrhythmias during pregnancy. *Postgrad Med J.* 2008;84:66-72.
4. Stiell IG, Clement CM, Symington C, et al. Emergency department use of intravenous procainamide for patients with acute atrial fibrillation or flutter. *Acad Emerg Med.* 2007;14:1158-64.
5. Kanji S, Stewart R, Fergusson DA, et al. Treatment of new-onset atrial fibrillation in noncardiac intensive care unit patients: a systematic review of randomized controlled trials. *Crit Care Med.* 2008;36:1620-4.
6. Schreibman DS, McPherson CA, Rosenfeld LE, et al. Usefulness of procainamide challenge for electrophysiologic arrhythmia risk stratification. *Am J Cardiol.* 2004;94:1435-8.
7. Procainamide hydrochloride. In: G McEvoy, GK ed. *AHFS Drug Information 2010.* Bethesda, MD: American Society of Health-System Pharmacists. Available at: http://online.statref.com/Document/Document.aspx?docAddress=BGLdJDuBloslpHqk2ipmdQ%3d%3d&Scroll=96&Index=0&SessionId=13349C2NWROGNLWX.
8. Klotz U. Antiarrhythmics: elimination and dosage considerations in hepatic impairment. *Clin Pharmacokinet.* 2007;46:985-96.
9. Christoff PB, Conti DR, Naylor C, et al. Procainamide disposition in obesity. *Drug Intell Clin Pharm.* 1983;17:516-22.
10. Coyle JD, Lima JJ. Procainamide. In: Evans WE, Schentag JJ, Jusko WJ, eds. *Applied Pharmacokinetics: Principles of Therapeutic Drug Monitoring.* 3rd ed. Vancouver, WA: Applied Therapeutics; 1992:22.1-.33.
11. Tisdale JE, Rudis MI, Padhi ID, et al. Disposition of procainamide in patients with chronic congestive heart failure receiving medical therapy. *J Clin Pharmacol.* 1996;36:35-41.
12. Procainamide. In: Phelps SJ, Hak EB, Crill CM eds. *Pediatric Injectable Drugs.* 9th ed. Bethesda, MD: American Society of Health-System Pharmacists; 2010:374-5.
13. Giardina EG, Dreyfuss J, Bigger JT, Jr., et al. Metabolism of procainamide in normal and cardiac subjects. *Clin Pharmacol Ther.* 1976;19:339-51.

14. Lessard E, Hamelin BA, Labbe L, et al. Involvement of CYP2D6 activity in the N-oxidation of procainamide in man. *Pharmacogenetics.* 1999;9:683-96.
15. Bauer LA, Black D, Gensler A, et al. Influence of age, renal function and heart failure on procainamide clearance and n-acetylprocainamide serum concentrations. *Int J Clin Pharmacol Ther Toxicol.* 1989;27:213-6.
16. Grasela TH, Sheiner LB. Population pharmacokinetics of procainamide from routine clinical data. *Clin Pharmacokinet.* 1984;9:545-54.
17. Moffett BS, Cannon BC, Friedman RA, et al. Therapeutic levels of intravenous procainamide in neonates: a retrospective assessment. *Pharmacotherapy.* 2006;26:1687-93.
18. Dutcher JS, Strong JM, Lucas SV, et al. Procainamide and N-acetylprocainamide kinetics investigated simultaneously with stable isotope methodology. *Clin Pharmacol Ther.* 1977;22:447-57.
19. Sherwin JE. Procainamide & N-Acetylprocainamide. In: Pesce AJ, Kaplan LA, eds. *Methods in Clinical Chemistry.* St Louis, MO: CV Mosby Company; 1987:922-6.
20. Singh S, Gelband H, Mehta AV, et al. Procainamide elimination kinetics in pediatric patients. *Clin Pharmacol Ther.* 1982;32:607-11.
21. Hasannejad H, Takeda M, Narikawa S, et al. Human organic cation transporter 3 mediates the transport of antiarrhythmic drugs. *Eur J Pharmacol.* 2004;499:45-51.
22. Lee W, Kim RB. Transporters and renal drug elimination. *Annu Rev Pharmacol Toxicol.* 2004;44:137-66.
23. Procainamide HCL. In: Wickersham RM, Novak KK, eds. *Drug Facts and Comparisons.* St. Louis, MO: Wolters Kluwer Health; 2010. Available at: http://online.factsandcomparisons.com/Monodisp.aspx?monoid=fandc-hcp1757&book=DFC.
24. Tisdale JE, Rudis MI, Padhi ID, et al. Inhibition of N-acetylation of procainamide and renal clearance of N-acetylprocainamide by para-aminobenzoic acid in humans. *J Clin Pharmacol.* 1995;35:902-10.
25. Brown JE, Shand DG. Therapeutic drug monitoring of antiarrhythmic agents. *Clin Pharmacokinet.* 1982;7:125-48.
26. Campbell TJ, Williams KM. Therapeutic drug monitoring: antiarrhythmic drugs. *Br J Clin Pharmacol.* 2001;52 Suppl 1:21S-34S.
27. Valdes R, Jr., Jortani SA, Gheorghiade M. Standards of laboratory practice: cardiac drug monitoring. National Academy of Clinical Biochemistry. *Clin Chem.* 1998;44:1096-109.
28. Gannon RH, Phillips LR. Metronidazole interference with procainamide HPLC assay. *Am J Hosp Pharm.* 1982;39:1966-7.
29. Koike Y, Mineshita S, Uchiyama Y, et al. Monitoring of Procainamide and N-Acetylprocainamide Concentration in Saliva After Oral Administration of Procainamide. *Am J Ther.* 1996;3:708-14.
30. Young DS, ed. *Effects of Pre-analytical Variables on Clinical Laboratory Tests.* 2nd ed. Washington, DC: AACC Press; 1997:3,441-443,445.
31. Young DS, ed. *Effects of Drugs on Clinical Laboratory Tests.* 5th ed. Washington, D.C.: AACC Press; 2000:3,653-659,660.
32. Vedove CD, Del Giglio M, Schena D, et al. Drug-induced lupus erythematosus. *Arch Dermatol Res.* 2009;301:99-105.
33. Rubin RL. Drug-induced lupus. *Toxicology.* 2005;209:135-47.
34. Weisbart RH, Yee WS, Colburn KK, et al. Antiguanosine antibodies: a new marker for procainamide-induced systemic lupus erythematosus. *Ann Intern Med.* 1986;104:310-3.
35. Procainamide Hydrochloride. Package labeling. Hospira: Lake Forest, IL. 2004.
36. Bauer LA, Black DJ, Lill JS, et al. Levofloxacin and ciprofloxacin decrease procainamide and N-acetylprocainamide renal clearances. *Antimicrob Agents Chemother.* 2005;49:1649-51.
37. Kimura N, Masuda S, Tanihara Y, et al. Metformin is a superior substrate for renal organic cation transporter OCT2 rather than hepatic OCT1. *Drug Metab Pharmacokinet.* 2005;20:379-86.
38. Kimura N, Okuda M, Inui K. Metformin transport by renal basolateral organic cation transporter hOCT2. *Pharm Res.* 2005;22:255-9.
39. Martin DE, Shen J, Griener J, et al. Effects of ofloxacin on the pharmacokinetics and pharmacodynamics of procainamide. *J Clin Pharmacol.* 1996;36:85-91.
40. Trujillo TC, Nolan PE. Antiarrhythmic agents: drug interactions of clinical significance. *Drug Saf.* 2000;23:509-32.
41. Koch-Weser J, Klein SW. Procainamide dosage schedules, plasma concentrations, and clinical effects. *JAMA.* 1971;215:1454-60.
42. Feldman S, Karalliedde L. Drug interactions with neuromuscular blockers. *Drug Saf.* 1996;15:261-73.
43. Tschuppert Y, Buclin T, Rothuizen LE, et al. Effect of dronedarone on renal function in healthy subjects. *Br J Clin Pharmacol.* 2007;64:785-91.

Chapter 20

Paul E. Nolan, Jr., Toby C. Trujillo, and Christy M. Yeaman

Quinidine (AHFS 24:04.04)

Quinidine is a class IA antiarrhythmic agent with cardiac electrophysiologic actions similar to those of procainamide and disopyramide.[1,2] Historically quinidine has been used to prevent recurrences of a variety of symptomatic supraventricular and ventricular arrhythmias as well as to convert paroxysmal atrial fibrillation to normal sinus rhythm.[1,2] However, in addition to mortality concerns with quinidine use, the emergence of more effective and better tolerated antiarrhythmic agents as well as non-pharmacological therapies has resulted in a reduced role for quinidine as an antiarrhythmic drug.[2-5] Quinidine is considered as the drug of choice for the treatment of severe, life-threatening malaria due to P. falciparum, and is used in treating uncomplicated malaria due to this organism.[1] In addition, a combination product containing dextromethrophan hydrobromide, 20 mg, and low-dose quinidine sulfate, 10 mg (Nuedexta®), was recently approved by the FDA for the treatment of pseudobulbar affect (PBA), a condition manifested by involuntary, sudden and frequent episodes of crying or laughing, and which occurs secondarily in several unrelated chronic neurological disorders.[6] This chapter will focus on the pharmacokinetics and pharmacodynamics of quinidine as it relates to its antiarrhythmic uses.

Monotherapy with quinidine is no longer routinely recommended to prevent recurrences of paroxysmal or persistent atrial fibrillation following non-pharmacologic or pharmacologic conversion to normal sinus rhythm.[3] However, the combination of quinidine plus verapamil appears as effective or superior to sotalol in preventing recurrences of paroxysmal or persistent atrial fibrillation and may produce fewer occurrences of torsade de pointes ventricular tachycardia.[2,3] As compared to several other selected antiarrhythmics, quinidine is only cautiously recommended for converting paroxysmal atrial fibrillation to normal sinus rhythm.[3] However, a recent large, uncontrolled patient series showed it to be both highly efficacious and safe for converting paroxysmal atrial fibrillation to normal sinus rhythm in patients following cardiac surgery or percutaneous coronary intervention.[7] If used for this indication however, quinidine must be combined with an agent such as digoxin, a beta-adrenergic antagonist, or a non-dihydropyridine calcium channel blocker such as verapamil or diltiazem, to prevent possible acceleration of the ventricular response that could occur with quinidine monotherapy.[3,7] Quinidine appears to cause more frequent adverse effects than flecainide when used to prevent recurrences of atrial flutter.[4] It is rarely used as prophylaxis to prevent recurrences of atrioventricular nodal reciprocating tachycardia (AVNRT), the most common form of paroxysmal supraventricular tachycardia (PSVT).[4] Interestingly quinidine appears to have an emerging role in the management of ventricular arrhythmias occurring in patients diagnosed with genetically acquired "channelopathies" such as Short QT syndromes (SQTS), Brugada syndrome, or loss-of-function mutations in the cardiac calcium channel.[5,8-11] Until recently there were three known genetic variants of SQTS, one of which involves a mutation in the KCNH2 gene (i.e., SQT1), the gene that encodes for the rapidly repolarizing, outwardly rectifying potassium current, IKr.[5,8] This gain-of-function mutation results in a significant increase in this repolarizing potassium current, which produces shortened atrial and ventricular effective refractory periods as well as a shortened QTc interval.[8] In patients with a mutation in the KCNH2 gene, quinidine can suppress inducibility of ventricular tachycardia/fibrillation during programmed electrical stimulation (PES) as well as restore the inverse linear relationship between the QT-interval and heart rate.[5,8] Quinidine also appears highly efficacious in preventing recurrences of a recently identified form of primary, recurrent ventricular fibrillation associated with inferolateral early repolarization.[9] The Brugada syndrome is characterized by an abnormal ECG generally consisting of ST segment elevation in leads V1 through V3 accompanied in some patients with a QRS complex resembling a right bundle branch block pattern.[5] Brugada syndrome occurs secondary to a mutation in the cardiac sodium channel gene (SCN5A), and is associated with a high risk for sudden cardiac death.[5] Quindine may prevent induction of ventricular fibrillation as well as spontaneously occurring ventricular arrhythmias in high-risk patients with Brugada syndrome.[5,10] A loss-of-function mutation in the cardiac calcium channel results in a clinical entity in which patients have a combination of ST-segment elevation in leads V1 through V3, a shorter-than-normal QT interval, and a history of sudden cardiac death.[11] Quinidine can prevent both PES-induced ventricular tachycardia and normalize the QT interval in patients with this cardiac calicium channel mutation.[11]

Lastly, although quinidine has been used in the management of fetal supraventricular or ventricular tachyarrhythmias via administration of quinidine to the mother (i.e., maternal transplacental therapy), more recent recommendations have excluded quinidine as a drug for treating fetal tachyarrhythmias.[12]

Usual Dosage Range in the Absence of Clearance-Altering Factors

Table 20-1 provides the usual dosage ranges for quinidine in the absence of factors that are known to alter clearance.

Quinidine is commercially available in two salt forms with differing salt fractions (S): gluconate (S = 0.62) and sulfate (S = 0.83). Quinidine dosages are usually expressed in terms of the particular quinidine salt.[1] Approximately 200 mg of quinidine sulfate is equivalent to 267 mg of quinidine gluconate.[1] Extemporaneously prepared oral solutions of 10 mg/ml of quinidine sulfate are stable for up to 60 days when refrigerated (5°C) or stored at room temperature (25°C).[13] The available dosage forms are listed in Table 20-2.

Table 20-1. Usual Dosage Range in Absence of Clearance-Altering Factors[1]

Salt Form	Route	Indication	Load	Maintenance
Gluconate	IV	Conversion	800 mg diluted in 40 mL of dextrose – 5% water (50 mL total volume). To be infused at 0.25 mg/kg/min; generally a total dose of 5 mg/kg or less is used in converting atrial fibrillation/flutter to normal sinus rhythm; however, up to a maximum of 10 mg/kg may be required[a]	N/A
	IM		No longer recommended because of potential for erratic absorption	
	Oral tablets (extended release)	Maintenance of normal sinus rhythm		324–660 mg/8–12 hr[b]
Sulfate	Oral tablets (regular or extended release)	Conversion of AF or maintenance of normal sinus rhythm	Regular release (for conversion of atrial fibrillation): 200 mg every 2 or 3 hr for 5–8 doses; alternatively 300 to 400 mg every 6 hours	Regular release: 200–400 mg/6–8 hr Extended release: 600 mg/8–12 hr.[b] Maximum dose: 3–4 g/day

[a]Intravenous doses have not been systematically evaluated for treating life-threatening ventricular tachyarrhythmias, but regimens similar to those described above have been used.
[b]Larger doses or more frequent administration only after evaluation of patient with ECG monitoring and quinidine concentration monitoring.

Table 20-2. Available Dosage Forms[1]

Dosage Form	Route/Dose	Quinidine Base Equivalent, mg	Product
Quinidine gluconate	Intravenous: 80 mg/mL	50 mg/mL	Quinidine gluconate injection
	Oral tablet: 324 mg extended-release[a]	202	Quinidine gluconate extended-release tablets
Quinidine sulfate	Oral tablet: 200 and 300 mg	166 and 249	Quinidine sulfate tablets
	Oral tablet: 300 mg extended-release[a]	249	Quinidine sulfate extended-release

[a]If necessary, extended-release tablets of quinidine may be broken in half in order to titrate dosages.[1]

General Pharmacokinetic Information

Accurate estimation of the pharmacokinetic parameters of quinidine is dependent on the analytical methods used to quantify quinidine concentrations.[14] Some older studies relied on relatively non specific assays. Specific assays such as HPLC can separate and/or distinguish quinidine from dihydroquinidine (a pharmacologically active contaminant found in all quinidine preparations) and the various metabolites of quinidine.[14]

Controversy exists regarding whether the pharmacokinetics of quinidine are dose-dependent. In two of the three investigations reporting no change in mean pharmacokinetic characteristics following dosage increases, only single intravenous[15] or oral[16] doses were administered. However, two of the four subjects in a third study exhibited a greater than proportional increase in AUC and steady state quinidine concentrations relative to the increase in dose.[17] Two other studies demonstrated dose-dependent pharmacokinetics for quinidine and both administered quinidine to steady state.[18,19] Possible causes of the dose-dependent pharmacokinetics include saturable first-pass hepatic removal or saturable renal secretion.[18,19] Clinicians should consider that greater than proportional increases in quinidine concentrations may occur in some patients as quinidine doses are increased.

Absorption

Quinidine, a weak base, is principally absorbed in the small intestine.[20] Rate and extent of absorption varies among quinidine formulations and salt forms and among study populations.

The extent of absorption is equivalent between commercially available quinidine sulfate tablets and quinidine sulfate solution.[21]

In patients with arrhythmias, but without clinical evidence of heart failure, hepatic disease, or renal dysfunction, peak quinidine concentrations occur within 2 hr following administration of quinidine sulfate.[22] Increased bioavailability occurs in these patients and may result from previous disease-mediated reductions either in hepatic blood flow or in hepatic microsomal enzyme activity and a subsequent decrease in hepatic first-pass metabolism.

The extent of absorption of a extended-release formulation of quinidine sulfate has been shown to be equivalent to that of a conventional-release formulation.[23] Maximum quinidine concentrations occur at approximately 3 hr for the extended-release formulation as compared to about 1–2 hr for the conventional-release preparation.

As would be expected, quinidine gluconate extended-release tablets are more slowly absorbed than quinidine sulfate conventional-release tablets.[24] Comparisons between extended-release sulfate and gluconate products suggest that the sulfate product produces less peak-to-trough fluctuations on 12-hr dosage schedules.[25]

Co-ingestion of either conventional-release or extended-release oral quinidine products with food generally alters the absorptive characteristics of quinidine.[26,27] The extent of quinidine absorption from an extended-release quinidine gluconate tablet is significantly enhanced when coadministered with either a low-fat or high-fat meal compated to fasting.[27] The rate of quinidine absorption is significantly increased following a low-fat meal compared to fasting or after a high-fat meal.

Bioavailability (*F*) of Dosage Forms

Irrespective of formulation or salt form, the bioavailability of quinidine is less than 100% due to first-pass hepatic metabolism.[20] Based on studies using appropriate assays, it appears that the bioavailability ranges from 70% to almost 90%. Table 20-3 provides the bioavailability of various dosage forms.

Table 20-3. Bioavailability of Dosage Forms (*F*)

Dosage Form	Route	*F* Comment
Quinidine gluconate	Intramuscular	77% (0.77) in healthy volunteers[28]
(S = 0.62)	Oral (extended release)	71% (0.71) (range 54%–88%) in healthy volunteers
Quinidine sulfate	Oral (immediate release)	87% (0.87) in arrhythmia patients[22]; 70% (0.7) (range
(S = 0.83)		51%–106%) in healthy volunteers[29]
	Oral (extended release)	85% (0.85) in healthy volunteers[23,a]

[a]The less specific assay used in this study may explain the increased bioavailability of the sulfate preparation relative to previous studies in healthy humans.

Distribution

The distribution of quinidine within the body is predominantly extravascular and is most often described by an open two-compartment model.[30] However, its distribution may also may be described by a three-compartment model.[31]

Elimination

Renal excretion

Renal excretion of unchanged quinidine accounts for only 13%–18% of an administered dose.[20,22] The renal elimination of quinidine occurs via glomerular filtration and active renal tubular secretion and is positively correlated with creatinine clearance.[32,33] Renal excretion varies inversely with urine pH.[34] Neither hemodialysis[35] nor peritoneal dialysis[36] has a clinically significant impact on systemic removal, although hemodialysis may remove some of the polar metabolites.[22]

Metabolism

Quinidine is eliminated from the body principally by oxidative hepatic metabolism.[20] Both *in vitro*[37] and *in vivo*[38] studies show that CYP3A4 is the hepatic microsomal P450 isoenzyme essentially responsible for quinidine oxidation. Isolated tissue, animal, and clinical studies suggest that the metabolites of quinidine, in addition to the contaminant dihydroquinidine, produce electrophysiologic effects that generally appear qualitatively similar to, but quantitatively less than or equal to, quinidine.[39-43] Given their pharmacodynamic and pharmacokinetic properties, it is likely that the metabolites and dihydroquinidine contribute to both the therapeutic and adverse effects attributed to the parent drug (see Table 20-4).[39–48]

Protein binding

In general, quinidine is extensively but variably bound to plasma proteins.[49] Protein binding assessments are highly dependent on the experimental conditions including temperature,[50] the presence of heparin, and blood collection techniques.[51] The major binding plasma proteins for quinidine are albumin and alpha1-acid glycoprotein (AAG).[52] Quinidine does not appear to bind significantly to circulating lipoproteins, so variations in lipoprotein levels should not alter unbound quinidine concentrations.[52] Protein binding averages 87% in normal subjects and is concentration-independent over a range of total quinidine concentrations of 1–5 mg/L.[52]

The protein binding of quinidine increases in trauma patients, following acute myocardial infarction or cardiac surgery,[53] in pre-hospital cardiac arrest,[54] and in atrial fibrillation and flutter,[55] because these clinical conditions produce increases in AAG. The protein binding of quinidine is decreased in chronic liver disease

Table 20-4. Quinidine Metabolites

Metabolites/ Dihydroquinidine	Activity[a]	Ratio[b]	t½
3-Hydroxyquinidine	Yes[39,40,44]	[c]	12.4 hr[41,d] 16.3 hr[42,e]
2′-Oxoquinidinone	Yes[40,44]	[c]	—
Quinidine 10,11-dihydrodiol	?[f]	0.13[45]	2.0 hr[45]
Quinidine *N*-oxide	Yes[39,40]	[c]	2.5 hr[41]
O-Desmethylquinidine	Yes[40,44]	≤0.10[48]	—
Dihydroquinidine[g,h]	Yes[39,40,44]	≤0.25[48]	11–24 hr[46]

[a]Electrophysiologic activity described in an in vitro, animal, or human study.
[b]Ratio of total (bound plus unbound) metabolite concentration to total quinidine concentration.
[c]The total or unbound concentration of each of these three metabolites may approach or exceed that of quinidine.[48]
[d]Results from healthy human volunteers.
[e]Results from patients with ventricular arrhythmias.
[f]? = activity unknown.
[g]Dihydroquinidine is a contaminant found in all commercial quinidine preparations.[42]
[h]Competes with quinidine for binding sites on plasma proteins.[45]

and with the coadministration of heparin.[51,56,57] Renal impairment in patients not undergoing hemodialysis may lead to similar, decreased, or increased protein binding relative to normal subjects, whereas quinidine binding tends to be decreased in uremic patients undergoing hemodialysis.[57,58] The protein binding of quinidine significantly increases in the postprandial state.[26]

Clearance (CL)

In healthy volunteers, the mean total body clearance averages 0.29 L/hr/kg with a range of 0.14–0.43 L/hr/kg.[29] In patients with arrhythmias, but without cardiac, renal, or hepatic dysfunction, the mean total body clearance is the same (0.29 L/hr/kg) but the interindividual range may be slightly larger (0.10–0.50 L/hr/kg).[22] Several factors, including comorbid disease and concomitant drug therapy, can affect the elimination of quinidine. These are specifically addressed in subsequent sections.

Volume of Distribution (*V*)

Table 20-5 presents the values for the volume of distribution of the central compartment (Vc) and the apparent volume of distribution (V_β) that have been established for select patient populations.

Half-Life and Time to Steady State

In healthy volunteers, the mean elimination half-life of quinidine is 5.7 hr (range of 4.5–7.2 hr) and time to steady state 23–36 hr (based on five half-lives of the range).[29] In patients with arrhythmias, but without cardiac, renal, or hepatic dysfunction, the half-life averages 7.8 hr (range of 4.8–11.8 hr).[22] Several factors including disease states and concomitantly administered drugs can affect the half-life of quinidine (see Pharmacokinetic Drug-Drug Interactions).

Therapeutic Range

Early development of the therapeutic range for quinidine was hampered by use of nonspecific assays.[14,59,60] An investigation using a specific HPLC procedure in patients with either unifocal, multifocal, or paired ventricular premature beats (VPBs) or nonsustained ventricular tachycardia suggested a therapeutic range of 2–6 mg/L, though some patients responded at concentrations of less than 2 mg/L.[61] In the treatment of either supraventricular or ventricular tachycardia, some patients required concentrations as high as 8 or 9 mg/L, respectively.[62] Prevention of PES-induced ventricular arrhythmias in patients with either SQTS syndrome or Brugada syndrome has occurred at concentrations (mean ± SD) of 2.1 ± 0.2 mg/L and 2.7 ± 1.0 mg/L, respectively.[8,9] On the other hand patients with Brugada syndrome not responding to quinidine were noted to have quinidine concentrations ranging from 1.5 to 8.0 mg/L.[9]

As a general guideline, quinidine concentrations of 2–6 mg/L should be considered the therapeutic range.

Table 20-5. Central (V_C) and Apparent (V_β) Volume Distribution

Population	Central Volume (Vc)[a]	Apparent Volume (V_β)[a]
Healthy volunteers	0.40 ± 0.34 L/kg[29]	2.53 ± 0.72 L/kg[29]
Patients with arrhythmias (without congestive heart failure)	0.91 ± 0.35 L/kg[30]	3 ± 1.41 L/kg[22]
Patients with hepatic dysfunction	NR[b]	3.8 ± 1.13 L/kg[56,c]
Patients with CHF	0.44 ± 0.12 L/kg[114]	1.81 ± 0.49 L/kg[114]

[a]Volume results reported as mean ± SD (SD reported or calculated from original reference).
[b]NR = not reported.
[c]Quinidine administered orally in this study.

Dosing Strategies

When selecting quinidine for a patient with an arrhythmia, the clinician should be cognizant of the following:

1. The therapeutic goal. Depending on the arrhythmia and accompanying symptoms, the therapeutic goal may be conversion to normal sinus rhythm or prevention or reductions in recurrences of symptomatic paroxysmal or persistent atrial fibrillation[1–3,60]; reductions in baseline, symptomatic, non-sustained ventricular ectopy by some percentage (e.g., 63%–95% reduction in baseline arrhythmia frequency)[63]; prevention of PES-induction or reductions in recurrences of sustained ventricular tachycardia or fibrillation[5,8-10]; or abolishment of a fetal supraventricular tachycardia.[12]
2. Patients frequently have comorbidities or other conditions that serve as contraindications, warnings, or precautions to the use of quinidine.[64]
3. Quinidine may modify the pharmacokinetics and possibly pharmacodynamics of other drugs (e.g., digoxin and propafenone).
4. Baseline PR, QRS, and QT intervals.
5. The cardiovascular and non-cardiovascular adverse effects associated with quinidine therapy.

Quinidine therapy is generally initiated either with maintenance or loading doses to produce estimated total serum or plasma concentrations of 3–4 mg/L. Maintenance doses of quinidine are usually administered orally, though intravenous dosing is sometimes used.[65,66] The hypotension that can accompany intravenous administration of quinidine may be related to the rate at which the dose is administered or the underlying clinical condition of the patient.[65,66] If an intravenous loading or maintenance dose (i.e., total dose of 3 to 10 mg/kg) of quinidine base is administered at a rate not greater than 0.3 to 0.5 mg/kg/min over 15 to 45 minutes, hypotension is generally mild and asymptomatic.[65,66] Continuous infusions of quinidine at rates ranging from 0.005 to 0.01 mg/kg/minute can be used with a low incidence of quinidine-associated hypotension.[66] Oral loading doses of quinidine may consist of a single dose of 600–1000 mg of conventional-release quinidine sulfate or 200–400 mg every 2 hours for a total of five doses.[59,67]

Prior to initiating quinidine therapy for the management of atrial fibrillation or atrial flutter, it is critical to administer an agent such as digoxin, diltiazem, verapamil, or a beta-blocker to control ventricular rate response.[1–4]

An individualized pharmacokinetic approach could consist of:

- an initial estimation of the total daily dose of oral, conventional-release quinidine sulfate, sustained-release quinidine sulfate, or sustained-release quinidine gluconate (or intravenous quinidine gluconate) using population clearance and,
- division of this total daily dose into two to four equal doses depending on the formulation to be used and patient clinical characteristics.

Regardless of the approach used, it is advisable to begin quinidine in a hospitalized, monitored setting for 2–3 days.[68]

Suggested Sampling Times and Effect on Therapeutic Range

Monitoring quinidine concentrations may be indicated:

- to establish baseline dose-concentration relationships.
- during quantitative evaluation of a patient's arrhythmia with Holter monitoring or during programmed electrophysiologic studies (PES) so that steady state concentrations can be targeted to those at which the arrhythmia was rendered either suppressed or noninducible.
- during or following recurrence of the arrhythmia after initial successful suppression.
- in the presence of conditions (drugs or disease states) that alter quinidine pharmacokinetics.
- for suspected cardiac or systemic toxicity.
- for suspected patient noncompliance.
- following a change in dose or dosage forms.
- when a patient's response at usual doses is abnormal or difficult to evaluate.

Steady state is generally achieved within 2 days for most patients taking quinidine. Therefore, a trough sample following 48 hours of continuous therapy would be an appropriate time to evaluate steady state dose-concentration relationships.

Pharmacodynamic Monitoring—Concentration-Related Efficacy

Twelve of fourteen (86%) patients with ventricular arrhythmias (i.e., unifocal, multifocal, or paired VPBs or unsustained ventricular tachycardia) evaluated by Holter monitoring demonstrated a therapeutic response at steady state quinidine concentrations ranging from 0.7 to 5.9 mg/L, though all but three responders required concentrations greater than 2.0 mg/L.[61] Thirty-eight patients with supraventricular tachycardia and 43 patients with ventricular tachycardia were administered quinidine and evaluated by PES.[62] Twenty-five (66%) with supraventricular tachycardia responded to quinidine when the mean (and range) quinidine concentration was 2.9 mg/L (1.0–8.3 mg/L). Only 8 (19%) patients with ventricular tachycardia responded, and the mean (range) concentration for responders was 3.9 mg/L (2.0–9.1 mg/L). For both groups of responders the concentrations were not significantly different than those reported for the nonresponders. Quinidine prevented PES-reinduction of ventricular fibrillation in 22 of 25 patients with Brugada syndrome at concentrations ranging from 1.3 to 5.2 mg/L.[9] In the 3 nonresponders quinidine concentrations were 1.5, 3, and 8 mg/L. Thus, quinidine concentrations must be evaluated in conjunction with careful clinical evaluation of the patient's response.

Pharmacodynamic Monitoring—Concentration-Related Toxicity

Quinidine produces concentration-dependent changes on the ECG.[69] With increasing quinidine concentrations there are decreases in interventricular conduction and delays in ventricular repolarization as evidenced by widening of the QRS interval and an increase in the QT interval, respectively. However, lengthening of the QT interval generally occurs at usual therapeutic quinidine concentrations and not uncommonly at concentrations below the lower limit of the therapeutic range.[68-70] Increases in the QRS interval infrequently occur at the usual therapeutic quinidine concentrations.[68,69]

Excessive prolongation of the QT interval may predispose approximately 2 to 4% of patients to developing quinidine-induced torsade de pointes (i.e., quinidine syncope), a potentially life-threatening ventricular tachycardia.[68-71] In order to minimize the risk for quinidine-induced torsade de pointes, the QT interval should be measured both prior to and following initiation of quinidine therapy (see Table 20-6).[72-74]

Risk factors for quinidine-induced torsade de pointes should be recognized and corrected if possible.[71,73-78] These include hypokalemia, hypomagnesemia, sinus bradycardia (<50 beats/minute), female gender, and the coadministration of other drugs that prolong ventricular repolarization. See Table 20-7 for the risk factors associated with developing torsade de pointes when using quinidine.

Table 20-6. Guidelines for Monitoring QT-Interval in Patients Receiving Quindine[72-74]

QT interval measurements should be:
Made manually from a 12-lead ECG.
Measured from beginning of QRS complex to the end of the T wave, preferably using one of the limb leads that best shows the end of the T wave.
Performed before administration of quinidine. If the patient's QTc interval (i.e., rate-corrected QT interval) in the absence of an interventricular conduction defect at baseline is > 450 milliseconds (ms) in males; > 470 ms in females; or > 460 ms in children aged 1 to 15 years of either gender, than quinidine should be avoided unless the baseline QTc prolongation is reversible (e.g., secondary to hypokalemia).
Averaged over 3 to 5 beats if the patient is in sinus rhythm and over 10 beats if the patient is in atrial fibrillation. Alternatively for atrial fibrillation the QT interval can be calculated by taking the average of the QT intervals with the shortest and longest R-R intervals on a 12-lead ECG tracing.
Prominent U waves should be included in the meaurement of the QT interval if they are large enough to merge into the T wave.
While the patient is receiving quinidine, the QT interval should be measured at the time of the estimated peak serum quinidine concentration.
QT interval should be adjusted for heart rate (i.e., QTc interval). The most commonly used formula for correcting the QT interval is the formula of Bazett: $QTc = QT/\sqrt{RR}$

Table 20-7. Risk Factors for Developing Quinidine-Induced Torsade de Pointes[71,73-78]

Electrolyte abnormalities

a. Hypokalemia
b. Hypomagnesemia

Other coadministered drugs

a. Digitalis glycosides
b. QT-prolonging drugs
c. Diuretics (loop diuretics and thiazide-like diuretics can deplete potassium and magnesium)
d. Drugs affecting quinidine pharmacokinetics (see Table 20-8 for details)

Clinical conditions

a. Congestive heart failure
b. Bradycardia
c. Baseline QT prolongation
d. Congenital long QT syndrome
e. Female gender
f. Possibly Caucasian race
g. Conditions affecting quinidine pharmacokinetics (see Table 20-9 for details)
h. Rapid rate of intravenous infusion with quinidine

Recent conversion from atrial fibrillation with quinidine

No established clinical guidelines presently exist for modifying quinidine dosing based upon changes in the QTc interval post-dose. However, dosing guidelines have been established for the class III antiarrhythmic agent, dofetilide, and these may be applicable to use with quinidine.[79] Therefore, if the post-dose QTc interval increases to more than 15% over baseline or exceeds 500 msec in the absence of an interventricular conduction delay, or 550 msec in the presence of an interventricular conduction delay, then the dose of quinidine should be reduced, perhaps by as much as 50%. If following the downward dose adjustment there is post-dose QTc prolongation exceeding 500 msec in the absence of an interventricular conduction delay, or 550 msec in the presence of an interventricular conduction delay, then discontinuation of quinidine should be considered. The QTc interval should be measured at a time corresponding to the predicted peak quinidine concentration, which is quinidine product-specific.

Although episodes of torsade de pointes may occasionally occur after months of uneventful treatment (usually in association with hypokalemia), most episodes occur within the first few days of quinidine therapy so it is generally advisable that initiation of quinidine therapy should occur on an inpatient basis.[68,69]

Quinidine-induced gastrointestinal adverse effects include diarrhea, nausea, vomiting, indigestion, and anorexia.[69,80] These adverse effects are common, affecting up to 30% of patients, and may be severe enough to require discontinuation of therapy. These effects appear to be dose- or concentration-related, although a reduction in dose may not alleviate diarrhea.[69,80] Initiation of quinidine therapy without a loading dose and the use of sustained-release quinidine preparations may reduce the frequency of these adverse effects.[69] Alternatively the coadministration of aluminum-containing antacids may reduce the severity of gastrointestinal distress or the use of cholestyramine resin may alleviate quinidine-induced diarrhea, permitting continued use of the antiarrhythmic.[69,80]

Additional concentration- or dose-related effects of quinidine may involve central nervous system (CNS) toxicity and elevated concentrations are associated with the syndrome of cinchonism.[69] Symptoms of cinchonism include tinnitus, vertigo, blurred vision, headache, and other CNS effects.

Most of the other adverse effects of quinidine appear unrelated to quinidine concentrations.[69] These include hypersensitivity reactions such as hepatitis, fever, rash, thrombocytopenia, and systemic lupus erythematosus.

Pharmacokinetic Drug-Drug Interactions

Drug-drug interactions associated with the use of quinidine are shown in Tables 20-8 and 20-9. Pharmacokinetic drug-drug interactions affecting quinidine generally are the consequence of either induction or inhibition

Table 20-8. Drug Interactions Altering Quinidine Concentrations

Interacting Drug	Change in Quinidine Concentrations	Clinical Impact
Amiodarone[84,85]	↑	Increased concentrations may lead to cardiac dysrhythmia; decrease quinidine dose by 30%–50%
Cimetidine[86,87]	↑	Increases quinidine concentration by 50%; decrease dose of quinidine by 33%
Verapamil[88–91]	↑	Decreased hepatic clearance and increased half-life; increased risk for hypotension; decrease dose of quinidine by 20%–50%
Ketoconazole fluconazole, and itraconazole[92-94]	↑	1.5- to 5-fold increase in quinidine concentrations due to CYP3A4 inhibition and decreased renal tubular secretion; monitor concentrations and adjust dose accordingly
Grapefruit juice[94,95]	↑	Delayed absorption of quinidine and inhibition of metabolism of quinidine to 3-hydroxyquinidine; the effects are variable in each patient; grapefruit juice should be avoided
Hydantoin and barbiturate anticonvulsants[96]	↓	CYP3A4 induction; adjust dose of quinidine accordingly
Rifampin[97]	↓	CYP3A4 induction; the change in $t½$ is not predictive of the change in quinidine concentration; adjust dose of quinidine accordingly
Nifedipine[98,99]	↑, ↓, or NC	CYP3A4 enzyme induction, inhibition, or no effect
Macrolides[93,94]	↑	Presumed CYP3A4 inhibition; monitor QTc; if QTc interval prolongation occurs, discontinuation of the macrolide may be required
Magnesium antacids[100]	↑	Monitor concentration and signs of toxicity of quinidine; adjust dose as required

NC = no change.

Table 20-9. Drug Interactions Caused by Quinidine

Interacting Drug	Change in Drug Concentrations	Clinical Impact
Warfarin[93]	↑	Anticoagulation effect is increased and bleeding may occur; monitor PT/INR and adjust warfarin as needed
Neuromuscular blocking agents[101]	↑	Effects of neuromuscular blocker can be enhanced, lower doses of neuromuscular blockers may be required
Digoxin[85,91,102-104]	↑	Increased effects of digoxin and 2- to 3-fold increases in digoxin concentrations; decrease digoxin dose according to concentration; also digoxin-quinidine combination may increase risk for quinidine-induced proarrhythmic effects
Procainamide[105,106]	↑	Increased procainamide and N-acetylprocainamide (NAPA) concentrations with possible increased toxicity; monitor procainamide and NAPA concentrations and ECG
Propafenone[107]	↑	Concentration can be increased in CYP2D6 extensive metabolizers; monitor ECG
Beta blockers[93]	↑	In CYP2D6 extensive metabolizers possible increased negative chronotropic and hypotensive effects; monitor BP and ECG
Tricyclic antidepressants[93]	↑	In CYP2D6 extensive metabolizers possible increased risk for developing tricyclic antidepressant adverse effects
Codeine[108]	↑	In CYP2D6 extensive metabolizers, there is a decrease in the analgesic effects of codeine due to impaired conversion of codeine to morphine
Chlorpheniramine[109]	↑	In CYP2D6 extensive metabolizers there may be prolonged antihistaminergic effects
Dextromethorphan[110]	↑	In CYP2D6 extensive metabolizers there are significant increases in dextromethorphan C_{max} and AUC with concomitant use of low-dose quinidine

of CYP3A4, the isozyme principally responsible for the metabolism of quindine.[37,38] Conversely, the effects of quinidine on the pharmacokinetics of other drugs appear to be generally limited to those agents that are substrates for CYP2D6, especially in patients characterized as CYP2D6 extensive metabolizers.[81,82] In addition, quinidine may increase the absorption and decrease the clearance of drugs that are substrates for p-glycoprotein (e.g., digoxin), an ATP-dependent efflux pump.[83] Nonetheless, many pharmacokinetic drug-drug interactions that occur are not clinically significant in that dose reductions or increases are not required across the board because the extent of the interaction may differ from one patient to another. Dosing recommendations are provided in the table where available. Clinical judgment and drug concentration measurements should dictate changes in dose when interactions may cause clinically significant changes in concentrations for some patients.

Pharmacodynamic Interactions

As previously discussed, quinidine has been implicated in causing torsade de pointes ventricular tachycardia.[68-71,73-78] The likelihood of torsade de pointes occurring in a patient is likely enhanced if quinidine is concurrently taken with drugs that prolong the QT interval like procainamide, dofetilide, sotalol, amiodarone, haloperidol, thioridazine, erythromycin, and methadone.[71,73-75] Coadministration of digoxin and diuretics may also increase the risk of proarrhythmic effects. The list of QT-prolonging drugs is constantly evolving and a maintained, internet-based database of these agents (www.qtdrugs.org) is available.[74] Careful monitoring of a patient's complete drug regimen, clinical profile, laboratory values especially electrolytes, and ECG is critical to minimizing the risk for developing quinidine-induced torsade de pointes.

Disease state interactions

Aging and various disease states can impact the pharmacokinetics of quinidine compared to normal adults. These are described in Table 20-10.

Table 20-10. Drug–Disease State or Clinical Condition Interactions

Clinical Condition	Interaction with Quinidine
Elderly[32,111,112]	There is an inverse relationship between age and clearance. Elderly patients have a longer half-life (9.7 hr) and diminished total body and renal clearances (0.16 and 0.06 L/hr/kg, respectively). There may be an accumulation of the active metabolite, hydroxyquinidine. No changes in protein binding.
Pediatrics[113]	Clearance decreases with increasing age.
CHF[104,114–117]	Total body clearance (0.19 L/hr/kg), volume of central compartment (V_c: 0.44 L/kg), V_b (1.81 L/kg), rate of absorption, and renal CL are decreased. There is no change in half-life because volume and clearance are decreased by the same proportion. When the ejection fraction (EF) is less than 30%, the efficacy of quinidine is diminished (<30%), and the risk of proarrhythmia is increased.
Hepatic disease[56,57]	Increased half-life (9 hours) and volume (V_b: 3.8 L/kg), similar oral clearance (0.31 L/hr/kg) to healthy controls, but decreased formation of metabolites. Unbound concentrations tend to be higher (36%) due to decreased protein binding.
Renal disease[32,44,117,118]	Quinidine metabolites may accumulate and half-life increase (11.7 hr). Dosing intervals for quinidine may be increased to 12 hr for creatinine clearances < 50 mL/min.
Female sex[76,77]	Greater propensity for quinidine-induced QT-prolongation in females.
Caucasian race[78]	Greater propensity for quinidine-induced QT-prolongation in Caucasians as compared to Koreans.
Pregnancy[11,12,119]	Risk Category C_M. No known reports linking the use of quinidine with congenital defects. Quinidine has been used relatively safely in pregnancy to treat either fetal or maternal tachyarrhythmias. Crosses placenta and achieves fetal serum concentrations similar to maternal values. Protein binding may be altered in pregnant patients and monitoring of concentrations may be indicated. Considered compatible with breast feeding by The American Academy of Pediatrics.

References

1. Quinidine Gluconate, Quinidine Sulfate. McEvoy GK, ed. In: *AHFS Drug Information 2010*. Bethesda, MD: American Society of Health-System Pharmacists; 2010:1640-6.
2. Yang F, Hanon S, Lam P, et al. Quinidine revisited. *Am J Med*. 2009;122(4):317-21.
3. Fuster V, Rydén LE, Cannom DS, et al. ACC/AHA/ESC 2006 guidelines for the management of patients with atrial fibrillation: a report of the American College of Cardiology/American Heart Association Task Force on Practice Guidelines and the European Society of Cardiology Committee for Practice Guidelines (Writing Committee to Revise the 2001 Guidelines for the Management of Patients With Atrial Fibrillation). *J Am Coll Cardiol*. 2006;48(4):e149-e246.
4. Blomström-Lundqvist C, Scheinman MM, Aliot EM, et al. ACC/AHA/ESC guidelines for the management of patients with supraventricular arrhythmias: a report of the American College of Cardiology/American Heart Association Task Force on Practice Guidelines and the European Society of Cardiology Committee for Practice Guidelines (Writing Committee to Develop Guidelines for the Management of Patients with Supraventricular Arrhythmias). *J Am Coll Cardiol*. 2003;42(8):1493-531.
5. Zipes DP, Camm AJ, Borgrefe M, et al. ACC/AHA/ESC 2006 guidelines for management of patients with ventricular arrhythmias and the prevention of sudden cardiac death. *J Am Coll Cardiol*. 2006;48(5):e247-e346.
6. http://www.nuedexta.com/NUEDEXTA_Full_Prescribing_Information-1.pdf. Accessed January 10, 2011.
7. Schwaab B, Katalinic A, Böge UA, et al. Quinidine for pharmacological cardioversion of atrial fibrillaiton:a retrospective analysis in 501 consecutive patients. *Ann Noninvasive Electrocardiol*. 2009;14(2):128-36.
8. Wolpert C, Schimpf R, Giustetto C, et al. Further insights into the effect of quinidine in Short QT Syndrome caused by a mutation in HERG. *J Cardiovasc Electrophysiol*. 2005;16(1):54-8.
9. Haïssaguerre M, Sacher F, Nogami A, et al. Characteristics of recurrent ventricular fibrillation associated with inferolateral early repolarization. *J Am Coll Cardiol*. 2009;53(7):612-9.
10. Belhassen B, Glick A, Viskin S. Excellent long-term reproducibility of the electrophysiologic efficacy of quinidine in patient with idiopathic ventricular fibrillation and Brugada syndrome. *Pacing Clin Electrophysiol*. 2009;32(3):294-301.
11. Antzelevitch C, Pollevick GD, Cordeiro JM, et al. Loss-of-function mutations in the cardiac calcium channel underlie a new clinical entity characterized by ST-segment elevation, short QT intervals, and sudden cardiac death. *Circulation*. 2007;115(4):442-9.
12. Strasburger JF, Wakai RT. Fetal cardiac arrhythmia detection and *in utero* therapy. *Nat Rev Cardiol*. 2010;7(5):277-90.
13. Allen LV. Erickson MA. Stability of bethanechol choloride, pyrazinamide, quinidine sulfate, rifampin, and tetracycline hydrochloride in extemporaneously compounded oral liquids. *Am J Health-Syst Pharm*. 1998;55(17):1804-9.
14. Guentert TW, Upton RA, Holford NHG, et al. Divergence in pharmacokinetic parameters of quinidine obtained by specific and nonspecific assay methods. *J Pharmacokinet Biopharm*. 1979;7(3):303-11.
15. Fremstad D, Nilsen OG, Storstein L, et al. Pharmacokinetics of quinidine related to plasma protein binding in man. *Eur J Clin Pharmacol*. 1979;15(3):187-92.
16. Gey GO, Levy RH, Pettet G, et al. Quinidine plasma concentrations and exertional arrhythmia. *Am Heart J*. 1975;90(1):19-24.
17. Russo J Jr, Russo ME, Smith RA, et al. Assessment of quinidine gluconate for nonlinear kinetics following chronic dosing. *J Clin Pharmacol*. 1982;22(5-6):264-70.
18. Bolme P, Otto U. Dose-dependence of the pharmacokinetics of quinidine. *Eur J Clin Pharmacol*. 1977;12(1):73-6.
19. Wooding-Scott RA, Smalley J, Visco J, et al. The pharmacokinetics and pharmacodynamics of quinidine and 3-hydroxyquinidine. *Br J Clin Pharmacol*. 1988;26(4):415-21.
20. Ueda CT, Williamson BJ, Dzindzio BS. Absolute quinidine bioavailability. *Clin Pharmacol Ther*. 1976;20(3):260-5.
21. Guentert TW, Upton RA, Holford NHG, et al. Gastrointestinal absorption of quinidine from some solutions and commercial tablets. *J Pharmacokinet Biopharm*. 1980;8(3):243-55.
22. Conrad KA, Molk BL, Chidsey CA. Pharmacokinetic studies of quinidine in patients with arrhythmias. *Circulation*. 1977;55(1):1-7.
23. Gibson DL, Smith GH, Koup JR, et al. Relative bioavailability of a standard and a sustained-release quinidine tablet. *Clin Pharm*. 1982;1(4):366-8.
24. Greenblatt DJ, Pfeifer HJ, Ochs H, et al. Pharmacokinetics of quinidine in humans after intravenous, intramuscular and oral administration. *J Pharmacol Exp Ther*. 1977;202(2):365-78.
25. Wright GJ, Melikian AP, Pitts JE, et al. Comparative quinidine plasma profiles at steady state of two controlled-release products and quinidine sulfate in solution. *Biopharm Drug Dispos*. 1987;8(2):159-72.
26. Woo E, Greenblatt DJ. Effect of food on enteral absorption of quinidine. *Clin Pharmacol Ther*. 1980;27(2):188-93.

27. Martinez MN, Pelsor FR, Shah VP, et al. Effect of dietary fat content on the bioavailability of a sustained release quinidine gluconate tablet. *Biopharm Drug Dispos.* 1990;11(1):17-29.
28. Mason WD, Covinsky JO, Velentine JL, et al. Comparative plasma concentrations of quinidine following administration of one intramuscular and three oral formulations to 13 human subjects. *J Pharm Sci.* 1976;65(9):1325-9.
29. Guentert TW, Holford NHG, Coates PE, et al. Quinidine pharmacokinetics in man:choice of a disposition model and absolute bioavailability studies. *J Pharmacokinet Biopharm.* 1979;7(4):315-30.
30. Ueda CT, Hirschfeld DS, Scheinman MM, et al. Disposition kinetics of quinidine. *Clin Pharmacol Ther*. 1976;19(1):30-6.
31. Ochs HR, Greenblatt DJ, Woo E. Clinical pharmacokinetics of quinidine. *Clin Pharmacokinet.* 1980;5(2):150-68.
32. Ochs HR, Greenblatt DJ, Woo E, et al. Reduced quinidine clearance in elderly persons. *Am J Cardiol.* 1978;42(3):481-5.
33. Notterman DA, Drayer DE, Metakis L, et al. Stereoselective renal tubular secretion of quinidine and quinine. *Clin Pharmacol Ther.* 1986;40(5):511-7.
34. Gerhardt RE, Knouss RF, Thyrum PT, et al. Quinidine excretion in aciduria and alkaluria. *Ann Intern Med.* 1969;71(5):927-33.
35. Woie L, Oyri A. Quinidine intoxication treated with hemodialysis. *Acta Med Scand.* 1974;195(3):237-9.
36. Hall K, Meatherall B, Krahn J, et al. Clearance of quinidine during peritoneal dialysis. *Am Heart J.* 1982;104(3):646-7.
37. Guengerich FP, Muller-Enoch D, Blair IA. Oxidation of quinidine by human liver cytochrome P-450. *Mol Pharmacol.* 1986;30(3):287-95.
38. Damkier P, Brøsen K. Quinidine as a probe for CYP3A4 activity: intrasubject variablility and lack of correlation with probe-based assays for CYP1A2, CYP2C9, CYP2C19, and CYP2D6. *Clin Pharmacol Ther.* 2000;68(2):199-209.
39. Kavanagh KM, Wyse DG, Mitchell LB, et al. Contribution of quinidine metabolites to electrophysiologic responses in human subjects. *Clin Pharmacol Ther.* 1989;46(3):352-8.
40. Thompson KA, Blair IA, Woosley RL, et al. Comparative in vitro electrophysiology of quinidine, its major metabolites and dihydroquinidine. *J Pharmacol Exp Ther.* 1987;241(1):84-90.
41. Vozeh S, Uematsu T, Guentert TW, et al. Kinetics and electrocardiographic changes after oral 3-OH-quinidine in healthy subjects. *Clin Pharmacol Ther.* 1985;37(5):575-81.
42. Ackerman BH, Olsen KM, Kennedy EE, et al. Disposition of 3-hydroxyquinidine in patients receiving initial intravenous quinidine gluconate for electrophysiology testing of ventricular tachycardia. *DICP.* 1989;23(5):375-8.
43. Ha HR, Vozeh S, Uematsu T, et al. Kinetics and dynamics of quinidine-N-oxide in healthy subjects. *Clin Pharmacol Ther.* 1987;42(3):341-5.
44. Drayer DE, Lowenthal DT, Restivo KM, et al. Steady state serum levels of quinidine and active metabolites in cardiac patients with varying degrees of renal function. *Clin Pharmacol Ther.* 1978;24(1):31-9.
45. Rakhit A, Holford NHG, Guentert TW, et al. Pharmacokinetics of quinidine and three of its metabolites in man. *J Pharmacokinet Biopharm.* 1984;12(1):1-21.
46. Ackerman BH, Olsen KM, Pappas AA. Disposition of dihydroquinidine among patients receiving parenteral quinidine. *Pharmacother.* 1990;10(3):245 (abstr).
47. Ueda CT, Makoid MC. Quinidine and dihydroquinidine interactions in human plasma. *J Pharm Sci.* 1979;68(4):448-50.
48. Thompson KA, Murray JJ, Blair IA, et al. Plasma concentrations of quinidine, its major metabolites, and dihydroquinidine in patients with torsades de pointes. *Clin Pharmacol Ther.* 1988;43(6):636-42.
49. Kates RE. Therapeutic monitoring of antiarrhythmic drugs. *Ther Drug Monit.* 1980;2(2):119-26.
50. Verme CN, Ludden TM, Harris SC. Effect of temperature on in vitro measurement of quinidine free fraction. *Clin Pharm.* 1988;7(2):142-6.
51. Kessler KM, Leech RC, Spann JF. Blood collection techniques, heparin and quinidine protein binding. *Clin Pharmacol Ther.* 1979;25(2):204-10.
52. Edwards DJ, Axelson JE, Slaughter RL, et al. Factors affecting quinidine protein binding in humans. *J Pharm Sci.* 1984;73(9):1264-7.
53. Garfinkel D, Mamelok RD, Blaschke TF. Altered therapeutic range for quinidine after myocardial infarction and cardiac surgery. *Ann Intern Med.* 1987;107(1):48-50.
54. Kessler KM, Lisker B, Conde C, et al. Abnormal quinidine binding in survivors of prehospital cardiac arrest. *Am Heart J.* 1984;107(4):665-9.
55. McCollum PL, Crouch MA, Watson SE. Altered protein binding of quinidine in patients with atrial fibrillation and flutter. *Pharmacotherapy.* 1997;17(4):753-9.
56. Kessler KM, Humphries WC, Black M, et al. Quinidine pharmacokinetics in patients with cirrhosis or receiving propranolol. *Am Heart J.* 1978;96(5):627-35.

57. Perez-Mateo M, Erill S. Protein binding of salicylate and quinidine in plasma from patients with renal failure, chronic liver disease and chronic respiratory insufficiency. *Eur J Clin Pharmacol.* 1977;11(3):225-31.

58. Kessler KM, Perez GO. Decreased quinidine plasma protein binding during hemodialysis. *Clin Pharmacol Ther.* 1981;30(1):122-6.

59. Sokolow M, Ball RE. Factors influencing conversion of chronic atrial fibrillation with special reference to serum quinidine concentration. *Circulation.* 1956;14(4 Part 1):568-83.

60. Byrne-Quinn E, Wing AJ. Maintenance of sinus rhythm after DC reversion of atrial fibrillation. A double-blind controlled trial of long-acting quinidine bisulphate. *Br Heart J.* 1970;32(3):370-6.

61. Carliner NH, Fisher ML, Crouthamel WG, et al. Relation of ventricular premature beat suppression to serum quinidine concentration determined by a new and specific assay. *Am Heart J.* 1980;100(4):483-9.

62. Berry NS, Bauman JL, Gallastegui JL, et al. Analysis of antiarrhythmic drug concentrations determined during electrophysiologic drug testing in patients with inducible tachycardias. *Am J Cardiol.* 1988;61(11):922-4.

63. Crawford MH, Bernstein SJ, Deedwania PC, et al. ACC/AHA guidelines for ambulatory electrocardiography. A report of the American College of Cardiology/American Heart Association Task Force on Practice Guidelines (Committee to Revise the Guidelines for Ambulatory Electrocardiography). Developed in collaboration with the North American Society for Pacing and Electrophysiology. *J Am Coll Cardiol.* 1999;34(3):912-48.

64. Humphries KH, Kerr CR, Steinbuch M, et al. Limitations to antiarrhythmic drug use in patients with atrial fibrillation. *CMAJ.* 2004;171(7):741-5.

65. Woo E, Greenblatt DJ. A reevaluation of intravenous quinidine. *Am Heart J.* 1978;96(6):829-32.

66. Allen LaPointe NM, Li P. Continuous intravenous quinidine infusion for the treatment of atrial fibrillation or flutter: a case series. *Am Heart J.* 2000;139(1 Pt 1):114-21.

67. Gaughan CE, Lown B, Lanigan J. Acute oral testing for determining antiarrhythmic drug efficacy. *Am J Cardiol.* 1976;38(6):677-84.

68. Roden DM, Woosley RL, Primm RK. Incidence and clinical features of the quinidine-associated long QT syndrome: implications for patient care. *Am Heart J.* 1986;111(6):1088-93.

69. Kim SY, Benowitz NL. Poisoning due to class IA antiarrhythmic drugs. Quinidine, procainamide and disopyramide. *Drug Safety.* 1990;5(6):393-420.

70. Roden DM, Thompson KA, Hoffman BF, et al. Clinical features and basic mechanisms of quinidine-induced arrhythmias. *J Am Coll Cardiol.* 1986;8(1 Suppl A): 73A-78A.

71. Gowda RM, Khan IA, Wilbur SL, et al. Torsade de pointes: the clinical considerations. *Int J Cardiol.* 2004;96(1):1-6.

72. Goldenberg I, Moss AJ, Zareba W. QT interval: how to measure and what is "normal." *J Cardiovasc Electrophysiol.* 2006;17(3):333-6.

73. Al-Khatib SM, Allen LaPointe NM, Kramer JM, et al. What clinicians should know about the QT interval. *JAMA.* 2003;289(16):2120-7. [Erratum, *JAMA.* 2003;290(10):1318.]

74. Gupta A, Lawrence AT, Krishmn K, et al. Current concepts in the mechanisms and management of drug-induced QT prolongation and torsade de pointes. *Am Heart J.* 2007;153(6):891-9.

75. Roden DM. Drug-induced prolongation of the QT interval. *N Eng J Med.* 2004;350(10):1013-22.

76. Benton RE, Sale M, Flockhart DA, et al. Greater quinidine-induced QTc prolongation in women. *Clin Pharmacol Ther.* 2000;67(4):413-8.

77. El-Eraky H, Thomas SHL. Effects of sex on the pharmacokinetic and pharmacodynamic properties of quinidine. *Br J Clin Pharmacol.* 2003;56(2):198-204.

78. Shin JG, Kang WK, Shon JH, et al. Possible interethnic differences in quinidine-induced QT prolongation between healthy Caucasian and Korean subjects. *Br J Clin Pharmacol.* 2006;63(2):206-15.

79. Dofetilide. McEvoy GK, ed. In: *AHFS Drug Information 2010.* Bethesda, MD: American Society of Health-System Pharmacists, Inc.; 2010:1685-7.

80. RuDusky BM. Cholestyramine therapy for quinidine-induced diarrhea. Case reports. *Angiology.* 1997;48(2):173-6.

81. Broly F, Libersa C, Lhermitte M, et al. Effect of quinidine on the dextromethorphan O-demethylase activity of microsomal fractions from human liver. *Br J Clin Pharmacol.* 1989;28(1):29-35.

82. Gibbs JP, Hyland R, Youdim K. Minimizing polymorphic metabolism in drug discovery: evaluation of the utility of in vitro methods for predicting pharmacokinetic consequences associated with CYP2D6 metabolism. *Drug Metab Dispos.* 2006;34(9):1516-22.

83. Fromm MF, Kim RB, Stein CM, et al. Inhibition of p-glycoprotein-mediated drug transport:a unifying mechanism to explain the interaction between digoxin and quinidine. *Circulation.* 1999;99(4):552-7.

84. Saal AK, Werner JA, Greene HL, et al. Effect of amiodarone on serum quinidine and procainamide levels. *Am J Cardiol.* 1984;53(9):1264-7.

85. Frietag D, Bebee R, Sunderland B. Digoxin-quinidine and digoxin-amiodarone interactions: frequency of occurrence and monitoring in Australian repatriation hospitals. *J Clin Pharm Ther.* 1995;20(3):179-83.

86. Hardy BG, Schentag JJ. Lack of effect of cimetidine on the metabolism of quinidine: effect on renal clearance. *Int J Clin Pharmacol Ther Toxicol.* 1988;26(8):388-91.

87. Hardy BG, Zador IT, Golden L, et al. Effect of cimetidine on the pharmacokinetics and pharmacodynamics of quinidine. *Am J Cardiol.* 1983;52(1):172-5.

88. Edwards DJ, Lavoie R, Beckman H, et al. The effects of coadministration of verapamil on the pharmacokinetics and metabolism of quinidine. *Clin Pharmacol Ther.* 1987;41(1):68-73.

89. Maisel AS, Motulsky HJ, Insel PA. Hypotension after quinidine plus verapamil. Possible additive competition at alpha-adrenergic receptors. *N Eng J Med.* 1985;312(3):1167-70.

90. Shibata K, Hirasawa A, Foglar R, et al. Effects of quinidine and verapamil on human cardiovascular alpha receptors. *Circulation.* 1998;97(13):1227-30.

91. Bauer LA, Horn JR, Pettit H. Mixed effect modeling for detection and evaluation of drug interactions: digoxin-quinidine and digoxin-verapamil combinations. *Ther Drug Monit.* 1996:18(1):46-52.

92. McNulty RM, Lazor JA, Sketch M. Transient increase in plasma quinidine concentrations during ketoconazole-quinidine therapy. *Clin Pharm.* 1989;8(3):222-5.

93. Michelats EL. Update: clinically significant cytochrome p-450 drug interactions. *Pharmacotherapy.* 1998;18(1):84-112.

94. Damkier P, Hansen LL, Brøsen K. Effect of diclofenac, disulfiram, itraconazole, grapefruit juice and erythromycin on the pharmacokinetics of quinidine. *Br J Clin Pharmacol.* 1999;48(6):829-38.

95. Min DI, Ku YM, Geraets DR. Effect of grapefruit juice on the pharmacokinetics of quinidine in healthy volunteers. *J Clin Pharmacol.* 1996;36(5):469-76.

96. Data JL, Wilkinson GR, Nies AS. Interaction of quinidine with anticonvulsant drugs. *N Eng J Med.* 1976;294(13):699-702.

97. Twum-Barima Y, Carruthers SG. Quinidine-rifampin interaction. *N Eng J Med.* 1981;304(24):1466-9.

98. Farringer JA, Green JA, O'Rourke RA, et al. Nifedipine-induced alterations in serum quinidine concentrations. *Am Heart J.* 1984;108(6):1570-2.

99. Munger MA, Jarvis RC, Nair R, et al. Elucidation of the nifedipine-quinidine interaction. *Clin Pharmacol Ther.* 1989;45(4):411-6.

100. Zinn MB. Quinidine intoxication from alkali ingestion. *Tex Med.* 1970;66(12):64-6.

101. Feldman S, Karalliedde L. Drug interactions with neuromuscular blockers. *Drug Safety.* 1996;15(4):261-73.

102. Rodin SM, Johnson BJ. Pharmacokinetic interactions with digoxin. *Clin Pharmacokinet.* 1988;15(4):227-44.

103. Hager WD, Fenster P, Mayersohn M, et al. Digoxin-quinidine interaction. Pharmacokinetic evaluation. *N Eng J Med.* 1979;300(22):1238-41.

104. Minardo JD, Heger JJ, Miles WM, et al. Clinical characteristics of patients with ventricular fibrillation during antiarrhythmic drug therapy. *N Eng J Med.* 1988;319(5):257-62.

105. Kim SG, Seiden SW, Matos JA, et al. Combination of procainamide and quinidine for better tolerance and additive effects for ventricular arrhythmias. *Am J Cardiol.* 1985;56(1):84-8.

106. Hughes B, Dyer JE, Schwartz AB. Increased procainamide plasma concentrations caused by quinidine: a new drug interaction. *Am Heart J.* 1987;114(4 Pt 1):908-9.

107. Funck-Brentano C, Kroemer HK, Pavlou H, et al. Genetically-determined interaction between propafenone and low dose quinidine: role of active metabolites in modulating net drug effect. *Br J Clin Pharmacol.* 1989;27(4):435-44.

108. Wilder-Smith CH, Hufschmid E, Thormann W. The visceral and somatic antinociceptive effects of dihydrocodeine and its metabolite, dihydromorphine. A cross-over study with extensive and quinidine-induced poor metabolizers. *Br J Clin Pharmacol.* 1998;45(6):575-81.

109. Yasuda SU, Zannikos P, Young AE, et al. The roles of CYP2D6 and stereoselectivity in the clinical pharmacokinetics of chlorpheniramine. *Br J Clin Pharmacol.* 2002;53(5):519-25.

110. Pope LE, Khalil MH, Berg JE, et al. Pharmacokinetics of dextromethorphan after single or multiple dosing in combination with quinidine in extensive and poor metabolizers. *J Clin Pharmacol.* 2004;44(10):1132-42.

111. Drayer DE, Hughes M, Lorenzo B, et al. Prevalence of high (3S)-3-hydroxyquinidine/quinidine ratios in serum, and clearance of quinidine in cardiac patients with age. *Clin Pharmacol Ther.* 1980;27(1):72-5.

112. Ackerman BH, Olsen KM. Accumulation of 3-hydroxyquinidine following chronic quinidine therapy. *DICP.* 1991;25(7-8):867-9.

113. Szefler SJ, Pieroni DR, Gingell RL, et al. Rapid elimination of quinidine in pediatric patients. *Pediatrics.* 1982;70(3):370-5.

114. Ueda CT, Dzindzio BS. Quinidine kinetics in congestive heart failure. *Clin Pharmacol Ther.* 1978;23(2):158-64.

115. Ueda CT, Dzindzio BS. Bioavailability of quinidine in congestive heart failure. *Br J Clin Pharmacol.* 1981;11(6):571-7.

116. Meissner MD, Kay HR, Horowitz LN, et al. Relation of acute antiarrhythmic drug efficacy to left ventricular function in coronary artery disease. *Am J Cardiol.* 1988;61(13):1050-5.

117. Kessler KM, Lowenthal DT, Warner H, et al. Quinidine elimination in patients with congestive heart failure or poor renal function. *N Eng J Med.* 1974;290(13):706-9.

118. Fattinger K, Vozeh S, Ha HR, et al. Population pharmacokinetics of quinidine. *Br J Clin Pharmacol.* 1991;31(3):279-86.

119. Briggs GG, Freeman RK, Yaffe SJ. Quinidine. In: *Drugs in Pregnancy and Lactation: A Reference Guide to Fetal and Neonatal Risk.* 8th ed. Philadelphia, PA: Lippincott Williams & Wilkins, a Wolters Kluwer business; 2008:1582-5.

Chapter 21

*John E. Murphy and Hanna Phan**

Theophylline (AHFS 86:16)

Introduction

Theophylline is a bronchial smooth muscle relaxant used in the treatment of asthma and other respiratory diseases. As methylxanthines, it and caffeine are also used to treat apnea, bradycardia, and weaning from the ventilator in neonates.[1] The use of theophylline has decreased considerably over the past 25 years due to the development and use of more effective treatments, particularly for asthma, though it still continues to have a role.[2] A series of reviews by the Cochrane Collaborative established that theophylline is an effective preventive treatment for childhood asthma, though less effective and with a higher side-effect profile than inhaled steroids and/or long-acting beta-2 agonists[3,4]; that it should not be used in the treatment of exacerbations of chronic obstructive pulmonary disease (COPD)[5]; that it does improve lung function and levels of oxygen and carbon dioxide in the blood of patients with COPD, who prefer it over placebo despite side effects;[6] that it is better than mask positive pressure for preterm infants with apnea[7]; that it is useful in extubating small preterm infants (<1000 g) in their first week of life[8]; and, though it has similar effects to caffeine for treating apnea in preterm infants, it has a narrower therapeutic range and shorter half-life and is thus potentially less useful once caffeine can be administered.[9] Although some evidence demonstrates its use in prevention of childhood asthma from the Cochrane Collaborative, theophylline is not a preferred treatment for asthma for all ages.[3,10] In fact, sustained-release theophylline (immediate release is not recommended) is considered a non-preferred alternative adjunctive maintenance treatment for asthma in older children (>5 years) and adults according to the National Asthma Education and Prevention Program.[3,10,11]

Usual Dosage Range in Absence of Clearance-Altering Factors[12]

The following dose recommendations are suggested to achieve theophylline concentrations of 5–10 mg/L in the neonate and approximately 10 mg/L in all other patient populations. Dosage adjustment should be based on an assessment of serum concentration and clinical status of the patient. For example, a concentration of 10 mg/L may be considered within normal limits; however, if a patient remains symptomatic, dosage increases may still be necessary to reach concentrations up to 15 mg/L for effect. Also, noteworthy is that additional care is advised in individualizing dosing for neonates due to greater potential for toxicity. Caution is required when dosing patients who are unhealthy, who smoke, or who are on other medications known to alter theophylline clearance (see drug-drug interactions and drug–disease state or condition interactions sections).

Loading dose[10-12]

The suggested loading dose of theophylline for patients without a history of theophylline use is 5 mg/kg (~6 mg/kg of aminophylline). If the patient has been receiving theophylline, it is advisable to first measure a concentration and then base the loading dose on the difference needed to achieve a desired concentration change. Generally, an increase of approximately 1 mg/L in concentration will occur with every 0.5 mg/kg of theophylline in a loading dose, based on ideal body weight. This generalization is based on a volume of distribution of 0.5 L/kg; however, note that volume of distribution varies based on age. Only rapid release products should be used for oral loading doses and IV doses are generally given over 20–30 minutes. The National Asthma Education and Prevention Program stated that in the emergency department "theophylline/aminophylline is not recommended because it appears to provide no additional benefit to optimal inhaled beta2-agonist therapy and may increase adverse effects."[11] Thus, at least for the emergency treatment of asthma, loading doses would not be warranted.

*Prior contributions to this chapter made by Edress H. Darsey are acknowledged and greatly appreciated.

Maintenance dose[12-14]

All doses in Table 21-1 are expressed in terms of anhydrous theophylline and should be converted to the proper dosage if aminophylline or another salt form is administered. The doses suggested represent the recommended starting and usual maximum dose. Further dosing should be individualized based on the patient's therapeutic response and measured steady state theophylline concentration. A patient's theophylline clearance can be calculated from a properly measured concentration and dosing history and a patient-specific dose can then be determined based on the actual clearance.

Dosage Form Availability[12,17]

Theophylline products are available in different salt forms and different delivery forms (IV, oral liquids including syrups and elixirs, regular release tablets and capsules, suppositories, and extended- and sustained-release tablets and capsules). When converting from one product to another, both bioavailability of the dosage form and theophylline salt equivalence must be considered (Table 21-2).

General Pharmacokinetic Information

Absorption

The bioavailability of theophylline depends on its formulation and route of administration.[12,17-19] With few exceptions, the bioavailability for most theophylline products is quite good (90%–100%). The absorption of theophylline can be delayed by intake of food; however, the extent of absorption is unchanged.[12] When a patient is changed from intravenous to oral therapy, the maintenance infusion should be stopped and oral

Table 21-1. Theophylline Maintenance Doses[a,b,c]

Age	IV Maintenance Dose Continuous Infusion (mg/kg/hr)	Oral/IV Starting and Usual Maximum Maintenance Dose
Neonates (PNA ≤24 days)	N/A[d]	1 mg/kg every 12 hr
Neonates (PNA >24–<28 days)	N/A[d]	1.5 mg/kg every 12 hr
Infants (4–52 weeks)		Total daily dose (mg) = [(0.2 × age in weeks) +5] × (weight in kg)
		PNA up to 26 weeks: administer total daily dose divided every 8 hr[e]
		PNA >26 weeks: administer total daily dose divided every 6 hr[e]
1–9 years	0.8–1 mg/kg/hr	Start with 10 mg/kg/day up to 16 mg/kg/day[f]
10–12 years	0.7 mg/kg/hr	Start with 10 mg/kg/day up to 16 mg/kg/day[f]
13–16 years	0.6 mg/kg/hr	Start with 10 mg/kg/day up to 16 mg/kg/day[f]
Adults	0.4 mg/kg/hr	10 mg/kg/day (usual maximum 800 mg/day)[f]
Young adult smokers[g]	0.7 mg/kg/hr	16 mg/kg/day[f]
Older patients and patients with cor pulmonale, congestive heart failure, or liver failure	0.2–0.3 mg/kg/hr	Start with 6 mg/kg/day (do not exceed 400 mg/day)[f]

[a]Use ideal body weight for obese patients.
[b]One study suggests that the maintenance doses required to achieve therapeutic concentrations in patients with asthma decreased over approximately 15 years, possibly due to the reduction in passive smoke inhalation by patients, a factor shown to increase clearance.[15,16] This might suggest more conservative dosing for the future.
[c]Adapted from reference 12.
[d]Not applicable; not usually dosed this way.
[e]Dosing interval refers to use of fast release oral product.
[f]Dosing interval in children and healthy adults can be divided and given every 8–12 hr with use of slow-release products.
[g]Cigarettes or marijuana.
PNA = postnatal age.

therapy should be begun immediately.[19] Table 21-3 provides the bioavailability percent, fraction of dose that is theophylline, and comments for various products.

Distribution

Theophylline is not distributed into fatty tissue; therefore, for obese patients, ideal body weight (IBW) should be used in the calculation of doses. Table 21-4 provides the population volumes of distribution for various age groups. Theophylline has been reported to distribute in the saliva with preliminary reports of saliva theophylline monitoring as part of treatment of apnea of prematurity.[20]

Protein binding

Theophylline is approximately 40% bound to plasma proteins in adults and 36% bound in neonates.[11,12] Due to the low percentage of theophylline bound to plasma proteins, changes in protein binding do not significantly affect theophylline clearance or volume of distribution.

Table 21-2. Theophylline Salt Equivalence (S)[a]

Drug	Anhydrous Theophylline Content (Mean ± SD)	S
Aminophylline anhydrous	85.7 ± 1.7	0.86
Aminophylline hydrous	78.9 ± 1.6	0.79
Theophylline monohydrate	90.7 ± 1.1	0.91

[a]Adapted from reference 12.
S = 1 for anhydrous theophylline.

Table 21-3. Bioavailability (F) of Dosage Forms[a]

Dosage Form	Bioavailability Comments
Intravenous aminophylline and theophylline	100% ($F = 1$)
Oral liquids	100% ($F = 1$)
Oral tablets and capsules (immediate release)	100% ($F = 1$); rate of absorption may be slowed when ingested with food or antacids
Oral tablets and capsules (enteric coated)	Incomplete and unpredictable, with no clinical indication for use
Oral tablets and capsules (extended release)	90%–100% ($F = 0.9$–1) with extent and rate of absorption dependent on particular products
Suppositories (cocoa butter)	Slow and erratic
Suppositories (PEG)	90%–100% ($F = 0.9$–1)
Rectal solution	90%–100% ($F = 0.9$–1)

[a]Generally, products taken once a day exhibit incomplete absorption when ingested with food. Theo-Dur Sprinkle absorption is markedly impaired. Theo-24 has resulted in rapid release of a potentially toxic amount of theophylline. Along with the route, form, and particular product of theophylline, its salt equivalence must be considered. The theophylline salt equivalence (S) for each salt, compared to anhydrous theophylline (S = 1), is found in Table 21-2.

Table 21-4. Volume of Distribution (V)

Age	Volume (L/kg)
Neonates (0–<4 weeks)	0.8
Infants (4 weeks–<1 year)	0.5–0.7
Children (≥1 year), adolescents, adults, and geriatrics	0.5

Metabolism and elimination

In adults, theophylline is 85%–90% metabolized by hepatic biotransformation into relatively inactive metabolites primarily via demethylation by the cytochrome P450 1A2 (CYP 450 1A2) pathway and hydroxylation by the CYP 450 2E1 pathway. The only active metabolite, 3-methylxanthine, forms more slowly than its rate of excretion and, therefore, exhibits no pharmacologic effects. Due to the small percent of a dose eliminated by renal excretion and the lack of significantly active metabolites, dosing adjustments are not required for renal dysfunction in adults.[11,13]

In neonates the N-demethylation pathway is absent, but this pathway is fully matured by 1 year of age. The CYP 450 pathways appear to be almost absent in neonates. Approximately 50% of a theophylline dose is excreted unchanged in the urine and 7%–10% of the dose is converted to caffeine in neonates. Caffeine, an active metabolite, has a considerably long half-life of approximately 100 hours, which leads to concentrations that are approximately 30% or more of theophylline concentrations. Dosing adjustments for renal dysfunction (urine output less than 2 ml/kg/hr) may be necessary in the neonate due to the higher fraction of unchanged theophylline excreted in the urine.[10,12]

Clearance (CL)[15,16]

The clearance values in Table 21-5 are for neonates, children, and healthy non-smoking adults. The drug–disease state or condition interactions section provides clearance values of other patient populations (Tables 21-6 and 21-7).

Half-life and time to steady state

The half-lives and estimated times to steady state for theophylline in neonates, children, and healthy non-smoking adults are listed in Table 21-8.

Dosing Strategies

The clearance of theophylline varies considerably among age groups and is affected by both drug and disease/condition interactions (Tables 21-5, 21-6, and 21-7). Furthermore, theophylline clearance has not been directly correlated to specific laboratory tests of liver function. Thus, most dosing approaches rely on use of the average dose or average clearance for age, disease state, or condition. When clearance is used, a dosage regimen can

Table 21-5. Clearance Relative to Age Groupings

Population	Mean (± SD) Clearance[a] (L/hr/kg)
Premature neonates	
PNA 1–30 days	0.02 (± 0.01)
PNA 25–57 days	0.04 (± 0.02)
Term infants	
PNA 1 week	~0.03 (± 0.01)
PNA 6 months	~0.06 (± 0.02)
PNA 9 months	~0.09 (± 0.02)
Children	
1–8 years	0.09 (± 0.03)
9–12 years	0.07 (± 0.02)
13–15 years	0.05 (± 0.02)
Adults (16–60 years) healthy, nonsmoking asthmatics	0.04 (± 0.01)
Elderly (>60 years) nonsmokers with normal cardiac, liver, and renal function	0.025 (± 0.01)

[a]Adapted from references 12, 13, 17, 21, and 22.
PNA = postnatal age.

Table 21-6. Impact of Select Drug-Drug Interactions on Theophylline Clearance (CL)[a,b]

Drug	Mechanism	CL Impact	CL Factor[c]
Allopurinol (≥600 mg/day)	(?) Inhibit metabolism	Decrease	0.8
Beta blockers (nonselective)	Inhibit metabolism	Decrease	0.7 Propranolol
Caffeine	Inhibit metabolism	Decrease	0.7
Calcium channel blockers	Inhibit metabolism	Decrease	0.5 Verapamil
Carbamazepine[d]	Induce metabolism	Increase	N/A
Charcoal	Adsorption	Increase	Up to 1.9
Cimetidine	Inhibit metabolism	Decrease	0.6 (0.5–0.8)
Clarithromycin	Inhibit metabolism	Decrease	N/A
Corticosteroids	Inhibit metabolism	Decrease	N/A
Disulfiram	Inhibit metabolism	Decrease	0.8
Erythromycin	Inhibit metabolism	Decrease	0.7
Fluvoxamine	Inhibit metabolism	Decrease	0.3
Interferon, human alpha 2-a and 2-b	Inhibit metabolism	Decrease	0.2 to 0.7
Loop diuretics (furosemide)[d]	Unknown	Decrease	0.7
Mexiletine	Inhibit metabolism	Decrease	~0.6
Moricizine	Induce metabolism	Increase	1.5
Phenobarbital	Induce metabolism	Increase	1.2
Phenytoin	Induce metabolism	Increase	1.6
Propafenone	Inhibit metabolism	Decrease	0.7
Rifampin	Induce metabolism	Increase	1.3 (to 1.8)
Quinolones (ciprofloxacin, enoxacin, etc.)	Inhibit metabolism	Decrease	0.7 (0.3–0.8)
Tacrine	Inhibit metabolism	Decrease	0.5
Terbinafine	Inhibit metabolism	Decrease	0.85
Ticlopidine	Inhibit metabolism	Decrease	0.65
Tobacco	Induce metabolism	Increase	1.6
Zafirlukast	Inhibit metabolism	Decrease	0.2
Zileuton	Inhibit metabolism	Decrease	0.5

[a]Adapted from references 13, 14, 17, 18, 36–38, 40, and 41.
[b]Many other pharmacokinetic and pharmacodynamic interactions have been reported with theophylline.
[c]Clearance factors represent the average change in studies of multiple patients or the clearance change in single patients in case reports. Wide variation should be expected when using these values to estimate the change in clearance that might occur with an interaction.
[d]May increase or decrease theophylline concentrations.

be developed based on a clinician's desired therapeutic range for the patient. In either case (i.e., use of average dose or average clearance), the initial dosing regimen chosen can be validated by follow-up with measured theophylline concentrations to ensure that a patient is in the desired range. If steady state concentrations are used, proportional changes in dosing should usually result in proportional concentration changes, unless the patient's condition changes.

When patients do not fit average clearances due to drug interactions or disease conditions, condition correction factors can be used to predict a patient's clearance. When population based clearance is known for a condition or interaction, it may be used as well. For example, Table 21-6 gives a clearance factor of 0.6 for patients on theophylline who are also receiving cimetidine. To estimate an adult patient's clearance, the clearance factor of 0.6 is multiplied times the average clearance of 0.04 L/h/kg to yield a predicted clearance of 0.024 L/h/kg.

One study evaluated the use of condition correction factors to predict theophylline clearance in patients with single and multiple conditions or drug interactions.[23] The authors found that when patients had single factors, the prediction of clearance was reasonable. As the numbers of conditions increased, the prediction of

Table 21-7. Impact of Drug–Disease State or Condition Interactions on Clearance (CL) and Half-Life (t½)[a]

Condition	Mean CL (L/hr/kg) (± SD)	Mean $t_{1/2}$ (hr) (± 1 SD)	CL Factor[b]
Otherwise healthy adult nonsmokers (reference value)	0.04	8	1
Acute pulmonary edema	0.02	19	0.5
COPD, stable elderly nonsmokers	0.03 (± 0.01)	11 (± 1)	0.8
COPD with cor pulmonale	0.03 (± 0.01)	—	0.8
CHF			0.4
Cystic fibrosis (14–28 years)	0.08 (± 0.02)	6 (± 2)	2
Fever associated with acute viral respiratory illness in (children 9–15 years)	—	7 (± 3)	0.5
Pneumonia	—	—	0.4
Liver disease			
Acute hepatitis	0.02 (± 0.01)	19 (± 1)	0.5
Cholestasis	0.04 (± 0.02)	14 (6–32)	1
Cirrhosis	0.02 (± 0.01)	32 (10–56)[c]	0.5
Child-Pugh Class B or C	—	23 (10)	—
Pregnancy			
1st trimester	—	9 (± 3)	
2nd trimester	—	9 (± 3)	
3rd trimester	—	13 (± 3)	
Sepsis with multiorgan failure	0.03	19 (± 3)	0.7
Thyroid disease			
Hypothyroid	0.02 (± 0.01)	12 (± 4)	0.6
Hyperthyroid	0.05 (± 0.01)	5 (± 1)	1.2
Children with Down syndrome	Decreased	—	
ECMO in neonates and infants	Decreased	—	
Smoking			
Moderate cigarette use	—	4.1 ± 1	
Heavy cigarette use	0.06 ± 0.02	5.4 ± 1	1.5
Marijuana use	0.07 ± 0.03	4.3 ± 1	1.8
Cigarette and marijuana use	0.09 ± 0.02	4.3 ± 1	2.3
Past cigarette use	0.05 ± 0.001	6.4 ± 1	1.3
Elderly smokers	0.04 ± 0.01	5.9 ± 1	1
Passive smoking (children)[12]	0.08 vs. 0.05 (in NS)	—	
Diet			
Low carbohydrate and high protein	—	5.2 ± 1	
High carbohydrate and low protein	0.05 ± 0.02	—	1.2
Charcoal-broiled beef (heavy consumption)	—	4.7 ± 0.4	
Caffeine	—	Increased	
Cabbage or Brussels sprouts (heavy consumption)	—	Decreased	

[a]Adapted from references 10, 13, 23, 38, 39, and 42–44.
[b]Compared to average adult clearance of 0.04 L/h/kg. Note that the clearance factor may not always have been based on head-to-head trials against average adults and variability may be considerable.
NS = children not exposed to passive smoking.

Table 21-8. Theophylline Half-Lives and Estimated Time to Steady State

Population	Mean (± SD) Half-Life[a] (hr)	Time to Steady State (hr)[b]
Premature neonates		
PNA 1–30 days	31 (± 12)	95–215
PNA 30–60 days	20 (± 5)	65–125
Term infants		
PNA 1 week	18 (± 1)	85–95
PNA 6 months	7 (± 1)	30–40
PNA 9 months	4 (± 1)	15–25
Children		
1–<9 years	3 (± 1)	10–20
9–15 years	4 (± 2)	10–30
Adults (16–60 years) healthy, nonsmoking asthmatics	8 (± 2)	30–50
Elderly (>60 years) nonsmokers with normal cardiac, liver, and renal function	10 (± 2)	40–60

aAdapted from references 12, 14, and 16.
[b]Assuming five half-lives to reach steady state and using ± one standard deviation of the half-life.
PNA = postnatal age.

clearance was not as accurate, no matter how the factors were combined (i.e., multiplied, averaged, etc.). This may be due to the effect of multiple factors leading to increased variability in clearance. Another study showed that the known interactions with theophylline of both cimetidine and ciprofloxacin are augmented when the two are used together with theophylline.[24] Thus, when correction factors are used to predict clearance or dose in patients with multiple conditions and/or drug-drug interactions, greater caution should be exercised.

One study examined dosing equations for use in infants up to 1 year of age and found that the following equation tended to produce concentrations in the 5–10 mg/L range, a reasonable place to start therapy in infants being treated for apnea, bradycardia, and asthma.[25]

$$\text{Dose (mg/kg/day)} = (0.2 \times \text{Postnatal age in weeks}) + 5 \qquad \text{Eq. 1}$$

As an example of developing a dosing strategy for apneic premature neonates receiving intravenous theophylline, the authors of one study used nonlinear mixed effects modeling to predict volume of distribution and clearance.[26] The resulting population predictors were:

$$V\text{ (L)} = 0.63 \times Wt \qquad \text{Eq. 2}$$

$$CL\text{ (L/h)} = 0.006 \times Wt^{0.75} \times P \qquad \text{Eq. 3}$$

Where Wt is weight in kg and P is 1.47 for babies with oxygen support and 1.0 without support. These parameters can then be used to develop a dosing regimen to produce desired concentrations in premature neonates.

Therapeutic Range[10-12,14,27-31]

For *asthma*, the therapeutic range was traditionally considered to be 10–20 mg/L. However, based on more recent data and the National Asthma Education and Prevention Program, a range of 5–15 mg/L enhances safety and gives up little, if any, therapeutic benefit. For *COPD*, the therapeutic range is also 5–15 mg/L. Since it is debatable whether theophylline increases diaphragmatic contractility in these patients, its efficacy is questionable. However, as discussed earlier, COPD patients prefer it to placebo and it improves lung function and levels of O_2 and CO_2 in the blood. Because COPD patients are usually elderly, may be on multiple medications, and their clinical status often changes in a manner that affects theophylline concentrations, concentrations should be monitored more frequently. One report described the anti-inflammatory activity of theophylline in low concentrations (i.e., 5–10 mg/L), which would reduce risk for adverse effects.[30] These actions enhance the anti-inflammatory effects of corticosteroids, making combination therapy potentially beneficial while reducing side effect potential at the lower concentrations.[31]

For *apnea or bradycardia in neonates*, the therapeutic range is 6–14 mg/L. Although a wide range of concentrations has been suggested, many neonates respond at low concentrations. Therapy should be started at low concentrations and can be increased in increments of approximately 3 mg/L as necessary to effect. For *ventilator weaning of neonates*, the therapeutic range is 5–20 mg/L. However, studies supporting the desired theophylline concentration for ventilator weaning are limited. Some authors suggest that concentrations greater than 8 mg/L are required to enhance diaphragmatic contractility and promote relaxation of respiratory muscles.

Therapeutic Monitoring

Per the National Asthma Education and Prevention Program, "routine serum concentration monitoring is essential due to significant toxicities, narrow therapeutic range, and individual differences in metabolic clearance."[11] How frequently monitoring should occur depends on the relative stability or instability of the patient, changes in concurrent drug therapy, their apparent response or signs of possible toxicity, and whether there is potential of non-compliance.

Suggested sampling times and effect on therapeutic range

Therapeutic reference ranges often refer to concentrations drawn as peaks.[11] Wherever concentration measurements are drawn in a dosing interval (e.g., peak, trough), it is important to be consistent with the timing of sampling on subsequent monitoring. One report showed circadian variation in theophylline clearance with nighttime clearance 13% higher than daytime, so altering between evening and morning may make changes in concentration more difficult to interpret.[32] There also appears to be diurnal variation in absorption rate (regular-release products) and extent (sustained-release products).[11] Sampling times for the various age groups, along with the reasons for the timing, are listed below:

Neonates

- 2 hr after the first loading dose to calculate the volume of distribution, if desired.
- Every 4–7 days to calculate clearance and evaluate need for dosage adjustment in this population whose clearance can change fairly quickly.

Infants, children, adults, and geriatrics

- 30 min after the first loading dose, if administered intravenously, to calculate the volume of distribution for any additional loading doses that might be needed.
- 12–24 hr after initiation of maintenance dose to determine if adequate concentrations are being maintained or if the drug is accumulating rapidly, if deemed necessary.
- 72 hr after initial dosing and then every 24 to 72 hr as needed to evaluate need for dosage adjustment in hospitalized patients.
- Every 4–7 days once hospitalized patients are stabilized, unless otherwise indicated, to evaluate need for dosage adjustment and determine if clearance is changing.
- Every 1–6 months in stable, ambulatory patients.
- When there are signs or symptoms of toxicity or lack of efficacy.
- In the emergency department, patients currently taking a theophylline-containing preparation should have a theophylline concentration measured to rule out theophylline toxicity.[10]

Pharmacodynamic Monitoring

Concentration-related efficacy

The following are useful indicators of theophylline efficacy:

Asthma or COPD

- Decrease in severity of wheezing and rales
- Respiration rate normalization
- Improvement of FEV_1
- Decrease in the ventilator support required

Apnea or bradycardia in neonates

- Decrease in number and depth of apneic and bradycardic episodes
- Heart rate normalization
- Decrease in the ventilator support required

Concentration-Related Toxicity

To reduce the potential for concentration-related toxicity, the following should be monitored when theophylline is used (see also Table 21-9):

- Liver function in patients receiving theophylline for asthma or COPD
- Liver and renal function in neonates receiving theophylline for apnea or bradycardia (urine output should be 2 ml/kg/hr or more)
- Drugs or disease states that may decrease theophylline clearance

Seizures and death induced by theophylline can occur in the absence of any other adverse effect; therefore, theophylline concentrations should be monitored. In neonates receiving theophylline for apnea, bradycardia, or ventilator weaning, the following adverse effects may indicate toxicity: tachycardia (heart rate of more than 180 beats/min), irritability, seizures, and vomiting (e.g., appearance like "coffee grounds").

Drug-Drug Interactions

Many drug interactions have been reported with the use of theophylline. Most are related to alterations in the clearance of theophylline, though some appear to have other mechanisms (Table 21-6).[33] As with most pharmacokinetic drug-drug interactions, some patients may experience adverse effects due to changes in a drug's clearance and concentration, while others may be unaffected. Only interactions reported as moderately or highly clinically significant are listed in Table 21-6. Caution is advised when an interaction has been reported, but other factors must be considered as well (e.g., older patients may start with lower clearance than younger patients and thus be at greater risk). Any drug that significantly inhibits or induces CYP 450 1A2 or CYP 450 2E1 should be suspect for potential impact on theophylline clearance and concentrations. In addition to drug-drug interactions, caution should be taken with concurrent use of selected herbal supplements, such as St. John's Wort, which has been reported to lead to reduced steady state theophylline concentrations.[34,35]

Drug–Disease State or Condition Interactions

Various disease states and conditions have been shown to alter theophylline clearance (Table 21-7). As seen with drug-drug interactions, there can be considerable variability in the impact of a given disease state or condition on theophylline clearance. Not only should one be aware of pharmacokinetic changes with the

Table 21-9. Concentration-Related Adverse Effects

Concentration	Adverse Effect
>20 mg/L	Nausea, vomiting, diarrhea, headache, irritability, insomnia, tremor[a]
>35 mg/L[b]	Hyperglycemia, hyperkalemia, hypotension,[c] cardiac arrhythmias, hyperthermia, seizures, brain damage, and death

[a]Effects have been reported with concentrations as low as 15 mg/L.
[b]Side effects that occur at lower concentrations may also occur at higher concentrations.
[c]May also occur due to too rapid an infusion; infusion rate should not exceed 20 mg/min.

presence of conditions (e.g., smoking), but also the cessation or improvement of such conditions as this will affect drug clearance.[43]

References

1. Schmidt B, Roberts RS, Davis P, et al. Caffeine therapy for apnea of prematurity. *N Eng J Med.* 2006;354(20):2112-21.
2. Wheeler DS, Jacobs BR, Kenreigh CA, et al. Theophylline versus terbutaline in treating critically ill children with status asthmaticus: A prospective, randomized, controlled trial. *Pediatr Crit Care Med.* 2005;6:142-7.
3. Seddon P, Bara A, Lasserson TJ, et al. Oral xanthines as maintenance treatment from asthma in children. The Cochrane Database of Systematic Reviews 2009 Issue 1. Date of Last Substantial Update: May 8, 2005. Available at: http://www.cochrane.org/reviews/en/ab002885.html. Accessed July 22, 2010.
4. Tee A, Koh MS, Gibson PG, et al. Long-acting beta2-agonists versus theophylline for maintenance treatment of asthma. Cochrane Database of Systematic Reviews 2009, Issue 3. Date of Last Substantial Update: November 14, 2007. Available at: http://www2.cochrane.org/reviews/en/ab001281.html. Accessed July 22, 2010.
5. Barr RG, Rowe BH, Camargo CA Jr. Methylxanthines for exacerbations of chronic obstructive pulmonary disease. The Cochrane Database of Systematic Reviews 2008 Issue 4. Date of Last Substantial Update: March 2, 2005. Available at: http://www.cochrane.org/reviews/en/ab002168.html. Accessed July 22, 2010.
6. Ram FSF, Jones PW, Castro AA, et al. Oral theophylline for chronic obstructive pulmonary disease. The Cochrane Database of Systematic Reviews 2009 Issue 4. Date of Last Substantial Update: April 16, 2002. Available at: http://www.cochrane.org/reviews/en/ab003902.html. Accessed July 22, 2010.
7. Henderson-Smart DJ, Subramaniam P, Davis PG. Continuous positive airway pressure versus theophylline for apnea in preterm infants. The Cochrane Database of Systematic Reviews 2009 Issue 1. Date of Last Substantial Update: March 31, 2005. Available at: http://www.cochrane.org/reviews/en/ab001072.html. Accessed July 22, 2010.
8. Henderson-Smart DJ, Davis PG. Prophylactic methylxanthines for extubation in preterm infants. The Cochrane Database of Systematic Reviews 2009 Issue 4. Date of Last Substantial Update: April 17, 2008. Available at: http://www.cochrane.org/reviews/en/ab000139.html. Accessed July 22, 2010.
9. Steer PA, Henderson-Smart DJ. Caffeine versus theophylline for apnea in preterm infants. The Cochrane Database of Systematic Reviews 2010 Issue 1. Date of Last Substantial Update: August 16, 2009. Available at: http://www.cochrane.org/reviews/en/ab000273.html. Accessed July 22, 2010.
10. Edwards DJ, Zarowitz BJ, Slaughter RL. Theophylline. In: Evans WE, Schentag JJ, Jusko WJ, eds. *Applied Pharmacokinetics: Principles of Therapeutic Drug Monitoring.* 3rd ed. Spokane, WA: Applied Therapeutics; 1992:13-1–13-38.
11. National Asthma Education and Education Program. Expert panel report III: guidelines for the diagnosis and management of asthma. 2007 July. Bethesda, MD: U.S. Department of Helath and Human Services; National Institutes of Health; National Heart, Lung, and Blood Institute. Available at http://www.nhlbi.nih.gov/guidelines/asthma/. Accessed July 29, 2010.
12. Theophyllines. In: McEvoy GK, ed. *AHFS Drug Information 2010.* Bethesda, MD: American Society of Health-System Pharmacists; 2010. Available at: http://online.statref.com/document.aspx?fxid=1&docid=1. Accessed July 22, 2010.
13. Hendeles L, Jenkins J, Temple R. Revised FDA labeling guideline for theophylline oral dosage forms. *Pharmacotherapy.* 1995; 15(4):409-27.
14. Taketomo CK, Hodding JH, Kraus DM. *Pediatric Lexi-Drugs Online.* Hudson, OH: http://online.lexi.com/crlsql/servlet/crlonline. Accessed July 30, 2010.
15. Asmus MJ, Weinberger MM, Milavetz G, et al. Apparent decrease in population clearance of theophylline: implications for dosage. *Clin Pharmacol Ther.* 1997;62:483-9.
16. Mayo PR. Effect of passive smoking on theophylline clearance in children. *Ther Drug Monit.* 2001;23:503-5.
17. Theophylline. Facts and Comparisons E-Answers. Wolters Kluwer Health Inc. http://online.factsandcomparisons.com/. Accessed July 30, 2010.
18. Murphy JE, Winter ME. Theophylline. In: Winter ME, ed. *Basic Clinical Pharmacokinetics.* 5th ed. Baltimore, MD: Wolters Kluwer: Lippincott Williams & Wilkins; 2010:403-41.
19. Hendeles L, Weinberger M. Theophylline, a state of the art review. *Pharmacotherapy.* 1983; 3:2-24.
20. Chereches-Panta P, Nanulescu MV, Culea M, et al. Reliability of salivary theophylline in monitoring the treatment for apnoea of prematurity. *J Perinatol.* 2007 Nov;27(11):709-12.
21. Islam SI, Ali ASS, Amal AF, et al. Pharmacokinetics of theophylline in preterm neonates during the first month of life. *Saudi Med J.* 2004;25(4):459-65.
22. Gilman JT, Gal P, Levine RS, et al. Factors influencing theophylline disposition in 179 newborns. *Ther Drug Monit.* 1986;8:4-10.
23. Haumschild MJ, Murphy JE. Prediction of theophylline condition correction factors. *Clin Pharm.* 1985;4:59-64.

24. Loi C, Parker BM, Cusack BJ, et al. Aging and drug interactions. III. Individual and combined effects of cimetidine and ciprofloxacin on theophylline metabolism in healthy male and female nonsmokers. *J Pharmacol Exp Ther.* 1997;280(2):627-37.

25. Hogue SL, Phelps SJ. Evaluation of three theophylline dosing equations for use in infants up to one year of age. *J Pediatric.* 1993;123:651-6.

26. duPreez MJ, Botha JH, McFadyen ML, et al. The pharmacokinetics of theophylline in premature neonates during the first few days after birth. *Ther Drug Monit.* 1999;21:598-603.

27. Moore ES, Faix RG, Banagale RC, et al. The population pharmacokinetics of theophylline in neonates and young infants. *J Pharmacokinet Biopharm.* 1989;17:47-66.

28. Self TH, Heilker GM, Alloway RR, et al. Reassessing therapeutic range for theophylline for laboratory report forms: the importance of 5–15 mg/L. *Pharmacotherapy.* 1993; 13(6):590-4.

29. Milsap RL, Krauss AN, Auld PA. Oxygen consumption in apneic premature infants after low-dose theophylline. *Clin Pharmacol Ther.* 1980; 28(4):536-40.

30. Barnes PJ. Theophylline in chronic obstructive pulmonary disease: New horizons. *Proc Am Thorac Soc.* 2005;2:334-9.

31. Cosio BG, Iglesias A, Rios A, et al. Low-dose theophylline enhances the anti-inflammatory effects of steroids during exacerbations of COPD. *Thorax.* 2009;64(5):424-9.

32. Nix DE, Di Cicco RA, Miller AK, et al. The effects of low-dose cimetidine (200 mg twice daily) on the pharmacokinetics of theophylline. *J Clin Pharmacol.* 1999;39:855-65.

33. Zucchero FJ, Hogan MJ, Sommer CD, et al. (eds). *Evaluations of Drug Interactions.* St. Louis, MO: First DataBank, Inc; 2003.

34. Morimoto T, Kotegawa T, Tsutsumi K, et al. Effect of St. John's wort on the pharmacokinetics of theophylline in healthy volunteers. *J Clin Pharmacol.* 2004;44:95-101.

35. Dasgupta A. Herbal supplements and therapeutic drug monitoring: focus on digoxin immunoassays and interactions with St. John's wort. *Ther Drug Monit.* 2008;30(2):212-7.

36. Upton RA. Pharmacokinetic interactions between theophylline and other medication (part I). *Clin Pharmacokinet.* 1991;20:66-80.

37. Upton RA. Pharmacokinetic interactions between theophylline and other medication (part II). *Clin Pharmacokinet.* 1991;20:135-50.

38. Hendeles L, Massanari M, Weinberger M. Theophylline. In: Evans WE, Schentag JJ, Jusko WJ, eds. *Applied Pharmacokinetics: Principles of Therapeutic Drug Monitoring.* 2nd ed. Spokane, WA: Applied Therapeutics; 1986:1105-209.

39. Stowe C, Phelps S. Altered clearance of theophylline in children with down syndrome: a case series. *J Clin Pharmacol.* 1999; 39:359-65.

40. Rasmussen BB, Jeppesen U, Gaist D, et al. Griseofulvin and fluvoxamine interactions with the metabolism of theophylline. *Ther Drug Monit.* 1997;19:56-62.

41. Katial RK, Stelzle RC, Bonner MW, et al. A drug interaction between zafirlukast and theophylline. *Arch Int Med.* 1998;158:1713-5.

42. Mulla H, Nabi F, Nichani S, et al. Population pharmacokinetics of theophylline during paediatric extracorporeal membrane oxygenation (ECMO) from routine monitoring data. *Br J Clin Pharmacol.* 2003;55:23-31.

43. Braganza G, Chaudhuri R, Thomson NC. Treating patients with respiratory disease who smoke. *Ther Adv Respir Dis.* 2008;2(2):95-107.

44. Edginton AN, Willmann S. Physiology-based simulations of a pathological condition: prediction of pharmacokinetics in patients with liver cirrhosis. *Clin Pharmacokinet.* 2008;47:743-52.

45. Granneman GR, Braeckman RA, Locke CS, et al. Effect of zileuton on theophylline pharmacokinetics. *Clin Pharmacokinet.* 1995;29 Suppl 2:77-83.

Chapter 22

Barry E. Gidal

Valproic Acid (AHFS 28:12.92)

Valproic acid (VPA) is a carboxylic acid-derivative anticonvulsant used in the management of partial and generalized seizures including absence, tonic-clonic, and myoclonic seizures. In addition, VPA is used in patients with bipolar-affective disorder as well as for prophylaxis of migraine headaches. For seizures, VPA may be used as monotherapy or in combination with other antiepileptic drugs.

Usual Dosage Range in the Absence of Clearance-Altering Factors

VPA is available in two salts, valproate sodium and divalproex sodium. Dosages of all salt forms are expressed in terms of VPA (mw = 144.2 g mol^{-1}, **S = 1**).[1] Table 22-1 provides usual dosage ranges in the absence of clearance-altering factors (other than age).

Table 22-2 provides information on available dosage forms of valproic acid.

Table 22-1. Usual Dosage Range in the Absence of Clearance-Altering Factors

Age Group	Dosage (Mean + SD)[a,b]
Neonates (<4 weeks)[2]	20 mg/kg/day
Infants (4 weeks –<1 year)[2]	34 ± 14 mg/kg/day
Children	
1 –<5 years	Not available[c]
5 –<10 years[3,4]	28 ± 10 mg/kg/day
10 –<15 years[3]	19 ± 6 mg/kg/day
Adults (18 –<60 years)[5]	13 ± 5 mg/kg/day
Geriatrics (≥60 years)[6]	11 ± 4 mg/kg/day

[a]Doses are for monotherapy to achieve mean Css_{av} of ~60–70 mg/L.
[b]Oral (capsules, tablets, and solution).
[c]Information on this specific age range not established.

Table 22-2. Dosage Form Availability[1]

Dosage Form	Product
Valproic acid	Depakene (various generic)
Oral capsules: 250 mg	
Divalproex sodium	
Oral capsules (coated particles): 125 mg	Depakote Sprinkle
Oral tablets (enteric coated, delayed-release): 125, 250, and 500 mg	Depakote (various generic)
Oral extended-release tablets: 500 mg	Depakote ER (various generic)
Valproate sodium	
Injection: 500 mg/5 ml[a]	Depacon
Oral solution: 250 mg/5 ml	Depakene syrup (various generic)

[a]Current labeling information suggests that intravenous VPA should be administered slowly (maximum rate = 20 mg/min). However, faster rates of administration have been safely employed (6–10 mg/kg/min) in both children and adults.[7–9] The parenteral formulation may be given intravenously only; intramuscular administration may result in tissue necrosis.

General Pharmacokinetic Information

Absorption

VPA is almost completely absorbed.[6,10] The bioavailability of capsules and enteric-coated tablets is similar, although more variability apparently exists with the enteric-coated form.[11] The rate of absorption depends on the dosage form.

It is important for the clinician to recognize that all the available oral formulations of valproic acid have very different absorption patterns and should not be considered interchangeable.[12] For example, valproic acid (Depakene) capsules and syrup are absorbed quickly. Due to their enteric coatings, divalproex delayed-release (Depakote) products exhibit both improved gastrointestinal (GI) tolerability and delayed absorption, the latter resulting in a shift of the area under the serum concentration–time curve (AUC) to the right.[11,13–15] Depakote tablets provide delayed, but not sustained-release. Depakote Sprinkles exhibit a sustained release profile and may be better tolerated due to decreased peak-trough variability compared to oral capsules and solution.

The delay in Depakote absorption may be 1–6 hr, with no change in the extent of absorption. This delay is dependent on gastric-emptying time and gastric pH with the lag phase for absorption differing significantly between fed and fasted patients. For both regular and coated preparations, food decreases the rate, but not extent of absorption. The time to achieve peak concentrations may be delayed to 3–8 hr due to dissolution rate changes. Once absorption starts, however, it is usually complete within 1–1.5 hr.[15]

Diurnal variations in VPA concentrations have been observed with the enteric-coated formulation, and may result in nighttime concentrations that are approximately 40% of daytime concentrations. This day-night variation does not seem to occur with the extended-release formulation.

An extended-release preparation (Depakote ER) is also commercially available as a generic product and offers the potential of once-daily administration. It is important to recognize that the extended-release product differs from enteric-coated, delayed-release divalproex sodium with respect to both rate and extent of absorption. Depakote ER is not bioequivalent to Depakote, however. Pharmacokinetic studies suggest that when converting a patient from the delayed-release enteric-coated product (Depakote) to the extended-release formulation (Depakote ER), an increase in the total daily dose of approximately 15% (14%–20%) is required to maintain equivalent AUC. In addition to once daily dosing, a potential advantage of this formulation is a reduction in valproate concentration fluctuations over the dosage interval. Mean peak to trough concentration fluctuations are substantially less than with Depakote following conversion.[16]

Conversion from standard-release to extended-release formulation (i.e., twice-daily Depakote to once-daily Depakote ER) may be accomplished all at once and does not appear to require a prolonged dosage titration or conversion period. In order to minimize excessive VPA concentration fluctuations, substitution of the extended-release formulation should begin within 12 hr of the last dose of Depakote. Conversion from standard, delayed-release formulation of divalproex (Depakote) to the extended-release formulation will reduce peak to trough fluctuations in VPA concentrations. While the ER formulation is acceptable for patients with epilepsy when given as a once daily regimen, less peak to trough fluctuation (~22% less) will be seen if Depakote ER is given on an every 12 hr basis as compared to once daily.[17] Whether this reduction in fluctuation is clinically meaningful in patients is unclear. An additional consideration for this formulation would be the impact of poor medication compliance. As would be expected, patients with missed doses of a once daily extended-release formulation are likely to display greater fluctuations in concentrations as compared to patients taking the extended-release formulation twice daily, or simply taking the standard, delayed-release preparation.[18] Pharmacokinetic simulations have suggested that missed doses of extended-release divalproex may be replaced up to 12 hr following a missed dose.[19]

The bioavailability of the various dosage forms is provided in Table 22-3.

Distribution

VPA is rapidly distributed into the central nervous system (CNS). VPA concentrations in cerebrospinal fluid (CSF) tend to be lower than unbound serum concentrations. Brain to total and unbound plasma concentration ratios are approximately 0.1 to 0.5, respectively, however significant interpatient variability may be noted. The precise mechanism involved in the transport of VPA into, as well as efflux from, the brain remains uncertain.

VPA distribution across the blood-brain barrier may be mediated by both passive diffusion and a carrier transport mechanisms, with transport of VPA into the brain apparently mediated by a fatty acid selective anion exchanger, while transport out appears to be mediated by a probenecid-sensitive active transport system.[11] VPA also distributes into breast milk, with typical serum concentrations in nursing infants ranging between 4%–12% of corresponding maternal concentrations.[11,20]

Estimating volume of distribution (V)

Table 22-4 provides volume of distribution values that can be assumed in the absence of disease or drug interactions when VPA is used in monotherapy. Single dose values were determined after a single dose and steady state volume determined under steady state conditions.

Protein binding

VPA is 90%–95% protein bound to albumin,[5,11,27–31] and its protein binding is saturable.[5,30,31] In adults, at total concentrations <75 mg/L, VPA percent unbound ranges between 7% and 10%. At total concentrations of 100–150 mg/L, however, percent unbound can be expected to increase to ~15% and 30%, respectively. This effect may be magnified in patients with significant hypoalbuminemia.[32] Therefore, although unbound concentrations may increase proportionally with dose, total concentrations may exhibit curvilinear kinetics (i.e., less than proportional increases in concentrations with dose changes).[33] The percent unbound fluctuates more than the total concentration due to fluctuations in free fatty acid concentrations in the morning and diurnal differences in unbound concentrations and total clearance.[5,34]

Elimination

VPA is primarily eliminated by the liver, with no clinically important first-pass metabolism. Since VPA is a low extraction drug, clearance is independent of blood flow. Only 3%–7% of a dose is excreted unchanged in the urine.

The metabolism of VPA in the liver is extensive. The three main metabolic pathways, in order of importance, are conjugation with glucuronic acid, β-oxidation, and Ω-oxidation.[11] The most abundant metabolite, VPA–glucuronide accounts for approximately 60% of the recovered dose in the urine and VPA may competitively inhibit the metabolism of other drugs that form glucuronide conjugates. Several glucuronyltransferase (UGT) isozymes have been identified as participating in VPA metabolism, and include UGT1A3, 1A4, 1A6, 1A8, and

Table 22-3. Bioavailability of Dosage Forms

Dosage Form	Bioavailability
Intravenous	100% (F = 1)
Intramuscular	IM injection is not recommended
Oral capsules and syrups	95%; range 90%–100% (F ~ 0.95)
Enteric-coated tablets (Depakote)	95%; range 90%–100% (F ~ 0.95)
Extended-release tablets (Depakote ER)	87% (F = 0.87)

Table 22-4. Volume of Distribution

Age Group	Single-Dose Volume (Mean ± SD)	Steady State Volume (Mean ± SD)
Neonates (<4 weeks)[2]	0.28 L/kg	Not available[a]
Infants (4 weeks –<1 year)[21,22]	Not available[a]	0.32 L/kg
Children (3–16 years)[3,23]	Not available[a]	0.22 ± 0.05 L/kg
Adults (18 –<60 years)[5,24,25]	0.12 ± 0.028 L/kg	0.15 ± 0.10 L/kg
Geriatrics (≥60 years)[25,26]	0.16 ± 0.02 L/kg	Not available[a]

[a]Data not available on this age range.

1A9. Cytochrome P450 isozymes involved in the oxidative metabolism of VPA include CYP2C9, CYP2A6, and CYP2B6.

Two of the desaturated metabolites, 2-ene-VPA and 4-ene-VPA may possess anticonvulsant activity. The 2-ene-VPA metabolite will accumulate in brain with chronic dosing.[35] One of VPA's potentially hepatotoxic metabolites, 4-ene, may be produced in larger quantities in patients on concomitant enzyme inducers, leading, in part, to the higher incidence of hepatotoxicity seen in children on polytherapy.[36] Both metabolites are generated via CYP isozymes, and therefore formation may be increased when VPA is given concomitantly with enzyme-inducing AEDs. CYP 2C9*1 appears responsible for the formation of 4-ene-VPA.[37] Unlike 4-ene-VPA, 2-ene-VPA does not appear to demonstrate embryoxicity or hepatotoxicity.

Clearance depends primarily on the age of the patient and concomitant medications. Newborns eliminate VPA slower than children or adults. While little is known in the elder population, in-vitro studies using human liver microsomes suggests no difference in VPA-glucuronide formation in elder vs. younger livers.[38] As discussed previously the diurnal fluctuation in VPA concentration–time profiles is great, so clinicians should be mindful when monitoring apparent "trough" concentrations at varying times of day.[34]

VPA exhibits concentration-related changes in apparent clearance, with lower clearance at higher concentrations. The lower apparent oral clearance of VPA at higher concentrations may reflect either saturable protein binding or partial saturation of intrinsic clearance. VPA is not removed efficiently by standard hemodialysis (<20%), but high-flux hemodialysis is effective.

The clearance values in Table 22-5 can be assumed in the absence of disease or drug interactions when VPA is used in *monotherapy* (i.e., no influence of enzyme inducers).

Half-life and time to steady state

The half-life ($t½$) values in Table 22-6 can be assumed in the absence of disease interactions when VPA is used in monotherapy. Some drug-drug interactions alter the half-life and time to steady state.

Table 22-5. Clearance by Age in the Absence of Clearance-Altering Factors

Age Group	Clearance at Steady State[a] (Mean ± SD or Range)
Neonates (<4 weeks)[2]	0.011 to 0.018 L/hr/kg
Infants (4 weeks –<1 year)[2,21,22]	0.019 ± 0.008 L/hr/kg
Children (3–16 years)[3,21,23]	0.018 ± 0.006 L/hr/kg
Adults (18 –<60 years)[5,24]	0.009 ± 0.005 L/hr/kg
Geriatrics (≥60 years)[11,25,26]	0.007 ± 0.005 L/hr/kg

[a]Use ideal body weight (IBW) in obese patients.

Table 22-6. Valproate Half-Life and Time to Steady State by Age Group

Age	Half-Life (Mean ± SD)	Time to Steady State[a]
Neonates (<4 weeks)[2]	17–20 hr	86–100 hr
Infants (4 weeks –<1 year)[2,22]	12.5 ± 2.8 hr	49–77 hr
Children (3–16 years)[3,4,23,39]	11 ± 4 hr	35–75 hr
Adults (18 –<60 years)[5,24]	11.9 ± 5.7 hr	31–88 hr
Geriatrics (≥60 years)[26]	15.3 ± 1.7 hr	68–85 hr

[a]Time to steady state based on + and – 1 SD of the mean half-life or range and assuming steady state reached in five half-lives.

Dosing Strategies

Initial dosing

The recommended initial target dose for VPA in adults is ~15 mg/kg/day. Typically, the VPA dose is gradually escalated in order to minimize initial adverse effects and enhance tolerability. A reasonable starting regimen would be VPA 250–500 mg once or twice daily. The dosage is gradually titrated upward (5–10 mg/kg/day) every 3–5 days. Eventual maintenance dosage depends primarily upon clinical response (efficacy versus toxicity) and also on the impact of concomitant medication interactions. Maintenance doses typically range between 15 and 60 mg/kg/day. When using Depakene or the enteric-coated formulation Depakote, the typical dosage frequency is twice to three times daily. The extended-release product Depakote ER may be given once or twice daily.

Oral loading doses of VPA may produce unacceptable GI side effects in some patients. For the treatment of acute seizures, larger intravenous loading doses have been used (~20–25 mg/kg), and are generally well tolerated at rapid infusion rates. Loading doses of intravenous VPA of 25 mg/kg have been reported to result in total peak concentrations of 80–200 mg/L.[7,8] Oral loading with the delayed-release formulation (Depakote) has been used in patients suffering from acute mania and in one small study was shown to be well tolerated.[40] Initial institution of Depakote ER following intravenous loading has also been employed in patients requiring prompt initiation of valproic acid therapy.[41]

Apparent oral clearance of VPA may correlate better with ideal body weight than with total body weight in obese patients. Thus, it may be prudent to use ideal body weight to estimate clearance and initial dosing needs in obese patients.

Dosage Adjustment

The simplest approach to dosage adjustment is based on the measurement of a trough concentration at steady state. Once this concentration is determined, VPA doses may be adjusted by a desired proportion, keeping in mind that as concentrations increase a curvilinear relationship between total concentration and dose is observed. Thus, at higher concentrations any given increase in the VPA dose results in proportional increases in the unbound concentration but less than proportional increases in the total VPA concentration. At higher measured total concentrations an unexpected degree of response or toxicity may be seen.

Therapeutic Range

Dose response to VPA is highly variable and dependent on the type and severity of seizure and an individual's pharmacokinetic parameters. Various seizure disorders or epileptic syndromes may require higher or lower average concentrations.

Studies correlating VPA concentrations with clinical response in patients with seizures have generally found that 40–50 mg/L is the minimum effective trough concentration for optimal seizure control. Seizure control tends to improve as the trough concentration increases from 40 to 120 mg/L. Monotherapy epilepsy trials suggest that higher concentrations (>80 mg/L) may be more effective than lower concentrations in treating complex-partial seizures.[42] Seizure control may improve with prolonged therapy independent of changes in concentrations.

Whether the optimal concentration ranges for conditions such as migraine headache or bipolar-affective disorder are different than that for seizures has not been clearly established. A consensus guideline from 2000 suggested that a similar range of trough VPA concentrations (~56–120 mg/L) may be effective for both acute mania and long-term maintenance.[43]

Depending on the clinical circumstances some patients may benefit from trough concentrations greater than 120 mg/L, and they may not exhibit adverse effects. However, the incidence of adverse effects such as tremor and thrombocytopenia may well increase at higher concentrations.[44] Increased CNS toxicity is generally seen when concentrations reach 175–200 mg/L.

An unbound VPA concentration range has not been established, though in some cases markedly elevated unbound concentrations have been associated with neurotoxicity. Determination of unbound VPA concentrations may be considered in patients with hypoalbuminemia.[32]

Typical adverse events associated with VPA treatment include tremor, weight gain, hair loss, hyperammonemia, GI distress, and decreased cognitive functioning.[36] Patients with these reactions must be closely monitored. Adverse reactions associated with elevated concentrations of VPA, such as thrombocytopenia and platelet dysfunction, may not be readily detectable by patient history or physical assessment. Thus, potentially toxic concentrations may be present but not apparent from other side effects.

Effect of Age and Pregnancy on Therapeutic Range

Elderly patients may display an increased percent unbound as a result of lower serum albumin concentrations and may have a reduced unbound clearance (~40%) as compared to younger subjects.[25,26] Measurement of unbound concentrations may therefore be reasonable in elderly patients, particularly for those with low serum albumin concentrations.

Alterations in VPA clearance and concentrations may also be expected in pregnancy. Total concentrations may begin to decline by the second trimester and can be expected to rise rapidly within 2–3 weeks postpartum. Unbound concentrations are however largely unchanged during pregnancy. These changes are likely due to changes in maternal protein binding. Therefore, as with elderly patients, monitoring of unbound concentrations may be warranted in pregnant patients.

One study suggests that VPA concentrations may vary in women as a function of menstrual cycle.[45] Whether these fluctuations are clinically meaningful is unclear.

Data from children (8–11 years of age) and adolescents (12–17 years of age) suggest that Depakote ER used as a once daily administration will result in relatively small fluctuations in concentrations across a 24-hour dosage period.[46]

Therapeutic Monitoring

Suggested sampling times and effect on therapeutic range

Because the diurnal fluctuation in VPA concentration–time profiles is great,[25,34] it is suggested that morning trough concentrations be used for monitoring. At a minimum, it is recommended that trough concentrations be consistently taken in the dosing interval (e.g., always before the morning dose or always before the afternoon dose). Trough VPA measurements should usually be obtained prior to a morning dose though, as these concentrations are the most consistent from day to day. Determination of peak concentrations is not typically employed. Timing of peak concentration measurements is highly dependent on the dosage form and the circumstances under which VPA is ingested. For example, the absorption of Depakote is highly dependent on administration in the fed or fasted state and Depakene can potentially produce large differences between peak and trough concentrations.[15] After any change in dosage or dosing interval, waiting 3 to 5 days prior to sampling should generally ensure that patients have achieved the new steady state.

With respect to optimal times for sampling VPA concentrations in patients receiving Depakote ER once daily in the morning, morning trough samples (21–24 hr following the previous dose) are typically considered to be the most reproducible. For patients taking this formulation in the evening, morning samples obtained 12–15 hr later can result in concentrations being 20%–25% higher than expected trough concentrations.[47] Therefore, timing of serum sampling as close to trough times would be the most reasonable approach and sampling around the expected peak time for this formulation (3–15 hr following dose administration) is unnecessary.

Initial and Follow-up Monitoring

Since VPA clearance at low concentrations may be significantly different than at higher steady state concentrations, VPA concentrations generally should not be determined following the initial dose. The most cost-efficient strategy involves achieving steady state conditions before determining VPA concentrations. If serum concentrations are obtained following IV loading, particularly if rapid infusion rates are employed (e.g., setting of acute seizures), then clinicians should be cognizant of the impact of concentration dependent protein binding. In this situation, percent unbound will decline as high initial peak concentrations decline.

Other indications for monitoring VPA concentrations include signs of toxicity, decreased seizure control, addition or withdrawal of antiepileptic or other interacting drugs, and suspected noncompliance.

Pharmacodynamic Monitoring—Concentration-Related Efficacy

Efficacy of VPA therapy is judged by a decrease in seizure activity. It may take several days to more than 1 week to achieve the full therapeutic effect at a given VPA concentration.[1] Little clinical or animal data exist to indicate specific synergistic or antagonistic pharmacodynamic interactions with other agents, though a potential synergistic effect of VPA and lamotrigine has been suggested in patients with refractory seizures resistant to pharmacotherapy.

The more common dose or concentration-related adverse effects of VPA therapy are GI in nature (e.g., nausea, vomiting, and diarrhea). Although hepatotoxicity has been reported in patients receiving VPA, a clear dose relationship is not established. Severe hepatotoxicity may be preceded by nonspecific symptoms such as loss of seizure control, malaise, and weakness.[1]

Thrombocytopenia, platelet aggregation defects, and tremor also appear to be concentration related. Evidence from clinical trials with the antiepileptic drug lamotrigine suggests that pharmacodynamic interactions between this agent and VPA exist and may lead to an increased incidence of tremor and rash.

Drug-Drug Interactions

Pharmacokinetic interactions with VPA are common and clinically important. VPA is an enzyme inhibitor and is subject to enzyme induction. The concomitant administration of drugs that utilize enzyme metabolism may affect the actions of these drugs and of VPA. For example, VPA decreases the elimination of carbamazepine epoxide (via inhibition of epoxide hydrolase),[48–51] phenobarbital (30%–50%),[52,53] and ethosuximide.[54] Because of protein binding displacement, phenytoin total concentrations can decline during co-medication with VPA, while unbound concentrations can increase secondary to inhibition of intrinsic clearance. Clearance of lamotrigine is also markedly inhibited by VPA, resulting in significant prolongations in lamotrigine half-life.[55] VPA is a potent inhibitor of lamotrigine metabolism, with near maximal inhibition occurring at VPA daily doses of 250–500 mg.[56] The combination of VPA and lamotrigine increases the risk for potentially serious rash. The mechanism for this apparent interaction is unknown. VPA also significantly reduces the clearance of lorazepam.[57] These interactions are presumably mediated via inhibition of glucuronyl transferase and can lead to clinically significant increases in serum concentrations of these compounds, with possible associated clinical toxicity. Enzyme inducers such as rifampin, phenytoin, carbamazepine, primidone, and phenobarbital increase the elimination of VPA, often requiring higher doses. Concomitant administration with AEDs such as gabapentin, pregabalin, levetiracetam, vigabatrin, or lacosamide would not be expected to result in significant pharmacokinetic interactions.

Co-administration of felbamate can reduce VPA clearance, possibly via inhibition of beta-oxidation. Through a similar mechanism, aspirin may also inhibit VPA metabolism.[58,59] Cimetidine and ranitidine do not affect the clearance of VPA.[60] Among the newer generation AEDs, VPA can increase rufinamide concentrations by up to 70%. Co-administration with oral contraceptives may decrease VPA concentrations, possibly as a result of UGT induction by ethinyl estradiol.[45]

Caution should be used when administering VPA concomitantly with CNS depressants, other anticonvulsants, monoamine oxidase inhibitors, and anticoagulants. It does not appear to alter the pharmacokinetics of oral contraceptive agents; however, VPA oral clearance is significantly increased in women taking oral contraceptive pills (21%–45% increase in total and unbound oral clearance, respectively), presumably due to induction of UDP-glucuronyl transferase by ethinyl estradiol.[61]

Co-administration with other highly protein bound drugs may result in protein binding displacement interactions. In one study, concomitant treatment with naproxen resulted in an approximate 20% increase in VPA total plasma clearance. Unlike aspirin, naproxen does not appear to alter VPA intrinsic clearance, so unbound VPA concentrations are not affected.[62]

Bidirectional interactions between VPA and several antiviral and antibiotic agents may also occur. For example, VPA may inhibit the metabolism of antiviral agents such as zidovudine while antibiotics in the carbapenem class have been shown to cause substantial reductions in concentrations of VPA, possibly via interference with its oral absorption.[63]

Table 22-7 shows a number of important drug-drug interactions between valproate and other antiepileptic drugs.

Table 22-7. Impact of Drug-Drug Interactions on the Concentrations of the Interacting Antiepileptic Drug (AED) and Valproic Acid (VPA)

AED	Effect on AED Concentration	Effect on VPA Concentration
Carbamazepine	Increased carbamazepine-epoxide	Decreased
Felbamate	Increased	Increased (≥35%)
Gabapentin, pregabalin	No effect	No effect
Levetiracetam	No effect	No effect
Lamotrigine	Increased	No effect/slight decrease
Lacosamide	No effect	No effect
Phenytoin	Decreased total phenytoin Increased unbound phenytoin	Decreased
Phenobarbital	Increased	Decreased
Primidone	Increased Increased phenobarbital	Decreased
Tiagabine	No effect	No effect/slight decrease
Topiramate	No effect/slight decrease	No effect
Vigabatrin	No effect	No effect

Drug–Disease State or Condition Interactions

In hepatic disease, renal impairment, and pregnancy, an increase in the volume of distribution and percent unbound can be expected due to changes in protein binding.[64] With hepatic cirrhosis, the percent unbound increases to 29%; in renal failure, the percent unbound increases to 18%.[11] Head trauma can also transiently increase VPA percent unbound and total clearance.[65]

References

1. Valproate sodium. In: McEvoy GK, ed. *AHFS Drug Information 2011*. Bethesda, MD: American Society of Health-System Pharmacists; 2011:2329-37.
2. Irvine-Meek JM, Hall KW, Otten NH, et al. Pharmacokinetic study of valproic acid in a neonate. *Pediatr Pharmacol.* 1982;2:317-21.
3. Chiba K, Suganuma T, Ishizaki T, et al. Comparison of steady-state pharmacokinetics of valproic acid in children between monotherapy and multiple antiepileptic drug treatment. *J Pediatr*. 1985;106:653.
4. Cloyd JC, Kriel RL, Fischer JH. Valproic acid pharmacokinetics in children. II. Discontinuation of concomitant antiepileptic drug therapy. *Neurology*. 1985;35:1623-7.
5. Bowdle TA, Patel IH, Levy RH, et al. Valproic acid dosage and plasma protein binding and clearance. *Clin Pharmacol Ther*. 1980;28:486-92.
6. Perucca E, Gatti G, Frigo GM, et al. Pharmacokinetics of valproic acid after oral and intravenous administration. *Br J Clin Pharmacol*. 1978;5:313-8.
7. Limdi NA, Knowlton RK, Cofield SS, et al. Safety of rapid intravenous loading of valproate. *Epilepsia*. 2007;48:478-83.
8. Ramsay RE, Cantrell D, Collins SD, et al. Safety and tolerance of rapidly infused Depacon. A randomized trial in subjects with epilepsy. *Epilepsy Res*. 2003;52:189-201.
9. Yu Kian-Ti, Mills S, Thompson N, et al. Safety and efficacy of intravenous valproate in pediatric status epilepticus and acute repetitive seizures. *Epilepsia*. 2003;44:724-6.
10. Chun AHC, Hoffman DJ, Friedmann N, et al. Bioavailability of valproic acid under fasting/ nonfasting regimens. *J Clin Pharmacol*. 1980;20:30-6.
11. Levy RH, Shen D, Abbott F, et al. Valproic Acid. Chemistry, biotransformation, and pharmacokinetics. In: Levy RH, Mattson RH, Meldrum BS, et al., eds. *Antiepileptic Drugs*. 5th ed. Philadelphia, PA: Lippincott-Williams & Wilkins; 2002:780-800.

12. Dutta S, Reed RC. Distinct absorption characteristics of oral formulations of valproic acid/ divalproex available in the United States. *Epilepsy Res*. 2007;73:275-83.

13. Wilder BJ, Karas BJ, Hammond EJ, et al. Twice daily dosing of valproate with divalproex. *Clin Pharmacol Ther*. 1983;34:501-4.

14. Levy RH, Cenraud B, Loiseau P, et al. Meal-dependent absorption of enteric coated sodium valproate. *Epilepsia*. 1980;21:273-80.

15. Fischer JH, Barr AN, Paloucek FP, et al. Effect of food on the serum concentration profile of enteric-coated valproic acid. *Neurology*. 1988;38(8):1319-22.

16. Dutta S, Zhang Y. Bioavailability of divalproex extended-release formulation relative to the divalproex delayed-release formulation. *Biopharm Drug Dispos*. 2004;25:345-52.

17. Reed RC, Dutta S, Cavanaugh JH, et al. Every 12 hour administration of extended-release divalproex in patients with epilepsy: impact on plasma valproic acid concentrations. *Epilepsy Behav*. 2006;8:391-6.

18. Ahmad AM, Douglas-Boudinot F, Barr WH, et al. The use of Monte Carlo simulations to study the effect of poor compliance on the steady-state concentrations of valproic acid following administration of enteric-coated and extended-release divalproex sodium formulations. *Biopharm Drug Dispos*. 2005;26:417-25.

19. Reed RC, Dutta S. Predicted serum valproic acid concentrations in patients missing and replacing a dose of extended-release divalproex sodium. *Am J Health-Syst Pharm*. 2004;61:2284-9.

20. von Unruh GE, Froescher W, Hoffmann F, et al. Valproic acid in breast milk: how much is really there? *Ther Drug Monit*. 1984;6:272-6.

21. Hall K, Otten N, Irvine-Meek J, et al. First dose and steady state pharmacokinetics of valproic acid in children with seizures. *Clin Pharmacokinet*. 1983;8:447-55.

22. Herngren L, Lundberg B, Negardh A. Pharmacokinetics of total and free valproic acid during monotherapy in infants. *J Neurol*. 1991;238:315-9.

23. Cloyd JC, Fischer JH, Kriel RL, et al. Valproic acid pharmacokinetics in children. IV. Effects of age and antiepileptic drugs on protein binding and intrinsic clearance. *Clin Pharmacol Ther*. 1993;53:22-9.

24. Herngren L, Negardh A. Pharmacokinetics of free and total sodium valproate in adolescents and young adults during maintenance therapy. *J Neurol*. 1988;235:491-5.

25. Bauer LA, Davis R, Wilensky A, et al. Valproic acid clearance: unbound fraction and diurnal variation in young and elderly adults. *Clin Pharmacol Ther*. 1985;37:697-700.

26. Perucca E, Grimaldi R, Gatti G, et al. Pharmacokinetics of valproic acid in the elderly. *Br J Clin Pharmacol*. 1984;17:665-9.

27. Riva R, Albani F, Franzoni E, et al. Valproic acid free fraction in epileptic children under chronic monotherapy. *Ther Drug Monit*. 1983;5:197-200.

28. Gugler R, Schell A, Eichelbaum M, et al. Disposition of valproic acid in man. *Eur J Clin Pharmacol*. 1977;12:125-32.

29. Patel IH, Levy RH. Valproic acid binding to human serum albumin and determination of free fraction in presence of antiepileptics and free fatty acids. *Epilepsia*. 1979;20:85-90.

30. Otten N, Hall K, Irvine-Meek J, et al. Free valproic acid: steady-state pharmacokinetics in patients with intractable epilepsy. *Can J Neurol Sci*. 1984;11:457-60.

31. Cramer JA, Mattson RH. Valproic acid: in vitro plasma protein binding and interactions with phenytoin. *Ther Drug Monit*. 1979;1:105-16.

32. Gidal BE, Collins DM, Deinlich B. Valproic acid neurotoxicity in a hypoalbuminemic patient. *Ann Pharmacother*. 1993;27:32-4.

33. Gidal BE, Maly MM, Spencer NM, et al. Relationship between valproic acid dosage, plasma concentration and clearance in adult monotherapy patients with epilepsy. *J Clin Pharm Ther*. 1995;20:215-9.

34. Bauer LA, Davis R, Wilensky A, et al. Diurnal variation in valproic acid clearance. *Clin Pharmacol Ther*. 1984;35:505-9.

35. Pollock GM, McHugh WB, Gengo FM, et al. Accumulation and washout kinetics of valproic acid and its active metabolite. *J Clin Pharmacol*. 1986;26:668-76.

36. Genton P, Gelise P. Valproic acid. Adverse effects. In: Levy RH, Mattson RH, Meldrum BS, Perucca E, eds. *Antiepileptic Drugs*. 5th ed. Philadelphia, PA: Lippincott-Williams & Wilkins; 2002:837-51.

37. Kiang TK, Ho PC, Anari MR, et al. Contribution of CYP2C9, CYP2A6 and CYP2B6 to valproic acid metabolism in hepatic microsome from individuals with the CYP2C9*1 genotype. *Toxicol Sci*. 2006;94:261-71.

38. Argikar UA, Remmel R. Effect of ageing on glucuronidation of valproic acid in human liver microsomes and the role of UDP-glucuronyltransferase UGT1A4, UGT 1A8 and UGT 1A10. *Drug Metab Dispos*. 2009;37:229-36.

39. Cloyd JC, Kriel RL, Fischer JH, et al. Pharmacokinetics of valproic acid in children: I. Multiple antiepileptic drug therapy. *Neurology*. 1983;33:185-91.

40. Miller BP, Perry W, Moutier CV, et al. Rapid oral loading of extended release divalproex in patients with acute mania. *Gen Hosp Psychiatry*. 2005;27:218-21.

41. Boggs JG, Preis K. Successful initiation of combined therapy with valproate sodium injection and divalproex sodium extended-release tablets in the epilepsy monitoring unit. *Epilepsia*. 2005;46: 949-51.

42. Beydoun A, Sackellares JC, Shu V. Safety and efficacy of divalproex sodium monotherapy in partial epilepsy: A double-blind, concentration-response design clinical trial. Depakote monotherapy for partial seizures study group. *Neurology*. 1997;48:182-8.

43. Treatment of Bipolar Disease. Available at http://www.psychguides.com/content/treatment-bipolar-disorder-2004. Accessed June 20, 2011.

44. Gidal BE, Spencer NW, Collins DM, et al. Valproate mediated disturbances of hemostasis: relationship to concentration and dose. *Neurology*. 1994;44:1418-22.

45. Herzog AG, Blum AS, Farina EL, et al. Valproate and lamotrigine level variation with menstrual cycle phase and oral contraceptive use. *Neurology*. 2009;72:911-4.

46. Dutta S, Zhang Y, Conway JM, et al. Divalproex-ER pharmacokinetics in older children and adolescents. *Pediatr Neurol*. 2004;30:330-7.

47. Reed RC, Dutta S. Does it really matter when a blood sample for valproic acid concentration is taken following once-daily administration of divalproex-ER? *Ther Drug Monit*. 2006;28:413-8.

48. Bowdle TA, Levy RH, Cutler RE. Effects of carbamazepine on valproic acid kinetics in normal subjects. *Clin Pharmacol Ther*. 1979;26:629-34.

49. McKauge L, Tyrer JH, Eadie MJ. Factors influencing simultaneous concentrations of carbamazepine and its epoxide in plasma. *Ther Drug Monit*. 1981;3:63-70.

50. Brodie MJ, Forrest G, Rappeport WG. Carbamazepine 10, 11 epoxide concentrations in epileptics on carbamazepine alone and in combination with other anticonvulsants. *Br J Clin Pharmacol*. 1983;16:747-50.

51. Levy RH, Moreland TA, Moreselli PL, et al. Carbamazepine/ valproic acid interaction in man and rhesus monkey. *Epilepsia*. 1984;25:338-45.

52. Patel IH, Levy RH, Cutler RE. Phenobarbital-valproic acid interaction. *Clin Pharmacol Ther*. 1980;27:515-21.

53. Suganuma T, Ishizaki T, Chiba K, et al. The effect of concurrent administration of valproate sodium on phenobarbital plasma concentration/dosage ratio in pediatric patients. *J Pediatr*. 1981;99: 314-7.

54. Pisani F, Narbone MC, Trunfio C, et al. Valproic acid-ethosuximide interaction: a pharmacokinetic study. *Epilepsia*. 1984;25:229-33.

55. Anderson GD, Yau MK, Gidal BE, et al. Bidirectional interaction of valproate and lamotrigine in healthy subjects. *Clin Pharmacol Ther*. 1996;60:145-56.

56. Gidal BE, Sheth RJ, Parnell J. Evaluation of the valproic acid-lamotrigine pharmacokinetic interaction: Relationship to valproate dose and serum concentration in healthy volunteers. *Neurology*. 2001;56:A331.

57. Anderson GD, Gidal BE, Kantor ED, et al. Lorazepam-valproate interaction: Studies in normal subjects and isolated perfused rat liver. *Epilepsia*. 1994;34:221-5.

58. Goulden KJ, Dooley JM, Camfield PR, et al. Clinical valproate toxicity induced by acetylsalicylic acid. *Neurology*. 1987;37:1392-4.

59. Orr JM, Abbott FS, Farrell K, et al. Interaction between valproic acid and aspirin in epileptic children: serum protein binding and metabolic effects. *Clin Pharmacol Ther*. 1982;31:642-9.

60. Webster LK, Mihlay GW, Jones DB, et al. Effect of cimetidine and ranitidine on carbamazepine and sodium valproate pharmacokinetics. *Eur J Clin Pharmacol*. 1984;27:341-3.

61. Galimberti CA, Mazzucchelli I, Arbasino C, et al. Increased apparent oral clearance of valproic acid during intake of combined contraceptive steroids in women with epilepsy. *Epilepsia*. 2006;47: 1569-72.

62. Addison RS, Parker-Scott SL, Hooper WD, et al. Effect of naproxen co-administration on valproate disposition. *Biopharm Drug Dispos*. 2000;21:235-42.

63. Patsalos PN, Perucca E. Clinically important drug interactions in epilepsy: Interactions between antiepileptic drugs and other drugs. *Lancet Neurology*. 2003;2:473-81.

64. Riva R, Albani F, Contin M, et al. Mechanism of altered drug binding to serum proteins in pregnant women: studies with valproic acid. *Ther Drug Monit*. 1984;6:25-30.

65. Anderson GD, Gidal BE, Hendryx RJ, et al. Decreased plasma protein binding of valproate in patients with acute head trauma. *Br J Clin Pharmacol*. 1994;37:559-62.

Chapter 23

Gary R. Matzke and Jeremiah J. Duby

Vancomycin (AHFS 8:12.28)

Vancomycin is a tricyclic glycopeptide antibiotic that is active against many Gram-positive organisms. It is used principally for the treatment of severe and/or resistant staphylococcal and enterococcal infections, but may also be used for moderate infections in patients who may be allergic to first-line antibiotics (e.g., penicillins). Vancomycin is bactericidal and acts by binding to the C-terminal D-alanyl-D-alanine residue of the pentapeptide cell wall building block, thereby inhibiting cell wall synthesis. Renal excretion is the primary route of elimination and kidney injury is the principle toxicity associated with vancomycin use. Therapeutic drug monitoring (TDM) of vancomycin is evolving as understanding and appreciation of the pharmacokinetic and pharmacodynamic characteristics of the agent evolve. Inter- and intra-patient variability in clearance compels careful consideration on an individual patient basis regarding the need for prospective dosage regimen design and monitoring. Moreover, the role of vancomycin as a mainstay of therapy for Gram-positive infections has been redefined over the past decade in part as the result of insidious changes in susceptibility. Optimizing the benefit and managing potential risks of intermediate and long-term exposure to vancomycin appear to be more important than ever.

Usual Dosage Range in Absence of Clearance-Altering Factors

Dosing weight

Actual body weight (ABW) appears to represent the anthropometric measure with the closest correlation to steady state volume of distribution and to total body clearance of vancomycin.[1] Weight-based dosing based on ABW is especially important for markedly obese patients as standard empiric dosing (e.g., 1 g IV every 12 hr) is likely to result in subtherapeutic exposure.[2] Increasing the frequency over which the empiric total daily dose is divided and extending the infusion time may be beneficial and necessary to assure that adequate concentrations are maintained for obese patients.

Loading dose

The primary advantage of a vancomycin loading dose is earlier attainment of desired concentrations. The potential benefit is likely greatest for patients with severe infections, critical illness, impaired renal function, and/or obesity.[3] A low daily maintenance dose (e.g., 500–1,000 mg/d) is likely to result in a pronounced delay (72–96 hours) in the achievement of target serum concentrations in patients with diminished clearance or an expanded volume of distribution. Loading doses of 25–30 mg/kg (ABW) are recommended for patients with normal renal function[4]; however, doses of 20–25 mg/kg may be appropriate for patients with stage 4 or 5 chronic kidney disease (CKD).

Empiric maintenance doses

Standard maintenance doses are shown in Table 23-1.[5-10]

Alternative method of administration: continuous infusion

Administration of vancomycin by continuous infusion would, in theory, be optimal since it appears to display concentration-independent bactericidal activity and a continuous infusion would maintain higher, sustained concentrations relative to the MIC of the pathogen. However, several studies have found no clinical or microbiological advantage associated with this dosing strategy, though cost savings were realized.[8–16] While a single study conducted in healthy volunteers found poorer tolerability of vancomycin when it was administered as a continuous infusion,[17] the majority of studies found comparable tolerability.[11-14] Continuous infusion may be advantageous for patients with very high clearance (e.g., burns, neurosurgery, trauma) or for whom relatively high doses of vancomycin (i.e. >4 g/d in adults) may be necessary. Pea and co-workers developed an equation

Table 23-1. Maintenance Doses and Dosing Intervals in Patients with Normal Renal Function for Age

Dosage Form	Maintenance Dosage (mg/kg)[a]	Interval (hr)
Intravenous		
Premature neonates[5,6]		
<27 weeks PCA,[b] and <0.8 kg	18	36
27–30 weeks PCA,[b] and 0.8–1.2 kg	18	24
31–36 weeks PCA,[b] and 1.2–2 kg	18	18
>36 weeks PCA,[b] and >2 kg	15	12
Full-term neonates[7]		
<2 kg		
0–7 days	12.5	12
8–28 days	15	12
>2 kg		
0–7 days	18	12
8–28 days	22	12
Infants (>1 week to <60 days of age)[8] with creatinine (mg/dl) of:		
≥1.7 kg	15	48
1.3–1.6	10	24
1.0–1.2	15	24
0.7–0.9	20	24
Infants and children (≥28 days – <16 years)[7]	10–15	6
Adults (≥16 –<65 years)[7]	15	12
Geriatrics (>65 years)[7]	10–15	12–24
Oral (treatment of pseudomembranous colitis only)[9]		
Children (<20 kg and ≥1–≤16 years)	12.5	6
Adults (>16–<65 years)	125–500 mg[c]	6–8
Intrathecal[10]		
Neonates, infants, and children (<16 years)	5–10 mg[c]	24
Adults (≥16–<65 years)	10–20 mg[c]	24

[a]Weight = actual body weight.
[b]PCA = Postconceptional age: the sum of the gestational age at birth and chronological age.
[c]Note dose in mg and not mg/kg.

to guide dosing based on target steady state concentrations and estimated creatinine clearance, below.[18]

$$\text{Infusion rate (g/24 hr)} = [0.029 \times \text{CrCl (ml/min)} + 0.94] \times [\text{target } Css_{av} \times (0.024)]$$

where infusion rate is expressed in g/24 hr, CrCl is the estimated creatinine clearance of the patient expressed in ml/min, and Css_{av} is the desired average steady state concentration.

Dosage Form Availability[19]

Vancomycin is available in oral and intravenous forms (see Table 23-2). Oral therapy is reserved for the treatment of pseudomembranous colitis and since systemic absorption is minimal, concentration monitoring is not warranted for most patients.

General Pharmacokinetic Information

Absorption

The absolute bioavailability of orally administered vancomycin is generally poor (<5%) in those with an intact gastrointestinal tract. However, elevated concentrations have been noted after oral dosing in patients with pseudomembranous colitis and/or severe renal failure.[20] Serum concentrations in the therapeutic range have been reported in these patients, so periodic monitoring should be considered, especially for patients receiving >2 g/day for ≥10 days. Table 23-3 provides the bioavailability for the dosage forms.

Volume of distribution (V)

The disposition of vancomycin after intravenous administration as an intermittent infusion (30–90 minute duration) is best characterized by a three-compartment pharmacokinetic model. The early distribution phases are generally not observed during clinical use due to the relatively long infusion rate. Blood samples are also usually obtained after distribution is complete for practical reasons (i.e., to facilitate calculations based on one-compartment model). The half-life of the initial distribution phase is approximately 7 min and that of the second phase is approximately 0.5–1 hr. Population volume of distribution values are highly variable, as shown in Table 23-4.[5,6,8,21-31]

Protein binding

The plasma protein binding of vancomycin ranges from 30% to 55% and is dependent on the patient's albumin concentration. In patients with hypoalbuminemia, the protein binding is lower. For example, in end-stage renal disease and burn patients, mean protein binding values of 19% and 29%, respectively, have been reported.[32,33]

Elimination

Vancomycin is primarily eliminated by glomerular filtration; approximately 80%–90% of an intravenously administered dose is recovered unchanged in the urine of adult patients with normal renal function.[20] Therefore, dosage adjustment is necessary for those with disease- and/or age-related alterations in renal function. The nonrenal clearance of vancomycin ranges from <5% to as high as 20% of total body clearance. Vancomycin undergoes biliary excretion, but the typical amount of drug eliminated in bile has not been established.[34] There are no active or inactive metabolites of vancomycin, but crystalline degradation products (CDP-1) have been noted to form in a time and temperature dependent manner (see Assay Issues for discussion of clinical relevance). Limited data in patients with hepatic impairment suggests that dosage adjustment is not warranted.

Clearance

Clearance values for various patient populations are shown in Table 23-5.[5,8,22-28,30,31,35] Renal function is the primary determinant of a patient's ability to clear vancomycin.

Half-life and time to steady state

The terminal elimination half-life ranges from 3 to 9 hr in adults with normal renal function (i.e., creatinine clearance of >80 ml/min/1.73 m^2). Table 23-6 shows the half-life values by age group and corresponding time to steady state values.[5,21,23-28,35]

Table 23-2. Available Dosage Forms

Dosage Form	Product (Manufacturer)
Powder for intravenous injection: 500 mg, 1 g, 5 g, and 10 g per vial	Vancomycin HCl (multiple)
Frozen premix in plastic container for injection: 500 mg/100 ml and 1 g/200 ml	Vancocin (Baxter Healthcare)
Oral capsules: 125 mg and 250 mg	Vancocin HCL (Viropharma)

Table 23-3. Bioavailability of Dosage Forms

Dosage Form	Bioavailability	Comments
Intravenous	100%	
Intramuscular (IM)	Not determined	Not recommended for IM use
Oral capsules and powder	<5%	Increased in pseudomembranous colitis

Table 23-4. Volume of Distribution by Age Grouping

Age	Volume L/kg (Mean ± SD)[a]
Premature neonates[5,6]	
27–30 weeks PCA[b]	0.55 ± 0.02
31–36 weeks PCA[b]	0.56 ± 0.02
>37 weeks PCA[b]	0.57 ± 0.02
Infants and full-term neonates[6,8,21]	0.69–0.79[c]
Infants (≥1 month – <1 year)[21]	0.69 ± 0.17
Children (2.5–11 years)[22]	0.63 ± 0.16
Adults (≥16 – <65 years)[23–28]	0.62 ± 0.15
Obese adults (>30% over IBW[d])[29]	0.56 ± 0.18
Adults with severe renal impairment[26,27]	0.90 ± 0.21
Geriatrics (≥65 years)[23]	0.76 ± 0.06
Critically ill[e] adults (42–76 years)[30,31]	1.69 ± 2.19

[a]Actual body weight.
[b]PCA = postconceptional age: the sum of the gestational age at birth and chronological age.
[c]Range rather than ± SD.
[d]IBW = ideal body weight.
[e]Medical intensive care unit patients.

Table 23-5. Average Clearance Values by Age Grouping

Age	Clearance L/hr/kg (Mean ± SD)
Premature neonates[5]	
27–30 weeks PCA[a]	0.06 ± 0.004
31–36 weeks PCA[a]	0.07 ± 0.004
>37 weeks PCA[a]	0.08 ± 0.004
Infants and full-term neonates[8]	0.07 ± 0.021
Children (2.5–11 years)[22]	0.11 ± 0.02
Adults (≥16 – <65 years)[23–28,35]	0.07 ± 0.025
Geriatrics (≥65 years)[23]	0.05 ± 0.003
Critically ill[b] adults (42–76 years)[30,31]	0.05 ± 0.037

[a]PCA = postconceptional age: the sum of the gestational age at birth and chronological age.
[b]Medical intensive care patients.

Dosing Strategies

A variety of approaches have been proposed for the dosing of vancomycin. These range from use of standard doses and little to no concentration monitoring, to dosing nomograms, to prediction of population pharmacokinetic parameters to initiate dosing, to full pharmacokinetic analysis. The use of therapeutic drug monitoring as part of dosing strategies is discussed later.

Population Pharmacokinetic Parameters

The approaches below allow prediction of clearance or half-life, which can then be matched with estimates of volume of distribution to develop initial dosage regimens designed to produce desired vancomycin concentrations. Follow-up with measured concentrations may be necessary to ensure that the desired concentrations are achieved.

A population pharmacokinetic and covariate analysis, conducted in 214 premature neonates with an average postconceptional age of 30.4 weeks, revealed that weight, postconceptional age, and renal function explained

Table 23-6. Half-Life and Time to Steady State by Age Grouping

Age	Half-Life (Mean ± SD)	Time to Steady State (hr)[a]
Premature neonates[5]		
27–30 weeks PCA[b]	6.6 ± 0.4 hr	31–35
31–36 weeks PCA[b]	5.6 ± 0.4 hr	26–30
>37 weeks PCA[b]	4.9 ± 0.4 hr	23–27
Full-term neonates[21]	6.7 hr	34
Infants (≥1 month–<1 year)[21]	4.1 hr	21
Children (2.5–11 years)[21]	5.6 ± 2.1 hr	18–39
Adults (≥16–<65 years)[23–28,35]	7.0 ± 1.5 hr	28–43
Adults with moderate to severe renal impairment (CrCl 10–60 ml/min)[26,27]	32 ± 19 hr	2.7–10.6 days
Geriatrics (≥65 years)[23]	12.1 ± 0.8 hr	57–65

[a]Time to steady state determined by assuming five half-lives was sufficient for steady state and using ± one SD of the mean t½.
[b]PCA = postconceptional age: the sum of the gestational age at birth and chronological age.

49.8%, 18.2%, and 14.1% of the variability observed in vancomycin clearance.[36] Several equations have been developed that relate vancomycin clearance to patient-specific variables in babies including postconceptional age, body weight, and CrCl.[8,37] For example, a population pharmacokinetic analysis of vancomycin concentration-time data obtained from 374 infants with a median postnatal age of 70 days and a median gestational age of 33.5 weeks, yielded the following equation.[8]

$$CL_{Vanc}\,(L/hr) = [W \times ((0.028/S_{cr}) + (0.000127 \times Age) + (0.0123 \times GA28))] + 0.006$$

where, W = weight (kg); S_{cr} = serum creatinine (mg/dl); Age = postnatal age (days) if S_{cr} <0.7 mg/dl (62 μmol/L in SI units) or Age = 0 if $S_{cr} \geq 0.7$ mg/dl (62 μmol/L); GA28 is 1 if gestational age >28 weeks and 0 if gestational age ≤ 28 weeks.

For adult patients, many investigators have evaluated the relationship between vancomycin clearance and CrCl, and several regression equations have been proposed for the prediction of pharmacokinetic parameters.[23,26,27,29,38-42] A comparison of seven published methods was conducted to determine which best predicted vancomycin serum concentrations that were measured in 189 patients of a community teaching hospital.[43] The method depicted below, which was determined using a one-compartment model,[26] performed the best, yielding the least bias [mean error (95%CI):–0.84(–1.70,0.02)] and best precision [root mean-squared error (95% CI) 6.05 (–3.77, 15.87)]. The authors cautioned that none of the methods were suitable to replace therapeutic drug monitoring in most patients:

$$CL_{Vanc}\,(ml/min) = 0.689(CrCl) + 3.66$$

where CrCl is in ml/min.

The elimination rate constant (*k*) of vancomycin can be predicted from the observed relationship with CrCl in adult patients with reduced renal function (CrCl <50 ml/min), as determined by numerous investigators. The following regression equation approximates the mean of the reported values and was determined using a one-compartment pharmacokinetic model[26]:

$$k\,(hr^{-1}) = 0.00083(CrCl) + 0.0044$$

where CrCl is in ml/min.

Such equations should be used with caution in patients with acute renal failure due to the unpredictable nonrenal clearance component (intercept term), though patients with severe chronic kidney disease and/or end stage renal disease do not appear to exhibit significant nonrenal clearance of vancomycin.

Therapeutic Range

Although a wide degree of interpatient variability is associated with vancomycin pharmacokinetics, concentration monitoring remains controversial because no clear relationship between serum concentrations and therapeutic response or toxicity is evident.[44-47] The peak concentration values reported in the literature are often confounded by the timing of the blood sample relative to the end of the infusion and vancomycin's multi-compartment pharmacokinetics. Conventional vancomycin therapy based on achieving peak concentrations of 30–40 mg/L and trough concentrations of less than 10–20 mg/L is based on empirical rather than scientific evidence. However, there is consensus that the monitoring of trough concentrations is prudent to ensure that they exceed the MIC of the pathogen in order to optimize efficacy and decrease the likelihood of resistance development.[15,46,48-50] Peak concentrations do not appear to correlate with safety or efficacy. The role of monitoring peaks is largely limited to estimating patient-specific pharmacokinetic parameters (i.e., k and V) for complex patients (e.g., those with critical illnesses, acute kidney injury, or stage 5 CKD). Peak concentrations should be drawn 1.5–2.5 hr after a 1-hr infusion or approximately 1 hr after a 2-hr infusion to allow for distribution, and the reference window for trough concentrations is within 30 minutes of the next scheduled dose. Table 23-7 provides the desired ranges for vancomycin trough concentrations.

Individualization of vancomycin therapy by means of concentration monitoring may be necessary for certain patient groups, including those with fluctuating renal function, patients receiving concurrent treatment with known nephrotoxins (e.g., aminoglycosides or furosemide), patients requiring higher than usual doses (>4 g/day), obese patients (those whose ABW is >30% over IBW), patients receiving dialysis, and pediatric patients (especially premature neonates).[44,45,51] Although there is some controversy regarding the need for concentration monitoring, vancomycin pharmacokinetics are unpredictable in these patient populations, so obtaining concentrations early in therapy will help ensure that trough concentrations are within the therapeutic range (i.e., above MIC). For patients with stable, normal renal function, obtaining a trough concentration after 3–5 days of therapy is usually adequate, if therapy is to be continued for 7–10 days or longer.[45] If the measured trough concentration is within 20% of the desired trough concentration, the patient may remain on the same regimen. If the concentration is not within the desired range, the dosing regimen should be adjusted proportionally. Vancomycin trough concentration monitoring should be repeated if there is a change in renal function (e.g., increase in serum creatinine of 0.5 mg/dl or 50%, whichever is greater) or a lack of therapeutic response despite documentation of the presence of a sensitive organism.

Due to the variability in vancomycin removal by dialysis with biocompatible membranes (non-cellulose-based dialyzers such as polysulfone and polymethylmethacrylate), blood samples for serum concentration

Table 23-7. Therapeutic Range[44,45,51]

Target Range and Indications for Monitoring	
Peak	
1.5–2.5 hours after infusion	No value recommended
Trough	
≤30 minutes before infusion	10–15 mg/L: conventional 15–20 mg/L: deep-seated infection, pneumonia, critical illness, dialysis
Indications for Monitoring	
↑ risk of treatment failure	Critical illness, severe sepsis/septic shock Deep-seated infections (i.e., CNS, osteomyelitis, endocarditis, pneumonia)
↑ risk of toxicity	Chronic kidney disease, acute kidney injury Critical illness Obesity (>30% above IBW) Concurrent nephrotoxin use (e.g., aminoglycosides, loop diuretics) High-dose therapy (>4 g/d) Pediatric patients (especially premature neonates)
Clinical course	Substantial changes in renal function Signs/symptoms of treatment failure Signs/symptoms of toxicity

determination should be obtained at least 2 hr after the end of dialysis, to allow for vancomycin redistribution from tissues.

The goal of treatment is to maximize the interaction between the drug and the pathogen by achieving adequate drug concentration at the site of infection. Vancomycin penetration to the lung, which is an important consideration in the treatment of Gram-positive pneumonia, is hindered because it is a large, polar molecule that is partially ionized at physiological pH and is 30% to 55% protein bound.[52] The mean serum to lung penetration ratio was found to be 6 to 1 in critically ill patients with MRSA pneumonia.[53] Therefore, when vancomycin is used to treat infections of the lung, dosage regimens should be designed to achieve trough concentrations at the higher end of the therapeutic range (15–20 mg/L) to maximize lung penetration.[50]

Pharmacodynamic Monitoring

Minimum inhibitory concentration (MIC) and efficacy

The Clinical and Laboratory Standards Institute (CLSI) changed the susceptibility breakpoint for the minimum inhibitory concentration (MIC) of vancomycin for *Staphylococcus aureus* from ≤4 mg/L to ≤2 mg/L in 2006.[54] Subsequent studies suggest substantially higher rates of treatment failure are associated with MICs above 1 mg/L. Sakoulas and colleagues identified a strong relationship with MICs of 1–2 mg/L and signs of clinical treatment failure of vancomycin for MRSA infections in a post hoc analysis of a prospective phase II/III trials.[55] In a similar study, Moise and co-workers demonstrated a 75% eradication rate of MRSA bacteremia for isolates with vancomycin MICs ≤1 mg/L, but a 79% treatment failure rate for those organisms with MICs of >1 mg/L but ≤2 mg/L. A 14.7 odds ratio for treatment failure was associated with MICs between 1 and 2 mg/L.[56] Lodise and colleagues demonstrated an association between an MIC breakpoint ≥1.5 mg/L and treatment failure.[57] The role of vancomycin for infections due to MRSA with MICs >2 mg/L appears to be limited, which is reflected in a practice guideline that recommends consideration of alternative therapy.[4]

Concentration-related efficacy

Historically, vancomycin has been classified as a concentration-independent or time-dependent killing agent, whereby the achievement of concentrations in excess of 4–5 times the minimum inhibitory concentration (MIC) of the pathogen do not result in an enhanced bactericidal effect.[58] Optimization of time-dependent killing agents relies upon maximization of the duration of time (T) the drug concentration exceeds the MIC of the pathogen (T > MIC). Vancomycin has been found to exhibit time-dependent killing in several in-vitro studies; however, other studies indicate a lack of association with the T > MIC.[59-63] These latter studies reveal that vancomycin activity may be more appropriately predicted by the AUC/MIC ratio, the pharmacodynamic parameter that indexes total drug exposure or the area under the concentration-time curve (AUC) to the MIC of the pathogen.[61,62]

Clinical studies evaluating vancomycin pharmacodynamics are rare and largely inconclusive. A relatively recent study conducted in 108 patients with MRSA pneumonia documented a superior clinical and bacteriological response to vancomycin therapy in those with a 24-hr AUC/MIC of ≥400 as compared to those with a 24-hr AUC/MIC <400. No association was found between T > MIC and response.[64] The 24-hr AUC/MIC value based on the estimated creatinine clearance of the patient, the 24-hr administration regimen, and the MIC value for the bacterial isolate is depicted below[27]:

$$AUC_{24} = \frac{D}{[(CrCl \times 0.79) + 15.4] \times 0.06}$$

where AUC_{24} is the 24-hr area under the curve expressed as mg × h/L, CrCl is the estimated creatinine clearance of the patient expressed in ml/min, and D is the vancomycin dosage in mg/24 hr. The calculated AUC is then divided by the MIC of the infecting organism.

Further well-designed pharmacodynamic studies are needed to fully elucidate the relationship of vancomycin concentration and patient outcomes. In the interim, since the routine determination AUC/MIC is not practical, the monitoring of trough concentrations seems prudent and consistent with current clinical practice guidelines.

The signs and symptoms of infection must also be used as an indicator to assess vancomycin efficacy. The patient's temperature and white blood cell count should be monitored daily for return to normal, and blood cultures should be repeated every 3 days until negative. The ratio of the minimal bactericidal concentration (MBC) to the MIC can also be used to monitor or predict the response to therapy; an MBC:MIC ratio of greater than 32:1 is associated with poor therapeutic response.[63] The MBC need not be determined routinely, but may be warranted in patients who are not responding to therapy or who have a serious infection (e.g., endocarditis and osteomyelitis).

Concentration-related toxicity

Although ototoxicity and nephrotoxicity have been historically associated with vancomycin therapy, the incidence is generally <2% and <5%, respectively. The original association of vancomycin with ototoxicity was based on two cases reported in 1958 of patients who experienced hearing loss and had a vancomycin concentration of greater than 80 mg/L. Additional case reports followed; however, evidence of a direct cause and effect relationship with vancomycin was lacking since most patients were receiving other agents known to be ototoxic such as aminoglycosides and erythromycin. These early reports are the foundational premise for the suspected relationship between attainment of peak concentrations of >30–50 mg/L and/or trough concentrations of >10–20 mg/L and ototoxicity. Later studies did not reveal an association with vancomycin concentration dose or duration of therapy and ototoxicity.[46,47]

Retrospective studies demonstrate an association between higher vancomycin trough concentrations and acute kidney injury, defined by increased serum creatinine.[65-68] Nevertheless, an emphasis on dosing to achieve higher target trough concentrations calls to question the risk-benefit of aggressive therapy. Two studies appear to circumvent the circular causality to provide reasonable estimations of risk based on stratification by dosing or exposure. Hidayat and colleagues investigated the effects of aggressive vancomycin dosing on treatment outcomes in patients with MRSA infections in a prospective cohort study.[69] Achievement of high trough concentration (15–20 mg/L) was associated with a superior clinical response and a substantially higher rate of nephrotoxicity. However, the observed difference was confounded by a higher concomitant use of nephrotoxic agents in the high trough group. Lodise and co-workers conducted a retrospective cohort study that stratified patients based on vancomycin exposure as measured by initial trough vancomycin concentrations.[70] The persuasive element of the design was the use of the highest initial trough concentration within the first 96 hours of treatment as the index of vancomycin exposure. The observed rates of nephrotoxicity were 5%, 21%, 20%, and 33% for patients with initial vancomycin trough concentrations of <10, 10–15, 15–20, and >20 mg/dL, respectively. Of note, there was no difference in the rates of nephrotoxicity for patients with levels of 10–15 and 15–20 mg/dl, and the mean AUC24 for patients that did not experience nephrotoxicity was nearly 900 mg x hr/L.

Common risk factors for nephrotoxicity include concomitant use of other nephrotoxins (e.g., aminoglycosides, amphotericin B), increased duration of therapy (>14 days), critical illness on initiation of therapy, and morbid obesity.[65-69] Early adjustment of vancomycin dosage to produce concentrations in the recommended therapeutic range may potentially minimize these toxicities.[20] Serum creatinine should be monitored every 3 days for patients with stable renal function and daily if the patient has unstable renal function or is receiving other nephrotoxic agents (e.g., aminoglycosides, loop diuretics, and amphotericin B).

Non-concentration-related toxicities

Intravenous administration of vancomycin may result in a histamine-like reaction characterized by flushing, tingling, pruritus, tachycardia, and an erythematous macular rash involving the face, neck, upper trunk, back, and arms. This adverse effect is often referred to as "red man syndrome." Systemic arterial hypotension or shock may also occur. This syndrome usually can be avoided by infusion of vancomycin at 15 mg/min or less or by pretreatment with an antihistamine. Eosinophilia, neutropenia, urticarial rashes, and drug fever also have been reported.[19,20]

Drug-Drug Interactions

No pharmacokinetic drug interactions have been reported with vancomycin. However, its concomitant use with other ototoxic and nephrotoxic drugs may increase the incidence of these toxicities. Data from several investigations indicate that vancomycin has the potential for producing nephrotoxicity, with the incidence ranging from 5% to 15%. When vancomycin was administered concomitantly with an *aminoglycoside* to adults, the incidence of nephrotoxicity increased in some, but not all, studies (range of 22%–35%).[20,71]

Concurrent use of a *loop diuretic* (e.g., furosemide) was associated with a 5-fold increase in the risk of developing nephrotoxicity; the risk may be greatest in individuals over 60 years of age.[72] Finally, concomitant amphotericin B was shown to increase the risk of nephrotoxicity by 6.7-fold.[72]

There is evidence to suggest that the elimination half-life of vancomycin is prolonged and clearance is decreased in neonates receiving indomethacin to induce closure of a patent ductus arteriosus. Thus, an empiric increase in the vancomycin dosing interval and concentration monitoring may be initially warranted.[6,37]

Drug–Disease State Interactions

The following disease states or conditions alter vancomycin disposition. Patients with *burn injuries* require more frequent doses of vancomycin to achieve similar target concentrations.[33,73,74] The total body clearance and renal clearance in these patients are highly correlated with CrCl,[61,62] and the increase in drug clearance appears to be due to a significant nonrenal component, as well as enhanced net tubular secretion.[46] Due to increased drug clearance, the half-life of vancomycin in burn patients averages 4 hours, so more frequent dosing (i.e., every 6 to 8 hours) may be necessary. The volume of distribution is unaltered.

Hepatic insufficiency has not been associated with any alteration in the elimination of vancomycin. The degree of protein binding, however, is reduced (to approximately 20%) and the unbound V increases by approximately 8% during serious infections.[75] The volume of distribution of vancomycin is increased in *critically ill* patients.[30,31] The larger volume may require the initial administration of higher than normal doses (i.e., >30 mg/kg/day in adults) in order to achieve therapeutic concentrations. Vancomycin therapy should be guided in these patients on the basis of their residual renal function (CrCl), volume status, and concentration monitoring may be warranted because of the marked variability in volume of distribution.

The impact of acute renal failure on the disposition of vancomycin is dependent on the severity and acuity of the insult. Nonrenal clearance of 0.96–1.2 L/hr is preserved for up to 7–10 days after injury, making the relationship between CrCl and CL_{Vanc} derived from patients with chronic kidney disease is not useful in projecting the degree of dosage adjustment.[76] Patients who are receiving intermittent hemodialysis (HD) with a high flux dialyzer or continuous renal replacement therapy (CRRT) require higher dosage regimens than those who are receiving HD with a low flux (cellulose, cellulose acetate, or cuprophane) dialyzer or no renal replacement therapy.[77,78] Furthermore, if the drug is given during CRRT or HD, the dosage may need to be increased further due to the enhanced rate of removal.[79,80]

Vancomycin clearance by the continuous venovenous hemofiltration (CVVH) is determined by the sieving coefficient (SC) and ultrafiltration flow rate (UFR) [$CL_{CVVH} = UFR \times SC$]. Vancomycin clearance by continuous venovenous hemodialysis (CVVHD) can be estimated by adding the filtration and dialytic clearances [$CL_{CVVHD} = (UFR \times SC) + (DFR \times SC)$], where DFR is the dialysate flow rate. Table 23-8 lists examples of sieving coefficients reported for vancomycin during CRRT.

Table 23-8. Examples of Sieving Coefficients During CRRT

Filter Membrane	Sieving Coefficient
AN69[77]	0.70
Polymethylmethacrylate[77]	0.86
Polysulfone[77,78]	0.68–0.80

Dosing and Concentration Monitoring in Hemodialysis Patients

Vancomycin is not significantly dialyzed by low-flux hemodialysis membranes made from cellulose acetate or cuprophane, but is significantly removed by high-flux membranes such as polysulfone, cellulose triacetate, and polymethylmethacrylate. Current guidelines suggest the maintenance of vancomycin trough concentrations of 15–20 mg/L and/or a 24-hour AUC/MIC ratio of greater than or equal to 400 for hemodialysis patients.[4]

The vancomycin concentrations for patients undergoing chronic intermittent hemodialysis will decrease during the dialysis session and then increase 3 to 6 hours after cessation of dialysis due to redistribution from tissues. In these patients, the blood samples for trough vancomycin concentration determination should be obtained immediately prior to the hemodialysis session and if it is within the desired range the current dosage regimen can be continued. If not, proportional dosage adjustments should be made.

Vancomycin use in chronic hemodialysis patients is complicated by the near absence of nonrenal clearance (residual of 0–0.24 L/hr) and the impact of the hemodialysis procedure. The dialytic clearance is dependent on the dialyzer membrane and the rate of blood flow through it.[80-84] The intradialytic clearance and $t\frac{1}{2}$ of vancomycin observed in chronic hemodialysis patients for some commonly used dialyzers are presented in Table 23-9. A more comprehensive listing of vancomycin clearance values for various dialysis filters can be found in a review.[84] When a high-flux hemodialysis membrane is used, an initial vancomycin dose of 20 mg/kg rounded to the nearest 100 mg should be administered. Vancomycin maintenance doses in this patient population typically range from 500 mg to 1 g (administered after dialysis) depending on the vancomycin concentration determined prior to dialysis.[80,85] A study conducted in 55 patients undergoing chronic intermittent hemodialysis with a high-flux polysulfone membrane found that a vancomycin dose of 500 mg administered with each dialysis session was superior to 20 mg/kg every second dialysis session in achieving and maintaining desired vancomycin concentrations.[86]

Table 23-9. Intradialytic Clearance and t½ for Commonly Used Dialyzers[84]

Dialyzer	CL (L/hr)	*t*½ (hr)
Cellulose/cellulose acetate	0.25–3.6	na[a]
Cuprophane	0.3–1	35.1
Cellulose triacetate	6.0	4.5
Polymethylmethacrylate	3.6–7.9	3.7–8.0
Polysulfone	3.8–7.8	4.7

[a]Not available.

Assay issues

Vancomycin concentrations can be determined by a variety of methods including enzyme multiplied immunoassay (EMIT), fluorescence polarization immunoassay (FPIA), high performance liquid chromatography (HPLC), and radioimmunoassay (RIA), with FPIA methods being used most often in clinical laboratories.[20] The FPIA methods used have similar reproducibility (precision), but differ significantly in accuracy due to cross-reactivity with inactive vancomycin crystalline degradation products (CDP-1).[87,88] All of the FPIA methods are based on polyclonal antibodies (pFPIA), except for the Abbott AxSYM system, which is based on a murine monoclonal antibody (mFPIA). Vancomycin spontaneously degrades into CDP-1 in a time and temperature dependent manner due to prolonged exposure to body temperature. CDP-1 accumulates in patients with renal impairment, particularly dialysis patients, and results in falsely elevated concentrations when measured by pFPIA methods.[88] The overestimation of vancomycin concentration can be large enough to impact dosing decisions; with typical overestimation of 36%–59%, but as high as 127% reported.[89-91] However, there is no cross reactivity with the AxSYM mFPIA method or EMIT methods, which are also based on a monoclonal antibody.[89-91]

References

1. Blouin RA, Bauer LA, Miller DD, et al. Vancomycin pharmacokinetics in normal and morbidly obese subjects. *Antimicrob Agents Chemother*. 1982;21(4):575-80.
2. Vance Bryan K, Guay DR, Gilliland SS, et al. Effect of obesity on vancomycin pharmacokinetic parameters as determined by using a Bayesian forecasting technique. *Antimicrob Agents Chemother*. 1993;37(3):436-40.
3. Wang JT, Fang CT, Chen YC, et al. Necessity of a loading dose when using vancomycin in critically ill patients. *J Antimicrob Chemother.* 2001;47(2):246.
4. Rybak MJ, Lomaestro BM, Rotschafer JC, et al. Vancomycin therapeutic guidelines: a summary of consensus recommendations from the Infectious Diseases Society of America, the American Society of Health-System Pharmacists, and the Society of Infectious Diseases Pharmacists. *Am J Health-Syst Pharm.* 2009;66:82-98.

5. McDougal A, Ling EW, Levine M. Vancomycin pharmacokinetics and dosing in premature neonates. *Ther Drug Monit.* 1995;17:319-26.

6. de Hoog M, Mouton JW, van den Anker J. Vancomycin pharmacokinetics and administration regimens in neonates. *Clin Pharmacokinet.* 2004;43(7):417-40.

7. Gilbert DN, Moellering RC, Eliopoulos GM, et al., eds. *The Sanford Guide to Antimicrobial Therapy 2010.* 36th ed. Sperryville, VA: Antimicrobial Therapy Inc; 2010:133.

8. Capparelli EV, Lane JR, Romanowski GL, et al. The influences of renal function and maturation on vancomycin elimination in newborns and infants. *J Clin Pharmacol.* 2001;41(9):927-34.

9. Malnick SDH, Zimhony O. Treatment of *Clostridium difficile*-associated diarrhea. *Ann Pharmacotherpy.* 2002;36:1767-75.

10. Luer MS, Hatton J. Vancomycin administration into the cerebrospinal fluid: a review. *Ann Pharmacotherapy.* 1993;27:912-21.

11. Di Filippo A, De Gaudio AR, Novelli A, et al. Continuous infusion of vancomycin in methicillin resistant staphylococcus infection. *Chemotherapy.* 1998;44(1):63-8.

12. Wysocki M, Thomas F, Wolff MA, et al. Comparison of continuous with discontinuous intravenous infusion of vancomycin in severe MRSA infections. *J Antimicrob Chemother.* 1995;35(2):352-4.

13. James JK, Palmer SM, Levine DP, et al. Comparison of conventional dosing versus continuous infusion vancomycin therapy for patients with suspected or documented gram-positive infections. *Antimicrob Agents Chemother.* 1996;40(3):696-700.

14. Wysocki M, Delatour F, Faurisson F, et al. Continuous versus intermittent infusion of vancomycin in severe Staphylococcal infections: prospective multicenter randomized study. *Antimicrob Agents Chemother.* 2001;45(9):2460-7.

15. Kitzis MD, Goldstein FW. Monitoring of vancomycin serum levels for the treatment of staphylococcal infections. *Clin Microbiol Infect.* 2006;12(1):92-5.

16. Vuagnat A, Stern R, Lotthe A, et al. High dose vancomycin for osteomyelitis: continuous vs. intermittent infusion. *J Clin Pharm Ther.* 2004;29:351-7.

17. Klepser ME, Patel KB, Nicolau DP, et al. Comparison of bactericidal activities of intermittent and continuous infusion dosing of vancomycin against methicillin-resistant Staphylococcus aureus and Enterococcus faecalis. *Pharmacotherapy.* 1998;18(5):1069-74.

18. Pea F, Furlanut M, Negri C, et al. Prospectively validated dosing nomograms for maximizing the pharmacodynamics of vancomycin administered by continuous infusion in critically ill patients. *Antimicrob Agents Chemother.* 2009;53:1863-7.

19. Vancomycin. In: *Drug Facts and Comparisons.* St. Louis, MO: Facts and Comparisons; 2007:1313.

20. Moise-Broder PA. Vancomycin. In: Burton ME, Shaw LM, Schentag JJ, et al., eds. *Applied Pharmacokinetics & Pharmacodynamics: Principals of Therapeutic Drug Monitoring.* Baltimore, MD: Lippincott Williams & Wilkins; 2006:328-40.

21. Schaad UB, McCracken GH, Jr., Nelson JD. Clinical pharmacology and efficacy of vancomycin in pediatric patients. *J Pediatr.* 1980;96(1):119-26.

22. Wrishko RE, Levine M, Khoo D, et al. Vancomycin pharmacokinetics and Bayesian estimation in pediatric patients. *Ther Drug Monit.* 2000;22(5):522-31.

23. Cutler NR, Narang PK, Lesko LJ, et al. Vancomycin disposition: the importance of age. *Clin Pharmacol Ther.* 1984;36(6):803-10.

24. Golper TA, Noonan HM, Elzinga L, et al. Vancomycin pharmacokinetics, renal handling, and nonrenal clearances in normal human subjects. *Clin Pharmacol Ther.* 1988;43(5):565-70.

25. Healy DP, Polk RE, Garson ML, et al. Comparison of steady-state pharmacokinetics of two dosage regimens of vancomycin in normal volunteers. *Antimicrob Agents Chemother.* 1987;31(3):393-7.

26. Matzke GR, McGory RW, Halstenson CE, et al. Pharmacokinetics of vancomycin in patients with various degrees of renal function. *Antimicrob Agents Chemother.* 1984;25(4):433-7.

27. Rodvold KA, Blum RA, Fischer JH, et al. Vancomycin pharmacokinetics in patients with various degrees of renal function. *Antimicrob Agents Chemother.* 1988;32(6):848-52.

28. Hurst AK, Yoshinaga MA, Mitani GH, et al. Application of a Bayesian method to monitor and adjust vancomycin dosage regimens. *Antimicrob Agents Chemother.* 1990;34(6):1165-71.

29. Ducharme MP, Slaughter RL, Edwards DJ. Vancomycin pharmacokinetics in a patient population: effect of age, gender, and body weight. *Ther Drug Monit.* 1994;16(5):513-8.

30. Del Mar Fernández de M, Gatta GM, Revilla N, et al. Pharmacokinetic/pharmacodynamic analysis of vancomycin in ICU patients. *Intensive Care Med.* 2007;33(2):279-85.

31. Llopis-Salvia P, Jimenez-Torres NV. Population pharmacokinetic parameters of vancomycin in critically ill patients. *J Clin Pharm Ther.* 2006;31(5):447-54.

32. Tan CC, Lee HS, Ti TY, et al. Pharmacokinetics of intravenous vancomycin in patients with end stage renal failure. *Ther Drug Monit.* 1990;12(1):29-34.

33. Zokufa HZ, Solem LD, Rodvold KA, et al. The influence of serum albumin and alpha 1-acid glycoprotein on vancomycin protein binding in patients with burn injuries. *J Burn Care Rehabil.* 1989;10(5):425-8.

34. Currie BP, Lemos-Filho L. Evidence for biliary excretion of vancomycin into stool during intravenous therapy: potential implications for rectal colonization with vancomycin-resistant enterococci. *Antimicrob Agents Chemother.* 2004;48(11):4427-9.

35. Garrelts JC, Peterie JD. Altered vancomycin dose vs. serum concentration relationship in burn patients. *Clin Pharmacol Ther.* 1988;44(1):9-13.

36. Anderson BJ, Allegaert K, van den Anker JN, et al. Vancomycin pharmacokinetics in preterm neonates and the prediction of adult clearance. *Br J Clin Pharmacol.* 2006;63(1):75-84.

37. Rodvold KA, Everett JA, Pryka RD, et al. Pharmacokinetics and administration regimens of vancomycin in neonates, infants and children. *Clin Pharmacokinet.* 1997;33(1):32-51.

38. Burton ME, Gentle DL, Vasko MR. Evaluation of Bayesian method for predicting vancomycin dosing. *Drug Intell Clin Pharm.* 1989;23:294-300.

39. Birt JK, Chandler MH. Using clinical data to determine vancomycin dosing parameters. *Ther Drug Monit.* 1990;12:206-9.

40. Leonard AE, Boro MS. Vancomycin pharmacokinetics in middle-aged and elderly men. *Am J Hosp Pharm.* 1994;51:798-800.

41. Rushing TA, Ambrose PJ. Clinical application and evaluation of vancomycin dosing in adults. *J Pharm Technol.* 2001;17:33-8.

42. Bauer LA. *Applied Clinical Pharmacokinetics.* 2nd ed. New York, NY: McGraw Hill, Medical Publishing Division; 2008:207-301.

43. Murphy JE, Gillespie DE, Bateman CV. Predictability of vancomycin trough concentrations using seven approaches for estimating pharmacokinetic parameters. *Am J Health-Syst Pharm.* 2006;63(23):2365-70.

44. Darko W, Medicis JJ, Smith A, et al. Mississippi mud no more: cost-effectiveness of pharmacokinetic dosage adjustment of vancomycin to prevent nephrotoxicity. *Pharmacotherapy.* 2003;23(5):643-50.

45. Karam CM, McKinnon PS, Neuhauser MM, et al. Outcome assessment of minimizing vancomycin monitoring and dosing adjustments. *Pharmacotherapy.* 1999;19(3):257-66.

46. Rybak MJ. The pharmacokinetic and pharmacodynamic properties of vancomycin. *Clin Infect Dis.* 2006;42(Suppl. 1):S35-S39.

47. Cantú TJ, Yamanaka-Yuen NA. Serum vancomycin concentrations: reappraisal of their clinical value. *Clin Infect Dis.* 1994;18:533-43.

48. Goldstein FW, Kitzis, MD. Vancomycin-resistant Staphylococcus aureus: no apocalypse now. *Clin Microbiol Infect.* 2003;9:761-5.

49. Hidayat LK, Hsu DI, Quist R, et al. High-dose vancomycin therapy for methicillin-resistant *Staphylococcus aureus* infections. *Arch Intern Med.* 2006;166:2138-44.

50. American Thoracic Society, Infectious Diseases Society of America. Guidelines for the management of adults with hospital-acquired ventilator associated and healthcare-associated pneumonia. *Am J Respir Crit Care Med.* 2005;171:388-416.

51. Miles MV, Li L, Lakkis H, et al. Special considerations for monitoring vancomycin concentrations in pediatric patients. *Ther Drug Monit.* 1997;19(3):265-70.

52. Kropec A, Daschner FD. Penetration into tissues of various drugs active against gram-positive bacteria. *J Antimicrob Chemother.* 1991;27 Suppl B:9-15.

53. Lamer C, de Beco V, Soler P, et al. Analysis of vancomycin entry into pulmonary lining fluid by bronchoalveolar lavage in critically ill patients. *Antimicrob Agents Chemother.* 1993;37(2):281-6.

54. CLSI. Performance standards for antimicrobial susceptibility testing. CLSI approved standard M100-S16. Wayne, PA: CLSI; 2006.

55. Sakoulas G, Moise-Broder PA, Schentag J, et al. Relationship of MIC and bactericidal activity to efficacy of vancomycin for treatment of methicillin-resistant Staphylococcus aureus bacteremia. *J Clin Microbiol.* 2004;42:2398-402.

56. Moise PA, Sakoulas G, Forrest A, et al. Vancomycin in vitro bactericidal activity and its relationship to efficacy in clearance of methicillin-resistant Staphylococcus aureus bacteremia. *Antimicrob Agents Chemother.* 2007;51(7):2582-6.

57. Lodise TP, Graves J, Evans A, et al. Relationship between vancomycin MIC and failure among patients with methicillin-resistant Staphylococcus aureus bacteremia treated with vancomycin. *Antimicrob Agents Chemother.* 2008;52:3315-20.

58. Craig WA. Pharmacokinetic/pharmacodynamic parameters: rationale for antibacterial dosing of mice and men. *Clin Infect Dis.* 1998;26(1):1-10;quiz 11-2.

59. Larsson AJ, Walker KJ, Raddatz JK, et al. The concentration independent effect of monoexponential and biexponential decay in vancomycin concentrations on the killing of *Staphylococcus aureus* under aerobic and anaerobic conditions. *J Antimicrob Chemother*. 1996;38(4):589-97.

60. Lowdin E, Odenholt I, Cars O. In vitro studies of pharmacodynamic properties of vancomycin against *Staphylococcus aureus* and *Staphylococcus epidermidis*. *Antimicrob Agents Chemother*. 1998;42(10):2739-44.

61. Ebert S. In vivo cidal activity and pharmacokinetic parameters for vancomycin against methicillin susceptible and -resistant *S. aureus* [abstract 439]. In: Program and abstracts of the 27th Interscience Conference on Antimicrobial Agents and Chemotherapy. Washington, DC: American Society for Microbiology; 1987:173.

62. Duffull SB, Begg EJ, Chambers ST, et al. Efficacies of different vancomycin dosing regimens against *Staphylococcus aureus* determined with a dynamic in vitro model. *Antimicrob Agents Chemother.* 1994;38:2480-2.

63. Sorrell TC, Packham DR, Shanker S, et al. Vancomycin therapy for methicillin-resistant *Staphylococcus aureus*. *Ann Intern Med.* 1982;97(3):344-50.

64. Moise-Broder PA, Forrest A, Birmingham MC, et al. Pharmacodynamics of vancomycin and other antimicrobials in patients with *Staphylococcus aureus* lower respiratory tract infections. *Clin Pharmacokinet*. 2004;43(13):925-42.

65. Cimino MA, Rotstein C, Slaughter RL, et al. Relationship of serum antibiotic concentrations to nephrotoxicity in cancer patients receiving concurrent aminoglycoside and vancomycin therapy. *Am J Med.* 1987;83(6):1091-7.

66. Rybak MJ, Albrecht LM, Boike SC, et al. Nephrotoxicity of vancomycin, alone and with an aminoglycoside. *J Antimicrob Chemother.* 1990;25(4):679-87.

67. Jeffres MN, Isakow W, Doherty JA, et al. A retrospective analysis of possible renal toxicity associated with vancomycin in patients with health care-associated methicillin-resistant Staphylococcus aureus pneumonia. *Clin Ther*. 2007;29(6):1107-15.

68. Lodise TP, Lomaestro B, Graves J, et al. Larger vancomycin doses (at least four grams per day) are associated with an increased incidence of nephrotoxicity. *Antimicrob Agents Chemother*. 2008;52(4):1330-6.

69. Hidayat LK, Hsu DI, Quist R, et al. High-dose vancomycin therapy for methicillin-resistant Staphylococcus aureus infections: efficacy and toxicity. *Arch Intern Med.* 2006;166(19):2138-44.

70. Lodise TP, Patel N, Lomaestro BM, et al. Relationship between initial vancomycin concentration-time profile and nephrotoxicity among hospitalized patients. *Clin Infect Dis*. 2009;49(4):507-14.

71. Farber BF, Moellering RC, Jr. Retrospective study of the toxicity of preparations of vancomycin from 1974 to 1981. *Antimicrob Agents Chemother.* 1983;23(1):138-41.

72. Vance-Bryan K, Rotschafer JC, Gilliland SS, et al. A comparative assessment of vancomycin associated nephrotoxicity in the young versus the elderly hospitalized patient. *J Antimicrob Chemother.* 1994;33(4):811-21.

73. Rybak MJ, Albrecht LM, Berman JR, et al. Vancomycin pharmacokinetics in burn patients and intravenous drug abusers. *Antimicrob Agents Chemother.* 1990;34(5):792-5.

74. Brater DC, Bawdon RE, Anderson SA, et al. Vancomycin elimination in patients with burn injury. *Clin Pharmacol Ther.* 1986;39(6):631-4.

75. Li L, Miles MV, Lakkis H, et al. Vancomycin-binding characteristics in patients with serious infections. *Pharmacotherapy.* 1996;16(6):1024-9.

76. Macias WL, Mueller BA, Scarim SK. Vancomycin pharmacokinetics in acute renal failure: preservation of nonrenal clearance. *Clin Pharmacol Ther.* 1991;50(6):688-94.

77. Joy MS, Matzke GR, Frye RF, et al. Determinants of vancomycin clearance by continuous venovenous hemofiltration and continuous venovenous hemodialysis. *Am J Kidney Dis.* 1998;31(6):1019-27.

78. Heintz, BH, Matzke GR, Dager WE. Antimicrobial dosing concepts and recommendation for critically ill patients receiving continuous renal replacement therapy or intermittent hemodialysis. *Pharmacotherapy.* 2009;29:562-77.

79. Scott MK, Macias WL, Kraus MA, et al. Effects of dialysis membrane on intradialytic vancomycin administration. *Pharmacotherapy.* 1997;17(2):256-62.

80. Foote EF, Dreitlein WB, Steward CA, et al. Pharmacokinetics of vancomycin when administered during high flux hemodialysis. *Clin Nephrol.* 1998;50(1):51-5.

81. Barth RH, DeVincenzo N. Use of vancomycin in high-flux hemodialysis: experience with 130 courses of therapy. *Kidney Int.* 1996;50(3):929-36.

82. Schaedeli F, Uehlinger DE. Urea kinetics and dialysis treatment time predict vancomycin elimination during high-flux hemodialysis. *Clin Pharmacol Ther.* 1998;63(1):26-38.

83. Welage LS, Mason NA, Hoffman EJ, et al. Influence of cellulose triacetate hemodialyzers on vancomycin pharmacokinetics. *J Am Soc Nephrol.* 1995;6(4):1284-90.

84. Matzke GR. Status of hemodialysis of drugs in 2002. *J Pharm Pract.* 2002;15(5):405-18.

85. Decker BS, Kays MB, Chambers M, et al. Vancomycin pharmacokinetics and pharmacodynamics during short daily

hemodialysis. *Clin J Am Soc Nephrol.* 2010;5:1981-7.

86. Harder C, Shalansky S, Werb R, et al. A comparison of two dosage regimens of intravenous vancomycin in high flux hemodialysis. *Pharmacotherapy.* 2002;22(10):1352.

87. Wilson JF, Davis AC, Tobin CM. Evaluation of commercial assays for vancomycin and aminoglycosides in serum: a comparison of accuracy and precision based on external quality assessment. *J Antimicrob Chemother.* 2003;52(1):78-82.

88. Somerville AL, Wright DH, Rotschafer JC. Implications of vancomycin degradation products on therapeutic drug monitoring in patients with end-stage renal disease. *Pharmacotherapy.* 1999;19(6):702-7.

89. Smith PF, Petros WP, Soucie MP, et al. New modified fluorescence polarization immunoassay does not falsely elevate vancomycin concentrations in patients with end-stage renal disease. *Ther Drug Monit.* 1998;20(2):231-5.

90. Smith PF, Morse GD. Accuracy of measured vancomycin serum concentrations in patients with end-stage renal disease. *Ann Pharmacotherapy.* 1999;33(12):1329-35.

91. Fitzpatrick F, McGaley T, Rajan L, et al. Therapeutic drug monitoring of vancomycin in patients receiving haemodialysis: time for a change. *J Clin Pathol.* 2006;59(6):666-7.

Chapter 24

Ann K. Wittkowsky

Warfarin (AHFS 20:12.04)

In 1939, Professor Karl Link at the University of Wisconsin, supported by a grant from the Wisconsin Alumni Research Foundation (WARF), isolated a coumarin derivative, dicumarol (bishydroxywarfarin), from spoiled sweet clover. This compound was found to have been responsible for hemorrhagic deaths in cattle in the Midwestern U.S. and Western Canada for over a decade. A similar compound, warfarin, was later synthesized and marketed as a rodenticide. By 1955, this compound was commercially available as an anticoagulant.[1]

Since then, warfarin has been established through clinical trials as a therapeutic agent for the prevention and treatment of venous and arterial thromboembolic disease. Unfortunately, a narrow therapeutic range and a vast array of drug, disease, and dietary interactions complicate safe use of warfarin. If not properly and respectfully used, this medication can lead to severe complications.

The antithrombotic effect of warfarin is the result of its interference with the hepatic synthesis of vitamin K dependent clotting factors II, VII, IX and X. In addition, it interferes with the synthesis of the anticoagulant proteins C and S. In order for these clotting factors to become biologically active, glutamic acid residues at the NH2-terminal region of clotting factor precursors must undergo gamma-carboxylation. This process requires the presence of vitamin KH2, a reduced form of vitamin K. In the process of gamma-carboxylation, vitamin KH2 is oxidized to vitamin KO, an inactive form of vitamin K which is then converted to vitamin K by vitamin K epoxide reductase (VKOR) and then to vitamin KH2 by vitamin K1 reductase. This vitamin K hepatic recycling process assures a continuous supply of vitamin KH2 for clotting factor synthesis.[2]

Warfarin inhibits VKOR and vitamin K1 reductase, resulting in accumulation of biologically inactive vitamin KO and thus a reduction in vitamin K dependent clotting factor synthesis. However, the biologic effects of warfarin are not apparent until the previously activated clotting factors are depleted. This depletion takes place according to the biologic half-life of each clotting factor (Table 24-1).[3] Thus, the full anticoagulant effect of warfarin does not occur for at least 3–7 days after beginning therapy or changing a dose. When warfarin therapy is discontinued, blood concentrations of the four vitamin K dependent clotting factors gradually return to pretreatment levels.

Warfarin is monitored not by drug concentration measurements but by therapeutic response to the presence of the drug in serum. The prothrombin time (PT) or protime, expressed as an international normalized ratio (INR), describes the time to clot formation. The goal of warfarin therapy is to extend this time sufficiently to prevent pathologic clotting while minimizing the risk of hemorrhagic complications. An INR of 2–3 is suggested for most indications, although higher INRs may be necessary in other situations such as mechanical valve replacement.[2] The safety and effectiveness of warfarin therapy can by improved by thorough knowledge of the pharmacokinetic and pharmacodynamic factors that influence its anticoagulant effect.

Table 24-1. Elimination Half-Lives of Vitamin K–Dependent Proteins

Factor	Half-Life
II	42–72 hr
VII	4–6 hr
IX	21–30 hr
X	27–48 hr
Protein C	8 hr
Protein S	60 hr

Usual Dosage Range in Absence of Clearance-Altering Factors

Warfarin doses required to reach a therapeutic INR vary considerably among individuals. Although the average dose to reach an INR of 2–3 is 4 to 5 mg once daily, doses may range from as little as 0.5 mg daily to 20 mg or more.[4] Numerous factors influence dosing requirements, including goal INR, interacting medications, dietary vitamin K intake, alcohol use, underlying disease states, age, genetic factors, and others.

A number of initiation and maintenance dosing strategies for adults and the elderly have been developed (see Dosing Strategies), all of which are based on assessment of INR response. Initiation therapy requires assessment of rate of increase in the INR after the first one to three doses of warfarin and until the INR reaches the lower limit of the therapeutic range, while maintenance therapy adjustments are based on an assessment of factors that may have led to changes in the INR. A weight-based loading protocol for infants and children has also been developed.[5] Infants and children appear to require lower warfarin doses than do adults.[6] A general description of dosing requirements is provided in Table 24-2.

Dosage Form Availability

Warfarin is currently available in both oral tablet and injectable form. Coumadin is the proprietary form of warfarin. Each dose strength of Coumadin is readily recognizable by its color (Table 24-3), and all Coumadin tablets are scored. The 10-mg tablet contains no dye and can be used to differentiate warfarin allergy from dye allergy in patients who present with mild allergic reactions after initiation of warfarin therapy.

Generic warfarin is available from many commercial sources. The various manufacturers of generic warfarin have generally continued the same color scheme for tablet size identifications, but there are a few color modifications as well as tablet shape and size changes. Practitioners should exercise appropriate caution when counseling patients based on color schemes of the doses.

The U.S. Food and Drug Administration has given generic warfarin products an AB bioequivalence rating, meaning that the 90% confidence intervals of the rate and extent of absorption of the generic product are within

Table 24-2. Usual Dosage Ranges

Age	Initiation Dose	Maintenance Dosage
Infants 1 mo–1 yr	0.2 mg/kg/day for 1–4 days	Average 0.33 mg/kg/day, based on INR response
Young children (1–6 years)	0.2 mg/kg/day for 1–4 days	Average 0.15 mg/kg/day, based on INR response
Children (6–13 years)	0.2 mg/kg/day for 1–4 days	Average 0.13 mg/kg/day, based on INR response
Teenagers (13–18 years)	0.2 mg/kg/day for 1–4 days	Average 0.09 mg/kg/day, based on INR response
Adults (18–70 years)	5–10 mg once daily for 1–4 days	5 mg (range 1–20 mg) once daily, based on INR response
Geriatrics (>70 years)	2.5–5 mg once daily for 1–4 days	2.5 mg (range 1–20 mg) once daily, based on INR response. Often lower than for adults

Table 24-3. Coumadin Color Scheme

Coumadin Dosage Size	Color
1 mg	Pink
2 mg	Lavender
2.5 mg	Green
3 mg	Tan
4 mg	Blue
5 mg	Peach
6 mg	Teal
7.5 mg	Yellow
10 mg	White

80% to 125% of the mean values of the innovator product.[7] Randomized controlled trials and observational studies have typically found no difference in stability of anticoagulant therapy or in the rate of adverse events when patients are switched from brand to generic warfarin.[8–12] Nevertheless, individual patients may experience changes in therapeutic response. Thus, patients should generally be treated with a single formulation of warfarin, and changes in product source should be considered when evaluating changes in therapeutic response.

General Pharmacokinetic Information

Warfarin is a racemic mixture of R and S enantiomers, optical isomers that differ significantly with respect to their pharmacokinetic and pharmacodynamic properties (Table 24-4).[13–15] S-warfarin is 2.7–3.8 more potent than R-warfarin, likely as a result of differences in receptor affinity to vitamin K reductase enzymes.[14,16,17]

Absorption

Warfarin is nearly 100% bioavailable (F = 1) when taken orally.[18] Both oral and intravenous formulations display similar pharmacokinetic characteristics.[19] The drug is rapidly and completely absorbed from the stomach and proximal small intestine with peak blood concentrations within 0.3 to 4 hr.[20] Food decreases the rate but not the extent of absorption.[21]

Distribution

Volume of distribution

The volume of distribution (V) for racemic warfarin ranges from 0.11–0.18 L/kg, similar to that of albumin.[22,23] The average V for both R and S warfarin is 0.15 L/kg.

Protein binding

Both R and S warfarin are highly (> 98%) bound to plasma proteins, primarily albumin.[24] Only the remaining free (unbound) concentration is pharmacologically active. The fraction of a given concentration that is unbound increases proportionately with decreasing plasma albumin concentrations and is accompanied by an increase in plasma clearance.[25,26] Stereoselective protein binding has been demonstrated, with a range of 98.9% to 100% for S warfarin compared to 98.7% to 99.9% for R-warfarin.[27] However, these differences are unlikely to be clinically significant.

Elimination

Warfarin displays stereoselective metabolism, involving both oxidation by cytochrome p450 enzymes in the liver parenchyma and reduction to diasteriomeric alcohols.[28–33] S-warfarin is approximately 90% oxidized, primarily by CYP2C9 to S-6-hydroxywarfarin and S-7-hydroxywarfarin formed in a 3:1 ratio, and to a lesser extent by CYP3A4 to S-4'-hydroxywarfarin and S-10-hdyroxywarfarin. R-warfarin is approximately 60% oxidized by CYP1A2 to R-6-hydroxywarfarin and R-7-hydroxywarfarin, by CYP3A4 to R-10-hydroxywarfarin and R-4'-hydroxywarfarin, and by CYP2C19 to R-8-hydroxywarfarin.

These inactive oxidative metabolites and reduced alcohol derivatives of warfarin are eliminated by urinary excretion. Approximately 50% of a dose of racemic warfarin administered orally is recovered in the urine over 9 days, with recovery of 31% of S-warfarin metabolites and 19% of R-warfarin metabolites and only trace amounts of unchanged drug.[31] Table 24-4 shows clearance values for S- and R- warfarin.[14,34]

A number of genetic variants of CYP2C9 have been identified.[35] In comparison to patients who are homozygous for the wild-type allele (CYP2C9*1*1), patients with a heterozygous (CYP2C9*1*2, CYP2C9*1*3, CYP2C9*2*3) or homozygous (CYP2C9*2*2, CYP2C9*3*3) presentation of a variant allele display significant reductions in the metabolism of S-warfarin to 7-hydroxywarfarin. In *in vivo* studies, the clearance of S-warfarin is 8% to 42% lower in CYP2C9*1/*2 heterozygotes compared to the homozygous wild-type, and subject with the CYP2C9*1/*3 genotype have 38% to 63% lower clearance. Comparatively, heterozygous *2/*3 patients had 70% to 77% lower clearance, and homozygous *2*2 and *3/*3 patients had 68% lower and 38% to 91% lower clearance rates, respectively.[36-40]

In response to reduced S-warfarin clearance, patients with variant expression of CYP2C9 have lower warfarin dosing requirements than patients with the wild-type allele.[41-43] Their risk of over-anticoagulation is higher during initiation therapy and during maintenance therapy, and they are more likely to experience bleeding complications of warfarin.[43-46]

The genetic expression of VKORC1 also influences warfarin dosing requirements. A number of single nucleotide polymorphisms of VKORC1 have been shown to be associated with interindividual and interethnic warfarin dosing requirements. The most significant of these are 1173C>T in intron 1 (expressed as CC, CT, or TT) and 3730G>A (expressed as GG, GA, or AA) in the 3' untranslated region, as well as -1639G>A (expressed as AA, AG, or GG).[47]

Initial work in 147 patients followed from initiation of warfarin therapy found that regardless of the presence of confounding variables, the mean adjusted daily dose of warfarin required to maintain a stable INR was higher (6.2 mg) among patients with the *VKORC1* 1173 CC genotype than patients carrying the CT (4.8 mg) or the TT genotype (3.5 mg).[48] Subsequently, 10 common noncoding *VKORC1* SNPs were identified, with 5 major haplotypes inferred in 368 patients (119 white, 96 of African descent, 120 of Asian descent), declaring a low-dose haplotype group (A) and a high-dose haplotype group (B).[49] The mean maintenance dose of warfarin for the 3 haplotype group combinations was 2.7 mg/d for A/A, 4.9 mg/d for A/B, and 6.2 mg/d for B/B. The A haplotype represents more warfarin sensitivity (i.e., less VKOR expressed), and the B haplotype represents less warfarin sensitivity. Asians had a higher proportion of group A haplotypes, and Africans had a higher proportion of group B haplotypes.

Half-life and time to steady state

The average elimination half-life of S warfarin is 29 hr and of R-warfarin is 45 hr.[13–15,23] Although it takes approximately five half-lives to reach steady state warfarin concentrations after initiation of therapy or dosage adjustments, therapeutic steady state is not achieved until the vitamin K-dependent clotting factors have also reached a new equilibrium.

Dosing strategies

Initiation dosing

Because of wide variability in dosing requirements among patients, the initial dosing of warfarin therapy is based on the presence or absence of factors that may influence dosing requirement and on the INR response to initial doses. Large fixed loading doses (10 mg–15 mg daily for several days) and loading doses based on body weight (1.5 mg/kg), although once favored, are no longer recommended as they increase the risk of both over-anticoagulation and hemorrhage.[50,51] Instead, two general methods for initiation with moderate warfarin doses are used. These are the "average daily dosing method" and "flexible initiation."

Average daily dosing method

In an evaluation of over 2000 patients taking stable doses of warfarin for a variety of indications, the geometric mean dose was 4.57 mg daily, and the arithmetic mean dose was 5.13 mg daily.[4] Patients who do not meet specific criteria that indicate either high or low sensitivity to the effects of warfarin can be initiated with a dose

Table 24-4. Pharmacokinetic and Pharmacodynamic Characteristics of the Enantiomers of Warfarin

	R-warfarin	S-warfarin
Bioavailability	95%–100%	95%–100%
Volume of distribution	0.12–0.22 L/kg	0.11–0.19 L/kg
Protein binding	98.7%–99.9%	98.9%– 100%
Elimination half-life	45 hr (20–70 hr)	29 hr (18–52 hr)
Hepatic metabolism	40% reduction 60% oxidation 1A2>3A4>2C19	10% reduction 90% oxidation 2C9>3A4
Clearance (single dose)	0.0005–0.0073 L/hr/kg	0.0009–0.0079 L/hr/kg
Clearance (multiple dose)	0.001–0.0052 L/hr/kg	0.0015–0.0131 L/hr/kg
Stereospecific potency	1.0 (reference)	2.7–3.8 × R warfarin

of 5 mg daily, with INR values checked within 3–5 days. Subsequent doses are based on the response to the INR and the INR is checked again in another 3–5 days. This pattern continues until the INR is above the lower limit of the therapeutic range, at which time a maintenance dose is selected based on the doses given to this point.

Patients who are expected to be more sensitive to the effects of warfarin are described in Table 24-5. In these patients, the average warfarin dosing requirement is likely to be reduced to 1–3 mg daily. Using the average daily dosing method, patients with any of these characteristics should be initiated with a lower dose (2.5 mg is often used), with subsequent dosing based on INR response as measured within 3–5 days.

Several algorithms have been developed to assist with dosing decisions after the first few doses of warfarin have been administered. After four doses of warfarin 5 mg daily, the INR on day 5 was used to predict weekly warfarin maintenance doses in a scheme by Pengo et al.[52] Siguret et al. administered warfarin 4 mg daily for three doses and used the INR on day 4 to predict maintenance dose in elderly patients.[53] Comparatively, the INR on day 15 after 2 weeks of warfarin 2 mg daily was used to predict maintenance dose requirements in elderly patients in a scheme by Oates et al.[54]

Two algorithms have been developed that use two INR values to predict warfarin maintenance dose. Tait et al. administered warfarin 5 mg daily for 4 days and used the INR on day 5 to select warfarin doses for days 5–7.[55] The subsequent INR on day 8 was then used to predict the maintenance dose. Kovacs et al. developed a similar algorithm using warfarin 10 mg daily for 2 days (Figure 24-1).[56] At day 3, the INR was used to guide dosing on days 3 and 4, and the INR on day 5 was used to guide the next 3 doses. In a study comparing this algorithm to a previously published 5 mg initiation algorithm, patients who received the 10 mg starting doses reached the therapeutic range more rapidly than those initiated with 5 mg starting doses, with no difference in the risk of major bleeding or overanticoagulation.[57] However, the patients in this study were relatively young and healthy outpatients with acute venous thrombosis. Warfarin initiation with 10 mg may lead to overanticoagulation and increased bleeding risk in older and less healthy patients with other indications for oral anticoagulation.[58] In addition, initiation with 10 mg can cause a rapid depletion of protein C, which may induce a relatively hypercoagulability.[59]

Each of these algorithms differs not only in method used to achieve stable dosing, but also in validation sample size, population studied, time to achieve a therapeutic INR, risk of under- and over-anticoagulation during initiation therapy, and success in predicting the maintenance dose. None is a "preferred method," but all demonstrate the importance of assessment of change in INR as a predictor of eventual warfarin maintenance dose requirement and the significance of evaluation of underlying factors that may influence warfarin dosing requirement in individual patients.

Flexible initiation. Hospitalized patients who are available for daily INR testing may benefit from flexible initiation of warfarin. Several flexible initiation algorithms have been developed, each of which considers the rate of increase in the INR on a daily basis to inform daily warfarin dose and to predict the maintenance dosing requirements.

The earliest nomogram by Fennerty et al. started with a 10-mg dose followed by daily INR and daily warfarin adjustments to reach a predicted maintenance dose by day 4.[60] This method was successfully applied in relatively young patients with thromboembolic disease (mean age 52) and in older patients with other indications for oral anticoagulation (mean age 66).[60,61] However, concerns about the use of 10-mg starting doses, particularly in the elderly, have persisted.

Table 24-5. Factors Likely to Increase Sensitivity to Warfarin

Age >75	Clinical congestive heart failure
Elevated baseline INR	Clinical hyperthyroidism
Fever	End stage renal failure
Diarrhea	Malignancy
Known CYP2C9 variant	Following heart valve replacement
Hypoalbuminemia	Hepatic disease
Malnutrition	Decreased overall oral intake
Drug-drug interactions	

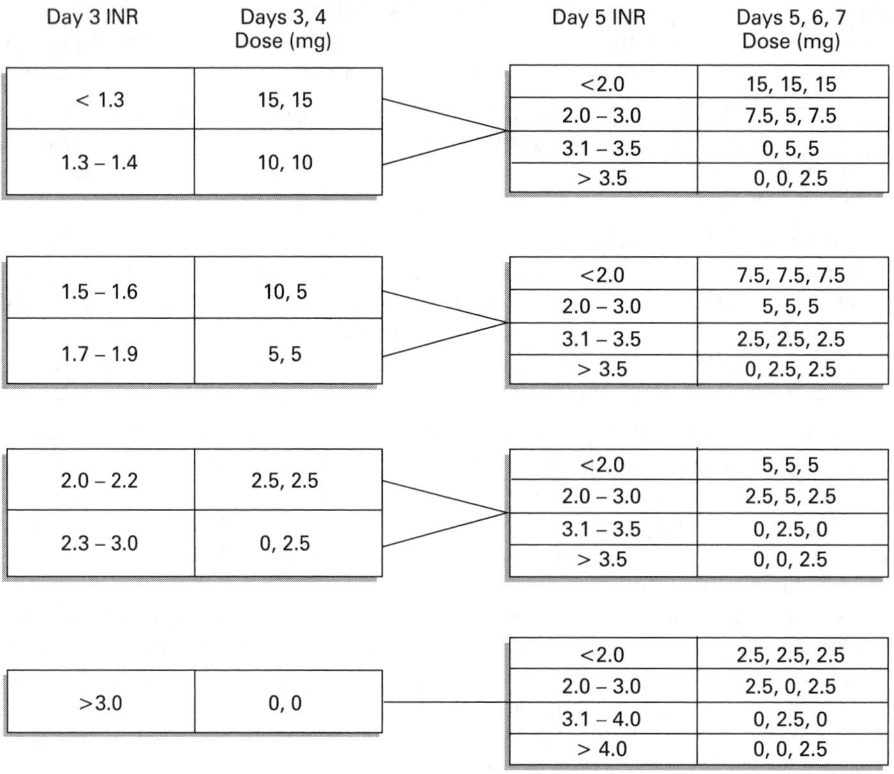

Day 3 INR	Days 3, 4 Dose (mg)	Day 5 INR	Days 5, 6, 7 Dose (mg)
< 1.3	15, 15	<2.0	15, 15, 15
1.3 – 1.4	10, 10	2.0 – 3.0	7.5, 5, 7.5
		3.1 – 3.5	0, 5, 5
		> 3.5	0, 0, 2.5
1.5 – 1.6	10, 5	<2.0	7.5, 7.5, 7.5
1.7 – 1.9	5, 5	2.0 – 3.0	5, 5, 5
		3.1 – 3.5	2.5, 2.5, 2.5
		> 3.5	0, 2.5, 2.5
2.0 – 2.2	2.5, 2.5	<2.0	5, 5, 5
2.3 – 3.0	0, 2.5	2.0 – 3.0	2.5, 5, 2.5
		3.1 – 3.5	0, 2.5, 0
		> 3.5	0, 0, 2.5
>3.0	0, 0	<2.0	2.5, 2.5, 2.5
		2.0 – 3.0	2.5, 0, 2.5
		3.1 – 4.0	0, 2.5, 0
		> 4.0	0, 0, 2.5

Figure 24-1. Warfarin initiation dosing algorithm based on starting with 10-mg doses on days 1 and 2.

Source: *Reprinted with permission from Kovacs MJ, Anderson DA, Wells PS. Prospective assessment of a nomogram for the initiation of oral anticoagulant therapy for outpatient treatment of venous thromboembolism.* Pathophysiol Haemost Thromb. *2002;32:131-133.*

A low-dose flexible initiation nomogram was associated with a lower risk of overanticoagulation in elderly patients (age >65) compared to a modification of the Fennerty nomogram.[62] More recently, an age-adjusted flexible warfarin initiation protocol was found to be superior to either the Fennerty nomogram or empiric dosing.[63] Further modifications of this age-adjusted flexible initiation protocol have since been published.[64]

Crowther et al. compared flexible initiation nomograms that started with either 5 mg or 10 mg starting doses followed by daily INR determination and prediction of the maintenance dose by day 6.[65,66] These authors concluded that the 10 mg initiation was more likely to result in overanticoagulation on each day that INR was evaluated. These popular algorithms are presented in Table 24-6.

Initiation nomograms that incorporate genetic information

Numerous algorithms that incorporate CYP2C9 and VKORC1 genetic information to predict warfarin dosing requirement have been published. In a homogenous, racially and ethnically diverse population, they explain only 37% to 55% of the variation in warfarin dose requirements.[67] During the first week of therapy, genotype alone accounts for 12% of therapeutic dose variability, but over the first several weeks of therapy becomes less relevant as INR and prior doses increasingly predict therapeutic dose, and genotype information.[68] In fact, much of the information provided by including genetic information in a dose-prediction model is captured by early INR response.[69]

A systematic review of small clinical trials that compared genotype-based warfarin dosing to a non-genotype strategy found no statistically significant difference in bleeding rates, time within therapeutic range, or time to

Table 24-6. Flexible Initiation Nomograms for Warfarin

Day	INR	5-mg Initiation Dose	10-mg Initiation Dose
1		5 mg	10 mg
2	< 1.5	5 mg	7.5 mg–10 mg
	1.5–1.9	2.5 mg	2.5 mg
	2.0–2.5	1.0– 2.5 mg	1.0–2.5 mg
	> 2.5	0	0
3	< 1.5	5–10 mg	5–10 mg
	1.5–1.9	2.5–5 mg	2.5–5 mg
	2.0–2.5	0–2.5 mg	0–2.5 mg
	2.5–3.0	0–2.5 mg	0–2.5 mg
	> 3.0	0	0
4	< 1.5	10 mg	10 mg
	1.5–1.9	5–7.5 mg	5–7.5 mg
	2.0–3.0	0–5 mg	0–5 mg
	> 3.0	0	0
5	< 1.5	10 mg	10 mg
	1.5–1.9	7.5–10 mg	7.5–10 mg
	2.0–3.0	0–5 mg	0–5 mg
	> 3.0	0	0
6	< 1.5	7.5–12.5 mg	7.5–12.5 mg
	1.5–1.9	5–10 mg	5–10 mg
	2.0–3.0	0–7.5 mg	0–7.5 mg
	> 3.0	0	0

Source: Adapted with permission from Crowther MA, Harrison L, Hirsh J. Warfarin: less may be better. *Ann Intern Med.* 1997;127:332-333.

achieve a stable warfarin dose.[70] Large scale, randomized controlled trials are underway to determine whether pharmacogenomic-based dosing will improve clinical outcomes. However, genotyping is unlikely to be cost-effective in most patients.[71]

Maintenance dosing

Once a patient has reached the lower limit of the therapeutic range and is at relative steady state, maintenance dosing adjustments are frequently required to maintain the INR within the therapeutic range. Numerous factors influence the stability of therapy, including drug and disease state interactions, dietary vitamin K intake, alcohol use, activity, stress and many others. These factors and the INR must be evaluated regularly. The frequency of monitoring and assessment is described in Table 24-7. Dosing adjustments are based on INR results and the presumed explanation for out of range INRs. For example, a transient cause of underanticoagulation, such as a missed dose, may be most appropriately managed by simply continuing the usual maintenance dose or giving a one-time "booster dose" (1.5–2 times the daily maintenance dose) to replace the missed dose. Comparatively, a more persistent cause of underanticoagulation such as the addition of an interacting enzyme inducer will require a more permanent dosing increase. Similarly, a transient cause of overanticoagulation such as acute illness may require holding a dose of warfarin without any change in the long-term maintenance dose. A more persistent cause of overanticoagulation such as addition of an interacting enzyme inhibitor will require a more permanent dosing reduction.

When dosing adjustments are required, they are generally in the range of 5% to 20% of the daily dose, or 5% to 20% of the total weekly dose.[72] The tablet size(s) available to the patient and the patient's own concerns regarding same daily dosing (e.g., 4 mg daily or 28 mg weekly) or alternate-day dosing (2.5 mg Mondays, Wednesdays, and Fridays, and 5 mg on all other days, or 27.5 mg/wk) must also be considered.[73]

A maintenance dosing guideline for a patient with a goal INR of 2–3 is presented in Table 24-8. However, it is imperative that the adjustments only be made in patients who have already reached the therapeutic range. The use of maintenance dosing adjustments (e.g., small 5% to 15% changes every 7 days rather than more aggressive initiation doses) during initiation therapy will significantly prolong the time to reach the lower limit of the therapeutic range.

Therapeutic Range

Many clinical trials evaluating the effectiveness and safety of warfarin have helped to establish specific INR ranges for the prevention and treatment of venous and arterial thromboembolism. The American College of Chest Physicians (ACCP) Conference on Antithrombotic and Thrombolytic Therapy meets every few years to summarize available literature and develop graded, evidence-based guidelines.[74] The therapeutic range for various indications, as recommended by the 8th ACCP Conference, are listed in Table 24-9.[2]

Therapeutic Monitoring

Warfarin therapy suppresses the vitamin K dependent clotting factors to different extents. In stable anticoagulated patients, factor II (mean activity 19%; range 9% to 54%) and factor X (mean activity 18%; range 9% to 45%) are suppressed to the greatest extent, compared to factor VII (mean activity 33%; range 16% to 57%) and factor IX (mean activity 48%; range 26% to 94%).[75] But despite considerable variability, mean activity of all clotting factors is highly predictive of INR.

The intensity of warfarin therapy is monitored by evaluation of the prothrombin time (PT), expressed as the INR.[76] The PT is prolonged by deficiencies in plasma concentrations of clotting factors II, V, VII, and X. It is measured by adding both calcium and a tissue thromboplastin to plasma, which accelerates activation of the extrinsic pathway of the clotting cascade. Time to clot formation is read in seconds using various technologies.

Thromboplastins are extracted from various tissue sources and prepared for use as commercial reagents. Because of lack of standardization among manufacturers of thromboplastins, each reagent is assigned an International Sensitivity Index (ISI) that describes its comparison to an international reference thromboplastin derived from human brain. The ISI is listed in the product information for each lot of thromboplastin.[77] The ISI is used to convert prothrombin time in seconds to the INR, using the formula:

$$INR = \left(\frac{PT_{patient}}{PT_{mean\ normal}} \right)^{ISI}$$

Table 24-7. Frequency of INR Monitoring and Patient Assessment

Initiation Therapy	
Flexible initiation method	Daily through day 4, then within 3–5 days
Average daily dosing method	Every 3–5 days until INR > lower limit of therapeutic range, then within 1 week
After hospital discharge	If stable, within 3–5 days; if unstable, within 1–3 days
First month of therapy	At least weekly
Maintenance Therapy	
Dose held today in patient with significant overanticoagulation	In 1–2 days
Dosage change today	Within 1–2 weeks
Dosage change made ≤2 weeks ago	Within 2–4 weeks
Routine follow-up of medically stable and reliable patients	Every 4–6 weeks
Routine follow-up of medically unstable or unreliable patients	Every 1–2 weeks

Table 24-8. Warfarin Dosing Adjustment Guidelines for INR Goal of 2–3

INR	Dosage Adjustment Guidelines
<1.5	• Consider a booster dose of 1.5–2 x daily maintenance dose • Consider resumption of prior maintenance dose if factor causing decreased INR is transient [e.g.: missed warfarin dose(s)] • If dosage adjustment needed, increase maintenance dose by 10%– 20%
1.5–1.8	• Consider a booster dose of 1.5–2 times daily maintenance dose • Consider resumption of prior maintenance dose if factor causing decreased INR is considered [e.g.: missed warfarin dose(s)] • If dosage adjustment needed, increase maintenance dose by 5%– 15%
1.8–2	• No dosage adjustment may necessary if the last 2 INRs were in range, if there is no clear explanation for the INR to be out of range, and if in the judgment of the clinician, the INR does not represent an increased risk of thromboembolism for the patient • Consider a booster dose of 1.5–2 x daily maintenance dose • Consider resumption of prior maintenance dose if factor causing decreased INR is transient [e.g.: missed warfarin dose(s)] • If dosage adjustment needed, increase maintenance dose by 5%– 10%
2–3	• Desired range
3–3.2	• No dosage adjustment may necessary if the last two INRs were in range, if there is no clear explanation for the INR to be out of range, and if in the judgment of the clinician, the INR does no represent an increased risk of hemorrhage for the patient • Consider continuation of prior maintenance dose if factor causing elevated INR is transient [e.g.: acute alcohol ingestion] • If dosage adjustment needed, reduce maintenance dose by 5%–10%
3.5–3.9	• Consider holding one dose • Consider resumption of prior maintenance dose if factor causing elevated INR is transient [e.g.: acute alcohol ingestion] • If dosage adjustment needed, decrease maintenance dose by 5%– 15%
>4	• Hold until INR < upper limit of therapeutic range • Consider use of mini dose (1.0–2.5 mg) oral vitamin K • Consider resumption of prior maintenance dose if factor causing elevated INR is transient [e.g.: acute alcohol ingestion] • If dosage adjustment needed, decrease maintenance dose by 5%– 15%

The mean normal PT is typically about 12 seconds for most thromboplastin reagents and is measured by averaging the PT of non-anticoagulated subjects. The INR is the value that would have been obtained if the reference preparation had been used in the test. In this way, results obtained at different laboratories can be compared and results from different lots of the same manufacturer of thromboplastin can also be compared.

Variations in thromboplastin sensitivity are due to differences in manufacturing, source, and method of preparation. More sensitive thromboplastins with ISI values close to 1.0 produces less rapid stimulation of factor X, resulting in greater prolongation of the PT for a given reduction in clotting factors.[78] Less sensitive thromboplastins activate residual factor X more rapidly and result in a less prolonged PT, despite a comparable reduction in clotting factors. ISI values range from 0.95 to 2.9, with a higher ISI number indicating a less sensitive reagent.

Although manufacturers carefully calibrate the ISI values of their thromboplastins, they do not, in most cases, provide ISI values that are specific to the instrumentation that will be used to measure INR at individual

Table 24-9. Optimal Therapeutic Range by Indication

Indication	Target INR (Range)
Atrial fibrillation	2.5 (2–3)
Atrial flutter	2.5 (2–3)
Cardioembolic stroke	2.5 (2–3)
Left ventricular dysfunction	2.5 (2–3)
Myocardial infarction	2.5 (2–3)
Venous thromboembolism	2.5 (2–3)
Valvular heart disease	2.5 (2–3)
Valve replacement, bioprosthetic	2.5 (2–3)
Valve replacement, mechanical	
Aortic, bileaflet	2.5 (2–3)
Aortic, other	3 (2.5–3.5)
Mitral, all	3 (2.5–3.5)

laboratories. One means of overcoming this problem is the use of calibrating plasma provided by reagent manufacturers.[79] By using plasma samples with carefully calculated INR values, a laboratory can verify the correct ISI value for its system.

Although PT is intended to be measured using plasma samples obtained by venipuncture, a number of point-of-care INR devices have been developed that use whole blood for rapid measurement of INR.[80] These test systems are used in anticoagulation clinics, physician offices, and hospital nursing units, and can be used for patient self-testing at home.[81]

Pharmacodynamic Monitoring

Patients treated with warfarin should be routinely monitored for signs and symptoms of the development, progression, or recurrence of venous or arterial thromboembolism. They should also be assessed regularly for the development of hemorrhagic complications to warfarin therapy. In addition, factors that influence the stability of the INR should be assessed on a regular basis. These include changes in dietary vitamin K intake, prescription and nonprescription medications and dietary supplements, underlying disease states, alcohol use, activity, the development of acute illness, and others.[2] Changes in any of these parameters can influence the intensity of anticoagulant therapy and increase the risk of hemorrhagic or thromboembolic complications.

INR-related efficacy

After initiation of warfarin therapy, initial elevations in the INR represent depletion of factor VII due to its short elimination half-life.[82] However, the antithrombotic effect of warfarin requires adequate depletion of factors II and X.[83] Since protein C also has a relatively short elimination half life, initial warfarin doses can induce a relative hypercoagulable state as the anticoagulant effect of protein C is depleted more rapidly than clotting factors II and X.[59] For these reasons, in addition to the known pharmacokinetic properties of warfarin, the antithrombotic effect of warfarin is delayed for 4–5 days after initiation. For treatment of acute venous thromboembolism, warfarin therapy must therefore be overlapped with heparin, a low molecular weight heparin, a direct thrombin inhibitor or an indirect factor Xa inhibitor during initiation therapy.[84] Current guidelines suggest that this overlap continue for a minimum of 5 days and until the INR is stable and above the lower limit of the therapeutic range.[85]

The INR is designed for monitoring long-term anticoagulation therapy and is less reliable during the induction phase of oral anticoagulant therapy. It is also less reliable for patients with significant liver dysfunction, hereditary factor deficiencies, or for screening for bleeding disorders. These conditions require evaluation of other measures of hemostasis.

The INR can be increased by the presence of heparin or low molecular weight heparin in the sample, as well as by direct thrombin inhibitors and factor Xa inhibitors.[86,87] The INR is also influenced by hemolysis and elevated hematocrit.[88,89] Specimens must be handled differently by laboratory personnel in each of these situations.

Antiphospholipid antibody (APA) syndrome is a condition associated with venous and arterial thromboembolism requiring chronic anticoagulation with warfarin and routine INR monitoring.[90] Since the INR is a phospholipid-dependent test, it may be invalid in patients with APA syndrome whether monitored by standard methodology or point-of-care testing.[91,92] In these patients an alternative monitoring strategy that is independent of phospholipids may be preferable. One option is the use of chromogenic factor X.[93] An INR of 2–3 is roughly equivalent to suppression of factor X to 35% of 45% of normal.

Time spent within the therapeutic range (time-in-therapeutic range; TTR) is a measure of the quality of anticoagulant control and is a predictor of both the efficacy and the safety of oral anticoagulation.[94] Increased TTR is associated with a reduction in both thromboembolic complications and hemorrhage. TTR can be measured as the fraction of INRs in range, as a cross section of INRs on a given day, or by a linear interpolation method.[95] Each method has advantages and limitations, but all allow an overall examination of the quality of anticoagulation control. The fraction of INRs in range is commonly used as a quality assurance measure in anticoagulation clinics, while linear interpolation of TTR is frequently used in clinical trials to describe the quality of anticoagulation control.

INRs below the therapeutic range are associated with an increased risk of thromboembolic events. The risk of stroke in patients with atrial fibrillation increases dramatically with INRs < 2.[96] Similarly, there is a steep increase in the risk of stroke at INRs < 2.5 in patients with mechanical heart valve replacement.[97] In patients with a first episode of idiopathic venous thromboembolism (VTE) treated for a minimum of 3 months, the risk of recurrent VTE in the 21 months following discontinuation of warfarin was lower in patients who spent more time within the therapeutic INR range of 2–3 and higher in patients who spent more time with an INR < 1.5.[98] Thus, the quality of oral anticoagulant control directly influences clinical outcomes.

INRs below the therapeutic range occur frequently during long term oral anticoagulation and may be the result of various dosing issues (initiation therapy, withholding warfarin for invasive procedures, noncompliance, response to dosing adjustments), or of interactions (with drugs, disease states, diet, alcohol, etc.).[99] However, up to 30% of INRs < 2 cannot be explained despite extensive patient assessment.

INR-related toxicity

Bleeding is the primary adverse effect associated with warfarin.[100] Bleeding is typically referred to as either minor or major depending on the site of bleeding, its clinical consequences, and/or the interventions required for control. The risk of bleeding is dependent on the intensity of anticoagulation, underlying patient characteristics, concomitant use of drugs that impact hemostasis, and the length of anticoagulant therapy.

Intensity of anticoagulation is a major determinant of the risk of major bleeding complications in patients taking warfarin. Outpatients taking warfarin who develop INRs > 6 are at a significantly greater risk of developing major bleeding within the next 2 weeks compared to patients with INRs within the therapeutic range of 2–3.[101] The risk of intracranial hemorrhage increases significantly when the INR is > 4.[97,102] Bleeding risk is also increased by variability in the INR, which is an indicator of poor management of warfarin therapy.[102,103]

When warfarin therapy is managed in a designated anticoagulation clinic setting the risk of major bleeding can be minimized in comparison to warfarin management by routine medical care.[104,105] However, advanced age appears to increase the risk of warfarin-related intracranial hemorrhage, even when patients are managed by anticoagulation clinics.[106,107]

Bleeding risk associated with warfarin therapy can be estimated by prediction methods that are based on the presence of risk factors for bleeding. One popular method assigns a point score (total 0–4 points) for the presence of age >65, history of stroke, history of gastrointestinal bleeding (1 point each) and any one of four other comorbid conditions (recent myocardial infarction, elevated serum creatinine >1.5 mg/dL, hematocrit <30% or diabetes) (1 point for any or all).[108] Application of this Bleeding Risk Index to warfarin patients managed in an anticoagulation clinic setting found that major bleeding occurred at a rate of 0.8%/patient-year in patients with a low risk score (0 points), 2.5%/patient-year in patients with an intermediate risk score (1–2 points), and 10.6%/patient yr in patient with a high risk score (3–4 points).[109]

Reversing INR-related toxicity

Reversal of over-anticoagulation is accomplished by withholding warfarin, administering vitamin K and/or administering blood products.[2] These strategies may be used alone or in combination, guided by the INR, the patient's bleeding risk and bleeding status, and the time needed for reversal. Blood products, such as fresh frozen plasma (FFP), act rapidly, have a short duration of effect, and are reserved for active bleeding. Prothrombin complex concentrates and recombinant factor VIIa have also been used to manage life-threatening warfarin induced bleeding. High dose vitamin K (10 mg by IV infusion) is often used in conjunction with blood products in patients who are bleeding. The onset of effect is relatively rapid and the duration of effect is prolonged, but can lead to extended warfarin resistance.

Lower doses of vitamin K can be used to reverse over-anticoagulation when no bleeding is present. The oral route is preferred as subcutaneous administration can lead to a delay in onset of effect and both subcutaneous and intramuscular administration can lead to hematoma formation.[110–113] Vitamin K doses in the range of 1–2.5 mg will reduce the INR back to within the therapeutic range within 24 hr without causing complete reversal or prolonged warfarin resistance.

There are currently two formulations of vitamin K_1 available in the United States, a scored 5-mg tablet (Mephyton) and an injectable preparation available as a 2-mg/ml or 10-mg/ml aqueous dispersion (Aquamephyton) that can be administered orally. When more rapid reversal is needed (for example, prior to invasive procedures), the intravenous route can be used. Rapid IV administration of vitamin K has been associated with anaphylactic reactions, so a prolonged infusion in 50–100 ml of diluent over 30–60 minutes is necessary.[114] Current recommendations for reversal of over-anticoagulation are listed in Table 24-10.[2]

Drug-Drug Interactions

Warfarin is highly susceptible to interactions with prescription and non-prescription drugs as well as with herbal and other natural products.[115] Through a variety of mechanisms these interactions may elevate or reduce the INR, increasing the risk of hemorrhagic or thromboembolic complications, respectively. Pharmacokinetic interactions are those that influence the absorption, distribution, metabolism, or excretion of warfarin. Pharmacodynamic interactions influence response to warfarin without altering its pharmacokinetics. Clinically significant warfarin drug interactions are listed in Table 24-11.[115–120] Clinically significant interactions between warfarin and dietary supplements are listed in Table 24-12.[115,120–124]

The impact of drug interactions on INR, bleeding risk, or risk of thromboembolism may be seen when interacting drugs are initiated, discontinued, or when there is a change in dose. Patient susceptibility to drug interactions is highly variable, as is the magnitude of the response, the time of onset, and the duration of the interaction once the interacting drug is discontinued.[125] These variables are influenced by numerous underlying patient characteristics that may influence clotting factor synthesis and degradation, the pharmacokinetics and/or pharmacodynamics of the interacting drug, and the pharmacokinetics and/or pharmacodynamics of the R and S enantiomers of warfarin.[126] Genetic expression of CYP2C9 influences warfarin dosing requirements and may also influence the risk and/or severity of warfarin drug interactions.[127]

Table 24-10. Current Recommendations for Reversal of Elevated INRs

INR	Strategy
< 5	Lower dose or omit dose
5–8.9	Omit one or two doses; or omit dose and give vitamin K ($\leq$1–2.5 mg orally). If more rapid reversal is required use $\leq$5 mg vitamin K orally. Repeat vitamin K (1–2 mg orally) if INR is still elevated at 24 hr.
≥ 9	Hold warfarin and give vitamin K (2.5–5 mg orally). Use additional vitamin K if necessary.
Serious bleeding with high INR	Hold warfarin and give vitamin K (10 mg slow IV infusion) supplemented with fresh frozen plasma, prothrombin complex concentrate, or recombinant factor VIIa. May repeat vitamin K every 12 hr if necessary.
Life-threatening bleeding (regardless of INR)	Hold warfarin and give fresh frozen plasma, prothrombin complex concentrates or recombinant factor VIIa supplemented with vitamin K (10 mg slow IV infusion). Repeat as necessary.

Table 24-11. Clinically Significant Warfarin Drug Interactions

Mechanism	Effect on INR	Drugs/Drug Classes
Increased synthesis of clotting factors	Decreased	vitamin K
Reduced catabolism of clotting factors	Decreased	methimazole propylthiouracil
Induction of warfarin metabolism	Decreased	alcohol (chronic use) aminoglutethimide aprepitant *Barbiturates* bosentan carbamazepine dicloxacillin ethchlorvynol fosphenytoin glutethimide griseofulvin mitotane nafcillin phenytoin primidone *Rifamycins* terbinafine
Reduced absorption of warfarin	Decreased	cholestyramine colestipol sucralfate
Unexplained mechanisms	Decreased	ascorbic acid azathioprine *Corticosteroids* cyclosporin mercaptopurine *Protease inhibitors* ribavirin
Increased catabolism of clotting factors	Increased	*Thyroid hormones*
Protein binding displacement	Increased	chloral hydrate
Decreased synthesis of clotting factors	Increased	*Cephalosporins* vitamin E
Impaired vitamin K production by gut flora	Increased	*Aminoglycosides* *Tetracyclines*

Table 24-11. (continued)

Mechanism	Effect on INR	Drugs/Drug Classes
Inhibition of warfarin metabolism	Increased	acetaminophen
		alcohol (acute use)
		allopurinol
		amiodarone
		Azole antifungals
		capecitabine
		celecoxib
		chloramphenicol
		cimetidine
		delavirdine
		disulfiram
		efavirenz
		Fluoroquinolone antibiotics
		fluorouracil
		fosphenytoin
		ifosfamide
		isoniazid
		leflunomide
		Macrolide antibiotics
		metronidazole
		omeprazole
		orlistat
		phenytoin
		propafenone
		quinidine
		quinine
		rofecoxib
		SSRIs
		Statins (not atorvastastin/ pravastatin)
		Sulfa antibiotics
		zafirlukast
Additive anticoagulant	Increased response	*Direct thrombin inhibitors*
		heparin
		Low molecular weight heparins
		Thrombolytic agents
	Unexplained mechanisms	acarbose
		Androgens
		carboplatin
		clofibrate
		Corticosteroids[a]

Table 24-11. (continued)

Mechanism	Effect on INR	Drugs/Drug Classes
		cyclophosphamide
		etoposide
		fenofibrate
		gefitinib
		gemcitabine
		gemfibrozil
		influenza virus vaccine
		isotretinoin
		mesalamine
		paclitaxel
		tamoxifen
		testosterone
		tolterodine
		tramadol
		trastuzumab
Increased bleeding risk	No effect	aspirin/acetylated salicylates
		clopidogrel/ticlopidine
		Glycoprotein IIb/IIIa inhibitors
		Non steroidal anti-inflammatory drugs
		prasugrel

Source: Adapted with permission from Wittkowsky AK. Drug interactions with oral anticoagulants. In: Colman RW, Marder VJ, Clowes AW, et al., eds. *Hemostasis and Thrombosis. Basic Principles and Clinical Practice.* 5th ed. Philadelphia, PA: Lippincott Williams & Wilkins; 2006.

Interacting drugs are not often strictly contraindicated in patients taking warfarin, though appropriate therapeutic alternatives with little or no interaction potential should be used when possible. When non-interacting alternatives are not available or not appropriate, the interacting drugs can be used concurrently as long as the frequency of INR monitoring and the dosing of warfarin are adjusted appropriately. These interventions should be guided by the pharmacokinetic and pharmacodynamic characteristics of warfarin and of the interacting drug, known characteristics of the interaction in similar patients, the expected time course associated with the known or presumed mechanism of the interaction, and the underlying thromboembolic or hemorrhagic risk of the patient involved. For example, enzyme inhibition interactions typically occur rapidly, so the INR should be checked 2–3 days after the interacting agent is added to warfarin therapy. Enzyme induction interactions tend to occur more slowly, so the INR should be checked within the first week after addition of the interacting drug. However, no guidelines for drug interaction management exist, and appropriately so, since each case must be handled individually due to expected variability in response.

Drug–Disease State or Condition Interactions

A number of disease states influence the therapeutic response to warfarin. The influence of these conditions should be considered during initiation of therapy when they may influence the starting dose of warfarin, as well as later in therapy when new onset, exacerbation, or improvement in these conditions may influence INR response and the maintenance dosing requirements for warfarin.

Table 24-12. Clinically Significant Interactions Between Warfarin and Dietary Supplements

Mechanism	Effect	Supplements
Inhibition of warfarin metabolism	Increased INR	Chinese wolfberry
		Cranberry juice
		Grapefruit juice
		Mango
Contain coumarin derivatives	Increased INR	Danshen/methyl salicylate
		Dong quai
		Boldo/fenugreek
Unknown	Increased INR	Curbicin
		Devil's claw
		Fish oil
		Glucosamine-chondroitin
		Melatonin
		Papaya extract
		Quilinggao
		Vitamin E
Inhibition of platelet aggregation	Increased bleeding	Garlic
		Ginger
		Ginkgo
Contain vitamin K/derivatives	Decreased INR	Avocado
		Coenzyme Q10
		Foods high in vitamin K
		Green tea
		Some multivitamins
		Sushi containing seaweed
Induction of CYP3A4	Decreased INR	St. John's wort
Unknown	Decreased INR	Ginseng
		Melatonin
		Soy

Source: Adapted with permission from Wittkowsky AK. Drug interactions with oral anticoagulants. In: Colman RW, Marder VJ, Clowes AW, et al., eds. Hemostasis and Thrombosis. Basic Principles and Clinical Practice. 5th ed. Philadelphia, PA: Lippincott Williams & Wilkins; 2006.

Advanced age

Warfarin dosing requirements decline with advanced age.[128] There do not appear to be differences in the pharmacokinetics of warfarin in young versus elderly patients, however.[129] The elderly may have reduced availability of vitamin K stores and lower plasma concentrations of vitamin K dependent clotting factors, both of which could contribute to this observation.[129,130] Age may be the most important readily available predictor of warfarin dosing requirement.[131]

Pregnancy and lactation

Warfarin is a teratogen and is associated with congenital abnormalities such as stippled calcifications and nasal cartilage hypoplasia, particularly when exposure occurs during weeks 6–12 of pregancy.[132] Other abnormalities as well as fetal hemorrhage can occur throughout pregnancy. Accordingly, warfarin is considered contraindicated in pregnancy. Alternative anticoagulants such as heparin and low molecular weight heparin should be used instead of warfarin in pregnant women. Warfarin is not excreted in breast milk and can be used safely post-partum by nursing mothers.[133]

Alcoholism

Acute alcohol ingestion can elevate the INR by inhibiting warfarin metabolism.[134] Patients who binge drink are at increased bleeding risk from overanticoagulation and from risk of falls. Conversely, chronic alcohol use is associated with CYP enzyme induction and causes higher warfarin dosing requirements in alcoholic patients. Patients taking warfarin should be encouraged to moderate their alcohol intake.

Liver disease

Hepatic disease is often accompanied by coagulopathy due to a reduction in clotting factor synthesis.[135] These patients may appear to be "auto-anticoagulated" with baseline elevated INRs. However, the degree of factor suppression in liver disease does not mimic that of patients treated with warfarin and thus these patients are not protected from thromboembolism.[136] Hepatic disease may reduce the clearance of warfarin.

Renal disease and hemodialysis

End stage renal disease is associated with reduced activity of CYP2C9, leading to lower warfarin dosing requirements.[137] Hypoalbuminemia associated with nephrotic syndrome increases the free fraction of warfarin, but there is also an associated increase in plasma clearance.[138] When INR is monitored in patients undergoing hemodialysis, blood draws should be taken from peripheral sites rather than from the dialysis graft as heparin can influence INR results.[139] It may also be necessary for the sample to be deheparinized with a heparin absorbent to eliminate any potential risk of contamination by heparin from the dialysis circuit.

Congestive heart failure

Exacerbations of heart failure can cause an increased responsiveness to warfarin and elevate the INR.[140] The likely mechanism of this effect is hepatic congestion leading to a reduction in warfarin metabolism.

Cardiac valve replacement

Patients commencing warfarin therapy after cardiac valve replacement appear to have increased response to warfarin.[141] This enhanced sensitivity diminishes over time and several weeks after surgery patients typically require higher doses than initially suspected. Hypoalbuminemia, age, diet, physical activity and reductions in clotting factor concentrations as a result of cardiopulmonary bypass all likely contribute to this phenomenon.

Nutritional status

Changes in dietary intake of vitamin K containing foods have a profound impact on warfarin dosing requirements and INR response.[124] Diets modified intentionally or as a result of disease, surgery, or other exogenous factors are likely to influence the therapeutic response to warfarin.

Thyroid disease

Hypothyroidism decreases the catabolism of clotting factors, leading to increased warfarin dosing requirements to maintain a therapeutic INR.[142] Conversely, hyperthyroidism increases sensitivity to warfarin.[143] Patient who start or stop thyroid replacement therapy or who undergo treatment for hyperthyroidism require careful INR monitoring and dosing adjustments to maintain safe and effective oral anticoagulation.

Smoking and tobacco use status

Constituents of cigarette smoke may induce cytochrome P450 enzymes, including CYP1A2, a minor contributor to the metabolism of R-warfarin.[144] Warfarin dosing requirements have been observed to decline after smoking cessation.[145] Chewing tobacco contains high quantities of vitamin K and can suppress INR response.[146]

References

1. Link KP. The discovery of dicumarol and its sequels. *Circulation.* 1959;19:97-107.
2. Ansell J, Hirsh J, Hylek E, et al. The pharmacology and management of the vitamin K antagonists. American College of Chest Physicians Evidence-Based Clinical Practice Guidelines (8th edition). *Chest.* 2008 (suppl 6);133:160s-98s.
3. Stirling Y. Warfarin-induced changes in procoagulant and anticoagulant proteins. *Blood Coag Fibrinolysis.* 1995;6:361-75.
4. James AH, Britt RP, Raskind CL, et al. Factors influencing the maintenance dose of warfarin. *J Clin Pathol.* 1992;45:704-6.
5. Streif W, Andrew M, Marzinotto V, et al. Analysis of warfarin therapy in pediatric patients: a prospective cohort study of 319 patients. *Blood.* 1999;94:3007-14.
6. Doyle JJ, Koren G, Cheng MY, et al. Anticoagulation with sodium warfarin in children: effect of a loading regimen. *J Pediatr.* 1988;113:1095-7.
7. Benet LZ, Goyan JE. Bioequivalence and narrow therapeutic index drugs. *Pharmacotherapy.* 1995;15:433-40.
8. Weibert RT, Yeager BF, Wittkowsky AK, et al. A randomized crossover comparison of warfarin products in the treatment of chronic atrial fibrillation. *Ann Pharmacotherapy.* 2000;34:981-8.
9. Witt DM, Tillman DJ, Evans CM, et al. Evaluation of the clinical and economic impact of a brand name-to-generic warfarin sodium conversion program. *Pharmacotherapy.* 2003;23:360-8.
10. Milligan PE, Banet GA, Waterman AD, et al. Substitution of generic warfarin for Coumadin in an HMO setting. *Ann Pharmacotherapy.* 2002;36:764-8.
11. Pereira JA, Holbrook AM, Dolovich L, et al. Are brand name and generic warfarin interchangeable? Multiple N-of-1 randomized crossover trials. *Ann Pharmacotherapy.* 2005;39:1188-93.
12. Paterson JM, Mamdani M, Juurlink DN, et al. Clinical consequences of generic warfarin substitution: an ecological study. *JAMA.* 2006;296:1969-72.
13. O'Reilly RA. Studies of the optical enantiomorphs of warfarin in man. *Clin Pharmacol Ther.* 1974;16:348-54.
14. Breckenridge A, Orme M, Wessling H, et al. Pharmacokinetics and pharmacodynamics of the enantiomers of warfarin in man. *Clin Pharmacol Ther.* 1973;15:424-30.
15. Hignite C, Uetriecht J, Tschanz C, et al. Kinetics of R and S warfarin enantiomers. *Clin Pharmacol Ther.* 1980;28:99-105.
16. Wingard LB, O'Reilly RA, Levy G. Pharmacokinetics of warfarin enantiomers: a search for intrasubject correlations. *Clin Pharmacol Ther.* 1973;15:424-30.
17. Choondara IA, Haynes BP, Cholerton S, et al. Enantiomers of warfarin and vitamin K1 metabolism. *Br J Clin Pharmacol.* 1986;22:729-32.
18. Stirling U, Howarth DJ, Stockley R, et al. Comparison of the bioavailabilities and anticoagulant activities of two warfarin formulations. *Br J Haematol.* 1982;51:37-45.
19. Breckenridge A, Orme M. Kinetics of warfarin absorption in man. *Clin Pharmacol Ther.* 1973;14: 955-61.
20. Pyoralak, K, Julssila J, Mustala O, et al. Absorption of warfarin from stomach and small intestines. *Scand J Gastroenterol.* 1971;6 (suppl 9):95-103.
21. Musa MN. Lyons LL. Absorption and disposition of warfarin: effects of food and liquids. *Curr Ther Res.* 1976;20:630-3.
22. O'Reilly RA, Welling PG, Wagner JG. Pharmacokinetics of warfarin following intravenous administration in man. *Thromb Haemost.* 1971;25:178-86.
23. Hewick DS, McEwen J. Plasma half-lives, plasma metabolites, and anticoagulant efficacies of the enantiomers of warfarin in man. *J Pharm Pharmacol.* 1983;25:458-65.
24. O'Reilly R. Interaction of the anticoagulant drug warfarin and its metabolites with human plasma albumin. *J Clin Invest.* 1969;48:193-202.
25. Yacobi A, Stoll RG, DiSanto R. Intersubject variation of warfarin binding in serum of normal subjects. *Res Commun Chem Pathol Pharmacol.* 1976;14:743-6.
26. Routledge PA, Chapman PH, Davies DM, et al. Pharmacokinetics and pharmacodynamics of warfarin at steady state. *Br J Clin Pharmacol.* 1979;8:243-7.
27. Cai WM, Hatton J, Pettigrew LD, et al. A simplified high performance liquid chromatographic method for direct determination of warfarin enantiomers and their protein binding in stroke patients. *Ther Drug Monit.* 1994;16:509-12.
28. Lewis RJ, Trager WF. Warfarin metabolism in man: identification of metabolites in urine. *J Clin Invest.* 1970;49:907-13.
29. Lewis RL, Trager WF, Chan KK, et al. Warfarin: stereochemical aspects of its metabolism and the interaction with phenylbutazone. *J Clin Invest.* 1974;53:1607-17.
30. Rettie AE, Korzekwa KR, Kunze KL, et al. Hydroxylation of warfarin by human cDNA expressed cytochrome p450: a role for P450-2C9 in the etiology of S-warfarin drug interactions. *Chem Res Toxicol.* 1992;5:54-9.
31. Toon S, Low LK, Gibaldi M, et al. The warfarin-sulfinpyrazone interaction: stereochemical considerations. *Clin Pharmacol*

Ther. 1986;39:15-24.

32. Lewis RL, Trager WF, Robinson AJ, et al. Warfarin metabolites: the anticoagulant activity and pharmacology of warfarin alcohols. *J Lab Clin Med.* 1973;81:925-31.

33. Chan KK, Lewis RJ, Trager WF. Absolute configurations of the four warfarin alcohols. *J Med Chem.* 1972;15:1265-70.

34. Chan E, McLachlan AJ, Pegg M, et al. Disposition of warfarin enantiomers and metabolism in patients during multiple dosing with rac-warfarin. *Br J Clin Pharmacol.* 1994;37:563-9.

35. Ingelman-Sunberg M, Daly AK, Nebert DW, et al. Human cytochrome P450 (CYP) Allele Nomenclature Committee (web site): http://www.imm.ki.se/CYPalleles/. Accessed November 2010.

36. Loebstein Y, Yonath H, Peleg D, et al. Interindividual variability in sensitivity to warfarin: nature or nurture? *Clin Pharmacol Ther.* 2001;70:159-64.

37. Scordo MG, Pengo V, Spina E, et al. Influence of CYP2C9 and CYP2C19 genetic polymorphisms on warfarin maintenance dose and metabolic clearance. *Clin Pharmacol Ther.* 2002;72:702-10.

38. Takahashi H, Kashima T, Nomizo Y, et al. Metabolism of warfarin enantiomers in Japanese patients with heart disease having different CYP2C9 and CYP2C19 genotypes. *Clin Pharmacol Ther.* 1998;63:519-28.

39. Takahashi H, Kashima T, Nomoto S, et al. Comparisons between in vitro and in vivo metabolism of S-warfarin: catalytic activities of cDNA-expressed CYP2C9, its Leu359 variant and their mixture versus unbound clearance in patients with the corresponding CYP2C9 genotypes. *Pharmacogenetics.* 1998;8:365-73.

40. Takahashi H, Wilkinson GR, Caraco Y, et al. Population differences in S-warfarin metabolism between CYP2C9 genotype-matched Caucasian and Japanese. *Clin Pharmacol Ther.* 2003;73:253-63.

41. Aithal GP, Day CP, Kesteven PJL, et al. Warfarin dose requirement and CYP2C9 polymorphisms. *Lancet.* 1999;353:1972-3.

42. Furuya H, Fernandez-Salguero P, Gregory W, et al. Genetic polymorphisms of CYP2C9 and its effect on warfarin maintenance dose requirement in patients undergoing anticoagulation therapy. *Pharmacogenetics.* 1995;5:389-92.

43. Higashi M, Veenstra DL, Kondo LM, et al. Influence of CYP2C9 genetic variants on the risk of overanticoagulation and of bleeding events during warfarin therapy. *JAMA.* 2002;287:1690-8.

44. Sanderson S, Emery J, Higgins J. CYP2C9 gene variants, drug dose, and bleeding risk in warfarin treated patients: a HuGEnet systematic review and meta-analysis. *Genet Med.* 2005;7:97-104.

45. Peyvandi F, Spreafico M, Siboni SM, et al. CYP2C9 genotypes and dose requirements during the induction phase of oral anticoagulation. *Clin Pharmacol Ther.* 2004;75:198-203.

46. Margaglione M, Colaizzo D, D'Andrea G, et al. Genetic modulation of oral anticoagulation with warfarin. *Thromb Haemost.* 2000;84:775-8.

47. Yang L, Ge W, Yu F, et al. Impact of VKORC1 gene polymorphism on interindividual and interethnic warfarin dosage requirement – a systematic review and meta-analysis. *Thromb Res.* 2010; 125:e159-e66.

48. D'Andrea G, D'Ambrosia RL, Di Perna P, et al. A polymorphism in the VKORC1 gene is associated with interindividual variability in the dose-anticoagulant effect of warfarin. *Blood.* 2005;105:645-9.

49. Rieder MJ, Peiner AP, Gage BF, et al. Effect of VKORC1 haplotypes on transcriptional regulation and warfarin dose. *New Engl J Med.* 2005;352:2285-93.

50. Schulman S, Lockner D, Bergstrom K, et al. Intensive initial oral anticoagulation and shorter heparin treatment in deep vein thrombosis. *Thromb Haemost.* 1984;52:276-80.

51. O'Reilly RA, Aggeler PM. Initiation of warfarin therapy without a loading dose. *Circulation.* 1968;38:169-77.

52. Pengo V, Biasiolo A, Pegoraro C. A simple scheme to initiate oral anticoagulant treatment in outpatients with nonrheumatic atrial fibrillation. *Am J Cardiol.* 2001;88:1214-6.

53. Siguret V, Gouin I, Debray M, et al. Initiation of warfarin therapy in elderly medical inpatients: a safe and accurate regimen. *Am J Med.* 2005;118:137-142.57.

54. Oates A, Jackson PR, Austin CA, et al. A new regimen for starting warfarin therapy in outpatients. *Br J Clin Pharmacol.* 1998;46:157-61.

55. Tait RC, Sefcick A. A warfarin induction regimen for out-patient anticoagulation in patients with atrial fibrillation. *Br J Haematol.* 1998;101:450-4.

56. Kovacs MJ, Anderson DA, Wells PS. Prospective assessment of a nomogram for the initiation of oral anticoagulant therapy for outpatient treatment of venous thromboembolism. *Pathophysiol Haemost Thromb.* 2002;32:131-3.

57. Kovacs MJ, Rodger M, Anderson DR, et al. Comparison of 10 mg and 5 mg warfarin initiation nomograms together with low molecular weight heparin for outpatient treatment of acute venous thromboembolism. *Ann Intern Med.* 2003;138:714-9.

58. Eckhoff CD, DiDomenico RJ, Shapiro NL. Initiating warfarin therapy: 5 mg versus 10 mg. *Ann Pharmacotherapy.* 2004;38:2115-21.

59. Harrison L, Johnston M, Massicotte MP, et al. Comparison of 5 mg and 10 mg loading doses in initiation of warfarin therapy. *Ann Intern Med.* 1997;126:133-6.

60. Fennerty A, Dolben J, Thomas J, et al. Flexible induction dose regimen for warfarin and prediction of maintenance dose. *Br J Med.* 1984;288:1268-70.

61. Cosh DG, Moritz CK, Ashman KJ, et al. Prospective evaluation of a flexible protocol for starting treatment with warfarin and predicting its maintenance dose. *Aust NZ J Med.* 1989;19:191-7.

62. Gedge J, Orme S, Hampton KK, et al. A comparison of a low-dose warfarin induction regimen with the modified Fennerty regimen in elderly inpatients. *Age Ageing.* 2000;29:31-4.

63. Roberts GW, Druskeit T, Jorgensel LE, et al. Comparison of an age adjusted warfarin loading protocol with empirical dosing and Fennerty's protocol. *Aust NZ J Med.* 1999;29:731-6.

64. Roberts GW, Helboe T, Nielsen CBM, et al. Assessment of an age-adjusted warfarin initiation protocol. *Ann Pharmacotherapy.* 2003;37:799-803.

65. Crowther MA, Ginsberg JB, Kearon C, et al. A randomized trial comparing 5 mg and 10 mg warfarin loading doses. *Arch Intern Med.* 1999;159:46-8.

66. Crowther MA, Harrison L, Hirsh J. Warfarin: less may be better. *Ann Intern Med.* 1997;127:332-3.

67. Lubitz SA, Scott SA, Rothlauf EB, et al. Comparative performance of gene-based warfarin dosing algorithms in a multiethnic population. *J Thromb Haemost.* 2010;8:1018-26.

68. Ferder NS, Eby CS, Deych E, et al. Ability of VKORC1 and CYP2C9 to predict therapeutic warfarin dose during the initial weeks of therapy. *J Thromb Haemost.* 2009;8:95-100.

69. Li C, Schwarz UI, Ritchie MD, et al. Relative contribution of CYP2C9 and VKORC1 genotypes and early INR response to the prediction of warfarin sensitivity during initiation of therapy. *Blood.* 2009;113:3925-30.

70. Neudoerffer K, Bent S, Nussbaum RL, et al. Genetic testing before anticoagulation? A systematic review of pharmacogenetic dosing of warfarin. *J Gen Intern Med.* 2009;24:656-64.

71. Eckman MH, Rosand J, Greenberg SM, et al. Cost-effectiveness of using pharmacogenetic information in warfarin dosing for patients with nonvalvular atrial fibrillation. *Ann Intern Med.* 2009;150:73-83.

72. Gage BF, Fihn SD, White RH. Management and dosing of warfarin therapy. *Am J Med.* 2000;109:481-8.

73. Wong WW, Wilson-Norton J, Wittkowsky AK. Same daily dosing of warfarin: Influence of regimen type on clinical and monitoring outcomes in stable patients in an anticoagulation management service. *Pharmacotherapy.* 1999;19:1385-91.

74. Hirsh J, Guyatt G, Albers G, et al. Executive Summary. Antithrombotic and Thrombolytic therapy: American College of Chest Physicians Evidence-based Clinical Practice Guidelines (8th Edition). *Chest.* 2008;133 (suppl 6):71s-105s.

75. Kumar S, Haight JRM, Tate G, et al. Effect of warfarin on plasma concentrations of vitamin K dependent coagulation factors in patients with stable control and monitored compliance. *Br J Haematol.* 1990;72:82-5.

76. Kitchen S, Preston FE. Standardization of prothrombin time for laboratory control of oral anticoagulant therapy. *Semin Thromb Hemost.* 1999;25:17-25.

77. WHO Expert Committee on Biological Standardization 28th Report. WHO Tech Rep Ser. 1977;610:4-16, 45-51.

78. Hirsh J, Poller L. The international normalized ratio. A guide to understanding and correcting its problems. *Arch Intern Med.* 1994;154:282-8.

79. Poller L, Triplett DA, Hirsh J, et al. The value of plasma calibrants in correcting coagulometer effects on international normalized ratios. *Am J Clin Pathol.* 1995;103:358-65.

80. Spinler SA, Nutescu ED, Smythe MA, et al. Anticoagulation monitoring Part 1: warfarin and parenteral direct thrombin inhibitors. *Ann Pharmacother.* 2005;39:1049-55.

81. Heneghan C, Alonso-Coello P, Garcia-Alamino JM, et al. Self-monitoring of oral anticoagulation: a systematic review and meta-analysis. *Lancet.* 2006;367:404-11.

82. Wessler S, Gitel SN. Warfarin: from bedside to bench. *New Engl J Med.* 1984;311:645-52.

83. Zivelin A, Roa LVM, Paraport SI. Mechanisms of the anticoagulant effect of warfarin as evaluated in rabbits by selective depression of individual procoagulant vitamin K dependent clotting factors. *J Clin Invest.* 1993;92:2131-40.

84. Wittkowsky AK. Why warfarin and heparin need to overlap when treating acute venous thromboembolism. *Dis Mon.* 2005;51:112-5.

85. Kearon C, Kahn S, Agnelli G, et al. Antithrombotic therapy for venous thromboembolic disease: American College of Chest Physicians Evidence-Based Clinical Practice Guidelines (8th edition). *Chest.* 2008;133 (suppl 6):454s-545s.

86. Tobu M, Iqbal O, Hoppensteadt D, et al. Anti-Xa and anti-IIa drugs alter international normalized ratio measurements: potential problems in the monitoring of oral anticoagulants. *Clin Appl Thromb Hemost.* 2004;10:301-9.

87. Phillips EM, Buchan DA, Newman N, et al. Low molecular weight heparin may alter point-of-care assay for international normalized ratio. *Pharmacotherapy.* 2005;25:1341-7.

88. Laga AC, Cheves TA, Sweeney JD. The effect of specimen hemolysis on coagulation test results. *Am J Clin Pathol.* 2006;126:948-55.

89. Marlar RA, Potts RM, Marlar AA. Effect of routine and special coagulation testing values of citrate anticoagulant adjustment in patients with high hematocrit values. *Am J Clin Pathol.* 2006;126:400-5.

90. Lim W, Crowther MA, Eikelboom JW. Management of antiphospholipid antibody syndrome. A systematic review. *JAMA.* 2006;295:1050-7.

91. Moll S, Oertel TL. Monitoring warfarin therapy in patients with lupus anticoagulants. *Ann Intern Med.* 1997;127:177-85.

92. Perry SL, Samsa GP, Oertel TL. Point-of-care testing of the international normalized ratio in patients with antiphospholipid antibodies. *Thromb Haemost.* 2005;94:1196-202.

93. Rosborough TK, Shepard MF. Unreliability of international normalized ratio for monitoring warfarin therapy in patients with lupus anticoagulant. *Pharmacotherapy.* 2004;24:838-42.

94. Veeger NJGM, Piersma-Wichers M, Tijssem JGP, et al. Individual time within target range in patients treated with vitamin K antagonists: main determinant of quality of anticoagulation and predictor of clinical outcome. A retrospective study of 2300 consecutive patients with venous thromboembolism. *Br J Haematol.* 2005;128:513-9.

95. Schmitt L, Speckman J, Ansell J. Quality assessment of anticoagulation dose management: comparative evaluation of measures of time-in-therapeutic range. *J Thromb Thrombolysis.* 2003;15:213-6.

96. Hylek E, Skates SJ, Sheehan MA, et al. An analysis of the lowest effective intensity of prophylactic anticoagulation for patients with nonrheumatic atrial fibrillation. *New Engl J Med.* 1996;335:540-6.

97. Cannegeiter SC, Rosendaal FR, Wintzen AR, et al. Optimal oral anticoagulant therapy in patients with mechanical heart valves. *New Engl J Med.* 1995;333:11-7.

98. Palareti G, Legnani C, Cosmi B, et al. Poor anticoagulation quality in the first 3 months after unprovoked venous thromboembolism is a risk factor for long-term recurrence. *J Thromb Haemost.* 2005;3:955-61.

99. Wittkowsky AK, Devine EB. Frequency and causes of overanticoagulation and underanticoagulation in patients taking warfarin. *Pharmacotherapy.* 2004;24:1311-6.

100. Schulman S, Beyth RJ, Kearon C, et al. Hemorrhagic complications of anticoagulant and thrombolytic treatment. American College of Chest Physicians Evidence-Based Clinical Practice Guidelines (8th edition). *Chest.* 2008;133(suppl 6):257s-98s.

101. Hylek EM, Chang YC, Skates SJ, et al. Prospective study of the outcomes of ambulatory patients with excessive warfarin anticoagulation. *Arch Intern Med.* 2000;160:1612-7.

102. Hylek EM, Singer DE. Risk factors for intracranial hemorrhage in outpatient taking warfarin. *Ann Intern Med.* 1994;120:897-902.

103. Fihn SD, McDonell M, Martin D, et al. Risk factors for complications of chronic anticoagulation. A multicenter study. Warfarin Optimized Outpatient Follow-Up Study Group. *Ann Intern Med.* 1993;118:511-20.

104. Witt DM, Sadler MA, Shanahan RL. Effect of a centralized clinical pharmacy anticoagulation service on the outcomes of anticoagulation therapy. *Chest.* 2005;127:1515-22.

105. Chiquette E, Amato MG, Bussey HI. Comparison of an anticoagulation clinic with usual medical care: anticoagulation control, patient outcomes, and health care costs. *Arch Intern Med.* 1998;158:1641-7.

106. Fihn SD, Callahan CM, Martin DC, et al. The risk for and severity of bleeding complications in elderly patients treated with warfarin. The National Consortium of Anticoagulation Clinics. *Ann Intern Med.* 1996;124:970-9.

107. Fang MC, Chang Y, Hylek EK, et al. Advanced age, anticoagulation intensity, and risk for intracranial hemorrhage among patients taking warfarin for atrial fibrillation. *Ann Intern Med.* 2004;141:745-52.

108. Beyth RJ, Quinn LM, Landefeld CS. Prospective evaluation of an index for predicting major bleeding in outpatients treated with warfarin. *Am J Med.* 1998;105:91-9.

109. Aspinall SL, DeSanzo BE, Trilli LE, et al. Bleeding Risk Index in an anticoagulation clinic. Assessment by indication and implications for care. *J Gen Intern Med.* 2005;20:1008-13.

110. Whitling AM, Bussey HI, Lyons RM. Comparing different routes and doses of phytonadione for reversing excessive anticoagulation. *Arch Intern Med.* 1998;158:2136-40.

111. Raj G, Kumar R, McKinney P. Time course of reversal of anticoagulant effect of warfarin by intravenous and subcutaneous phytonadione. *Arch Intern Med.* 1999;159:2721-4.

112. Crowther MA, Douketis JD, Schnurr T, et al. Oral vitamin K lowers the international normalized ratio more rapidly than subcutaneous vitamin K in the treatment of warfarin-associated coagulopathy. *Ann Intern Med.* 2002;137:251-4.

113. DeZee KJ, Shimeall WT, Douglas KM. Treatment of excessive anticoagulation with phytonadione (vitamin K). *Arch Intern Med.* 2006;166:391-7.

114. Martin JC. Anaphylactoid reactions and vitamin K (letter). *Med J Aust.* 1991;155:851.

115. Wittkowsky AK. Drug interactions with oral anticoagulants. In: Colman RW, Marder VJ, Clowes AW, et al., eds. *Hemostasis*

and Thrombosis. Basic Principles and Clinical Practice. 5th ed. Philadelphia, PA: Lippincott Williams & Wilkins; 2006.

116. Tatro DS, ed. *Drug Interaction Facts*. St. Louis, MO: Wolters Kluwer; 2010.
117. Hansten P, Horn J. Principals of oral anticoagulant drug interactions. In: *Drug Interactions and Updates Quarterly*. Vancouver, WA: Applied Therapeutics; 1993.
118. Wells PS, Holbrook AM, Crowther NR, et al. Interactions of warfarin with drugs and food. *Ann Intern Med*. 1994;121:676-83.
119. Harder S, Thurmann P. Clinically important drug interactions with warfarin. An update. *Clin Pharmacokinet*. 1996;30:416-44.
120. Holbrook AM, Periera JA, Labiris R, et al. Systematic overview of warfarin and its drug and food interactions. *Arch Intern Med*. 2005;165:1095-1106.
121. Heck AM, DeWitt BA, Lukes AL. Potential interactions between alternative therapies and warfarin. *Am J Health-Syst Pharm*. 2000;57:1221-7.
122. Greenblatt DJ, von Moltke LL. Interaction of warfarin with drugs, natural substances, and foods. *J Clin Pharmacol*. 2005;45:127-32.
123. Vaes LP. Chyka PA. Interactions of warfarin with garlic, ginger, ginkgo and ginseng: nature of the evidence. *Ann Pharmacother*. 2000;34:1478-82.
124. Nutescu EA, Shapiro NL, Ibrahim S, et al. Warfarin and its interactions with foods, herbs, and other dietary supplements. *Expert Opin Drug Saf*. 2006;5:433-51.
125. Hansten P, Horn J. *Drug Interactions Analysis and Management*. St. Louis, MO: Wolters Kluwer; 2010.
126. Wittkowsky AK. Warfarin drug interactions: detection, prediction, prevention. *J Thrombosis Thrombolysis*. 1996;2:295-9.
127. Daly AK, Aithal GP. Genetic regulation of warfarin metabolism and response. *Semin Vasc Med*. 2003;3:231-7.
128. Gurwitz JH, Avorn J, Ross-Degnan D, et al Ageing and the anticoagulant response to warfarin therapy. *Ann Intern Med*. 1992;116:901-4.
129. Sheperd AMM, Hewick DS, Moreland TA, et al. Age as a determinant of sensitivity to warfarin. *Br J Clin Pharmacol*. 1977;4:315-20.
130. Hodges SJ, Pilkington MJ, Schearer MJ, et al. Age-related changes in the circulating levels of congeners of vitamin K2, menaquinone-7 and menaquinone-8. *Clin Sci*. 1990;78:63-6.
131. Garcia D, Regan S, Crowther M, et al. Warfarin maintenance dosing patterns in clinical practice. Implications for safer anticoagulation in the elderly population. *Chest*. 2005;127:2049-56.
132. Bates SM, Ginsberg GS. Anticoagulants in pregnancy. Fetal effects. *Baillieres Clin Obstet Gynaecol*. 1997;11:479-88.
133. Clark SL. Porter TF, West FG. Coumarin derivatives and breast feeding. *Obstet Gynecol*. 2000;95 (6 pt 1):938-40.
134. Fraser AG. Pharmacokinetic interactions between alcohol and other drugs. *Clin Pharmacokinet*. 1997;33:79-90.
135. Mammen EF. Coagulation abnormalities in liver disease. *Hematol Oncol Clin North Am*. 1992;6:1247-57.
136. Deitcher SR. Interpretation of the international normalized ratio in patients with liver disease. *Lancet*. 2002;359:47-8.
137. Dreisbach AW, Japa S, Gebrekal AB, et al. Cytochrome P4502C9 activity in end stage renal disease. *Clin Pharmacol Ther*. 2003;73:475-7.
138. Ganeval D, Fischer AM, Barre J, et al. Pharmacokinetics of warfarin in the nephrotic syndrome and effect on vitamin k-dependent clotting factors. *Clin Nephrol*. 1986;25:75-80.
139. Leech BF, Carter CJ. Falsely elevated INR results due to the sensitivity of a thromboplastin reagent to heparin. *Am J Clin Pathol*. 1998;109:764-8.
140. Self TH, Reaves AB, Oliphant CS, et al. Does heart failure exacerbation increase response to warfarin? A critical review of the literature. *Curr Med Res Opin*. 2006;22:2089-94.
141. Rahlman M, BinEsmael TIM, Payne N, et al. Increased sensitivity to warfarin after heart valve replacement. *Ann Pharmacother*. 2006;40:397-401.
142. Stephens MA, Self TH, Lancaster D, et al. Hypothyroidism: effect on warfarin anticoagulation. *South Med J*. 1989;82:1585-6.
143. Kellett HA, Sawers JS, Boulton FE, et al. Problems of anticoagulation with warfarin in hyperthyroidism. *Q J Med*. 1986;58:43-51.
144. Zevin S, Benowitz NL. Drug interactions with tobacco smoking. An update. *Clin Pharmacokinet*. 1999;36:425-38.
145. Evans M, Lewis GM. Increase in International Normalized Ratio after smoking cessation in a patient receiving warfarin. *Pharmacotherapy*. 2005;25:1656-9.
146. Kuykendall JR, Houle MD, Rhodes RS. Possible warfarin failure due to interaction with smokeless tobacco. *Ann Pharmacother*. 2004;38:595-7.

Appendix A

Therapeutic Ranges of Drugs in Traditional and SI Units[a]

Drug	Traditional Range	Conversion Factor[b]	SI Range
Acetaminophen	>5 mg/dL toxic	66.160	>330 μmol/L toxic
N-Acetylprocainamide	4–10 mg/L	3.606	14–36 μmol/L
Amitriptyline	75–175 ng/mL	3.605	180–720 nmol/L
Carbamazepine	4–12 mg/L	4.230	17–51 μmol/L
Chlordiazepoxide	0.5–5.0 mg/L	3.336	2–17 μmol/L
Chlorpromazine	50–300 ng/mL	3.136	150–950 nmol/L
Chlorpropamide	75–250 μg/mL	3.613	270–900 μmol/L
Clozapine	450–? ng/mL	0.003	1.38–? μmol/L
Cyclosporine	100–200 ng/mL[c]	0.832	80–160 nmol/L
Desipramine	100–160 ng/mL	3.754	170–700 nmol/L
Diazepam	100–250 ng/mL	3.512	350–900 nmol/L
Digoxin	0.9–2.2 ng/mL	1.281	1.2–2.8 nmol/L
Disopyramide	2–6 mg/L	2.946	6–18 μmol/L
Doxepin	50–200 ng/mL	3.579	180–720 nmol/L
Ethosuximide	40–100 mg/L	7.084	280–710 μmol/L
Fluphenazine	0.5–2.5 ng/mL	2.110	5.3–21 nmol/L
Glutethimide	>20 mg/L toxic	4.603	>92 μmol/L toxic
Gold	300–800 mg/L	0.051	15–40 μmol/L
Haloperidol	5–15 ng/mL	2.660	13–40 nmol/L
Imipramine	200–250 ng/mL	3.566	180–710 nmol/L
Isoniazid	>3 mg/L toxic	7.291	>22 μmol/L toxic
Lidocaine	1–5 mg/L	4.267	5–22 μmol/L
Lithium	0.5–1.5 mEq/L	1.000	0.5–1.5 μmol/L
Maprotiline	50–200 ng/mL	3.605	180–720 μmol/L
Meprobamate	>40 mg/L toxic	4.582	>180 μmol/L toxic
Methotrexate	>2.3 mg/L toxic	2.200	>5 μmol/L toxic
Nortriptyline	50–150 ng/mL	3.797	190–570 nmol/L
Pentobarbital	20–40 mg/L	4.419	90–170 μmol/L
Perphenazine	0.8–2.4 ng/mL	2.475	2–6 nmol/L
Phenobarbital	15–40 mg/L	4.306	65–172 μmol/L
Phenytoin	10–20 mg/L	3.964	40–80 μmol/L
Primidone	4–12 mg/L	4.582	18–55 μmol/L
Procainamide	4–8 mg/L	4.249	17–34 μmol/L
Propoxyphene	>2 mg/L toxic	2.946	>6 μmol/L toxic
Propranolol	50–200 ng/mL	3.856	190–770 nmol/L
Protriptyline	100–300 ng/mL	3.797	380–1140 nmol/L
Quinidine	2–6 mg/L	3.082	5–18 μmol/L
Salicylate (acid)	15–25 mg/dL	0.072	1.1–1.8 mmol/L
Theophylline	10–20 mg/L	5.550	55–110 μmol/L
Thiocyanate	>10 mg/dL toxic	0.172	>1.7 mmol/L toxic
Valproic acid	50–100 mg/L	6.934	350–700 μmol/L
Warfarin	1–3 mg/L	3.243	3.3–9.8 μmol/L

[a] Source: Traub SL. Interpreting Laboratory Data. 2nd edition. Bethesda, MD: American Society of Health-System Pharmacists; 1996:p. 397.
[b] Traditional units are multiplied by conversion factor to get SI units.
[c] Whole blood assay.

Appendix B

Nondrug Reference Ranges for Common Laboratory Tests in Traditional and SI Units[a]

Laboratory Test	Reference Range Traditional Units	Conversion Factor	Reference Range SI Units	Comment
Alanine aminotransferase (ALT)	0–30 IU/L	0.01667	0–0.50 μkat/L	SGPT
Albumin	3.5–5 g/dL	10.00	35–50 g/L	
Ammonia	30–70 μg/dL	0.587	17–41 μmol/L	
Aspartate aminotransferase (AST)	8–42 IU/L	0.01667	0.133–0.700 μkat/L	SGOT
Bilirubin (direct)	0.1–0.3 mg/dL	17.10	1.7–5 μmol/L	
Bilirubin (total)	0.3–1.0 mg/dL	17.10	5–17 μmol/L	
Calcium	8.5–10.8 mg/dL	0.25	2.1–2.7 mmol/L	
Carbon dioxide (CO_2)	24–30 mEq/L	1.000	24–30 mmol/L	Serum bicarbonate
Chloride	96–106 mEq/L	1.000	96–106 mmol/L	
Cholesterol (HDL)	>35 mg/dL	0.026	>0.91 mmol/L	desirable
Cholesterol (LDL)	<130 mg/dL	0.026	<3.36 mmol/L	desirable
Creatine kinase (CK)	40–200 IU/L	0.01667	0.667–3.33 μkat/L	males
	35–150 IU/L		0.583–2.50 μkat/L	females
Serum creatinine (SCr)	0.7–1.5 mg/dL	88.40	62–133 μmol/L	
Creatinine clearance (CrCl)	90–140 mL/min/1.73 m^2	0.017	1.53–2.38 mL/sec/1.73 m^2	
Folic acid	≥3.3 ng/dL	2.212	>7.3 nmol/L	
γ-glutamyl transpeptidase	0–30 U/L (but varies)	0.01667	0–0.50 μkat/L (but varies)	GGTP
Globulin	2–3 g/dL	10.00	20–30 g/L	
Glucose (fasting)	70–110 mg/dL	0.056	3.9–6.1 mmol/L	fasting
Hemoglobin (Hgb)	14–18 g/dL	0.622	8.7–11.2 mmol/L	males
	12–16 g/dL		7.4–9.9 mmol/L	females
Iron	50–150 μg/dL	0.179	9–26.9 μmol/L	
Iron-binding capacity	250–410 μg/dL	0.179	45–73 μmol/L	TIBC
Lactate dehydrogenase	100–210 IU/L	0.01667	1.67–3.50 μkat/L	LDH
Serum lactate (venous)	0.5–1.5 mEq/L	1.000	0.5–1.5 mmol/L	Lactic acid
Serum lactate (arterial)	0.5–2.0 mEq/L	1.000	0.5–2.0 mmol/L	
Magnesium	1.5–2.2 mEq/L	0.500	0.75–1.1 mmol/L	
5′ Nucleotidase	1–11 U/L (but varies)	0.01667	0.02–0.18 μkat/L (but varies)	
Phosphate	2.6–4.5 mg/dL	0.329	0.85–1.48 mmol/L	
Potassium	3.5–5.0 mEq/L	1.000	3.5–5.0 mmol/L	
Sodium	136–145 mEq/L	1.000	136–145 mmol/L	
Total serum thyroxine (T_4)	4–12 μg/dL	12.87	51–154 nmol/L	Total T_4
Triglycerides	<200 mg/dL	0.0113	<2.26 mmol/L	
Total serum triiodothyronine (T_3)	78–195 ng/dL	0.0154	1.2–3.0 nmol/L	Total T_3
Urea nitrogen, blood	8–20 mg/dL	0.357	2.9–7.1 mmol/L	BUN
Uric acid (serum)	3.4–7 mg/dL	59.48	202–416 μmol/L	

[a] Source: Traub SL. Interpreting Laboratory Data. 2nd edition. Bethesda, MD: American Society of Health-System Pharmacists; 1996:p. 399. Note that some laboratories are maintaining traditional units for enzyme tests.

INDEX

A

AB-rated generic cyclosporine, 159
absorption
age-dependent difference in, 34
  geriatric, 46–48
  pediatric intramuscular, 30–31
  pediatric oral, 30
  pediatric percutaneous, 31
  pediatric rectal, 31
acetaminophen, 139
acquired immunodeficiency syndrome (AIDS), 38–39, 283
actual body weight (ABW), xxxi, 3–4, 5–6
acute myocardial infarction, 238
acyclovir, 108, 166
adherence, to drug regimen, 15
adjusted body weight (ABW), 19, 22, 25
adolescence, antidepressants, 129
advanced age. *See also* geriatric patient
  lidocaine, 238
  warfarin, 366
adverse drug reactions/events (ADEs), 46
albumin, 31–32
alcoholic liver disease, 129
alcoholism
antidepressants, 129
  warfarin, 367
American Academy of Neurology, 150, 151
American Academy of Pediatrics, 239
American College of Chest Physicians, 203, 210, 216, 358
American College of Clinical Pharmacology, xxxii
American Epilepsy Society, 150
American Psychiatric Association, 244
amikacin, 36, 38, 92–94, 99, 102
amiloride, 1
aminoglycosides, 2, 13, 344
  absorption, 93
  assay issues, 105–6
  bioavailability, 94
  children dosing, 101
  clearance, 95, 97
  concentration measurement frequency, 103–4
  concentration-related efficacy, 106
  disease state/condition interactions, 108–9
  distribution, 93, 94
  dosage form availability, 92–93
  dosage interval, 87
  dosing strategies, 95–102
  dosing weight and volume of distribution, 96–97
  drug concentration measurement, 15
  drug disposition factors, 36, 37, 38
  drug-drug interactions, 108
  elimination, 95, 98
  follow-up concentration measurements, 104
  geriatric dosing, 102
  half-life, time to steady state, 95, 96, 97
  hemodialysis, 81
  initial concentration measurement, 104–6
  LDEI, 91, 92, 98–103, 107, 110
  loading dose, 91–92
  maintenance dose, 92
  monitoring approaches, 105
  neonate dosing, 100–101, 102
  once-daily dosing, 99, 101
  pharmacokinetic monitoring, 106–8
  protein binding, 94
  renal clearance, 23
  sampling times, 103
  SDSI, 91, 92, 98, 102, 104, 105, 106, 110
  therapeutic monitoring, 103–6
  therapeutic ranges, 102–3, 105
  toxicity, 106–8
  usual dosage range, 91–92
  volume of distribution, 95, 96–97
amitriptyline, 121, 122, 125, 126
amphotericin B, 108, 344, 345
ampicillin, 30
amputations, creatinine clearance estimation, 7
Anderson, Douglas M., 263–72
angiotensin converting enzyme inhibitors (ACEIs), 45, 292
antacids, 138, 165
antibiotics, 333
anticoagulants, 333
anticonvulsants, 46, 333
antidepressants, 52, 119
  disease state/condition, 129–32
  dosage form availability, 121–22
  dosing strategies, 123–25
  drug-drug interactions, 128–29, 130–31
  metabolism, 124
  pharmacokinetic parameters, 122–23
  therapeutic monitoring, 128
  therapeutic range, 125–27
  usual dosage range, 119–20
antidiabetic agents, 46
antiepileptic drugs, 178
  dosage forms, 136
  felbamate, 135–37
  gabapentin, 137–38
  generic substitutions, 151
  lacosamide, 147–48
  lamotrigine, 138–40
  levetiracetam, 142–43
  newer, 150–51
  oxcarbazepine, 143–45
  pregabalin, 146–47
  rufinamide, 148–49

tiagabine, 140
topiramate, 141–42
vigabatrin, 149–50
antihypotensive agents, 52
antiparkinson drugs, 52
antiplatelet agents, 212
antipsychotic agents, 52
antirejection agents
absorption, 161
disease state/condition interactions, 166–67
distribution, 161–62
dosage form availability, 159, 160
dosage range, 159
dosing recommendations, 159, 160
drug-drug interactions, 165–66
elimination, 162
half-life, time to steady state, 162–63
pharmacodynamic monitoring, 164–65
protein binding, 162
sampling times, 164
therapeutic range, 163
antiretroviral agents, 39
arbekacin, 92
ascites, aminoglycosides, 108
asphyxia, 36
aspirin, 333
asthma, 315, 323
atorvastatin, 165, 166
average steady state concentration (Css_{av}), xxxi–xxxii

B

bacitracin, 108
Bainbridge, Jacquelyn L., 135–57, 169–83, 197–201
Banzel, 148–49
barbiturates, 49, 52, 200
Bayesian analysis, 96, 103
Beers Criteria, 52
benzodiazepines, 49, 52
bepridil, 77
beta-adrenergic antagonist, 299
beta-agonists, 52
beta-blockers, 49, 52, 304
beta-lactam antibiotics, 32
bilirubin, 32
binding, of medication, 22, 23
body
composition, 19, 21
mass index, 22
size descriptor equations, 20, 21, 22
surface area (BSA), 33
weight, creatinine clearance estimation, 5–6
breast milk, lithium, 255
bupropion, 122, 125, 126, 128, 129, 131
burns, aminoglycosides, 108

C

C, xxxii
Calcium, 47
calcium channel blockers, 49, 52
capreomycin, 108
carbamazepine
absorption, 170–71
antiepileptic drugs, 136, 139, 142–45, 148–49, 151
clearance based on age, 173
disease state/condition interactions, 177–78
distribution, 171–72
dosage form availability, 170
dosage form bioavailability, 171, 173
dosage forms, 170
dosing strategies, 174
drug-drug interactions, 176–77, 178
elimination, 172–73
ethosuximide, 200
half-life, time to steady state, 173
pharmacodynamic monitoring, 175–76
protein binding, 172
therapeutic monitoring, 175
therapeutic range, 174
usual dosage range, 169–70
volume of distribution, 173
carbamazepine epoxide, 333
carbapenem antibiotics, 333
Carbatrol, 145, 171, 173
carbidopa, 47
carboplatin, 108
cardiac disease, antidepressants,129
cardiac valve replacement, warfarin, 367
Carson, Stanley W., 243–62
cefazolin, 2
cefoperazone, 108
ceftazidime, 37
cephalosporins, 13, 77, 108
chloramphenicol palmitate, 30
chlordiazepoxide, 49
chlorpromazine, 176
chronic kidney disease
clinical assessment of renal function, 73
commonly used drug pharmacokinetic parameters, 79–80
drug dosing strategies, 77–78
drug hemodialyzability factors, 81
gastrointestinal absorption, 76
metabolism, 75–76
renal drug elimination, 74
renal drug transporters, 74–75
volume of distribution, 76–77
chronic obstructive pulmonary disease (COPD), 321, 323
chronic renal insufficiency, 7
C_i, xxxii
cidofovir/probenecid, 75
cimetidine, 1, 7, 75, 138, 333
ciprofloxacin, 46
ciprofloxacin/azlocillin, 75
cirrhosis, 108, 282
citalopram, 126, 127
CL, xxxiii
clindamycin, 30
Clinical and Laboratory Standards Institute (CLSI), 106, 343

clomipramine, 176
clorazepate, 47, 49
clotting factors, 351
cloxacillin, 37–38
C_{max}, xxxii
CNS depressants, 333
CNS depression, 281
Cochrane Collaborative, 315
Cockcroft/Gault equation, 2–4, 5, 7, 8–9, 23, 24, 73
colchicine, 166
colistin, 108
College of American Pathologists, 210
concentration verification, xxx–xxxi
congestive heart failure, 237, 367
continuous infusion unfractionated heparin, 219
continuous renal replacement therapies (CRRT), 73, 78, 81–85, 345
continuous venovenous hemodiafiltration (CVVHDF), 82–85
continuous venovenous hemofiltration (CVVH), 82–85, 345
corticosteroids, 31, 322
Coumadin, 352
coumarin, 351
CrCl, xxxiii
creatine, 1
creatinine assay
    interference compounds, 2
    standardization, 2
creatinine clearance (CrCl), 1
    chronic kidney disease, 73
    geriatric patient, 51
    obese/overweight patient, 23–24
    pediatric, 32
creatinine clearance estimation
    adult formulas, 2–5
    amputations, 7
    assay standardization, 2
    body weight in, 5–6
    chronic renal insufficiency, 7
    dialysis, 7
    geriatric patients, 6
    glomerular filtration rate factors in, 1–2
    liver disease, 7
    pediatrics, 7–8
    spinal cord injury, 7
    unstable renal function, 8, 9
creatinine concentration, time to steady state serum, 8–9
critically ill patient, 283
Css, xxxii
Css_{av}, xxxiii
Css_{max}, xxxiii
Css_{min}, xxxiii
cyclosporine, 159–67
cystic fibrosis (CF), 37–38, 102, 108

D

D, xxxiii
Dager, William E., 203–227
dalteparin, 220
Δt, xxxiv
Depakene, 328, 331
Depakote, 328, 331
Depakote ER, 328, 331, 332
desipramine, 122, 125, 126
desmethylsertraline, 122
dialysis, 342–43. *See also* hemodialysis
    regimen, 78, 81
    aminoglycosides, 109
    creatinine clearance estimation, 7
    lithium, 254
diazepam, 31, 33, 49
dicumarol, 351
diflunisal, 48
digitalis glycosides, 46
digoxin
    antiepileptic drugs,148
    antirejection agents, 166
    assay issues, 189–90
    bioavailability of dosage forms, 187
    clearance, 187, 188
    CrCl-based maintenance doses, interval adjustments, 186
    disease/condition interactions, 192
    dosage form availability, 186
    dosing strategies, 187–89
    drug-drug interactions, 191–92
    half-life, time to steady state, 188
    loading/maintenance doses, 186
    pediatric dosing, 30, 32, 37
    pharmacodynamic monitoring, 190–91
    pharmacokinetic parameters, 187
    procainamide, 291, 299
    quinidine, 304, 308
    renal dosing, 76
    sampling times, 189
    therapeutic monitoring, 189–90
    therapeutic range, 189
    usual dosage range, 185
    volume of distribution, 187, 189
Dilantin, 274
diltiazem, 299, 304
disopyramide, 77, 299
diuretics, 291
divalproex, 328
donepezil, 46
dosage
    adjustments, xxxi
    proportionality, 25, 26
    titrating down, 16–17
    titrating up, 16
Dowling, Thomas C., 73–87
drug concentration monitoring
    decision making process, 14
    dosing approaches, 15–17
    measurements outside predicted range, xxix–xxx
    need evaluation, 13–15
drug disposition
    age-dependent differences in, 34
    pediatric patient factors, 36–39

Drug Reaction with Eosinophilia and Systemic Syndrome (DRESS), 140
drug selection, 13–14
Duby, Jeremiah J., 337–50
duloxetine, 128

E

efficacy, 14–15
Egeberg, Michael D., 135–57, 169–83
EMLA (eutectic mixture of lidocaine and prilocaine), 31
end-stage renal disease (ESRD), 73, 76
enfuvirtide, 39
enoxaparin, 220
Erstad, Brian. 19–28
escitalopram, 122
estimating equations
 body mass index, xxxv
 ideal body weight in children 1–18, xxxiv–xxxv
 lean or ideal body weight in adults, xxxiv
 surface area in square meters, xxxv
estradiol, 48
ethacrynic acid, 108
ethanol, 147, 200
ethinyl estradiol, 139
ethosuximide, 333
 absorption, 197–98
 bioavailability of dosage forms, 198
 clearance, 198
 disease state/condition interactions, 200–201
 distribution, 198
 dosage form availability, 197
 dosing strategies, 199
 drug-drug interactions, 200
 elimination, 198
 half-life, time to steady state, 199
 maintenance dosages, 197
 metabolism, 198
 pharmacodynamic monitoring, 200
 protein binding, 198
 therapeutic monitoring, 199–200
 therapeutic range, 199
 usual dosage range, 197
 volume of distribution, 198
exchange transfusion, 36
extended-spectrum penicillins, 108
extracorporeal membrane oxygenation (ECMO), 36–37

F

F, xxxiii
famotidine, 7
felbamate, 135–37
febrile neutropenia, aminoglycosides, 109
felbamate, 46, 333
Felbatol, 135–37
fentanyl, 48
fetal exposure, lithium, 255
Finley, Patrick R., 119–34
flecainide, 299
fluoroquinolone antibacterials, 46
fluoxetine, 122, 125, 127, 128
fluvastatin, 165
fluvoxamine, 128, 236
folic acid, 47
fondaparinux, 205
 dosage form availability, 221
 dosage range, 221
 drug-condition interactions, 222
 pharmacokinetic information, 221–22
 reversing effect of, 222
 therapeutic monitoring, 222
Formea, Christine, 159–68
fosphenytoin, 46
 dosage form availability, 274
 usual dosage range, 273
frailty, 45
furosemide, 77, 108, 345

G

gabapentin, 46, 137–38, 146, 147, 268, 333
Gabitril, 140
galantamine, 46
Garnett, William R., 135–57, 169–83, 197–201
gastric emptying rate, 30
gastric pH, 30
gentamicin, 36–37, 92–94, 99, 102, 106, 108
geriatric patient
 aminoglycosides, 102
 aminoglycosides dosing weight/volume of distribution, 96–97
 antidepressants, 129
 creatinine clearance estimation, 6
 drug elimination, 49, 51
 drug monitoring, 45–46
 drugs with increased bioavailability, 48
 explicit criteria for inappropriate medication orders, 53–54
 increased free fractions, 48–49
 lean body weight to fat ratio, 49
 pharmacodynamic changes influencing drug response, 51–52
 pharmacokinetic parameters, average drug dose commonly used, 55–67
 physiologic changes in, 46–49
 protein binding, 48–49, 50
 theophylline, 322
Ghibellini, Giulia, 243–62
Gidal, Barry E., 327–36
glomerular filtration rate (GFR), 1–2
 geriatric patient, 51
 obese/overweight patient, 24
 pediatric patient, 32–33
glyburide, 166
glycoprotein IIb/IIIa inhibitors, 212

H

haloperidol, 200
halothane, 52
hemodialysis, 78, 81–82, 84–85, 345. *See also* dialysis

aminoglycosides, 109
dosage recommendations, 83–84
dosage regimen adjustment for, 81–82
principles of, 78, 81
vancomycin, 345–46
warfarin, 367
hemodialyzability, 81
heparin
body composition and, 21
reversing effect of, 213
toxicities related to, 214
unfractionated, 203–16
hepatic disease, 238, 282
hepatic dysfunction/insufficiency
aminoglycosides, 109
antidepressants, 131
hexachlorophene solution, 31
HMG-CoA reductase inhibitors, 45, 166
human immunodeficiency virus (HIV), 38–39
hydroxybupropion, 122
hydroxyzine, 52
hypothermia (therapeutic), 109

I

ibuprofen, 38
ideal body weight (IBW), xxxii, 3–4, 5–6
imipenem, 75
imipramine, 49, 122, 125, 126
indomethacin, 37
infants, theophylline, 322
inflammatory disease states, antidepressants, 131
inhaled corticosteroids, 13
insulin, 52
intensive care patient, aminoglycosides, 109
international normalized ratio, 351, 355, 356
adjustment guidelines, 359
efficacy, 360–61
frequency of, 358
reversing toxicity, 362
toxicity, 361
inulin clearance, 7, 24
iron, 47
isoniazid, 200
isotope dilution mass spectrometry (IDMS), 2, 8, 24
itraconazole, 30
itraconazole/cimetidine, 75
itraconazole/digoxin, 75
itraconazole/quinidine, 75

J

Jaffe method assay, 1, 7–8
Jelliffe equation, 2–4
Johnson, Sarah L., 135–57, 169–83, 197–201

K

κ, xxxiii
κ_a, xxxiii
Karlix, Janet, 159–68
Keppra, 142–43
K_m, xxxiii

L

lacosamide, 147–48, 176, 333
lactation, 238–39, 283, 366–67
Lamictal, 138–40
lamivudine, 39
lamotrigine
antiepileptic drugs, 138–40, 144, 148, 149
carbamazepine, 176
ethosuximide, 201
geriatric patient, 46
valproic acid, 333
large dose-extended interval (LDEI), 91, 92, 98–`01
lean body weight (LBW), xxxii, 49
levetiracetam
antiepileptic drugs, 142–43
carbamazepine, 176
ethosuximide, 201
geriatric patient, 46
phenobarbital, 268
valproic acid, 333
levodopa, 47
levofloxacin, 46
lidocaine, 48, 49, 273
bioavailability of dosage forms, 231
clearance, 233
disease state/condition interactions, 237–39
distribution, 231
dosage form availability, 229, 230
dosing strategies, 233–35
drug-drug interactions, 236–37
elimination, 232
half-life, time to steady state, 233, 234
hydrochloride dosing methods, 235
metabolite formation, activity, 232
pharmacodynamic monitoring, 236
protein binding, 232
sampling times, 235–36
therapeutic range, 235–36
usual dosage range, 229
ventricular arrhythmia dosage ranges, 230
volume of distribution, 231
life-threatening illness dosing, 15–16
linezolid, 31
Link, Karl, 351
lipophilicity, 22–23
lipophilics, 31
lithium, 46
absorption, 244–45
assay issues, 252
bioavailability of dosage forms, 245
clearance by age, 246
concentration measurement frequency, 250–51
concentration-related toxicity, 254
disease state interactions, 253–56
distribution, 245–46
dosage form availability, 244

dosage prediction by a priori demographics, 248
dosage prediction by population pharmacokinetics, measured concent, 248–49
dosage prediction by renal clearance estimation, 248
dosage prediction by traditional pharmacokinetics, 247–48
dose prediction methods, 247
dosing strategies, 247–49
drug-drug interactions, 252–53, 255
elimination, 246
half-life, time to steady state, 247
maintenance dosing recommendations, 244
pharmacodynamic monitoring, 252
sampling times, 249–50
therapeutic monitoring, 249–52, 253
therapeutic range, 249
therapeutic response sequence, 253
usual dosage range, 243–44
volume of distribution by age, 246
liver disease
creatinine clearance estimation, 7
warfarin, 367
loop diuretics, 344, 345
lorazepam, 49, 147, 333
lovastatin, 165
low molecular weight heparin (LMWH), 205, 206, 216–17
assay issues, 218
disease state dosing, 217
disease state/condition interaction, 220
dosage form availability, 217
dosing strategies, 218
dosing, monitoring summary, 221
drug-drug interactions, 220
pharmacodynamic monitoring, 219
pharmacokinetic information, 217–18
pharmacokinetic, pharmacodynamic parameters, 216
reversing effect of, 219–20
therapeutic monitoring, 218
therapeutic range, 218
usual dosage range, 217
loxapine, 200
Lyrica, 146–47

M

malabsorption, 283
malnutrition
aminoglycosides, 109
antidepressants, 131
mannitol, 108
Mathias, Kathryn R., 91–118
Matzke, Gary R., 73–87, 337–50
McCormack, James P., 13–17
mechanical ventilation (postoperative), aminoglycosides, 109
meningitis, aminoglycosides, 109
meperidine, 48, 49
Mephyton, 362
metabolism
phase I enzymes and age, 35
phase II enzymes and age, 35
metformin, 148
methicillin, 37, 38
metoclopramide, 52
midazolam, 36–37
Miller, Susan W., 45–71
mirtazapine, 128
Modification of Diet in Renal Disease (MDRD) study/equations, 4–5, 24, 73
moexipril, 45
monitoring frequency, xxxi
monoamine oxidase inhibitor, 121, 122, 333
mono-hydroxylated derivative (MHD), 143–44
morbid obesity, 238
morphine, 45
Murphy, John E., xxix–xxxvii, 91–118, 289–98, 315–25
mycophenolate mofetil, 166

N

n-acetylprocainamide (NAPA), 292
clearance, 293
dose, 293
pharmacodynamic monitoring, 294–96
sampling, 294
therapeutic range, 293
Nahata, Milap C., 29–44
nalidixic acid, 30
naproxen, 48, 333
narcotic analgesics, 49, 52
National Asthma Education and Prevention Program, 315, 321, 322
National Institutes of Health (NIH), 2
National Kidney Disease Education Program (NKDEP), 2, 4
neonates
aminoglycosides, 100–101, 102
theophylline, 322
Neoral, 159
nephrotoxicity, aminoglycosides, 107
neuromuscular toxicity, aminoglycosides, 108
Neurotonin, 137–38
nevirapine, 39
New York Heart Association, 291
nifedipine, 166
Nolan, Jr., Paul E., 229–42, 299–313
non-renal clearance, 24–25
nonsteroidal anti-inflammatory drugs (NSAIDs), 46, 48
norepinephrine reuptake inhibitors, 119
norfluoxetine, 122, 126, 128
norgestrel/ethinyl estradiol, 166
nortriptyline, 49, 122, 125, 126
Nuedexta, 299
nutritional status, warfarin, 367
nystagmus, 281

O

obese/overweight patients
accurate weight, 19
body composition, 19, 21

dose proportionality, 25, 26
dosing recommendations, 25–26, 27
pharmacokinetic considerations, 22–25
size descriptors, 22
obesity, 5–6, 22, 109, 283
o-desmethylvenlafaxine, 122
opioids, 45
oral contraceptives, 148, 149, 333
orlistat, 166
oseltamivir/probenecid, 75
otoxicity, aminoglycosides, 107–8
oxazepam, 49
oxcarbazepine, 46, 143–45, 201
oxycodone, 147

P

Pachorek, Robert F., 1–12
Page II, Robert L., 185–95, 289–98
Pai, Vinita B., 29–44
pancreatitis, aminoglycosides, 109
paroxetine, 127, 128
patent ductus arteriosus (PDA), 37
aminoglycosides, 109
peak aminoglycoside concentration, 103
peak concentration (C_{peak}), xxxii
pediatric patient
absorption—intramuscular, 30–31
absorption—oral, 30
absorption—percutaneous, 31
absorption—rectal, 31
age groupings and birth age, 29
age-dependent differences in drug disposition, 34–35
age-dependent differences in phase I metabolizing enzymes, 35
age-dependent differences in phase II metabolizing enzymes, 35
aminoglycosides dosing, 100–101
creatinine clearance estimation, 7–8
dosing, 29
drug disposition factors, 36–39
drug distribution, 31–32, 34
elimination, 32–33
metabolism, 33
pharmacokinetic information, 30–31
renal elimination, 32–33, 34
penicillin derivatives, 38
penicillins, 74, 77
peritoneal dialysis, aminoglycosides, 109
Phan, Hanna, 315–25
pharmacokinetic equations, xxxv–xxxvii
pharmacokinetic monitoring factors, xxix
pharmacokinetic symbols, xxxii–xxxiii
phenelzine, 122
phenobarbital, valproic acid, 333
phenobarbital, 36
absorption, 264
antiepileptic drugs, 136, 139, 148, 149
assay considerations, 266–67
bioavailability, 264
clearance, 265
conditions altering pharmacokinetics, 270
CYP enzymes, drugs with reduced concentrations in presence, 269–70
distribution, 264
dosage form availability, 264
drug-drug interactions, 268
drugs affecting concentrations, 268
half-life, time to steady state, 265–66
loading, maintenance doses, 263
pharmacodynamic monitoring, 267–68
protein binding, 265
sampling times, 267
therapeutic range, 266, 267
usual dosage range, 263
valproic acid, 333
volume of distribution, 265
phenothiazines, 49, 52, 200
phenytoin, 13, 15
absorption, 274–75
antiepileptic drugs, 136, 139, 142, 145, 148, 149
assay techniques, 279–80
carbamazepine, 176
clearance, 277
disease state/condition interactions, 282–83
distribution, 275–77
dosage form availability, 274, 275
drug-drug interactions, 281, 282
elimination, 277–78
ethosuximide, 200
geriatric patient, 46, 49
half-life, time to steady state, 278–79
hemodialysis, 77
loading dose, 273
maintenance dose, 273
non-concentration side effects, 281
pediatric patient, 33
pharmacodynamic monitoring, 280–81
pharmacogenomics, 277–78
protein binding, 276–77
sampling times, 279–80
therapeutic monitoring, 279–80
therapeutic range, 279
usual dosage range, 273
valproic acid, 333
volume of distribution, 275–76
piperacillin-tazobactam, 108
plasma protein binding. *See* protein binding
pneumonia, 102
postpartum, aminoglycosides, 109
potassium, 165
pravastatin, 165
prednisolone, 166
pregabalin, 146–47, 333
pregnancy
aminoglycosides, 109
lidocaine, 238–39
lithium, 254
phenytoin, 283
warfarin, 366–67
prematurity, aminoglycosides, 109

primidone, 139, 149, 200, 333
procainamide, 299
  absorption, 289
  assays, 294, 295
  bioavailability of dosage form, 290
  clearance, 291, 292–93
  concentration toxicities, 295–96
  disease state/condition interactions, 297
  distribution, 289–90
  dosage form availability, 290
  dosing strategies, 292
  drug-drug interactions, 296
  elimination, 292
  half-life, time to steady state, 291
  metabolism, 290–91
  NAPA and, 292
  pharmacodynamic monitoring, 294–96
  sampling times, 294
  therapeutic monitoring, 293–94
  usage dosage range, 289, 290
  volume of distribution, 291
Prograf, 159
propafenone, 304
propranolol, 48, 52
protamine, 222
protamine sulfate, 213, 215
protein binding, xxx, 31, 77
  antidepressants, 122
  carbamazepine, 172
  geriatric patient, 48–49, 50
prothrombin time, 351, 359–60
proton-pump inhibitors, 45
protriptyline, 128

Q

QT-interval monitoring, 305
Quetelet's index, 23
quinidine, 299–300
  absorption, 301
  available dosage forms, 300
  bioavailability of dosage forms, 301
  clearance, 303
  disease state/condition interactions, 308
  distribution, 302
  dosing strategies, 304
  drug-drug interactions, 306–8
  elimination, 302
  gluconate, 301, 304
  half-life, time to steady state, 303
  metabolism, 302
  metabolites, 302
  pharmacodynamic monitoring, 305–6
  protein binding, 302–3
  renal excretion, 302
  sampling times, 304–5
  sulfate, 301, 304
  therapeutic range, 303
  usual dosage range, 300
  volume of distribution, 303

R

R_0, xxxiii
raloxifene, 46
ranitidine, 7, 30, 333
Rapamune, 159
renal clearance
  drug elimination, 74
  drug transporters, 74–75
  excretion, narrow therapeutic range drugs, 51
  geriatric patient, 51
  obese/overweight patient, 23–24
renal disease/insufficiency, 238
  antidepressants, 131
  warfarin, 367
renal failure, 282–83
renal function, clinical assessment, 73
rifampin, 139, 333
rivastigmine, 46
  tobacco use, warfarin, 367
Roberts, A. Joshua, 203–227
ropinirole, 46
rufinamide, 148–49, 333

S

S, xxxiii
Sabril, 149–50
Salazar-Corcoran equation, 6, 23–24
salicylate, 1, 48
Sandimmune, 159
Sawchuk-Zaske techniques, 96
S_{Cr}, xxxiii
selective estrogen receptor modulators (SERMs), 45–46
selective serotonin reuptake inhibitors, 119, 120, 122, 124, 125, 129
selegiline, 121, 122, 176
serotonin norepinephrine reuptake inhibitors, 119, 124, 131
sertraline, 46, 122, 126, 127, 128
severe trauma, 238
simvastatin, 165
sirolimus, 159–67
small dose–short interval (SDSI), 91, 92, 98
smoking
  antidepressants, 131
  warfarin, 367
spinal cord injury, creatinine clearance estimation, 7
spironolactone, 1
St. John's Wort, 323
Staphylococcus aureus, 343
statins, 166
stavudine, 39
steady state, xxxii
sulfamethoxazole/trimethoprim, 166
sulfonamides, 32

T

t, xxxiii
T, xxxiv

t', xxxiii
$t_{1/2}$, xxxiii–xxxiv
$t_{1/2a}$, xxxiv
tacrine, 46
tacrolimus, 159–67
Tallian, Kimberly B., 263–72
tamoxifen, 46
τ, xxxiv
Tegretol–XR, 145, 171, 173
temazepam, 49
testosterone, 48
theophylline, 13, 16
  absorption, 316–17
  bioavailability of dosage forms, 317
  carbamazepine,176
  clearance, 318
  clearance age groupings, 318
  disease state/conditions, 320, 323–24
  distribution, 317
  dosage form availability, 316
  dosing strategies, 318–19, 321
  drug-drug interactions, 319, 323
  elimination, 318
  geriatric patient, 46, 49, 52
  half-life, time to steady state, 318, 321
  loading dose, 315
  maintenance dose, 316
  metabolism, 318
  pediatric patient. 36, 37
  pharmacodynamic monitoring, 322–23
  protein binding, 317
  renal drug dosing, 77
  salt equivalence, 317
  sampling times, 322
  therapeutic monitoring, 322
  therapeutic range, 321–22
  usual dosage range, 315–16
  volume of distribution, 317
therapeutic range, xxxii
therapy initiation
  concentration verification, xxx–xxxi
  dosage adjustments, xxxi
  monitoring frequency, xxxi
  pharmacokinetic monitoring factors, xxix
  population mean values, xxix
  protein binding issues, xxx
thiamine, 47
thioridazine, 49
thrombolytic agents, 212
thyroid disease
  antidepressants, 132
  warfarin, 367
tiagabine, 46, 140
ticarcillin, 37–38
ticlopidine, 46
tinzaparin, 220
tissue sensitivity, 47
tobacco use, warfarin, 367
tobramycin
  aminoglycosides, 92–94. 99. 102., 106
  pediatric patient, 36, 38
Topamax, 141–42
topiramate, 46, 141–42
toremifene, 46
torsade de pointes, 305, 306
toxicity, 15
t_{peak}, xxxiii
trandolapril, 45
tranylcypromine, 122
trazodone, 129
triamterene, 1
triazolam, 149
tricyclic antidepressants
  antidepressants, 119, 122, 125, 126, 129
  ethosuximide, 200
  geriatric patient, 49
Trileptal, 143–45
trimethoprim, 1
trough, xxxiii
trough aminoglycoside concentration, 103
Trujillo, Toby C., 229–42, 299–313

U

unfractionated heparin
  absorption, 204
  aPTT and weight–based dosing adjustment, 207
  assay issues, 212
  bioavailability of routes of administration, 204
  coagulation tests, 211
  disease state/condition interactions, 209, 215
  distribution, 204–5
  dosage adjustment protocol, 207
  dosage form availability, 204
  dosing strategies, 205–10
  dosing/monitoring summary, 215–16
  drug-drug interactions, 214, 215
  elimination, 205
  outcomes, 208
  pharmacodynamic monitoring, 212–213
  pharmacokinetic dosing approaches, 207–10
  protein binding, 205
  reversing effect of, 213
  sampling times, 212
  therapeutic monitoring, 211–12
  therapeutic range, 210–11
  usual dosage range, 203–4
University of Wisconsin, 351
unstable renal function, creatinine clearance estimation, 8, 9
urea, 108

V

V, xxxiv
vaccines, attenuated live, 165
valproate, 139, 149, 176
valproic acid, 13
  absorption, 328
  antiepileptic drugs, 136, 139, 142, 145
  bioavailability of dosage forms, 329

carbamazepine, 176
clearance, 330
disease state/condition interactions, 334
distribution, 328–29
dosage adjustment, 331
dosage form availability, 327
dosing strategies, 331
drug-drug interactions, 333–34
elimination, 329–30
ethosuximide, 200
half-life, time to steady state, 330
initial, follow-up monitoring, 332
pharmacodynamic monitoring, 333
phenytoin, 276
pregnancy and, 332
protein binding, 329
therapeutic monitoring, 332
therapeutic range, 331–32
usual dosage range, 327
volume of distribution, 329
vancomycin
absorption, 338–39
aminoglycosides, 108
assay issues, 346
bioavailability of dosage forms, 340
clearance, 338, 340
continuous infusion, 337–38
disease state interactions, 345
dosage form availability, 338, 339
dosing strategies, 340
dosing weight, 337
drug concentration measurements, 15
drug-drug interactions, 344–45
elimination, 339
half-life, time to steady state, 338, 341
hemodialysis and, 345–46
loading dose, 337
maintenance doses, 337, 338
obese/overweight patient, 23, 25
pediatric patient, 36, 37
pharmacodynamic monitoring, 343–44
pharmacokinetic parameters, 340–41
protein binding, 339
renal drug dosing, 81
therapeutic range, 341–43
usual dosage range, 337–38
volume of distribution, 339
volume of distribution by age, 340
venlafaxine, 122, 126–28
venous thromboembolic disease, 205–7
verapamil, 299, 304
vigabatrin, 149–50, 333
Vimpat, 147–48
vitamin K agonists, 215
vitamin K intravenous, 362
V_{max}, xxxiv
volume of distribution, 22–23

W

warfarin
absorption, 353
average daily dosing, 354–55
dietary supplements interaction, 366
disease state/condition interactions, 365–67
distribution, 353
dosage form availability, 352–53
dosing adjustment guidelines, 359
dosing strategies, 354–58
drug-drug interactions, 362–65
elevated INR reversal recommendations, 362
elimination, 353–54
enantiomers of, 354
factors likely to increase sensitivity, 355
flexible initiation, 354, 355, 357
genetic information, 356–57
geriatric patient, 46, 52
half-life, time to steady state, 354
half-lives of Vitamin K-dependent proteins, 351
initiation dosing, 354–56, 358
maintenance dosing, 357–58
optimal therapeutic range, 360
pediatric patient, 32
pharmacodynamic monitoring, 361–62
protein binding, 353
therapeutic monitoring, 358–60
therapeutic range, 358
unfractionated heparin, 205, 215
usual dosage range, 352
vancomycin, 351
volume of distribution, 353
Winter, Michael E., 273–287
Wisconsin Alumni Research Foundation, 351
Withering, Sir William, 185
Wittkowsky, Ann K., 351–72

Y

Yeaman, Christy M., 299–313

Z

zidovudine, 333
Zonegran, 145–46
zonisamide, 145–46

Notes